14.50

John W. R-Love M.D.
Chestnut Lodge - 424-8300
Rockville Md 20850
500 W. Montgomery Ave

PSYCHOPHARMACOLOGY

"... It is fundamentally wrong, and naive, to expect that drugs can present the mind with gratis gifts—put into it something which is not already there. Neither mystic insights, nor philosophic wisdom, nor creative power can be provided by pill or injection. The psychopharmacist cannot *add* to the faculties of the brain—but he can, at best, *eliminate* obstructions and blockages which impede their proper use. He cannot aggrandise us—but he can, within limits, normalise us; he cannot put additional circuits into the brain, but he can, again within limits, improve the coordination between existing ones, attenuate conflicts, prevent the blowing of fuses, and ensure a steady power supply. That is all the help we can ask for—but if we were able to obtain it, the benefits to man-kind would be incalculable. . . ."

(Koestler, 1967)

PSYCHOPHARMACOLOGY

Thomas Ban, M.D.

Associate Director of Research, Douglas Hospital, Verdun, Quebec; Assistant Professor of Psychiatry, McGill University, Montreal, Quebec; Psychiatric Research Consultant, Hôpital-des-Laurentides, L'Annonciation, Quebec; Psychiatric Research Consultant, Lakeshore General Hospital, Pointe Claire, Quebec

THE WILLIAMS & WILKINS COMPANY • BALTIMORE 1969

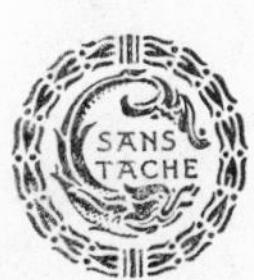

Made in the United States of America

Library of Congress Catalog Card Number 69-16711

Composed and printed at the
Waverly Press, Inc.
Mt. Royal and Guilford Aves.
Baltimore, Md. 21202, U.S.A.

Foreword

Whenever a new scientific discipline reaches a certain stage of development it becomes essential to make its accumulated information, its still unsolved problems and its practical applications available in a single place. This can best be achieved in a book written by an expert who is an active worker in the field and who, in addition to knowing his subject matter and having personally struggled with its problems, is also capable of using his own enthusiasm as a pedagogic tool.

Dr. Ban is such an expert who has written such a book. His book covers the numerous aspects of psychopharmacology in an authentic, detailed and usable manner. It is a book for the clinician with an interest in the theory and practice of comprehensive psychopharmacology who needs a sophisticated guide and a reliable source of references. It is also a textbook for the medical student who needs an uncluttered introduction to psychopharmacology. The nonclinical researcher—pharmacologist and psychologist—will appreciate the clear and honest exposition of the many problems existing at the interface between research and clinical application of the results of research. (Among the many problems dealt with in this book—above and beyond the obvious problems of methodology and semantics—are the perplexing legal and ethical dilemmas of psychopharmacology.) And for physicians in practice, there are several chapters which could serve as a vademecum of applied therapeutics.

I doubt that a similarly comprehensive one-volume, one-man library on psychopharmacology can ever be written again. I doubt it because the rapidly accelerating expansion of knowledge in this field will probably soon mean the emergence of new subdivisions. These might include experimental and clinical psychopharmacology in healthy humans, psychopatho-pharmacology, *i.e.*, psychopharmacology in psychopathological conditions, psychopharmacodiagnosis, behavioral pharmacology in animals and theoretical psychopharmacology, involving submolecular processes. On the other hand, several of today's problems of psychopharmacology, *e.g.*, the legal and ethical aspects as well as the methodological questions which puzzle us now, conceivably will some day be solved by widely accepted new definitions, regulations and practices.

For the time being it is still possible to grasp all of the essentials of psychopharmacology in one expansive and well coordinated effort and to assemble them between the covers of one book. It is astounding that the new science of psychopharmacology—hardly fifteen years old since its inception at the halfway mark of the century—has already grown to the dimensions outlined in this considerable volume. This young and vigorous science is growing at such a rapid rate that a brief look at the historical context in which it developed is indicated. Two other new developments of modern medicine and engineering made the rapid growth of psychopharmacology possible: the techniques of modern social psychiatry and the electronic computers.

When psychopharmacology first came into being its empirical roots found fertile ground in clinical psychiatry. It was preceded by a decade and one-half of the physiological (coma and convulsive) therapies which had marked the first successful application of any physical treatment of the functional psychoses. Large-scale clinical acceptance of psychopharmacology coincided with the establishment and acceptance of the open-door mental hospital, relaxed discharge policies and the widespread adoption of other progressively oriented principles in the care of the mentally ill.

There has been, and there continues to be, a heated debate on which factors "really" accounted in the mid-fifties for the striking reduction of patients in residence in mental hospitals—the new drug or the new social therapies. I cannot see the point for either side in trying to "win" this argument, since there is probably no psychiatrist living today who would want to part either with the new drugs or the new social treatment measures. Both are undoubtedly responsible to a considerable extent for the progress we have achieved in the care of the mentally ill when we compare today's sustained therapeutic results and successes in rehabilitation with those of the late 1940's. It is clear that both factors interacted significantly since the new liberal treatment policies would almost certainly have been doomed to fail without the help of the new drugs, as they had, in fact, failed more than two generations ago when they were first tried. On the other hand, the true therapeutic potential of the new drug could not have been adequately exploited in the rigidly restricted environment of mental hospitals prior to the introduction of the new social therapies. In a way, one might compare the role of the new psychopharmaceuticals in relation to modern community psychiatry to the role of anesthesia in relation to surgery—one development closely linked to the other.

Another fortunate coincidence in the history of the early stages of psychopharmacology was the development of electronic computers, which made it possible to employ statistical techniques of hitherto undreamed-of complexity in the evaluation of psychopharmacological data. Man is a very difficult behavioral system to study because of his almost limitless complexity and because of the obvious restrictions which ethics imposes on the control of many experimental factors in dealing with human subjects. Faced with this complexity and the relative lack of controls, a researcher must attempt to compensate for the unavoidable inadequacies in the design of his experiments by careful randomization of his sample and sophisticated statistical evaluation of his observations. But the quantitative processing of behavioral observations in man, which is such an essential requirement for the psychopharmacologist, became practical as a routine experimental procedure only with the development of electronic computers and computer programing.

The future course of psychopharmacology appears bright and exciting, and the promising outlook for the new science is reflected in this book which is both a landmark on the road traveled and a signpost pointing toward new directions.

Heinz E. Lehmann, M.D.

Preface

Psychopharmacology is a new scientific discipline which encompasses all the aspects and interactions between psychoactive drugs and biological systems. It evolved in the course of systematic studies with psychoactive substances of increasing specificity.

In addition to their therapeutic impact, psychopharmacological substances have become instrumental in elucidating many biochemical, physiological, behavioral and psychological mechanisms involved in psychopathology. The psychopharmacological method has opened new vistas for psychiatric progress, heralded a new era in psychiatry, and is now considered by some to be the first step toward a new psychiatry.

This book is divided into three parts. The first, General Psychopharmacology, deals with the basic interdisciplinary research which constitutes the science of psychopharmacology. Following this, Systematic Psychopharmacology reviews the available information on the most important groups of psychoactive drugs. Part Three, Applied Psychopharmacology, discusses the therapeutic implications.

Thomas Ban, M.D.

Acknowledgments

Many people, far more than can be mentioned by name, assisted in preparing this book. To all of them I am very grateful.

In particular, I am indebted to Dr. H. E. Lehmann for the confidence he displayed in my ability to perform this task; to Dr. D. Silver for the conscientious editing of the manuscript throughout its various stages; to Dr. J. D. F. Leith for the reading of the final script prior to submission; to Dr. S. Debow for assisting in the preparation of the references; and to Mr. E. Zelenak, Editor, The Williams and Wilkins Company.

I also wish to thank Arthur Koestler and his publishers, The MacMillan Company and the Hutchison Publishing Group Ltd., for allowing me to quote from their book *The Ghost in the Machine*; and *Applied Therapeutics* for permitting me to use material freely from my articles on clinical psychopharmacology.

To the Staff of the Research Department of the Douglas Hospital I wish to express my sincere appreciation for their untiring efforts throughout the two years this book was in preparation.

THOMAS BAN

Contents

Chapter Twenty

General Therapeutic Principles 373

Chapter Twenty-One

Treatment of Psychiatric Disorders 391

APPENDIX

Appendix One

Vademecum Psychopharmacologicum 432

Part One

GENERAL PSYCHOPHARMACOLOGY

One
General Principles

Psychopharmacology, a new scientific discipline, developed as a result of empirical observations that various chemical substances can differentially influence the higher psychological functions of the nervous system.

In the not so distant past the majority of psychoactive drugs were obtained from naturally occurring minerals, plants and animals. Only very few were made synthetically. The physician had the difficult task of selecting, through his knowledge of botany, for example, the proper plants from which to make his crude drug preparations. With advancing chemical technology, the picture has changed. At present not only are we replacing naturally occurring drugs by synthetically manufactured substances, but also most of our therapeutic chemicals are no longer found in nature. The physician no longer relies upon his own resources but upon the products of the pharmaceutical industry. Today, it is his curiosity rather than his need which stimulates the physician to acquire some knowledge of the active ingredients used in the manufacturing of drugs. Consequently, another major change has taken place. For the physician of the past each single physical and chemical datum that he discovered, usually with great difficulty, about his crude drug preparation was essential before applying the drug in treatment. In the modern era, the conveniently supplied manufactured substances are specifically prepared for therapeutic application, and all the necessary considerations have already been given to the relevant pharmacognostic data.

The numerous pharmacological and clinical investigations resulting from the ever increasing number of new psychoactive substances have revealed many drugs with common pharmacological characteristics and similar clinical effects. These common pharmacological characteristics are not only important in predicting clinical applicability of other newly developed drugs, but they are also of great heuristic value in helping to understand the underlying mechanisms of the psychopathological manifestations.

Basically, there are four major approaches employed in the search for new psychotherapeutic drugs (Vane, 1964).

First, there is the rational approach. This approach is based on the established knowledge of the fundamental pathology involved. Essentially this approach attempts to discover drugs which will correct the underlying pathological process. In the absence of any well established fundamental knowledge of either the structural or the functional basis of most of the psychopathologies, the rational approach has very limited application at present.

A second approach is to isolate the active principle of naturally occurring substances which has been found, empirically, to be therapeutically useful. The isolation of psychoactive Rauwolfia alkaloids and consequently their chemical synthesis are a good example of this approach.

A third approach is based on attempts to

"imitate" chemicals which are already therapeutically well established. The psychoactive thioxanthene and dibenzoazepine drugs are results of this kind of research endeavor.

Finally, there is the random screening of various preparations in an attempt to find therapeutic substances. The benzodiazepines, a widely used group of drugs, were discovered in this manner.

For all practical purposes, the search for new psychoactive substances is based on the last three approaches. However, in the course of developing new psychoactive chemicals with well defined physical and chemical properties and with systematically explored neurochemical and neurophysiological effects, the possible relationships between chemical structure and psychopharmacological activity and between pharmacodynamic (and toxic) actions in animals and therapeutic (and adverse) effects in humans are constantly being revealed.

By investigating the effects of psychoactive substances and the mechanisms by which they produce or counteract psychopathological phenomena, psychopharmacological research provides a method which not only unselectively extends the information of the behavioral, psychophysiological, neurophysiological and neurochemical correlates of clinical symptoms but also is instrumental in directing attention to the functional pathology involved.

A. STRUCTURE AND ACTIVITY

The idea that there might be a relationship between the chemical structure and the activity of various pharmacological substances is not new. The first attempts to correlate chemical structure and biological activity were made by Blake (1869, 1870) and Brown and Fraser (1868). However, it was almost 20 years later that the publication of the now classical paper of Blake (1884) on structure and activity relationships established this particular area of pharmacological research.

The notion of structure-activity relationship was originally based on the assumption that some kind of a chemical interaction occurred between a given drug and specific tissues of the organism. This implies that chemically similar compounds will likely show similar pharmacological activity. More recently, this theory has been refined. It is now postulated that cell surfaces have a variety of receptor sites which can be occupied only by the appropriate activating drug, and it is a specific chemical interaction which occurs between the drug and the cell receptor which is responsible for the characteristic pharmacological and biological actions (Grollman, 1965). In the same frame of reference, the reaction of any drug with a receptor depends upon the chemical configuration of both. This implies that the affinity between the drug and the receptor is higher for a particular "key drug" than for any other substance. Furthermore, since "key drugs" occupy their particular receptors, the responses evoked are not only proportional to the numbers of receptors involved but also specific to the properties of the occupied receptors.

Paton (1961) has suggested another possibility which he considered particularly applicable to psychoactive substances. In contrast to the former hypothesis, drug action is considered to be independent of the properties of the receptor sites. In Paton's theory it is the "rate of association" of a drug with the cellular receptor in the brain and the "speed of their dissociation" which determine pharmacodynamic and, consequently, clinical effects. He maintains that rapid dissociation is responsible for psychostimulant properties and slow dissociation for psychosedative effects. This is supported by the findings that compounds with the same electronic configuration, dipole moment, resonance energy, tautomerism and chelating action have similar effects on the organism. Although these physical properties of a compound are dependent on its chemical structure, the specificity of biological activity is determined primarily by the size and shape of the molecule configuration rather than by its chemical properties (Grollman, 1965).

In 1962 Szent-Györgyi proposed an entirely different notion regarding structure and biological activity of substances. According to this hypothesis, the activity of some of the psychoactive compounds may be

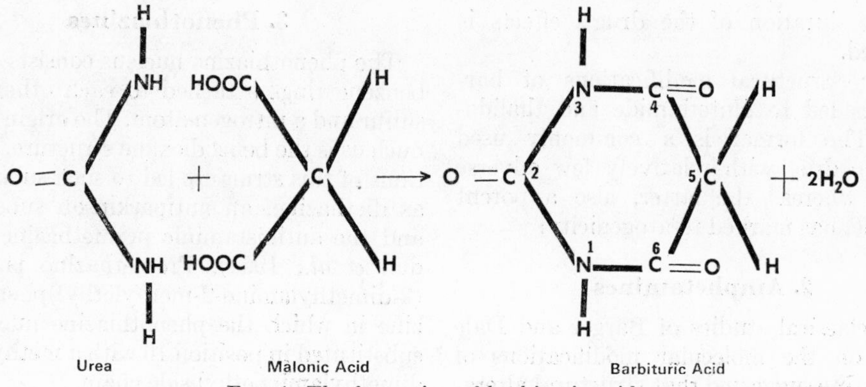

Urea + Malonic Acid ⟶ Barbituric Acid $+ 2H_2O$

FIG. 1. The formation of barbituric acid

better understood in terms of the "charge transfer" phenomenon, which is also referred to as the "redox reaction."

The "charge transfer" phenomenon was recognized through the discovery that, when specific carbon atoms with a high electron density touch other specific carbon atoms which are electron deficient, an electron may be transferred from the highest filled orbit (of the donor molecule) to the deficient orbit (of the acceptor molecule). The "redox reaction" takes place in two steps, in the course of which an electron is given up by the donor molecule (first step) and taken on by the acceptor molecule (second step). In the first step energy is "lost," whereas in the second step, energy is "gained."

Szent-Györgyi's (1962) hypothesis was based on the finding that chlorpromazine, the first known antipsychotic (or psychotostatic) substance, was the most active electron donor known among the stable molecules (Karreman *et al.*, 1959). It was therefore assumed that the action of chlorpromazine "was most probably related to its ability to transfer charges onto nerve cell molecules for which it had a specific affinity." This hypothesis was further substantiated by Cotzias and Borg (1962) and Bolt and Forrest (1966). Whether this new concept will become more generally applicable remains to be seen. It has certainly opened new vistas and offers understanding beyond the classical molecular theory.

Although not nearly as scientifically sophisticated as the above theories, two complementary pragmatic approaches are currently employed in studying the relationship between structure and activity. These are the use of isosterism, *i.e.*, the exploration of possible substitutions in the molecule of the drug without essential changes in its physiochemical and biological properties, and the systematic exploration of specific physiochemical structural changes in substances which correlate with specific biological effects (Ariëns, 1964). Applying these techniques, some characteristic patterns of structure-activity relationships were revealed within (and across) the seven categories of psychoactive drugs most widely used in clinical medicine.

1. Barbiturates

The derivatives of the psychopharmacologically inactive barbituric acid (the condensation product of urea and malonic acid) are called barbiturates.

Substitution of the hydrogen atoms in position 5 by alkyl or aryl groups in the barbituric acid molecule resulted in barbiturate substances with sedative and hypnotic properties. The hypnotic activity was further increased by substitution of the carbonyl oxygen in position 2 with a sulfur atom; by methylation of the nitrogen atom in position 3; and by an increase in the length of the alkyl side chains to a maximum total of six or seven carbon atoms in position 5. With the increase of hypnotic potency there is a shortening of the latency period, *i.e.*, a decrease in the time lapse between the drug administration and the onset of action; and also the duration of the drug's effects is decreased.

Other structural modifications of barbiturates led to glutethimide and thalidomide. The former is a commonly used hypnotic drug with relatively few adverse effects, whereas the latter, also a potent hypnotic, has marked teratogenicity.

2. Amphetamines

The classical studies of Barger and Dale (1910) on the molecular modifications of epinephrine suggested that structural alterations may lead to quantitative or even qualitative changes in the biological activity of the substance. As a result of their experiments, they established the importance of the phenylethylamine skeleton in the production of sympathomimetic effects.

It was only seventeen years later that Alles (1927) synthesized and discovered amphetamine, the α-methyl derivative of the sympathomimetic parent substance, which combined adrenergic effects with central stimulating properties.

Systematic investigations with amphetamine and comparison with epinephrine suggested that the absence of hydroxyl radicals on the benzene ring is probably responsible for the more prolonged action of the former compound. It was also revealed that saturating the benzene ring eliminates, whereas substitution on the first carbon atom increases, the central stimulating effects of the substance.

Molecular modifications of the amphetamine structure led to the synthesis of pipradrol and methylphenidate, both selectively stimulant drugs with relatively few adverse effects.

The substitution of the phenyl ring of amphetamine with an indole nucleus resulted in the virtual elimination of the psychomotor stimulant effect, replacing it with euphoriant or antidepressant properties paired with monoamine oxidase enzyme-inhibiting action (Biel, 1964). The α-methyl derivative of these substances (MP-809) was recognized to have psychotopathic actions, whereas the α-ethyl analogue (etryptamine) had toxic effects on the hemopoietic system.

3. Phenothiazines

The phenothiazine nucleus consists of two benzene rings attached to each other by a sulfur and a nitrogen atom. The origin of this nucleus is the benzodioxane structure. Variations of this structure led to such substances as diethazine, an antiparkinson substance, and the antihistaminic promethazine (Gordon *et al.*, 1964). Promethazine is a 10-(2-dimethylamino-2-methylethyl)phenothiazine in which the phenothiazine nucleus is substituted in position 10 with a methylated, dimethylaminoethyl side chain.

In the course of therapy with promethazine, sedation was noted to be a prominent side-effect. In the attempt to enhance this sedative effect a large number of molecular modifications of promethazine were synthesized and studied. This work resulted in the synthesis of chlorpromazine by Charpentier *et al.* (1952), in which the dimethylaminoethyl side chain of promethazine was replaced by a dimethylaminopropyl side chain and a chlorine atom was substituted in position 2 of the phenothiazine nucleus. These modifications not only greatly enhanced the sedative effect of the moiety but, as was later discovered, also added tranquilizing and antipsychotic (or psychotostatic) properties to the compound.

Further research was directed toward discovering changes in pharmacological activity in general or psychotropic activity in particular through various modifications of the chlorpromazine molecule. Systematic

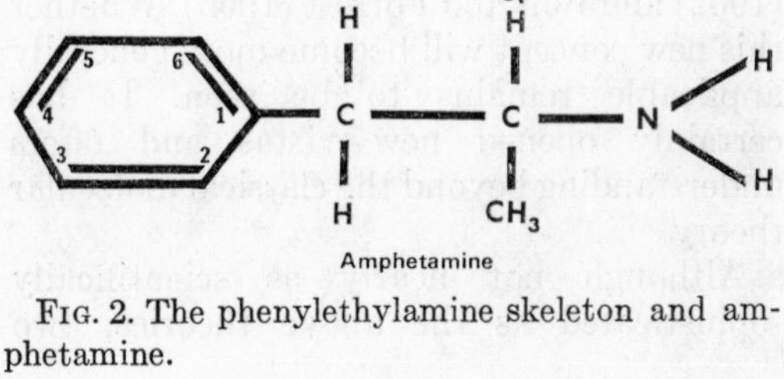

Phenylethylamine Skeleton

Amphetamine

FIG. 2. The phenylethylamine skeleton and amphetamine.

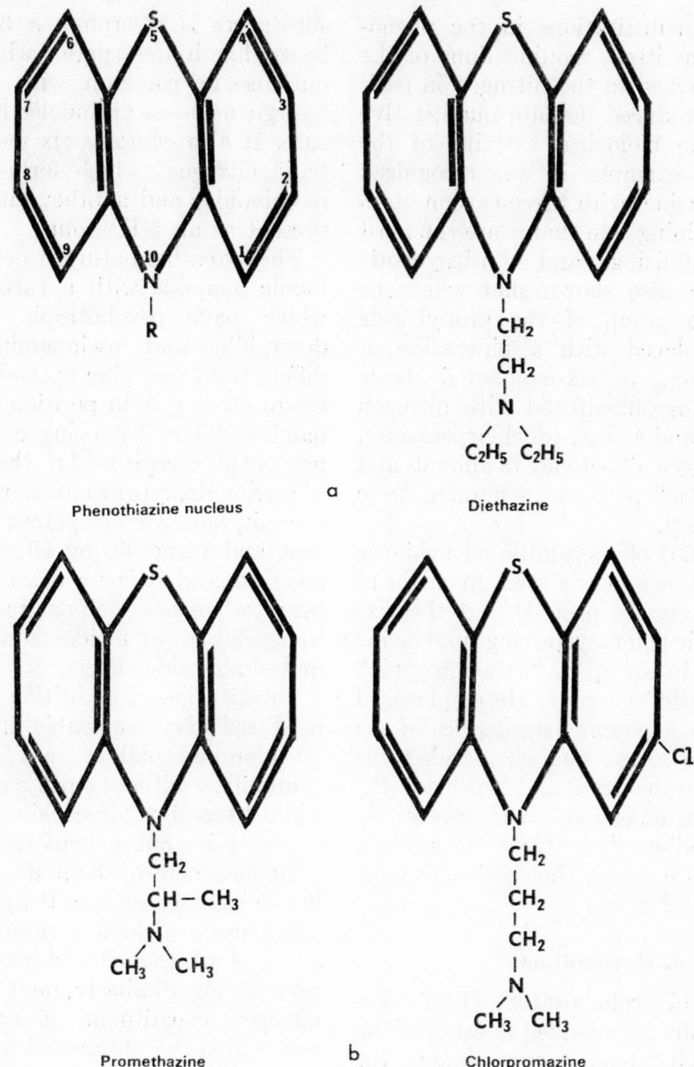

FIG. 3. *a*, The phenothiazine nucleus and diethazine. *b*, Promethazine and chlorpromazine

exploratory work revealed that replacement or substitution of the phenothiazine nucleus in positions 1, 3, 4, 6, 7, 8 and 9 resulted only in a marked diminution of psychotropic properties. Whereas substitution of the chlorine atom in position 2 by a hydrogen atom (promazine) decreased the "cataleptogenic" potential in animals, replacement by a trifluoromethyl group in the same position (triflupromazine) increased not only the "cataleptogenic" potential in animals but also the psycholeptic (and neuroleptic) effects in man.

Another striking example of structure-activity relationship was shown by substituting a sulfur atom in position 5 of the chlorpromazine molecule by two methylene groups (ethylene linkage). The outcome of this modification, the iminodibenzyl, imipramine, was devoid of antipsychotic activity but became instead a most useful antidepressant drug. Finally, replacing the nitrogen in position 10 by a carbon atom led to chlorprothixene (a thioxanthene derivative), which has a somewhat weaker antipsychotic effect than chlorpromazine but which has equal tranquilizing and probably even stronger sedating properties.

Besides the substitutions in the phenothiazine nucleus itself, modifications of the side chain attached to the nitrogen in position 10 also produced definite quantitative changes in the biological activity of the molecule. For example, it was recognized that phenothiazines with three-carbon atom (propyl) containing side chains are the most potent tranquilizing and antipsychotic agents. It was also shown that when the dimethylamino group of the propyl side chain was replaced with a piperazine or piperidine ring, a six-membered basic heterocyclic ring substituted with nitrogen in positions 1 and 4 (*e.g.*, prochlorperazine), the "cataleptogenic" potency in animals and the "neuroleptic" potency in humans were greatly increased.

Janssen (1966) offers additional evidence for the importance of the straight chain of three carbon atoms (propyl) and the six-membered basic heterocyclic ring (piperazine or piperidine) in regard to "cataleptogenic" and "neuroleptic" potency. He emphasized that in the most potent neuroleptics of the butyrophenone series, *e.g.*, haloperidol (the chlorpromazine analogue) and triperidol (the triflupromazine analogue), both essentially 4-phenylpiperidine derivatives, a straight propylene chain links the basic nitrogen with the benzoyl group.

4. Rauwolfias

Shore and his collaborators (1957) discussed the problems involved in establishing structure-activity relationships among the various Rauwolfia preparations while working with a series of alkaloids derived from *Rauwolfia serpentina*. They found that in spite of their chemical similarities only some had a depressant and tranquilizing action. Nevertheless, it was recognized that compounds with characteristic psychotropic effects had cerebral monoamine-releasing properties, whereas those lacking this property had little or no monoamine-liberating potential (Sourkes, 1962).

Among the various Rauwolfia preparations, only tertiary indole alkaloids with a carbocyclic ring E have so far yielded drugs with characteristic antihypertensive and psychotropic effects. The prototype of these substances is reserpine, a 3,4,5-methoxybenzoylmethylreserpate with the basic nucleus—in common with serotonin and lysergic acid—of an indoleethylamine structure. It also contains six methyl groups, a basic nitrogen (which forms a quaternary methiodide) and another nitrogen which is present as an NH group.

The two other naturally occurring tertiary indole akaloids with a carbocyclic ring E which have psychotropic properties are deserpidine and rescinnamine. Deserpidine differs from reserpine by lacking a methoxy group on ring A in position 11, and rescinnamine differs by being a trimethoxycinnamate of reserpic acid methyl ester (instead of a trimethoxybenzoate as reserpine is). As a result, both are less potent in their depressant and tranquilizing effects. Deserpidine has a somewhat faster onset of action, however, whereas rescinnamine has both a somewhat lower incidence and intensity of undesirable side-effects.

Substitutions in position 10 on ring A produced very noticeable alterations. Thus 10-chlorodeserpidine was found to be a tranquilizer without antihypertensive action, while 10-methoxydeserpidine has only antihypertensive but no tranquilizing properties.

Replacement of the hydrogen atom of the indole nitrogen on ring B by a methyl or an alkyl group yielded a reserpine antagonist and a pharmacologically inactive substance, respectively. Similarly, quaternization of the nitrogen constituent of rings C and D neutralized the pharmacological effects.

5. Tricyclic Antidepressants

The iminodibenzyl nucleus, the basic constituent of the tricyclic antidepressant compounds, was synthesized by Thiele and Holzinger (1899). It consists of two benzene rings attached to each other by a nitrogen atom and an ethylene bridge (the latter differentiates it from the phenothiazine nucleus).

Imipramine was the first of the tricyclic antidepressants. In this compound the iminodibenzyl nucleus is substituted in position 5 with a dimethylaminopropyl side chain. The replacement of the nitrogen atom (of imipramine) in position 5 by a carbon

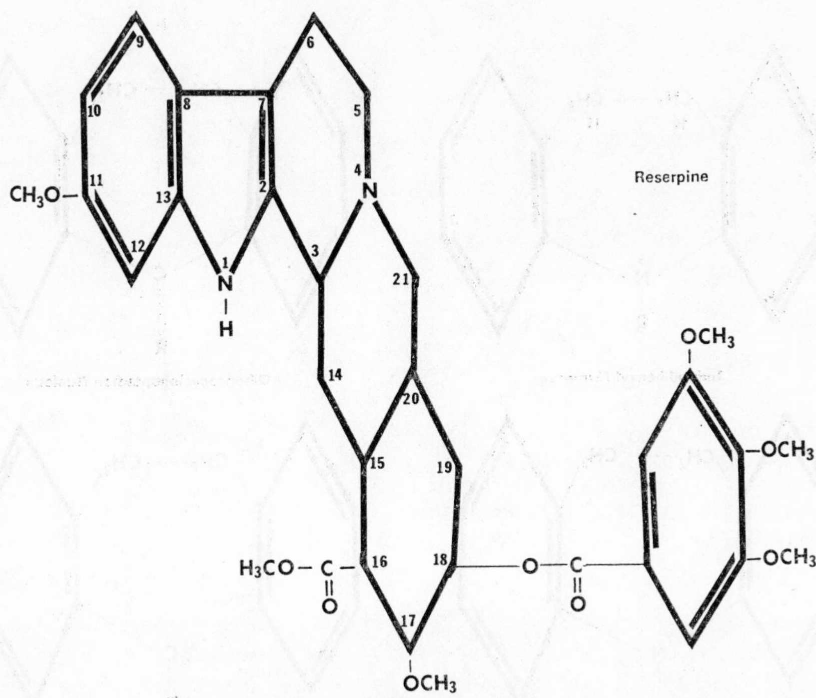

FIG. 4. The structural formula of reserpine

atom resulted in amitriptyline. The latter is a dibenzocycloheptene derivative in contrast to imipramine, which is a dibenzoazepine. It has similar potent antidepressant properties but with somewhat less pronounced anticholinergic effects. Amitriptyline also has a definite sedative action.

Desmethylation of imipramine and amitriptyline lead to desipramine and nortriptyline, respectively. The antidepressant effects are maintained in both of these new substances, and in addition they appear to have a somewhat faster onset of action, clinically, than their parent compounds (Ban and Lehmann, 1962).

The structural similarities between the tricyclic antidepressants (thymoleptics) and the phenothiazine antipsychotics (neuroleptics) were compared by Petersen and Nielsen (1967). They pointed out that from a chemical point of view there are different criteria for optimal thymoleptic and neuroleptic activity among the tricyclic compounds. According to them, substitution in one benzene ring in position 2 increases neuroleptic (but not thymoleptic) activity; a double bond between the nucleus and the side chain is in favor of neuroleptic (but not of thymoleptic) properties; a tertiary configuration is essential for neuroleptic effects, while a secondary amine configuration is optimal for thymoleptic action; and the basic amino (piperazine) group which is optimal for neuroleptics is disadvantageous for thymoleptics.

6. Monoamine Oxidase Inhibitor (MAOI) Antidepressants

The common characteristic of this group of substances is their monoamine oxidase enzyme-inhibiting action, which seems to parallel euphorizing and/or mood-lifting effects. Chemically, they are either hydrazines or substituted phenylethylamine derivatives.

The parent substance of iproniazid, the first hydrazine MAOI antidepressant drug, is nicotinic acid (Valentine, 1962). On the other hand, the parent substance of the phenylethylamine-derivative MAOI antidepressants is amphetamine.

Systematic studies with the hydrazine type of MAOI antidepressants revealed that among the various subgroups of this category

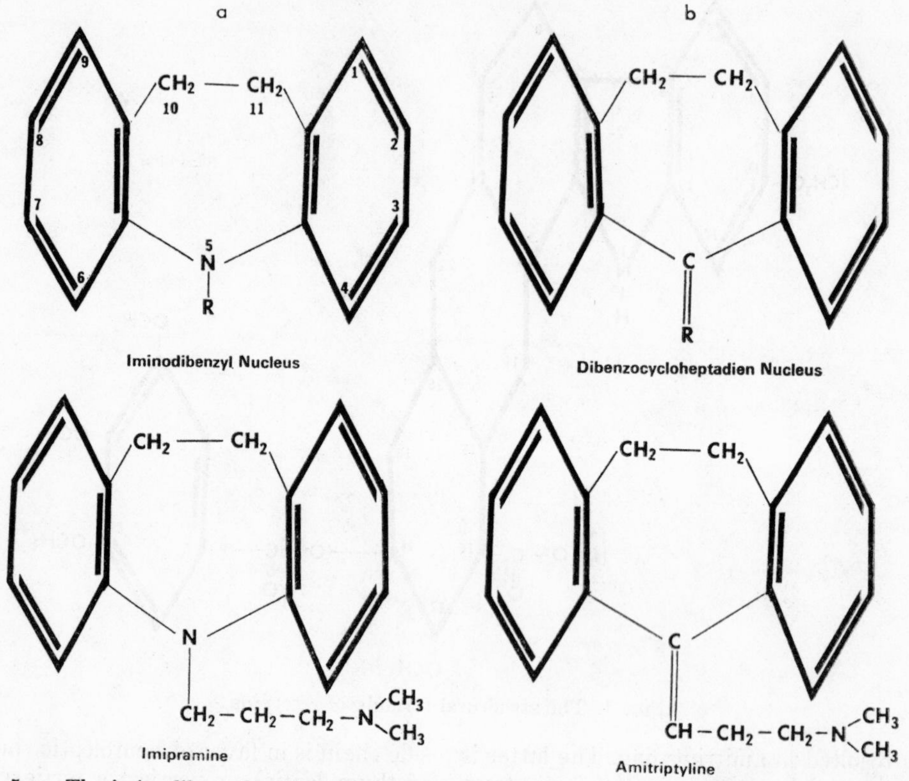

FIG. 5. *a*, The iminodibenzyl nucleus and imipramine. *b*, The dibenzocycloheptadien nucleus and amitriptyline.

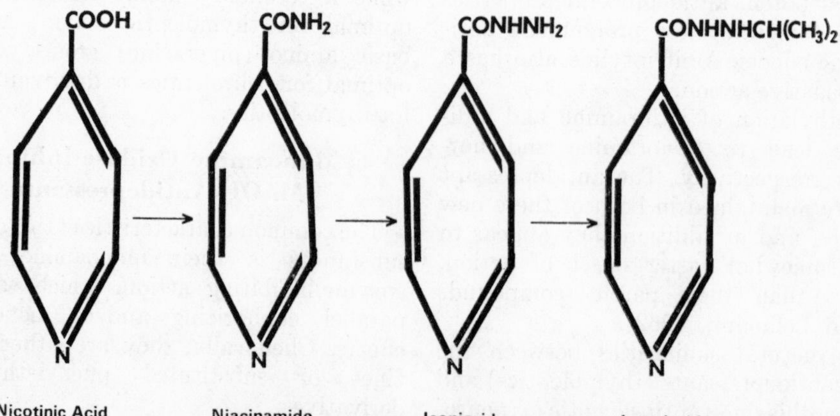

FIG. 6. Evolvement of iproniazid from nicotinic acid

the aralkyl derivatives display a stronger affinity for brain enzymes than the alkyl or aminoalkyl derivatives. Clinically, they also display a more reliable psychotropic—euphorizing—effect. Further investigations revealed that the toxicity of these substances can be greatly decreased and a more specific organ selectivity achieved by acylating the various psychoactive hydrazine type of MAOI drugs.

In comparing the two major groups of MAOI antidepressants, it was revealed that hydrazine derivatives have a rather delayed onset of action (euphoria followed by hyper-

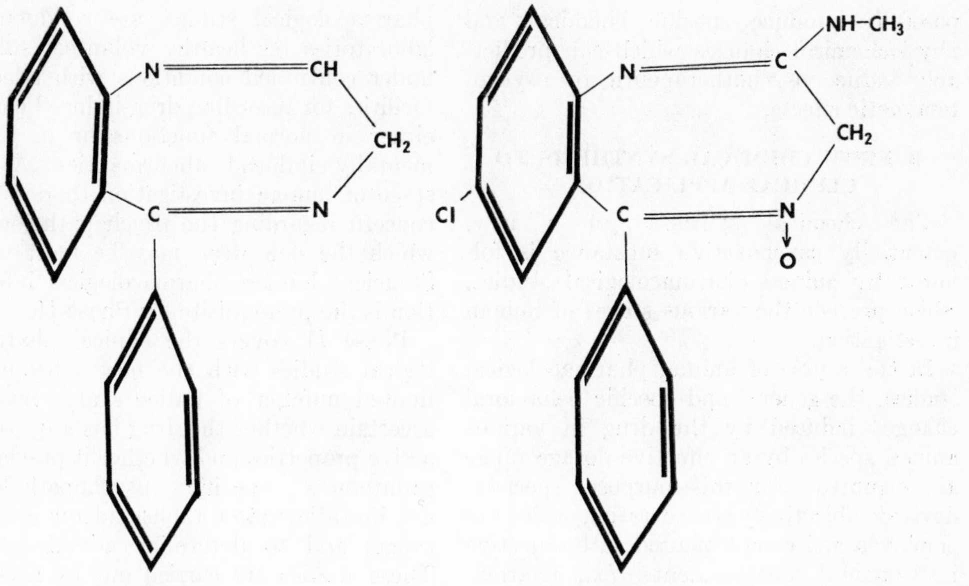

Benzodiazepine Nucleus

Chlordiazepoxide

FIG. 7. The benzodiazepine nucleus and chlordiazepoxide

thymia) in contradistinction to the substituted phenylethylamines, where an almost immediate psychomotor stimulation precedes the euphorizing and mood-lifting effects.

7. Benzodiazepines

The benzodiazepine nucleus originates from the benzoxadiazepine structure, the first member of which was described by Auwers and Meyenburg in 1891. Other benzoxadiazepines were described by Bischler (1893), Auwers (1924), Meisenheimer and Diedrich (1924) and Dziewonski and Sternbach (1935).

It was Sternbach *et al.* (1964) who prepared the first pharmacologically active compound of the benzodiazepine series. His continuous work with these substances led to the discovery of chlordiazepoxide, the first psychoactive benzodiazepine. The basic constituent of chlordiazepoxide is the benzodiazepine nucleus, which consists of a benzene nucleus and a seven-membered ring with a nitrogen atom in positions 1 and 4.

A common characteristic of benzodiazepine derivatives is the substitution of a phenyl or pyridyl ring in position 5.

Chlordiazepoxide, the parent compound, has a methylamino group attached to the carbon atom of the benzodiazepine nucleus in position 2, two hydrogens in position 3, an *N*-oxide group in position 4 and a chlorine atom in position 7. Diazepam, another benzodiazepine derivative, differs from chlordiazepoxide in having a methyl group in position 1, a carbonyl (instead of the methylamino) in position 2 and no *N*-oxide (oxygen) in position 4. This structural change resulted in a substance which is generally more effective than chlordiazepoxide, particularly in controlling agitation. On the other hand, by attaching a hydrogen atom in position 1 and replacing the chlorine atom in position 7 by an NO_2 group, nitrazepam was produced. This drug is much more useful for night sedation, especially for sleep induction, in contrast to the other benzodiazepines, which are primarily anxiolytic-sedative (minor tranquilizer) drugs.

In spite of the various theoretical formulations, the work on structure-activity relationships is primarily based on empirical observations. Irrespective of the numerous structure-activity correlations and relationships, the stage of development has not been reached whereby the investigator can purposefully produce specific chemical and physiochemical changes which can predictably induce psychotherapeutic or psychotomimetic effects.

B. FROM CHEMICAL SYNTHESIS TO CLINICAL APPLICATION

The chemical synthesis of a new, potentially psychoactive substance is followed by animal pharmacological studies, which precede the various stages of human investigation.

In the course of animal pharmacological studies, the general and specific behavioral changes induced by the drug in various animal species by an effective dosage range are explored. For this purpose, specially devised subjectively scored rating scales are employed and complemented with objective instrumental measurements, *i.e.*, pharmacological tests. Whereas rating scales and pharmacological tests reveal the action of the drug on a number of "static" behavioral variables, conditioning procedures provide information on its effect on the different "dynamic" stimulus-response constellations. Since the conditional reflex is a behavioral phenomenon and a functioning pattern of the central nervous system, conditioning studies are the connecting link between the induced overt behavioral changes and the neurophysiological substrates. Finally, an attempt is made to reveal the neurochemical basis of the changes, *i.e.*, the chemical interaction which triggers the particular neurophysiological activity reflected in conditional reflex variables and overt behavior.

Human investigations with a new psychoactive drug commence upon completion of the animal pharmacological studies and are carried out in three successive phases. These are human pharmacology (Phase I), clinical pharmacology (Phase II), and clinical investigation (Phase III) (Beaulnes, 1964).

Phase I, or human pharmacology, begins when a new drug is used for the first time in man. The main purpose at this stage is to establish the compound's general and specific pharmacodynamic actions, its safe dosage range, its toxicity and the different possible routes of administration. Human pharmacology is an essential part of both general and comparative pharmacology. Human pharmacological studies are conducted in laboratories on healthy volunteer subjects under controlled conditions with adequate facilities for recording drug-induced changes either in normal functions or in experimentally induced abnormalities. At this stage of human investigation there is little concern regarding the psychopathology for which the new drug may be most useful. Sufficient human pharmacological information is the prerequisite for Phase II.

Phase II covers the clinical pharmacological studies with the new substance. A limited number of patients are chosen to ascertain whether the drug has any psychoactive properties and whether it prevents or counteracts specific psychopathological manifestations; to establish adequate dosage range; and to determine adverse effects. These studies are carried out by a clinical pharmacologist, *i.e.*, a clinical psychiatrist trained in pharmacological methods. The information he provides is essential for the clinical investigator.

Phase III, or clinical investigation, is designed to establish the optimal treatment schedules of the investigational drug in the various clinical conditions and to determine the incidence and type of different adverse reactions which may occur in the course of treatment. Thus, the clinical investigator is primarily interested in the therapeutic effectiveness and potential adverse reactions of the new drug. In this phase, the drug trials are conducted on hospitalized or ambulant patients under a variety of circumstances.

The three well structured consecutive stages of human investigation are presented in an "ideal" form in the third, fourth and fifth chapters of this book. In the course of human pharmacology, the effects of the experimental substance on the corresponding variables studied in animals are explored in healthy human volunteers, whereas in clinical pharmacology the action of the new drug on psychopathological symptoms and its psychological, psychophysiological, neurophysiological and neurochemical correlates are investigated. Finally, verification of the data is carried out in the clinical investigation.

Prior to any "human studies" with a new

drug, there are a number of legal and ethical aspects to consider. These have to be reviewed and the investigation justified to avoid any subsequent difficulties.

C. LEGAL AND ETHICAL CONSIDERATIONS

1. General Aspects

Human experiments have been instrumental in the development of medical skill. For many centuries they were not controlled by legislation but were bound essentially by the code of approval-dependence of the scientific fraternity (Alexander, 1966). In the middle of the nineteenth century, Bernard (1865) asserted that "physicians conduct therapeutic experiments daily." He felt that "it is the duty and the right of the physician to perform an experiment on man whenever it can save his life, cure him, or gain him some personal benefits." He did not think in terms of legal jurisdiction but spoke of "the principle of medical and surgical morality," which "consists of never performing on man an experiment which might be harmful to him to any extent, even though the result might be highly advantageous to science, *i.e.*, to the health of others." He stressed, however, that performing experiments exclusively for the patient's own advantage does not prevent it from turning out profitably to science (Ladimer and Newman, 1963).

It is interesting to note that the very first systematic presentation on the legal aspects of human experiments was documented in the Nuremberg Code (1947). This was done to protest and prevent the kind of criminal brutality that the former German National Socialist Government sanctioned by law, which encouraged and led to indiscriminate experiments on human beings. Thus the first legal formulation of ethics of human experiments was drawn up by the Nuremberg Military Tribunal (1947).

The now famous Nuremberg Code consists of ten laws which were incorporated into a formal judgment. These are: (1) the subject must give voluntary consent prior to the experiment; (2) the experiment should be such as to yield fruitful results for the good of society (the results should be unprocurable by other methods or means of study, and the procedures should neither be random nor unnecessary in nature); (3) the experiments must be based on the results of prior animal studies and a knowledge of the natural history of the disease and should be so designed that the anticipated results will justify their performance; (4) the experiment should be conducted in a manner which will avoid all unnecessary physical and mental suffering or injury; (5) no experiment should be conducted where there is an *a priori* reason to believe that death or disabling injury will occur; (6) the degree of risk involved should never exceed that determined by the humanitarian importance of the problem to be solved; (7) proper preparations should be made and adequate facilities provided to protect the experimental subject against even remote possibilities of injury, disability or death; (8) all phases of the experiment should be conducted by scientifically qualified persons only, and the highest degree of skill and care should be rendered through all stages of the experiment by all those engaged in the investigation; (9) during the course of the experiment, the human subject should be at liberty to bring the experiment to an end if he has reached a physical or mental state where continuation of the experiment seems to him to be undesirable; (10) during the course of experiments the scientist in charge must be prepared to terminate the experiment at any stage if he has probable cause to believe, in the exercise of the good faith, superior skill and careful judgment required of him, that continuation of the experiment is likely to result in injury, disability, or death to the experimental subject.

The Rules of the Nuremberg Code were adopted in the United States by the American Medical Association. They emphasized particularly three of the ten articles, *i.e.*, voluntary participation, prior animal experiments and proper medical protection. The French Academy of Science stressed the necessity of true volunteers and qualified investigators.

The principles expressed in the Nuremberg Code were revived by the United Nations Third Committee on Social, Humanitarian, and Cultural Questions in 1955. In their draft covenants on civil and political rights, they adopted many of the points of the Nuremberg Code based on the spirit of the Nuremberg trials. Two of the main points were that "no one shall be subjected to torture or to cruel, inhuman, or degrading treatment or punishment" and that "in particular no one shall be subjected without his free consent to medical or scientific experimentation."

The most recent guiding principles on human experimentation were incorporated in the Declaration of Helsinki (1964). This is based partly on the Declaration of Geneva of the World Medical Association, according to which the health of the patient has to be the physician's first consideration, and partly on the International Code of Medical Ethics, which declares that "any act or advice which could weaken physical or mental resistance of a human being may be used only in his interest."

The five basic principles of the Helsinki declaration are as follows: (1) clinical research must be based on laboratory and animal experiments or other scientifically established facts; (2) it must be conducted under the supervision of a qualified medical man; (3) it is essential to evaluate the importance of the objective in proportion to the inherent risk involved to the subject; (4) it should be preceded by the assessment of inherent risks and foreseeable benefits; and (5) special caution must be exercised in cases in which the personality of the subject is liable to be altered by drugs or experimental procedures.

The basic principles of the Helsinki declaration are complemented by special recommendations, according to which, in therapeutic clinical research, "the doctor must be free to use a new treatment measure if in his judgment it offers hope of saving life, reestablishing health, or alleviating suffering." However, the document states that "if at all possible (*i.e.*, not excluded by the patient's mental state), the doctor should obtain the patient's freely given consent after the patient has been given a full explanation." Furthermore, "in case of legal incapacity, consent should also be procured from the legal guardian; and that in case of physical incapacity the permission of the legal guardian replaces that of the patient."

For nontherapeutic clinical research, the Helsinki document maintains that even here it is "the duty of the doctor to remain the protector of the life and health of that person on whom clinical research is being carried out" and stresses that "the nature, the purpose and the risk of this research must be explained to the subject by the doctor." The Declaration emphasizes the necessity of free consent in nontherapeutic clinical research. For this it is essential that the experimental subject should be in "such a mental, physical and legal state as to be able to exercise fully his power of choice." In spite of any consent, however, the "responsibility for clinical research always remains with the research worker," and "it never falls on the subject." The last paragraph of the Declaration emphasizes that the "investigator must respect the right of each individual to safeguard his personal integrity," and consequently at any time during the course of clinical research the subject or his guardian should be free to withdraw permission for the research to be continued. This is independent of the obligation that "the investigating team should discontinue the research if in their judgment, it may if continued be harmful to the individual."

Since 1964 the Declaration of Helsinki has been endorsed by several nations and numerous medical associations. The Judicial Council of the American Medical Association recommended its adoption at the American Medical Association's 1966 Annual Convention.

2. Special Aspects

Not too long ago, and even now in certain parts of the world, the protection of the public from the toxic effects of drugs was entirely a moral-ethical problem between the patient and his physician. But with the change from the use of the physician's own preparations and small pharmacy to the establishment of the big pharmaceutical houses, there was a gradual shift toward the view that this protection should be provided by legal jurisdiction. At present, in the majority of civilized countries the release of drugs for general distribution is under some sort of government control. In certain countries, moreover, *e.g.*, the United States and Canada, there are regulations which also control the release of compounds for investigational purposes. These controls are exercised in the United States by the Food and Drug Administration (FDA) (1964), in Canada by the Food and Drug Directorate (FDD) (1964), in England by the Dunlop committee (which is not a legal body but consists of representatives of the medical profession, the pharmaceutical industry and the Government), in the USSR by a special committee and in France by a specially appointed committee for each single drug in question.

In the United States, Congress made its first attempt to exert some control on drugs by passing the first Pure Food and Drug Act in 1906. An amendment in 1912 gave the government the authority to prosecute any false therapeutic claims if fraudulent intent was involved (Da Silva, 1966).

In 1937 sulfanilamide was distributed in the United States in liquid form, with the use of diethylene glycol as a dissolving agent, which caused the death of over 100 persons before it could be removed from the market. This stirred the United States Congress, which took action to safeguard and prevent similar catastrophies. The Federal Food and Cosmetic Act, finally enacted in 1938, made provisions which required that the manufacturer not only test the safety of his drug but also report on this safety to the FDA before marketing the product (Kessenich, 1960).

In 1951 the Humphrey-Durham Amendment was enacted, which distinguished for the first time between drugs which required a medical prescription and those which could be sold without a prescription. The following year, in its final report to the United States Congress, the Delaney Committee expressed the opinion that "chemicals have been utilized without adequate and sufficient testing of their long-range, injurious effects." They recommended that the public be safeguarded by making it absolutely compulsory to have adequate tests done before an article reaches the market.

However, it was not until 10 years later (1962), subsequent to the thalidomide crisis, when a therapeutically useful substance was found to be responsible for the birth of deformed babies, that the Kefauver-Harris Drug Amendment was enacted. According to the Kefauver-Harris Act, (1) the effectiveness as well as the safety of a new drug has to be determined; (2) the distribution and the use of the investigational drug have to be adequately controlled; (3) the procedures for approving and withdrawing approval of a new drug must follow the recommendations of the Act; (4) drugs can be produced only in accordance with sound manufacturing practices; (5) provision has to be made for keeping records and reporting on the distribution of approved drugs by the manufacturer so that an ineffective or unsafe drug can be removed from the market or its directions for use revised; and (6) prescription drug advertising must conform to government approval.

At the same time, the three successive phases of drug investigation were formulated. According to this, Phase I starts when the new drug is first introduced into man, with the purpose of determining human toxicity, metabolism, absorption, elimination, preferred routes of administration and its safe dosage range. Phase II includes the initial trials on a limited number of patients for specific disease control or prophylactic purposes, and Phase III provides for the assessment of the drug's safety, effectiveness and optimum dosage schedules for a particular diagnosis and for therapy or prophylaxis for groups of subjects "victimized by a given condition or disease." Consequently, it was established that, besides the required New Drug Application, an obligatory Notice of Claimed Investigational Exemption for a new drug must also be submitted prior to the introduction of any drug for human use. In the American regulations, the filing of this application is sufficient to begin using the drugs on humans (even though the application may later be rejected), but in Canada, a drug cannot be used in humans before official permission is granted.

The steadily growing number of pharmacological substances, particularly for psychotherapeutic use, resulted in the passing of a resolution by the National Advisory Health Council of the United States in December, 1965. A directive was formulated, the gist of which is that Public Health Service (PHS)-supported research should be reviewed by the grantee's institutional associates to ensure the safety of humans involved in the investigation. The National Institutes of Health (NIH) broadened the requirements of this directive by asking for the establishment of a review committee within the investigator's institution charged with approving his judgment. Furthermore, the NIH also asked for the consent of human experimental subjects, unless the investigator exercising his professional judgment deems this not feasible or contrary to the best interest of the subjects (Da Silva, 1966).

In February, 1966, the Surgeon-General of the United States issued a policy statement in which various methods to safeguard humans involved in PHS-supported clinical research were listed. In this, it is clearly established that any experiment on a normal, healthy person which causes grievous bodily harm is a criminal offence unless the subject has voluntarily consented to the experiment. However, "the same experiment on an infirm person who might benefit directly from its performance would not give rise to an action, criminal or civil, providing that the procedure was carried out with the exercise of due care by the subject's personal physician" independent of whether consent for the experiment was given. All this, of course, does not imply "that the physician is released from the legal obligation to show due skill and care."

Special policies were formulated on the same issues by the Surgeon-General for controlled experiments. In these it was clearly expressed that, "when one has voluntarily submitted himself to a physician for diagnosis and treatment, it will be presumed, in the absence of evidence to the contrary, that what the physician did was either expressly, or by implication, authorized." If the design of the experiment is such that the physician at random selects alternate patients for treatment "a" or treatment "b," no written consent is necessary nor is the experimenter obliged to disclose that a controlled study is being undertaken.

Furthermore, controlled experiments on humans were classified into five grades in accordance with the degree of risk or litigation which might be involved. Grade I covers the controlled experiment which is conducted as a part of a treatment for an illness, in the course of which the experimental subject (patient) is given an established remedy for comparison with either another established remedy, a placebo or a nonestablished remedy. For this procedure it has been explicitly stated that no written consent is necessary and the experiment need not be discussed with the patient. Grade II covers the events whereby the experiment is also carried out as a part of treatment, but in contradistinction to Grade I it is for an illness for which there is as yet no established remedy. Although no written consent is necessary even in these cases, the subject should be informed that a new remedy is being tried, although he does not need to be informed that there is no alternate remedy of any value. Grade III still includes experiments which are conducted as part of the treatment for an illness for which there is an established remedy. However, in these experiments, instead of the established remedy either a placebo or a nonestablished remedy is given. In Grade III, written consent and informing the patients that a new remedy is being tried are advised. In contradistinction to the first three grades, in Grades IV and V the experiments are not part of treatment but serve as a control to a physiological, pharmacological or surgical experiment, which in the case of Grade IV is not dangerous or in the case of Grade V is dangerous to the patient's life. In either case, written consent is advised. In the last two grades the experimental subjects have to be aware of the dangers (or lack of danger) involved, and a "written release should be signed by the subject barring him from taking legal action should damages ensue, and witnessed as to explanation of the dangers."

In consideration of all of these, the experimental subject, to succeed in a legal action against the experimenter, has to prove that he suffered a pecuniary loss; that the experimenter was willingly reckless; that there was a causal connection between the loss and the experiment; that he did not consent to the risk and therefore was not a party to the experiment. On the other hand, the likelihood of litigation involving the experimenter may be minimized, in general, by conducting the experiment as part of treatment; by arranging for the experimental treatment to be prescribed by the personal physicians from whom the subject sought help; and by obtaining a written consent and explaining the dangers of the experiment if it is not conducted as part of treatment and if it is not prescribed by the personal physician.

The United States FDA has recently amended its regulations with a statement of policy formulated by Goddard (1966) regarding consent for use of investigational new drugs on humans. The essence of this amendment is that whenever an investigational drug is used on human beings the investigators should obtain consent from the subjects (or their representatives) except where it is deemed not feasible or, in the investigator's professional judgment, is contrary to the best interest of the subject.

This is the state of affairs to date, and it cannot be overemphasized how important it is for anyone involved in psychopharmacological studies to be aware not only of the legal but also of the ethical and moral implications of experimenting on humans.

REFERENCES

ALEXANDER, L.: Limitations in experimental research on human beings. Lex et Scientia, *3:* 8 (1966).

ALLES, G. A.: Comparative physiological action of phenylethanolamines. J. Pharmacol. Exp. Ther., *32:* 121 (1927).

AMERICAN MEDICAL ASSOCIATION JUDICIAL COUNCIL: Annual report on the first national congress on medical ethics. J.A.M.A., *198:* 445 (1966).

ARIËNS, E. J. (ed.): Molecular pharmacology. (Academic Press, New York, 1964.)

ARIËNS, E. J., *et al.*: A molecular approach to general pharmacology. In: Molecular pharmacology (ed., Ariëns, E. J.). (Academic Press, New York, 1964.)

AUWERS, K.: Zur Constitution der Acyl-indazole. Ber. Deutsch. Chem. Ges., *57:* 1723 (1924).

AUWERS, K., AND MEYENBURG, F.: Über eine neue Synthese von Derivaten des Isindazols. Ber. Deutsch. Chem. Ges., *24:* 2370 (1891).

BAN, T. A., AND LEHMANN, H. E.: Clinical trials with desmethylimipramine (G-35020)—a new antidepressive compound. Canad. Med. Ass. J., *86:* 1039 (1962).

BARGER, G., AND DALE, H. H.: Chemical structure and sympathomimetic action of amines. J. Physiol. (London), *41:* 19 (1910).

BEAULNES, A.: The place of clinical pharmacology in academic medicine. In: Conference on human pharmacology (eds., Murphy, C. W., and Parker, J. M.). (The Canadian Foundation for the Advancement of Therapeutics, Ste. Adele-en-Haut, 1964.)

BERNARD, C.: Introduction to the study of experimental medicine. (Baillière, Paris, 1865.)

BIEL, J. H.: Some rationales, for the development of antidepressant drugs. In: Molecular modification in drug design (ed., Gould, R. F.). (American Chemical Society, Washington, 1964.)

BISCHLER, A.: Zur Kenntnisse der Phenmiaziendederivate. Ber. Deutsch. Chem. Ges., *26:* 1891 (1893).

BLAKE, J.: On the action of the salts of iron when introduced directly into the blood. J. Anat., *3:* 24 (1869).

BLAKE, J.: On the action of the inorganic substances when introduced directly into the blood. J. Anat., *4:* 201 (1870).

BLAKE, J.: On the connection between physiological action and chemical constitution. J. Physiol. (London), *5:* 124 (1884).

BOLT, A. G., AND FORREST, I. S.: Charge transfer reactions between melanin and chlorpromazine. (Presented at the 152nd American Chemical Society meeting, New York, 1966.)

BROWN, A. C., AND FRASER, T. R.: On the connection between chemical constitution and physiological action. Trans. Roy. Soc. (Edinburgh), *25:* 1 (1868).

CHARPENTIER, P., *et al.*: Recherches sur les diméthylaminopropyl-*N*-phénothiazines substituées. C. R. Acad. Sci. (Paris), *235:* 59 (1952).

COTZIAS, G. C., AND BORG, D. C.: Phenothiazines and manganese. In: The ultrastructure and metabolism of the nervous system (eds., Korey, S. R., Pope, A., and Robins, E.). (Williams and Wilkins, Baltimore, 1962.)

DA SILVA, T.: Personal communication (Letter, Ottawa, 1966).

DECLARATION OF HELSINKI: World Med. J., *11:* 281 (1964).

DZIEWONSKI, K., AND STERNBACH, L. H. (1935): In: Sternbach, L. H., *et al.:* 1,4-Benzodiazepines. In: Psychopharmacological agents (ed., Gordon, M.). (Academic Press, New York, 1964.)

FDA: Investigational drug circular No. 1. (U.S.

Dept. Health, Education and Welfare, Washington, 1964.)

FDA: Investigational drug circular No. 2. (U.S. Dept. Health, Education and Welfare, Washington, 1964.)

FDA: Investigational drug circular no. 3. (U.S. Dept. Health, Education and Welfare, Washington, 1964.)

FDD: Guide for completing a preclinical submission on investigational drugs under section C. 08 005 of the Food and Drug Regulations. (Dept. National Health and Welfare, Ottawa, 1964.)

Goddard, J. L.: Consent for use of investigational new drugs on humans: statement of policy. (Federal Register, Washington, 1966.)

Goddard, J. L.: Consent for use of investigational new drugs on humans: statement of policy. Psychopharmacol. Serv. Cent. Bull., *4:* 46 (1966).

Gordon, M., Craig, P. N., and Zirkle, C. L.: Molecular modification in the development of phenothiazine drugs. In: Molecular modification in drug design (ed., Gould R. F.). (American Chemical Society, Washington, 1964.)

Grollman, A.: Pharmacology and therapeutics. (Lea and Febiger, Philadelphia, 1965.)

Janssen, P. A. J.: The chemical anatomy of neuroleptic drugs. Sartryck ur Farmacevtisk Rev., *65:* 272 (1966).

Janssen, P. A. J.: The pharmacological and clinical mode of action of neuroleptic drugs. Clin. Trials J., *2:* 370 (1966).

Karreman, G., *et al.:* On the mechanism of action of chlorpromazine. Science, *130:* 1191 (1959).

Kessenich, W. H.: The challenge of new drugs to the Food and Drug Administration. In: Antibiotic Annual 1959–1960 (ed., Martin-Ibanez, F.). (Antibiotica, New York, 1960.)

Koestler, A.: The ghost in the machine. (Hutchison, London, 1967.)

Ladimer, I., and Newman, R. W. (eds.): Clinical investigation in medicine: legal, ethical and moral aspects. (University Law Medicine Research Institute, Boston, 1963.)

Meisenheimer, J., and Diedrich, A.: Über die Isomeren Acyl-indazole von K. von Auwers. Ber. Deutsch. Chem. Ges., *57:* 1715 (1924).

Nuremberg Military Tribunal: United States versus Karl Brandt *et al.* "The medical case." Trials of War Criminals, *2:* 181 (1947).

Paton, W. D. M.: A theory of drug action based on the rate of drug-receptor combination. Proc. Roy. Soc. (Biol.), *154:* 21 (1961).

Petersen, P. V., and Nielsen, I. M.: Chemical configuration and pharmacological action of thymoleptic drugs with special reference to a new group of bicyclic compounds. In: Antidepressant drugs (eds., Garattini, S., and Dukes, M. N. G.). (Excerpta Medica Foundation, Amsterdam, 1967.)

Shore, P. A., *et al.:* On the physiologic significance of monoamine oxidase in brain. Science, *126:* 1063 (1957).

Sourkes, T. L.: Biochemistry of mental disease. (Hoeber Medical Division, Harper and Row, New York, 1962.)

Sternbach, L. H., Randall, L. O., and Gustafson, S. R.: 1,4-Benzodiazepines (chlordiazepoxide and related compounds). In: Psychopharmacological agents (ed., Gordon, M.). (Academic Press, New York, 1964.)

Szent-Györgyi, A.: On the possible role of quantum phenomenon in normal and abnormal mental function. In: Ultrastructure and metabolism of the nervous system (eds., Korey, S. R., Pope, E., and Robins, E.). (Williams and Wilkins, Baltimore, 1962.)

Thiele, J., and Holzinger, O.: Über *o*-Diamidodibenzyl. Ann. Chem. (Justus Liebigs), *305:* 96 (1899).

U.N. Third Committee on Social, Humanitarian and Cultural Questions. (Draft international covenants on human rights, New York, 1955.)

Valentine, M.: An introduction to psychiatry. (Livingstone, Edinburgh, 1962.)

Vane, J. R.: A plan for evaluating potential drugs. In: Evaluation of drug activities: pharmacometrics (eds., Laurence, D. R., and Bacharach, A. L.) (Academic Press, London, 1964.)

World Medical Association: Aspects of human experimentation. World Med. J., *7:* 84 (1960).

World Medical Association: Draft code of ethics on human experimentation. Brit. Med. J., *2:* 1119 (1962).

Two

Animal Pharmacology

Animal pharmacology is the scientific study of the effect of drugs on the animal organism. The animal pharmacological information in this chapter will, however, be restricted to the methods, techniques, procedures and results pertinent to psychoactive substances.

A preliminary step in the animal pharmacological investigation is to establish an effective dosage range for the new substance. This is followed by pharmacodynamic and toxicity studies.

Experiments to establish the effective dosage range are carried out on conscious (*i.e.*, nonanesthetized), nonrestricted (*i.e.*, nonparalyzed) animals (usually rodents). At the same time, the dose-response curves are obtained by administering single doses of the drug in increasing amounts. The dose-response curve is based on continuous and careful observations and recordings for at least 24 hours. This is followed by regular, repeated observations for a week to detect any possible delayed effects. During this time particular attention is paid to any changes in behavior, central nervous system activity, autonomic functions, cardiovascular and neurovascular effects.

It is most important to recognize the smallest dose which produces any detectable effect and the ED_{50} (*i.e.*, the dosage which produces a particular effect in 50 per cent of the animals tested) as well as to reveal the time span between the appearance and the disappearance of any of the induced manifestations. It is also essential to detect the smallest amount of the drug which produces either an irreversible impairment or a lethal effect and to establish the LD_{50}, *i.e.*, the dose which kills 50 per cent of the animals tested.

At this point the therapeutic index, *i.e.*, the ratio between the lethal dose (LD_{50}) and the effective dose (ED_{50}), is calculated. A high therapeutic index, *i.e.*, a wide discrepancy between the LD_{50} and the ED_{50}, is one of the prerequisites of further exploratory work with the substance. With all this data in hand, pharmacodynamic investigations may commence.

A. PHARMACODYNAMICS

Pharmacodynamics is one of the youngest of the medical sciences. It is the study of general and specific behavioral changes induced by a drug in an organism.

The ultimate goal of pharmacodynamic investigations in animals is to enable the investigator to predict the possible clinical usefulness of a particular drug. The various testing procedures used in this area of research are many, but essentially there are four major approaches. These are: (1) rating scales; (2) pharmacological tests; (3) conditioning studies; and (4) attempts to establish the (*a*) neurochemical and (*b*) neurophysiological sites of action of the experimental substance.

1. Rating Scales

Subjectively scored rating scales are used in animal pharmacological studies not only to reveal and measure drug-induced behavioral changes but also as investigational tools to predict potential clinical therapeutic profiles. For the latter purpose, scales consisting of behavioral characteristics, such as wakefulness, drives, discrimination, time-sense, memory, mood and the acquisition or extinction of certain behavioral patterns, all of which are present in both animal and man, are particularly useful (Irwin, 1966).

There are many rating scales available for assessing the "psychological" effects of drugs in animals. One of the most extensively used is that constructed by Irwin (1959, 1962). Irwin's rating scale (for the rat and mouse) consists of three major categories with which the behavioral, neurological and autonomic profiles of the chemical can be assessed. The three major categories are further subdivided into subcategories, *i.e.*, (1) awareness; (2) mood; (3) motor activity (components of the behavioral profile); (4) central nervous system excitation; (5) posture; (6) motor incoordination; (7) muscle tone; (8) reflexes (components of the neurological profile); (9) autonomic measurements; and (10) miscellaneous.

Furthermore, each subcategory is rated on the basis of several quantifiable manifestations. Thus, (1) awareness is considered to be the composite of four traits: alertness, visual placing, passivity and sleeping. (2) Mood is scored on the basis of five characteristics: grooming, vocalization, restlessness, irritability (aggression) and digging (in the cage). (3) Motor activity is rated on four subfunctions: spontaneous activity, environmental reactivity, touch response and pain response. (4) Central nervous system excitation is measured by the startle response, tremors, twitches and convulsions. (5) Posture is assessed on the basis of body posture and limb positions. (6) Motor incoordination is assessed by abnormal gait and the righting reflex. (7) Muscle tone is assessed through limb tone, grip strength, shiver, body tone and abdominal tone. (8) Reflexes are measured through the pinna, corneal, scratch and righting reflexes. (9) Autonomic activity is assessed through breathing, pupil size, palpebral opening, piloerection, retching, skin color, defecation and respiratory rate. (10) Miscellaneous covers other properties which are not included under any of the headings but which are seen under the influence of the experimental substance, *e.g.*, dehydration, fits, etc.

All the measurable effects are scored on an arbitrary scale from 0 to 8. Four is assigned to a characteristic which is usually present under normal circumstances. The degree to which this characteristic is altered is scored from 4 to 8 if it is increased and 4 to 0 if it is decreased. Manifestations which are normally absent but are observed only after drug administration are scored 1 to 8.

Irwin's (1959) rating scale was found to be quite effective in assessing drugs which may be potentially useful clinically as autonomic, analgesic, muscle relaxant and psychotherapeutic substances. In the last group it may differentiate among psychomotor stimulants, psychomotor depressants, antidepressants, tranquilizers, etc.

Another very useful scale for screening potentially psychoactive drugs is that developed by Norton (1957). The Norton scale (for hamster, cat and monkey) consists of 25 rating scale items which are grouped into five categories: sociability; contentment; excitement; defensive hostility; and aggressive hostility. Each category on the Norton (1957) scale consists of a number of items which are rated by the observer. For example, the fifth category, aggressive hostility, is measured by squatting, pulling, chasing, biting and rearing (alone) in the hamster and by pouncing, rearing, biting, clawing and squatting in the cat.

Characteristic drug effects have been established on this scale for chlorpromazine (antipsychotic), chlordiazepoxide (anxiolytic), methamphetamine (psychomotor stimulant) and lysergic acid diethylamide (psychotomimetic substance). Consequently, the Norton scale has been found quite reliable in differentiating antipsychotic, anxiolytic, stimulant and psychotomimetic drugs.

It has been suggested that the higher the species phylogenetically, the wider the range of behavioral effects which can meaningfully be studied (Irwin, 1966). Thus Norton and deBeer (1956), Norton (1957) and Irwin (1964) indicated that the cat is superior to rodents in evaluating the behavioral effects of drugs, despite the major disadvantage that it is unable to metabolize certain compounds (Irwin, 1964). This was further supported by Kinnard *et al.* (1967). In the search for methods to evaluate antidepressant activity in animals, he found the cat observational techniques more satisfactory than the rat observational techniques. He also considered the former better for the purpose of clearly identifying the antidepressant activity of imipramine-like compounds.

The Kinnard scale (for cat) consists of 32 rating scale items which group into nine factors: social interaction; reaction to observer; general activity; depressive syndrome; agitation; sleep; self-care; anxiety; and hostility. Each factor consists of a number of positive and negative signs. For example, positive signs for the fourth factor (depressive syndrome) are ataxia, relaxation of the nictating membrane, crying and indifference, and the major negative sign of the same factor is grooming.

On the basis of five prototype psychotropic compounds (amphetamine, pentobarbital, imipramine, chlorpromazine and perphenazine), distinctive profiles for drugs with stimulant, sedative, antidepressant and antipsychotic properties were established which can be used for screening new potentially psychoactive drugs.

It should be noted that evaluating behavior by rating scales is based on the subjective judgment of human observers. Thus the recorded scores are subject to degrees of error which may be expected whenever personal judgment and subjectivity are involved in rating a particular item. In spite of this and other shortcomings, however, rating scales have become extremely useful "tools" for screening and predicting potential psychoactive drugs.

2. Pharmacological Tests

In the pharmacological tests the subjective rating scale technique is replaced by objective, instrumental measurements. Consequently, pharmacological tests are aimed not at substituting but rather at complementing rating scales in assessing drug-induced changes.

One of the first systematic pharmacological test procedures for psychoactive agents was described in the late nineteenth century when Stewart (1898) explored the effects of alcohol on rats. Since then, pharmacological test procedures have been continuously improved and refined. In the course of this progress it was learned that not only the simultaneous measurements of a drug's multiple effects (*i.e.*, the drug-response profile) but also the measurements of a drug's single specific effects in increasing doses (*i.e.*, the drug-response curve) are of crucial importance. It has also been shown that the drug-response profiles and drug-response curves differ with a single dose of the compound compared with chronic administration.

In pharmacological tests, the same activity is often measured by two entirely different means, and conversely, the same means are frequently used to measure different activities. However, common characteristics of pharmacological tests are that they require a particular situation in which the animal performs a demonstrable and measurable activity. It is important to realize that, although a pharmacological test must be sensitive enough to detect even minute changes induced by molecular modifications in a psychoactive substance, it should not be so sensitive, on the other hand, that it does not pick up the similarities among compounds. This was very well elucidated by Vernier (1966), who summed up the desirable features of a pharmacological test or test battery for screening potentially psychoactive drugs.

According to Vernier (1966), a predictive criterion should be sensitive enough for the drug effect to be picked up at low doses; it should confer qualitative specificity so that it should detect and differentiate (preferably) all known clinically effective standard agents; it should be simple; and it should be sufficiently general to apply to a complete range of active drugs.

In general, pharmacological tests can be divided into two major categories: direct testing and indirect testing. In direct testing it is the effect of the psychoactive substance on a particular activity which is measured.

On the other hand, in indirect testing the effect of the drug is tested on an activity which has been induced by either a chemical or a physical stimulus.

a. Direct Testing

The aim of direct testing is to establish objective and quantifiable criteria of psychotropic action and differential characteristics for psychoactive drugs which exert clinically different effects. There are a great many direct pharmacological tests available for detecting psychotropic properties in an investigational substance. Even more, there are reliable procedures for the immediate differentiation of their central nervous system stimulant or depressant action. Tests to discriminate among sedative, anxiolytic and antipsychotic substances or between stimulants and antidepressants, however, are less reliable. For detection of psychotropic properties, some of the frequently employed direct pharmacological tests are the jiggle cage, actophotometer, runway, revolving cylinder, rotating rod, inclined screen and swimming survival tests.

In differentiating between central nervous system (CNS) depressants and stimulants, three tests proved to be particularly useful: the jiggle cage, the actophotometer and the runway tests (Turner, 1965). It was found that CNS depressants reduce spontaneous motor activity (Jacobsen, 1964) and, in most cases, also voluntary motor activity. The reduction of spontaneous motor activity, regardless of the nature of the body movement, can be measured in the jiggle cage (Chen, 1964) or, if restricted to the measurement of walking and running activity, by an actophotometer (Kuhn and Van Maanen, 1961). The decrease of voluntary motor activity is reflected in the diminished performance of thirsty rats to obtain water on the runway test. Further differentiations among the various CNS depressants were achieved by using other techniques.

It has been found that sedatives, *e.g.*, barbiturates, characteristically interfere with motor coordination. For example, they interfere with the animals' usual ability to cling to the screened side of a revolving cylindrical cage (Hassert *et al.*, 1961). Similarly, sedatives cause the animals to fall off a rotating rod (Boissier *et al.*, 1961; and Mason, 1964).

Generally, motor coordination is less impaired with anxiolytic drugs than with the sedatives. The former may, however, interfere with motor control. They may also exert a taming effect. Interference with motor control by anxiolytic drugs was found particularly characteristic of the muscle relaxant substances, *e.g.*, propanediols. This is measured by placing the animal on a slightly inclined screen. Normally the animal would have no difficulty resting on this slight incline. But under the influence of these drugs, it cannot prevent itself from sliding down (Friedman and Ingalls, 1960). The taming effect particularly characteristic of the benzodiazepines was revealed by a decrease in "defensive aggression" (Jacobsen, 1964).

An important aspect of the effects of the drugs discussed thus far is that they produce a "shift" in behavior; *i.e.*, the observed behavior which is present under the experimental conditions can be seen to a lesser or greater extent under normal conditions as part of the animals' usual behavioral repertoire. Some drugs, however, produce a "change" in behavior; *i.e.*, they induce a pattern of behavior that is never seen under normal conditions. Such changes can be seen, for example, with phenothiazines or butyrophenones, etc.

The third group of CNS depressants are the neuroleptics with antipsychotic effects, *e.g.*, phenothiazines, which produce a change that is alien to the animal's normal behavioral repertoire. The characteristic altered state induced by these antipsychotics is called catalepsy, which can be divided into a number of steps and measured by various means.

Catalepsy can be divided into four stages of severity. In the first stage the animal appears "disinclined" to move, whereas in the second stage it does not move even if prodded. In the third stage, the animal can be placed with its forelegs on a high platform, and in the fourth stage the animal can be placed sitting on its hind legs with one foreleg on a high platform, while the other foreleg hangs in the air without support (Jacobsen, 1964).

In contrast to drugs which depress the CNS in various ways, stimulants, *e.g.*, amphetamines, share the common characteristic of increasing spontaneous motor activity. This can be shown by the jiggle cage or actophotometer tests (Turner, 1965). They also improve performance on the runway test, and most of them increase the spontaneous displacement of sand (Siegmund and Wolf, 1952).

Although there are many pharmacological tests for investigating potential stimulants, there is no simple pharmacological test to date which will recognize potential antidepressant drugs with any certainty. There are indications, however, that improvement of swimming survival in a hopeless survival contingency (Irwin, 1966) may turn out to be a good measure of potential clinical antidepressant properties, although the improved performance by antidepressants on this test is shared by narcotics.

The use of the swimming survival test for screening antidepressant drugs is based on the notion that prolonged stress situations in man sometimes lead to exhaustive depression (Kielholz, 1960). The neurochemical mechanisms involved in such situations were studied in animals by Matussek *et al.* (1967).

Another possibly useful test for potential antidepressants is the "increased natatory exhaustion time" (Jacob and Michaud, 1961). Whether this test will reveal antidepressant action with reasonable consistency still remains to be seen.

b. Indirect Testing

The aim of indirect testing is to detect psychotropic properties and the differential effects of psychoactive drugs which cannot be revealed by direct testing methods. The test procedures in indirect testing are so designed that the effects of prevention, counteraction or potentiation of artificially induced changes can be studied.

The prototype scheme of indirect testing is the following: The animal is given a drug with a known pharmacological action before or after administration of the investigational substance. Consequently, the chemical antagonism or synergism is recorded, and the possible psychopharmacological potentials are assessed.

The indirect tests most commonly used in screening for psychoactive substances are the barbiturate or amphetamine "potentiation" or "antagonism" tests, which were also found useful for differentiating between CNS stimulants and CNS depressants. Characteristically, CNS stimulants antagonize barbiturate-induced changes and potentiate amphetamine actions, whereas CNS depressants produce the opposite effects.

There are more specific tests, which appear to be significantly correlated with anxiolytic, antipsychotic and antidepressant actions. For example, potential anxiolytic effects may be detected by the amphetamine group toxicity test. It was observed that amphetamine toxicity is considerably greater when the drug is given to a group of mice kept in the same cage than when animals are kept separately, in individual cages (Chance, 1947). This increased amphetamine toxicity in animals kept in crowded conditions is reversed by drugs which exert an anxiolytic effect in humans (Vane, 1964). Among the various groups of anxiolytic drugs, the benzodiazepines were found to have a blocking effect on strychnine, pentetrazol and electroshock-induced seizures. Of the propanediols, meprobamate and mephenesin have a particularly antagonizing effect on pentetrazol and strychnine-induced convulsions, respectively.

Antipsychotic drugs appear to inhibit caffeine-induced increased motor activity. They also simultaneously decrease (lower) the threshold for cerebral seizures. This was found to be particularly so with reserpine or related compounds (Bein, 1959). More recently, it was found that the β-β-iminodipropionitrile-induced ECC syndrome (excitement, choreiform head movements and circling behavior) is effectively counteracted by reserpine and significantly decreased by chlorpromazine administration. Although the lysergic acid diethylamide-induced ECC syndrome can be counteracted only by chlorpromazine and not by reserpine, it is generally agreed that the antagonism of the chemically induced ECC syndrome is related to the antipsychotic action of drugs (Gabay, 1966)

Antidepressant drugs were found to potentiate the action of both 5-hydroxytryptophane (5-HTP) and 3,4-dihydroxyphenylalanine (dopa). They antagonize the effects of reserpine (a Rauwolfia alkaloid) and tetrabenazine (a benzoquinolizine). Thus, antidepressant drugs potentiate monoamine (*e.g.*, serotonin, norepinephrine) precursors and antagonize monoamine releasers. Many pharmacological tests show these actions. For example, pretreatment with a monoamine oxidase inhibitor (MAOI) type of antidepressant increases some of the central effects of 5-HTP in animals, such as head twitching, excitation and pyrexia (Corne *et al.*, 1963). The same applies to the central effects (excitation, pyrexia) of dopa (Chen, 1964). Also, after pretreatment with an MAOI antidepressant, reserpine (for a longer period) and tetrabenazine (for a shorter period) did not cause sedation, miosis, hypothermia or hypotension, but induced stimulation, mydriasis, hyperthermia and hypertension. Similarly, after pretreatment with a tricyclic antidepressant, the sedative and hypothermic effects of monoamine releasers were antagonized as well as their enhancing action on barbiturate and ethanol anesthesia (Pletscher, 1965). Other characteristic interactions which have been revealed were that antidepressants, particularly of the tricyclic type, enhanced the psychomotor-stimulating effect of amphetamine and 2-benzylpiperidines and potentiated the reserpine-antagonism of dopa. The dibenzoazepine derivatives (*e.g.*, imipramine) were found to have a particularly strong antagonistic action against the centrally mediated increase in parasympathetic activity induced by reserpine. The dibenzocycloheptene derivatives (*e.g.*, amitriptyline) were observed to counteract some of the central effects induced by such cholinergic agents as tremorine and/or arecoline, whereas antidepressants in general were found to raise the threshold for cerebral seizures.

Another approach, which uses both direct and indirect pharmacological tests, was proposed by Petersen and Nielsen (1967). This appears to be valuable in screening for and differentiating between neuroleptic (antipsychotic) and thymoleptic (antidepressant) drugs. Petersen and Nielsen proposed a battery of tests which may successfully differentiate between these two groups of differentially active tricyclic substances.

According to Petersen and Nielsen (1967), the effects of a tricyclic neuroleptic are characterized by the following: reduction of motor activity, cataleptogenic action, facilitation of reserpine-induced changes, anti-apomorphine potential and antagonism of noradrenaline, serotonin and acetylcholine effects. On the other hand, the effects of tricyclic thymoleptics are characterized by facilitation of apomorphine-induced vomiting, potentiation of noradrenaline effects, interference with reserpine-produced changes and antagonism of tremorine, acetylcholine and serotonin effects.

A battery of direct and indirect tests was recommended by Janssen (1965) for the recognition of neuroleptic (antipsychotic) action. With the use of this battery, he described a "typical" neuroleptic-induced behavioral profile.

According to Janssen (1965), under the influence of a typical neuroleptic drug at low dose levels, operant behavior as a whole tends to disappear, whereas spinal reflexes remain normal. At the same time, exploratory behavior—as seen in the Open Field Test—decreases, conditioned responses are blocked and the animal responds less or more slowly to a variety of visual, tactile or auditory environmental stimuli. Discriminatory ability, however, remains normal. Natural, environmental or amphetamine-induced agitation or hyperactivity disappears rapidly. With higher doses, cataleptic immobility is the characteristic feature, when the animal "allows" its body to be placed in a variety of abnormal postures. Spontaneous motor activity is abolished, and the animal is indifferent to most environmental stimuli. Paradoxically, it is still capable of performing complicated acts. Muscular tone is usually increased; muscular tremors, restlessness, neurodysleptic movements and signs of CNS-excitation may be present (in monkeys, cats, sheep and cattle). With high doses, prostration, loss of righting reflex, ataxia, convulsions, palpebral ptosis and other symptoms of CNS-depression usually occur. Almost all neuroleptic drugs are powerful antiemetic agents and prevent the emetic effect produced by apomorphine. They are also typical adrenolytic substances of the alpha-receptor blocking type. As a consequence, they produce adrenaline reversal, reduce the pressor effects of noradrenaline, protect against toxic doses of catecholamines, dilate the arterial system, increase peripheral blood flow, decrease peripheral resistance and produce orthostatic hypotension. Some neuroleptics also have antihistaminic activity and a body-temperature lowering effect (*e.g.*, chlorpromazine), whereas others may produce gastric ulceration (*e.g.*, reserpine) or have weak anticholinergic properties (*e.g.*, chlorprothixene).

Finally, a battery of direct and indirect tests was recommended by Vernier (1966) for the recognition of antidepressant action. Vernier's (1966) battery for the recognition of antidepressant action consists of six groups of tests. According to this, antidepressant drugs prevent tetrabenazine and RO4-1284 induced ptosis and sedation (Vernier *et al.*, 1962; and Sulser *et al.*, 1962); produce an increased rate of lever pressing on a Sidman avoidance schedule (1953, 1956, 1959, 1963) after tetrabenazine, *d*-amphetamine and cocaine administration and an increase of spontaneous motor activity after RO4-1284 (Scheckel and Boff, 1964; and Sulser *et al.*, 1964); antagonize reserpine-induced hypothermia, ptosis, reduced spontaneous motor activity and facilitation of pentetrazol-induced "toxic extensor seizures" (Costa *et al.*, 1960; Vernier *et al.*, 1962; Askew, 1963; Garattini *et al.*, 1962; Metysova and Metys, 1965; Halliwell *et al.*, 1964; Chen and Bohner, 1961; and Domenjoz and Theobald, 1959); potentiate *d*-amphetamine-induced increase in spontaneous motor activity, self-stimulation and avoidance (Vernier *et al.*, 1962; Halliwell *et al.*, 1964; Frommel *et al.*, 1960; Stein, 1961; Carlton, 1961; and Weissman, 1961); shorten the duration of the loss of righting reflex after reserpine and ethanol administration (Sulser *et al.*, 1962; and Halliwell *et al.*, 1964); and block yohimbine-induced mortality in mice (Quinton, 1963; and Halliwell *et al.*, 1964).

3. Conditioning Procedures

Rating scales and pharmacological test results supply important data on drug-induced changes in animal behavior but give no information regarding the effect of the compound on the different stimulus-response constellations. This kind of information can only be provided by employing various conditioning procedures.

Conditioning is primarily a behavioral method, and as such it is based on developing specific behavioral (including autonomic) responses to formerly unspecific stimuli. The stimuli (and the responses) are well defined and measurable in the experimental situation. The method of conditioning is based on the conditional reflex, a behavioral phenomenon which is also one of the functioning patterns of the nervous system. Thus the behavioral conditioning method is closely linked to neurophysiology.

In assessing presently available psychoactive drugs, there are three basically different stimulus-response constellations (reflexes) which are frequently examined. These are the unconditional reflex, which is an innate specific response to a particular stimulus; the conditional reflex, which is an acquired specific response to a formerly unspecific stimulus; and the orienting reflex, originally conceived of as a startle response that interferes with conditioned responses.

a. Unconditional Reflex

Pavlov's (1928) conceptualization of the unconditional reflex (UR) was derived from his observation that food in close connection with the sensory end organs of the oral cavity consistently elicited salivary secretion. He called the food an unconditional stimulus (US) of alimentary salivation and the resulting salivary secretion a UR to food. Consequently, he defined the UR as a predictable obligatory response elicited by a specific stimulus which assumes an innate stimulus-response constellation. Thus in the UR, the direction taken by the impulse (or excitation) as it leaves the sense organ is determined solely by the nature of the impulse itself and follows its own through routes in the nervous system until the response (muscular, vascular, visceral or glandular) is produced. Other examples of UR's studied in animal pharmacology are the pupillary constriction to a light stimulus; vasodilation to hot temperature; withdrawal of the front paw to an electric shock, etc.

Two of the frequently used procedures for testing UR activity in animals under the influence of psychoactive drugs are to use the "jumping box" (a soundproof cage with a grill floor which provides for the unconditional—electric shock—stimulus which elicits the unconditional motor—escape—response) and to lightly touch the animal's nose, an even simpler procedure. To the latter US, under normal conditions, rats respond by head withdrawal.

UR activity is differentially influenced by psychoactive drugs, particularly by psychostimulant and psychosedative substances. Thus psychostimulant drugs in general have a facilitating (strengthening) effect on the motor component of the responses to US's. If the stimulant drug is a sympathomimetic, there is a similar marked (increased) response of the autonomic nervous system. On the other hand, sedatives (and also hypnotics) were found to have an inhibiting influence on UR's. This was recently confirmed by Killam and Killam (1965), who, using rather sophisticated instrumentation, were able to demonstrate that a sedative barbiturate (pentobarbital) depressed not only the electroencephalographic but also the behavioral responses to the unconditional direct-central stimulation of the reticular activating system.

Although Corson *et al.* (1963) found that meprobamate, an anxiolytic propanediol substance, abolished unconditional antidiuretic (and also electrolytic) responses, the effect of anxiolytic, antidepressant and antipsychotic drugs in general on UR behavior remains inconsistent. One possible cause for the inconsistent findings is the difference in the procedures used. For example, whereas Bambas *et al.* (1956) found that chlorpromazine has an inhibitory effect on the UR to a peripheral US, the same substance in Killam and Killam's (1965) experiment did not exert any effect on the electroencephalographic or behavioral UR's when the US was a direct, central stimulus.

b. Conditional Reflex

The effects of psychoactive drugs on conditional reflex (CR) activity can be studied by three different experimental paradigms. These are the classical or Pavlovian conditioning paradigm; the instrumental conditioning paradigm (Konorski and Miller, 1937; and Skinner, 1935, 1937); and the "experimental neurosis" model.

i. Classical Paradigm. An illustrative example of CR formation in the frame of reference of the classical conditioning paradigm is the frequently quoted experiment of Pavlov (1928). In this experiment the presentation of a metronome beat preceded the feedings of the animal on several occasions. After pairing the auditory stimulus with feeding a number of times, the metronome beat "acquired" the property to elicit salivary secretion. Thus the metronome beat became a conditional stimulus (CS) of salivation and salivation a CR to the metronome beat. Accordingly, the CR was defined as an acquired response in which a formerly unspecific stimulus becomes effective in triggering off a formerly specific response. Thus in the CR the direction taken by the CS-produced impulse (or excitation) as it leaves the sense organ is determined by the US and follows the through routes of the latter stimulus in the nervous system.

There are several routinely applied procedures for testing CR activity under the influence of psychoactive drugs. Besides acquisition or CR formation, the testing of CS discrimination and CR extinction is also frequently used.

By CS discrimination (or differentiation) Pavlov (1928) understood the phenomenon whereby the CR becomes limited to its particular CS. Differentiation follows a period of generalization during which a nonreinforced stimulus with similar but not identical qualities to the CS also elicits the CR. He defined extinction as cessation of CR's that occurs if reinforcement is withheld.

Pavlov (1928) postulated that two fundamental processes—the excitatory and the inhibitory processes—are the basis of CNS activity. He maintained that CR formation (or acquisition) is due to the excitatory process, whereas CS discrimination and CR extinction are due to the (internal) inhibitory process.

In animal psychopharmacological studies all three phenomena, *i.e.*, CR formation, extinction and CS discrimination, have been systematically investigated. For this purpose, the motor and the autonomic, *e.g.*, heart rate, components of the conditional withdrawal (escape) response and the autonomic, *e.g.*, salivary secretion, and the motor components of the conditional food reflex have been most frequently studied. As a result, differential patterns with the various psychoactive groups have been revealed.

It was demonstrated that stimulants, *e.g.*, caffeine and amphetamines, generally facilitate CR formation. They have a strengthening effect on the excitatory process, cause a moderate loss of CS differentiation (Gantt, 1957, 1959) and delay the extinction of the CR; *i.e.*, they have a weakening effect on the (internal) inhibitory process.

On the other hand, sedatives, *e.g.*, barbiturates, were found to interfere with CR formation only in such doses which also interfered with the UR. Thus, in Killam and Killam's experiments (1965), pentobarbital not only depressed the unconditional electroencephalographic and behavioral responses to the unconditional direct stimulation of the brain stem reticular formation but also depressed the electroencephalographic and behavioral responses to the auditory CS. One may infer from this that it produced a weakening of the excitatory process.

No consistent CR patterns within the classical paradigm have been recognized to date with antidepressant drugs. There are controversial findings whether or not they block conditional withdrawal (escape) reactions. However, Savchuk (1960) maintains that they interfere with CS differentiation, *i.e.*, that they weaken internal inhibition (Astrup, 1966).

Anxiolytic drugs were found to produce a dissociation (schizokinesis) among the various components of the CR. They appear to have only little or no effect on the motor component of the conditional withdrawal (escape) reaction, as demonstrated with meprobamate and phenaglycodol (Fink and Swinyard, 1962), whereas they diminished the autonomic (cardiac) component of the same reaction (Gliedman and Gantt, 1956; Gantt, 1962). Furthermore, with benzodiazepines, *e.g.*, chlordiazepoxide or diazepam, the behavioral components (tension manifested in the raised tail, arched back and immobility of the animal) of the conditional withdrawal (escape) reaction are alleviated.

In an extensive conditioning study with anxiolytic substances, Corson (1966) revealed that meprobamate eliminated or markedly inhibited all the conditioned antidiuretic, cardiac, respiratory and salivary responses but had no significant influence on classical motor defense reflexes or on discrimination-avoidance responses. He obtained similar results with diazepam and phenobarbital (although the latter substance appeared to depress the general alertness too). Corson's (1966) findings were confirmed by Newton (1966).

The effect of various antipsychotic drugs on CR behavior has been extensively explored. It was recognized that the phenothiazine, chlorpromazine, has a marked inhibitory effect on the motor component of the conditional withdrawal (escape) reflex (Courvoisier, 1956), whereas it affects the concomitant autonomic (cardiac) components to a much lesser extent (Tedeschi *et al.*, 1961). This finding was further supported by Killam and Killam (1965), who found that chlorpromazine selectively blocked the behavioral response to the conditional auditory stimulus of direct reticular activating system stimulation, leaving the electroencephalographic response to the CS unaffected. Similar inhibitory effects on the motor components of the withdrawal (escape) reaction were revealed by other antipsychotic phenothiazines.

Tedeschi *et al.* (1961) demonstrated that the selective inhibition of the motor components of the CR was greater with the aminoalkylphenothiazines than with the piperazinylalkyl-derivatives. The selective inhibition was stronger with methotrimeprazine than with chlorpromazine in the former group and weakest with prochlorperazine and thioproperazine in the latter group.

The same pattern of selective inhibition that is seen with antipsychotic phenothiazines appears to be true for other antipsychotic drugs, *e.g.*, chlorprothixene (a thioxanthene) and reserpine (a Rauwolfia alkaloid). (Even more, it also applies to mescaline, a psychotomimetic substance as recognized by Bridger and Gantt in 1956.)

Since concomitant with the interference of CR formation there is also a facilitation of extinction of the CR (and also of CS differentiation under certain conditions), it was suggested that antipsychotic drugs have a weakening effect on the excitatory process while they strengthen internal inhibition (Kaminsky and Savchuk, 1956; Sklyarova, 1960).

More recently, the effect of ribonucleic acid (RNA) on CR behavior of the rat was examined (Cameron *et al.*, 1963). It was found that RNA, a drug which may affect "memory" beneficially, increased CR formation and decreased the rate of the extinction.

ii. Instrumental Paradigm. In contradistinction to the classical paradigm in which the association of the CS with the US is the prerequisite to establish a CR, in the instrumental paradigm it is the association of the response with a motivational factor (reward or punishment) which is most important for "acquisition."

The usual procedure employed in the instrumental conditioning paradigm is carried out in a Skinner Box (Skinner, 1937). When the animal performs the task that is to become the CR, *e.g.*, lever pressing, it is rewarded, for example, with a pellet of food. Instead of receiving a reward, the animal may be conditioned to avoid punishment, *e.g.*, an electric shock, by the same procedure. Thus the reinforcing feature may be either a reward or the avoidance of punishment. When the animal receives a reward directly for a particular response, it is called approach conditioning, and when the animal receives a reward indirectly, *i.e.*, by avoiding punishment by a particular response, it is called avoidance conditioning.

Free operant conditioning techniques are a variation of the instrumental conditioning paradigm. In some instances every lever pressing is rewarded, while in others different schedules of reward are employed. Among the different schedules the most commonly used are the fixed ratios, the fixed intervals and the variable intervals.

In the course of psychopharmacological experiments in which the instrumental conditioning paradigm was used, it has been found that stimulants, *e.g.*, caffeine, amphetamines and 2-benzylpiperidines, enhance operant avoidance and approach reactions, although the amphetamines, because of their anorexic action, decrease operant food responses. On the other hand, sedatives, *e.g.*, barbiturates, were revealed to have a decreasing effect on operant behavior.

The effect of barbiturates on operant behavior was clearly demonstrated in the classical experiments by Miller (1961, 1964). In six varied but related experimental designs he trained rats to run to the end of a runway or press a lever to obtain either food or water, *i.e.*, the reward. The results revealed that animals given a small dose of amobarbital did not run as fast and pressed the lever less often than the control group (Steinberg, 1965).

The effect of antidepressants on operant behavior has been studied by a great number of investigators. Differential effects on operant avoidance and operant approach behavior were revealed.

Lever pressing avoidance responses, with the use of the Sidman avoidance schedule (Sidman, 1959), were shown to be increased under the influence of thymoleptic (antidepressant) drugs (Gatti and Bovet, 1963), an effect resembling that seen with some anticholinergic substances, *e.g.*, hyoscine, benactyzine (Jacobsen, 1963). Similar results were obtained by Dews (1962) and Vaillant (1964), who investigated the effects of tricyclic antidepressants on various patterns of operant behavior. Their results indicate that doses of imipramine up to 10 mg./kg. may increase the over-all response rate of pigeons. Carlton (1961) also reported that imipramine increased the facilitating effect of amphetamine in an operant, shock-avoidance situation (Valzelli *et al.*, 1967).

Hanson (1961) compared the effects of amitriptyline and imipramine on squirrel monkeys with the Sidman avoidance conditioning schedule (Sidman, 1959). He used doses of 5, 10 and 20 mg./kg. of both drugs. At the two lower doses, a progressive decrease in response rate with an increase in the number of shocks was observed. This was similar to the effect of antipsychotic phenothiazines (Plotnikoff, 1963; and Cook and Catania, 1964). However, with amitriptyline at the highest dose levels, an increase in over-all response rate occurred, without a reduction in the number of shocks the animal received. The same dose of imipramine did not cause a similar increase in responses (Dureman and Henriksson, 1967).

Similarly to lever pressing avoidance responses, operant approach behavior was decreased under the influence of antidepressant drugs in squirrel monkeys. Thus when Hanson (1961) compared amitriptyline and imipramine (40, 80 and 160 mg./kg.) on a multiple fixed interval-fixed ratio schedule, amitriptyline showed no effect after the first dose, caused a decrease of over-all response rate with some disruption of the fixed interval schedule after the second dose and produced a complete cessation of responses at the highest dose, with loss of even the fixed ratio responses. Imipramine had no effect at the lowest dose, produced a slight decrease in response rate after the middle dose and finally caused a marked drop in response rate at the highest dose with some disruption of the fixed interval performance but maintenance of the fixed ratio response (Vernier, 1961).

Among the anxiolytic substances, propanediols show no effect on operant behavior below such doses which do not interfere with UR's. More recently, however, an increment in lever pressing avoidance responses was found after administration of benzodiazepine compounds, *e.g.*, chlordiazepoxide (Gatti and Bovet, 1963).

The prevailing characteristic of drugs with antipsychotic properties in the instrumental conditioning paradigm is their ability to depress operant behavior. The same applies to the "morphiomimetic" and psychotomimetic substances (Jacobsen, 1963). Although phenothiazines in general and chlorpromazine in particular have a stronger action in this respect on avoidance and a lesser influence on approach responses, Rauwolfia alkaloids, particularly reserpine, have the opposite effect (Hecht *et al.*, 1960; and Hecht, 1963). It is usually the interference with operant avoidance responses, however, and not with the operant approach responses, which is considered to be correlated with antipsychotic properties.

A comparative study with ten antipsychotic drugs on avoidance behavior was conducted by Gatti (1957, 1966). The substances included in the experiment were chlorpromazine, prochlorperazine, perphenazine, triflupromazine, trifluoperazine, fluphenazine (all phenothiazines), haloperidol, triperidol, R-2028 (butyrophenones) and chlorprothixene (a thioxanthene). A modification of the continuous Sidman type of lever pressing discrimination-avoidance procedure (Sidman, 1959), was used. Shocks of 1.5 A. and 2 seconds duration were given at 30-second intervals with the light turned on if the rats did not press the lever. Each response turned off the light and started a response-shock interval (*i.e.*, 30 second) which consisted of a dark period of 18 seconds, followed by a period of 12 seconds in which the light was turned on as a warning stimulus. Shocks could be avoided by responding during the first (dark) period, which postponed both the presentation of the warning stimulus and the shock, or by responding during the second (lighted) period, which turned off the light and led to the avoidance of the shock. It was found that chlorprothixene and the butyrophenones differed from phenothiazines in having a relatively higher proportion of responses during the first section of the response-shock interval. Furthermore, with increasing dosages the proportion of these responses was reduced by chlorpromazine, while it was enhanced by haloperidol. Among the phenothiazines, the three chlorinated derivatives equally depressed responses to the warning stimulus (CS). The differences in responses to shock (US) were accounted for by a slightly greater proportion of presignal avoidance responses with chlorpromazine. The trifluoromethyl phenothiazines depress responses to light (CS) and to shock (US) differentially. The former are better preserved with fluphenazine, more affected by triflupromazine, whereas the results with trifluoperazine are in an intermediate position.

iii. Experimental Neurosis. Experimental neurosis is a term which means behavior disturbances produced in an animal by experimental procedures which resemble the symptoms observed in human neuroses. The concept of experimental neurosis developed in Pavlov's (1928) laboratory while CR experiments were being carried out on animals. In the classical experiment the dog was conditioned to respond to the presentation of a circle but not to an ellipse. As the experiment went on, the ellipse was made to resemble the circle more and more. Soon the dog began to encounter increasing difficulty in discriminating between the two objects. After a certain time of failing to discriminate its behavior suddenly changed. Unlike its former behavior, the dog now struggled to avoid entering the experimental room for the succeeding tests; instead of standing quietly waiting for the CS, it appeared restless, howled and attempted to bite indiscriminately. At the same time, the already established CS discrimination disappeared. In other similar experiments, the "experimental neurosis" manifested itself in an inhibited type of behavior in contrast to the excited state described above.

The interaction of pharmacological agents with experimentally induced neuroses was first described by Pavlov (1928). He recognized that rest brought about complete cure of most of the experimental neuroses. However, neuroses with predominantly excitatory manifestations could be "treated" only by sedatives (*e.g.*, bromides) in addition to rest. On the other hand, in those neuroses with prevailing inhibitory manifestations where rest alone remained ineffective, the administration of caffeine, a stimulant, seemed to be quite useful. When the "neurosis" manifested itself in a mixed, *i.e.*, inhibitory and excitatory, form, the simultaneous administration of the two substances, *i.e.*, caffeine and bromide, was required.

On the basis of these findings it was formulated that sedatives, particularly inorganic bromide salts, facilitate the restitution of the inhibitory process and particularly of internal, *i.e.*, differential, delayed and extinctive, inhibitory functions (Astrup, 1966); whereas stimulants, *e.g.*, caffeine, promote the restitution of the excitatory process, *i.e.*, conditional reflex formation. Gantt (1966) stressed the importance of the interaction between the underlying constitutional factors and the drug's pharmacological action. He suggested regulating the dose according to the temperament and studied the possible change of reactivity caused by the drug through some as yet unknown processes, which he called autokinesis.

More recently, the effect of various psychoactive substances has been systematically explored on experimental neuroses. For these investigations Masserman's (1943) experimental procedure was usually followed. In this procedure the "conflict" is produced when the formerly rewarded lever pressing response is "unexpectedly" associated with a concomitant "punishment," *e.g.*, electric shock. Findings with stimulants and antidepressants in this experimental procedure are inconsistent, but antipsychotic drugs decrease the number of shocks an animal receives while pressing a lever to get food. On the other hand, anxiolytic drugs, especially the benzodiazepines (also propanediols), in contradistinction to the antipsychotics, increase the number of shocks the animal receives.

In Miller's (1961 and 1964) experiments, while amobarbital significantly reduced lever pressing to obtain a reward in the original experimental setting, the same substance in a conflictual situation, when the rats could obtain the rewards only if they sometimes received punishment (by means of electric shock), had a different effect. In this constellation the performance of undrugged controls fell off markedly, whereas the performance of rats under the influence of the drug was little affected.

In other experiments rats were trained to give themselves injections, by pressing a bar, with a solution of amobarbital, and it was found that the rate of self-injection decreased. When, under the same conditions, they were given electric shocks and were presumably "frightened," the rate of self-injection increased (Steinberg, 1965).

c. *Orienting Reflex*

The concept of the orienting reflex originated from an incidental observation during Pavlov's (1928) early work in conditioning. During one of the experiments in which a CR salivary secretion was established to a metronome beat, a strong sound occurred following the CS but preceding the CR. The animal turned in the direction of the new sound and did not respond with salivary secretion to the already conditioned stimulus. The phenomenon was conceptualized by Pavlov (1928) as "external inhibition;" *i.e.*, the strong sound produced a startle reaction which temporarily interfered (by external inhibition) with the already established CR (Ban, 1964).

More recently, in a modern neurophysiological frame of reference, Gastaut (1956, 1957, 1958) summarized the role of different morphological structures in orienting behavior. According to him, the application of a stimulus prior to any conditioning procedure results in a startle response with its visceral effects and generalized desynchronization of the electroencephalogram. This corresponds with the activation of the brain stem reticular formation. The startle response is followed by a reaction of attention (orienting response) in which Gastaut (1956) pointed out the additional influence of the intralaminar and thalamic reticular nuclei with their more localized desynchronizing effect on the electroencephalogram. Thus Gastaut (1956) contrasted the primitive, undifferentiated signal (emotional) quality of the startle response with the more appropriately attentive recognition of the orienting reflex.

Orienting behavior has been investigated in psychopharmacological studies. The inhibitory effect of CNS depressants and the facilitating effect of CNS stimulants (*i.e.*, substances with a primary effect on arousal function, which is related to brain stem reticular formation structures) on the orienting reflex have been reported. Antidepressant and anxiolytic drugs (*i.e.*, compounds with a primary effect on affectivity, which is related to limbic lobe, visceral brain structures) do not seem to exert any characteristic influence on the OR. The effect of antipsychotics (*i.e.*, drugs which act on integrational processes, which are primarily related to the activity of the cerebral cortex) generally seems to resemble the CNS depressant, and the effect of psychotomimetic drugs in general is similar to the CNS stimulant pattern. The depressant effects of antipsychotics on the OR were demonstrated by Gantt (1957). In his experiments both chlorpromazine and reserpine diminished the motor (centrally mediated skeletal muscle) and cardiac (autonomic) components of the orienting reflex.

Since CR phenomena are overt behavioral manifestations which reflect the functioning of their morphological substrates, the effect of psychoactive substances on CR variables can provide meaningful indications in regard to the site of action of these drugs.

4. Site of Action

a. *Neurophysiological Correlates*

Since central nervous system (CNS) structures are intimately related with psychological, and consequently psychopathological, processes, the accumulating information on the neurophysiological correlates of psychotropic drug action in animals may hopefully lead to an early indication of their therapeutic action in men.

The role of the various CNS structures in psychological processes was succinctly presented by Smythies (1966). According to the classical view, the prevailing importance of the cerebral cortex in general and of the association areas in particular was stressed.

In this frame of reference the sensory input was considered to be transmitted via the thalamus, a shunt of nervous impulses, to the grey matter of the cerebral hemispheres. Here the various "messages" are integrated and selectively channelled to the precentral-frontal-motor areas, resulting in skeleto-muscular actions, and to the hypothalamus, evoking appropriate affective responses and their autonomic concomitants. To this point, the role of the basal ganglia is limited to the refinement of motor activity, and the prevailing function attributed to the rhinencephalic structures is the sense of smell.

The classical view on the functional role of various brain structures in higher nervous activity was gradually replaced, after 1936, by newer concepts. The recognition of the functional importance of the reticular formation by Magoun and Rhines (1946) and the demonstration of the essential role of brain stem reticular formation structures in the complex psychological function of consciousness by Moruzzi and Magoun (1949) were two important contributions which brought about major changes in our concepts of various functions of the CNS. Another important contribution was the recognition of the intralaminar and thalamic nuclei, a part of the thalamic reticular system, and their role and effects in attention (Gastaut, 1958).

The discovery of the functional importance of the reticular formation together with the findings by electroanatomical and physiological studies renewed interest in the limbic system (MacLean, 1949). These developments provided additional support for Papez's (1937) assertion that the strongly developed fiber connections between certain parts of the rhinencephalon, namely the hippocampus, mammillary bodies, anterior thalamus and cingulate gyrus, suggested "a functional circuit largely concerned with emotion and its expression."

Further investigations revealed that the limbic system, the reticular formation and other related structures (for example, the hypothalamus and the septal nuclei) form a complex and integrated system (with connections to the extrapyramidal motor system, thalamic nuclei and the cerebral cortex) which is closely connected with the various aspects of psychological functioning (Smythies, 1966).

In view of the relationships between various brain structures and psychic activity, it appeared desirable to reveal the influence of the various psychopharmacological substances on various well defined areas of the nervous system in animal experiments. Furthermore, since psychotropic drugs are defined as substances which have a prevailing effect on the higher function of the CNS, an integral part of pharmacodynamics of the known psychoactive compounds is to reveal their action on the different "hierarchical levels" of the nervous system.

The actions of psychopharmacological substances on the following structures have been explored (in ascending order): autonomic nervous system, spinal cord, medulla oblongata, brain stem reticular formation, hypothalamus, thalamus, septum, amygdala, hippocampus and the cerebral cortex. Direct information on the changes in the electrical activity of these structures following psychoactive drug administration can be obtained by implanted electrode techniques. By this method the drug-induced changes on the spontaneous electrical activity of any particular section of the brain can be revealed, and the electrical after-effects of direct stimulation can be studied.

i. Autonomic Nervous System. Autonomic nervous system (ANS) responses are intimately related to "affectivity" in general and "emotions" in particular. The effect of various psychoactive drugs on ANS functioning can be recognized by behavioral observations or revealed by pharmacological testing. To determine whether the effects are central or peripheral in origin, psychopharmacological procedures are employed.

α. Behavioral Observations. Much information on the action of psychoactive drugs on the two functional aspects (sympathetic and parasympathetic) of the autonomic nervous system has been collected through behavioral observations. For example, the size of pupils (sympathicotonia: mydriasis; parasympathicotonia: miosis) and the body temperature (sympathicotonia: hyperthermia; parasympathicotonia: hypothermia) were found to be reliable indicators of psychoactive drug effects on the ANS.

β. Pharmacological Tests. Behavioral observations are complemented by pharmacological tests in assessing the influence of psychoactive drugs on autonomic functions. For example, adrenaline antagonism was found useful in the detection of sympatholytic effects (Turner, 1965) and antisialagogue activity, *i.e.*, the blockade of salivation, in the detection of parasympatholytic action (Issekutz, 1917). (A reduced number of ulcerations in the stomach was also found to be a sensitive indicator of the parasympatholytic action of psychoactive drugs, as revealed by the Shay ulcer test, in which the flow of gastric juice is stopped by ligation of the pylorus) (Shay *et al.*, 1945).

γ. Psychopharmacological Procedures. Psychopharmacological procedures are used to indicate whether the autonomic changes induced by a psychoactive drug were the result of central (hypothalamic) or peripheral effects of the substances. For example, the morphine-atropine test can distinguish between central (counteracts morphine- but not atropine-induced mydriasis) and peripheral (counteracts atropine- but not morphine-induced mydriasis) parasympatholytic actions of psychoactive drugs. On the other hand, the strychnine test distinguishes between peripheral (does not potentiate strychnine effect) and central (potentiation of strychnine effect) sympathotonic actions.

Of the various psychoactive drugs it has been found that the sedatives, *e.g.*, barbiturates, have an inhibiting effect on parasympathetic ganglia. More recently, it has been revealed that they also exert an inhibitory action on the transmission of impulses in the sympathetic ganglia. Stimulants, *e.g.*, amphetamines, on the other hand, produce characteristic sympathotonic changes.

Similarly, the stimulant MAOI antidepressants were recognized as central sympathotonic drugs, although more recently their inhibitory or blocking effect on ganglionic transmission has also been observed. In contradistinction to the MAOI's, tricyclic antidepressants are known for their strongly parasympatholytic action. Although anxiolytic drugs, *e.g.*, benzodiazepines, are only weak sympatholytics, antipsychotic phenothiazines were early characterized as being strongly sympatholytic substances. Similarly, the antipsychotic Rauwolfias were found to interfere (via central mechanisms) with sympathetic nervous system activity.

In spite of these findings, however, the exact relationship between psychostimulant and sympathotonic, antidepressant and parasympatholytic and antipsychotic and sympatholytic activity still remains to be proven.

ii. Spinal Cord. The action of psychoactive substances on the spinal cord was seen in their effects on the monosynaptic front-leg reflex (knee jerk) and the polysynaptic hind-limb reflex.

With sedative barbiturates, an inhibitory effect on both the mono- and polysynaptic reflexes was observed. The polysynaptic pathways appear to be more susceptible to these effects. On the other hand, stimulant amphetamines have long been recognized as having a facilitating effect on these reflexes.

Although antidepressant and antipsychotic drugs do not show any consistent action, anxiolytic benzodiazepines (and also propanediols) have an inhibitory effect on the monosynaptic (and also polysynaptic) reflex functions. This inhibitory action of benzodiazepines and propanediols on the knee jerk is counteracted by strychnine, whereas strychnine-induced convulsions are counteracted by substances belonging to either of these two groups of anxiolytic drugs.

iii. Medulla Oblongata. The action of psychoactive drugs on the medullary centers *in vivo* has been detected primarily by their effect on the vomiting center. Since a number of vital centers, *e.g.*, respiratory and cardiovascular, are also located in this region, the effects of psychoactive substances on these centers are a sensitive indicator of medullary action.

It has been recognized that sedative barbiturates in toxic doses paralyze the cardiovascular center and that morphine depresses the respiratory center. Both of these actions were found to be counteracted, at least in part, by stimulants, *e.g.*, amphetamine drugs.

The trigger zone sensitivity threshold of the vomiting center shows changes under the influence of a great many psychoactive drugs. The antiemetic strength of various psychotropic substances can be tested by the antiapomorphine test. This test measures the dose (increased or decreased) of apomorphine required to induce vomiting after administration of the substance under investigation. Whereas anxiolytic benzodiazepines were found to have an inconsistent effect in this test, tricyclic antidepressants have consistently shown a mild antiemetic action. A moderate to strong antiapomorphine effect was found to be characteristic of antipsychotic drugs, particularly phenothiazines.

iv. Brain Stem Reticular Formation. The complex psychological function consciousness is related to the activity of the brain stem reticular formation structures in humans. These structures provide for the coordination of the different levels of the central nervous system. For this reason the action of psychopharmacological substances on the brain stem reticular formation is one of the most extensively explored areas of research.

The brain stem reticular formation consists of grey (cellular) masses in the tegmentum of the medulla, pons and midbrain. Whereas the descending reticular system is considered a part of the extrapyramidal system, the ascending reticular system is considered to be part of the sensory pathways of the central nervous system. The impulse from an environmental stimulus is transmitted in part through the lemniscal system to a localized area in the cortex and in part through the side branches of the reticular system, diffusely, to the whole cortex. Both indirect environmental stimulation and direct stimulation of the brain stem reticular formation by implanted electrodes produce an electroencephalographic arousal reaction. This is seen on the surface electroencephalogram as desynchronized activity of low amplitude and fast rhythm, the opposite of that observed in deep sleep.

Psychoactive drugs were recognized to have a differential effect on the arousal reaction, which is intimately related to the functioning of these structures. Among the various psychoactive drugs it was found that sedative barbiturates have a particularly strong depressant effect on the brain stem reticular activating system. It was shown that they produce an increased threshold to direct electrical stimulation in these structures and depress evoked potentials to a variety of peripheral sensory stimuli.

In contrast to sedatives, Bradley and Key (1958) demonstrated that stimulant amphetamines lower the electroencephalographic and behavioral thresholds for arousal. This applies to both environmental and direct stimulation, which means that, besides lowering the threshold of sensory impulses from the periphery, amphetamines also have a direct stimulating action on the brain stem.

The effect of anxiolytic substances on these structures is equivocal. For example, whereas propanediols, *e.g.*, meprobamate, did not seem to have an effect on the brain stem, benzodiazepines, *e.g.*, chlordiazepoxide, were found to have a biphasic effect. The latter substance in low doses "sensitizes" brain stem reticular formation structures with a concomitant facilitation of transmission of afferent nerve impulses, whereas in high doses it has a blocking effect.

There is a differential effect of the two major groups of antidepressant drugs on brain stem reticular formation structures. The MAOI's were recognized to have a stimulating (arousal) effect on brain stem reticular activity as reflected in the "alerting" electroencephalographic response, in contrast to the tricyclic antidepressant drugs, which were found to have an inhibitory "suppressant" action (acute block) at first, which later is replaced by "chronic arousal" (Himwich, 1965).

It was thought for some time that the crucial effect of antipsychotic phenothiazine drugs is their influence on the brain stem reticular formation function. More recently, however, when arousal to peripheral stimulation was differentiated from the arousal produced by direct stimulation through implanted electrodes, it was learned that under the influence of phenothiazines the arousal reaction was diminished to peripheral stimulation only, which implies that their action is mainly on the afferent pathways to the reticular formation.

Not all antipsychotic drugs exert the same effect on brain stem reticular formation functions. A distinctly different action on these structures is shown by the antipsychotic Rauwolfia preparations, *e.g.*, reserpine, which in small doses exert a stimulating effect on brain stem reticular formation activity and induce a facilitation of the transmission of impulses in these areas and only in high doses produce an inhibitory effect.

Because of the differential effects of antipsychotic phenothiazines and Rauwolfias on these structures, it was surmised that chlorpromazine might exert its antipsychotic actions by reducing the excessive transmission of unselected sensory information (stimuli), which might explain the sleep-inducing properties of this drug, without a blockade of all sensory communication (input) (Killam and Killam, 1960). On the other hand, it is considered that reserpine might exert its antipsychotic effects by reducing excessive inhibition and thus by "exposing the patient to conditioning by external stimuli."

Although much is yet to be learned about the functions of the reticular system and even more about the way it responds to the effects of psychoactive drugs, for practical purposes it is generally accepted that sedative barbiturates in certain dosages inhibit the arousal syndrome, while simultaneously lowering the state of consciousness. Anti-acetylcholine drugs, *e.g.*, hyoscine, atropine, benactyzine and diphenhydramine, as well as tricyclic antidepressants, initially have a blocking effect on the arousal system without, however, affecting consciousness. On the other hand, it is well established that stimulant amphetamines, phenylethylamine derivatives in general (including adrenaline, pipradrol, etc.), acetylcholine and MAOI antidepressant drugs have a stimulating effect on the "arousal system" with concomitant observable behavioral effects.

It was noted that when arousal to peripheral stimulation was differentiated from the arousal produced by direct stimulation through implanted electrodes, in the case of barbiturates or amphetamines, the arousal effect to both peripheral and direct stimulation was equally altered (inhibited or facilitated, respectively), whereas in the case of chlorpromazine and LSD_{25}, the arousal effect was significantly changed (inhibited or facilitated, respectively) to peripheral stimulation only (Bradley, 1958).

v. Hypothalamus. The primary functions of the hypothalamus are regulatory in nature. This structure is the central regulator of the sympathetic nervous system, endocrine glands and body temperature. Its activity is intimately associated with emotional responses. The controlling effect of the cerebral cortex on hypothalamic activity has been known for a long time. According to more recent information, however, its functioning is more specifically under the inhibitory influence of certain septal areas and under the stimulating influence of the amygdala.

The effect of various psychoactive drugs on the hypothalamus can be inferred from behavioral observations in the intact animal and by their effects on "sham rage," produced by decortication. However, it is the effects of psychotropic chemicals on "self-stimulation," *i.e.*, on the positive and negative motivational centers present in the hypothalamus, which are most extensively studied.

The action of drugs on hypothalamic motivational mechanisms was studied by the self-stimulation technique of Olds and Milner (1954). In self-stimulation the animal delivers electrical stimulation to its own brain (*e.g.*, hypothalamus) via implanted microelectrodes by performing an arbitrarily selected response, *e.g.*, lever pressing. The animal may respond at rates of up to 8000 per hour until exhaustion. For the purpose of psychopharmacological studies, these high rate performances are unsuitable, and therefore other devices have been developed to lower the rate of self-stimulation. In one of these devices the self-stimulation rate is lowered by reducing the intensity of the electrical stimulation to very low values, near or just below the threshold of reinforcement. In another device the baseline rate is lowered by decreasing the number of opportunities for reinforcement; *e.g.*, responses are reinforced with brain stimulation only at variable intervals according to a random schedule (Stein, 1967).

With the use of the Olds and Milner (1954) technique in psychopharmacological studies, it was revealed that self-stimulation is selectively facilitated by psychostimulants, especially by the amphetamines and also to a lesser extent by cocaine (but not by strychnine, picrotoxin and nicotine). It was also noted that tricyclic antidepressants increased self-stimulation only when electrodes were placed in the lateral hypothalamic nuclei, whereas they potentiated the methamphetamine-induced increment in the rat also with electrodes placed in the posterior hypothalamic region. In contradistinction to psychostimulants and antidepressants, it was found that self-stimulation is selectively inhibited with electrodes placed in the ventral posterior hypothalamus by antipsychotic and depressant drugs, *e.g.*, phenothiazine derivatives and butyrophenones, or the monoamine depleters, such as the Rauwolfia alkaloid reserpine and the benzoquinolizine tetrabenazine, respectively. Anxiolytic and sedative substances, such as the propanediols, benzodiazepines and/or barbiturates have no effect on self-stimulation below the doses which severely impair motor functions (Stein, 1967).

Other effects of psychoactive drugs on the hypothalamus are as follows. Sedative barbiturates do not seem to act directly on hypothalamic centers, although it is still maintained that one of the effects of these drugs is on the sleep areas of the diencephalon (Grollman, 1965). On the other hand, the stimulant amphetamines appear to stimulate the medial and lateral regions of the hypothalamus. It has been suggested that as a consequence they stimulate the inhibitory and depress the excitatory "feeding centers" located in the medial and lateral portions of the hypothalamus, respectively, and thereby exert their anorexigenic effects.

Although anxiolytic benzodiazepines were found to have an inhibitory effect on the hypothalamic centers which control pituitary prolactin secretion and also on the sympathetic nuclei of the posterior hypothalamus, indirect evidence, *e.g.*, sympathicotonic manifestations in general and hyperthermia in particular, suggests that MAOI antidepressants have the opposite, *i.e.*, stimulating, effect on the latter structures.

The effects on the hypothalamus of antipsychotic drugs in general and the phenothiazines in particular are even more complex. Investigations suggest that "sham rage" can be controlled by chlorpromazine and reserpine. This implies that these antipsychotic drugs may have a controlling effect on some hypothalamic centers. Furthermore, the characteristic ptosis and miosis produced with reserpine and to a lesser degree with chlorpromazine, the inhibitory effect of these two drugs on central heat regulation and their effect on endocrine functions strongly suggest a definite hypothalamic action.

In 1959 systematic studies began on the evaluation of the biological effects of a group of synthetic derivatives of plant regulator acids. The result of this work was the discovery of the psychoactive properties of centrophenoxine, which is the dimethylamine-ethyl ester of *p*-chlorophenoxyacetic acid. This auxin derivative, which has stimulant and alerting properties and, according to some investigators, has a beneficial effect on organic confusional states, acts principally on the hypothalamus and induces (via the hypothalamic structures) increased hypophyseal secretion (Thuillier, 1961).

vi. Thalamus. It was long believed that the thalamus is the "reservoir" of all of the sensory input wherefrom the various unspecific impulses were selectively transmitted to the specific cortical centers. Consequently, a role in the affective—emotional—responses was attributed to the thalamic structures. More recently, the function of selective attention was suggested to be intimately related to the intralaminar and thalamic nuclei.

The effect of various psychoactive drugs on the thalamus is most frequently investigated today by implanted electrode techniques. Thus the action of the substance on spontaneous electrical activity, on the after-effects of direct stimulation and on recruiting responses can be studied. It has been found that direct electrical stimulation of the anterior thalamic part of the reticular formation results in a successive increase in amplitude of electroencephalographic responses in the corresponding cortical areas. Because the number of neurons involved in this response successively increases, this response is usually called a recruiting response.

The effects of psychoactive drugs on the thalamus are as follows. Stimulants, *e.g.*, amphetamines, are seen to decrease the recruiting activity of the thalamic intralaminary system, as opposed to sedatives, *e.g.*, barbiturates, which enhance this activity (Monnier and Krupp, 1959).

Although antidepressants did not seem to exert a consistent effect on thalamic structures, antipsychotics in general and phenothiazines in particular, *e.g.*, chlorpromazine, in small doses produced an enhancement of the recruiting response similar to that seen with barbiturates. In high doses, however, the same drug, as well as reserpine, was found to exert an inhibitory effect similar to that seen with the amphetamines. Anxiolytic benzodiazepines produce a general inhibitory effect on thalamic functions. This was primarily recognized in an increased threshold to stimulation, in a diminished responsivity, *i.e.*, low amplitude, and in a shortened duration of after-discharges.

Simultaneous surface and depth recordings of electrical activity revealed that synchronization of the electrical activity after administering meprobamate, an anxiolytic propanediol drug, starts from the thalamus and from there it spreads to the cerebral cortex. Thus, at least in the case of this substance, the primary target area of action is considered to be in the thalamic centers.

vii. Septum. Certain septal areas have an inhibitory influence on brain stem reticular formation structures and on hypothalamic centers. To a certain extent they control behavioral arousal and emotional output.

In psychopharmacological studies with implanted electrode techniques, Schallek and Kuehn (1960) revealed that tricyclic antidepressants, particularly imipramine, had a depressant effect on inhibitory septal areas. This was reflected in increased threshold to electrical stimulation, with suppression of after-discharges, and in hypothalamic release phenomena.

Anxiolytic drugs, *e.g.*, propanediols or benzodiazepines, also shorten the duration of after-discharges from the same septal areas. Furthermore, benzodiazepines slow the spontaneous electrical activity of the septum and control irritability produced by septal lesions.

viii. Amygdala. Whereas certain septal areas inhibit, the amygdala has a facilitating effect on hypothalamic activity and concomitantly on emotional output. It also appears to play a role in conditioning and learning. In psychopharmacological studies, Schallek (1960) showed that MAOI antidepressants enhance the excitability of this structure, *i.e.*, lower the threshold to electrical stimulation and prolong the time of after-discharges. Tricyclic antidepressants were found to have a similar effect but to a lesser degree. This suggests an amygdala-septum-hypothalamus "system," in which the stimulating, inhibiting and conducting functions are carried out by the amygdala, certain septal areas and the hypothalamus, respectively.

Anxiolytics in general suppress the activity of the amygdala. This was demonstrated in the elevated threshold for electrical stimulation and in the shortened duration of after-discharges under the influence of anxiolytic drugs. Benzodiazepines were shown to slow the spontaneous electrical activity recorded by implanted electrodes, whereas diazepam controlled the effect of cocaine-induced seizures, which spread from the amygdala to other central nervous system structures. It has been suggested that the anxiolytic effect of benzodiazepines is related to their effects on the amygdala.

Antipsychotic phenothiazines were shown to shorten the duration of characteristic seizure-like discharges from the amygdala. Furthermore, Ursin (1962) demonstrated that chlorpromazine not only blocks the afferent influences from the periphery but also blocks the influences from the amygdala to the other CNS structures.

ix. Hippocampus. Recent memory and "active" forgetting appear to be functionally related to the hippocampus.

In psychopharmacological studies with implanted electrode techniques, it is possible to show that stimulant amphetamines which have an excitatory effect on brain stem reticular formation structures transiently suppress the activity of the hippocampus. On the other hand, sedative barbiturates which depress the brain stem reticular formation are seen to exert a transient excitatory effect on this structure. A relationship between the brain stem and hippocampal functions in arousal was suggested. It is thought that there is a brain stem-hippocampus axis in which the former represents the excitatory and the latter the inhibitory endpoint.

MAOI and tricyclic antidepressants have a differential effect on hippocampal functions. Although MAOI's were found to have an inhibitory influence, manifested in suppressed after-discharges to direct electrical stimulation without an actual change in the threshold of stimulation, tricyclic antidepressants induced a convulsant brain wave pattern originating in the hippocampal region.

Anxiolytic benzodiazepines slow the spontaneous electrical activity and depress hippocampal after-discharges to direct stimulation. On the other hand, antipsychotic Rauwolfias induce a regular, continuous electrical activity of the hippocampus. More recently, it has been shown that magnesium pemoline, a substance with a possible beneficial effect on memory disturbances, facilitates evoked potentials not only in the sensory motor cortex, similar to the stimulant amphetamines, but also in the hippocampus (Gallant and Bishop, 1967).

x. Cerebral Cortex. According to the classical view, the frontal cortex is concerned with motor and social integration, the parietal lobes with sensory and spatial functions and the temporal lobes with complex sensory integration and emotions. More recently, on the basis of Penfield and Jasper's (1954) work, it has been suggested that the temporal lobes are also involved in the interpretation of experience and possibly in the "laying down" of permanent memory stores.

Differential effects of various psychoactive drugs on the cerebral cortex were demonstrated by surface electroencephalographic recordings. With sedative barbiturates there is at first a fast wave (15 to 35 cycles per second) activity, which spreads from the frontal areas to the parietal and occipital cortex, corresponding to the disinhibitory state produced by these drugs. This disinhibitory state is followed by a lowering of the level of alertness concomitant with a slow (2 to 8 cycles per second) frequency and characteristically large amplitude waves, *i.e.*, increased voltage. Paradoxically, atropine was found to induce excitement simultaneously with high amplitude, slow wave activity, similar to that seen in barbiturate-induced sleep.

Stimulants in general increase the frequency and decrease the voltage of the electroencephalogram. Thus the characteristic amphetamine effect is manifest in fast wave and low voltage activity, which may lead to desynchronization. More recently, however, the amphetamine-produced desynchronization was found to be restricted to the frontal cortex (in rabbits), while at the same time it was possible to depict through the occipital leads slow waves of high voltage activity. It was noted that physostigmine also induces low voltage fast waves without manifesting behavioral stimulation.

Antidepressants do not show any uniform action on the electroencephalogram. The effects of these drugs are reflected by desynchronization (aralkylhydrazines and tricyclics), sleep spindles or seizure-like discharges (hydrazides) and increased theta rhythm and fast beta activity (tricyclics). Anxiolytics, *e.g.*, benzodiazepines, produce a shift toward fast activity and synchronization, while the effect of antipsychotic phenothiazines and Rauwolfias is characterized by protraction (slowing) of the basal rhythm, increased delta activity and induction of spontaneous seizure discharges.

The characteristic neurophysiological action profiles of psychotropic drugs in animals have been summarized by Himwich (1965). He described the effects of seven prototype psychoactive drugs in a systematic manner on the medullary (respiratory) centers, mesodiencephalic (midbrain reticular formation and thalamic projections) activating systems (MDAS), limbic structures and the neocortex. According to him, prototype sedatives, *e.g.*, barbiturates, depress the activity of medullary respiratory centers, have a blocking effect on the MDAS, inhibit limbic structures and depress the neocortex. The central actions of sedatives are distinctly different from those of the anxiolytics or antipsychotics. Neither of the latter groups has any effect on the respiratory centers or on the neocortex. Of the anxiolytics, benzodiazepines have a diphasic (facilitates in low doses and blocks in high doses the transmission of nerve impulses) effect and propanediols have no effect on the MDAS, whereas both these groups have an inhibitory influence on limbic structures. Of the antipsychotics, the Rauwolfia alkaloid reserpine first produces an early arousal and later a blocking of the MDAS, while the phenothiazines induce an acute block and chronic arousal with inhibition of limbic structures. Acute block and chronic arousal of the MDAS with limbic lobe stimulation characterizes tricyclic antidepressants, while MDAS arousal without an effect on limbic structures is typical of MAOI antidepressants.

b. Neurochemical Correlates

The first attempts to reveal the neurochemical correlates of psychopharmacological properties was directed toward investigating their effect on the "over-all energy metabolism of the CNS." By this approach, important information was obtained, but the main differential features among psychoactive substances could not be delineated. To date there is no evidence of a differential effect of various psychoactive drugs on the over-all energy metabolism of the CNS. This is partly due to the fact that, on the basis of the oxygen consumption of the brain, one can differentiate only between states of full consciousness and coma.

In regard to the various aspects of energy metabolism, the following was learned. In the mitochondria the energy produced in the oxidation of glucose is used to phosphorylate adenosine diphosphate (ADP) to adenosine triphosphate (ATP). Since sedative barbiturates and antipsychotic phenothiazines were both found to interfere with (or inhibit) oxidative phosphorylation, this process did not provide for differentiation between these two groups of psychoactive drugs. Furthermore, on the basis of their interference with oxidative phosphorylation, it was expected that phenothiazines and barbiturates would lead to reduced ATP levels in the brain. Instead, the administration of these drugs led to an increase in ATP levels. This was due to the decreased ATP utilization in the CNS. Another effect encountered was enhancement of glycolysis or an increase in glycogen stores in the CNS after MAOI antidepressant or antipsychotic Rauwolfia drug administration, respectively. An inhibitory effect on oxygen uptake with a short lasting increase in glucose concentration in the CNS was found also with anxiolytic benzodiazepine compounds.

Because of the rather limited findings from energy metabolism studies and the relative absence of differential effects in the exploration of the neurochemical correlates of psychotropic drug action, other means had to be employed. Another approach was based on Quastel and Wooldridge's (1928) fundamental findings on the competitive inhibition of enzymes and the theory of chemical transmission of nervous impulses, *i.e.*, the chemical counterpart of Ramon y Cajal's (1909) "neuron" concept.

On the basis of the theory of the chemical transmission of nerve impulses, it was assumed that there are chemical transmitters in the CNS, continually formed and inactivated by specific enzymes. It was also assumed that under physiological conditions there is a balance among the chemical transmitter substances; that the action of psychoactive drugs may be correlated with a change in this balance; and that this change of balance is an outcome of interference (competitive inhibition) with one or the other of the specific enzymes responsible for the formation or inactivation of the chemical transmitter substances by the psychoactive compound.

The immediate problem which arose was to define a neurochemical transmitter substance. According to Elkes (1958), and Eccles (1964), neurochemical transmitter substances fulfill four essential criteria: they must be identifiable by chemical and biological tests; an enzyme system responsible for their synthesis and destruction must be present in those areas of the CNS where the transmitter substance is found; the inhibition of any of these specific enzymes by specific drugs or antimetabolites has to be reflected in a corresponding disturbance in function, which is clearly discernible in both chemical and functional terms; and the administration of the transmitter substance into the CNS has to be reflected in a corresponding functional disturbance.

At present there are five substances which at least partially fulfill these criteria. These are acetylcholine, serotonin, norepinephrine, γ-aminobutyric acid and substance P.

There are several ways of collecting information on the effects of psychoactive drugs on CNS transmitters. A common method is to sacrifice the animal after a certain period of drug administration and then establish either the total brain content of the transmitter substance (or substances) in question or, less often, the amount of the substance in a specific area. More recently, with bioassay techniques it has become possible to measure directly the effects of a drug on particular enzymes.

i. Acetylcholine. Acetylcholine is the result of the esterification of choline by acetic acid. The enzyme which catalyzes the formation of acetylcholine is known as choline acetylase. According to Nachmansohn (1958), acetylcholine is usually present in protein-bound form in the organism and is released in small amounts to receptor sites situated on the effector organ. The free acetylcholine is then destroyed by hydrolysis. The enzyme catalyzing this reaction is known as acetylcholine esterase.

The discovery that acetylcholine was the transmitter substance at the synaptic junctions of the peripheral nervous system led Dale *et al.* (1936) to suggest that the substance might have a similar function in the CNS. About the same time Quastel *et al.* (1936) and Stedman and Stedman (1937) discovered that brain homogenates were able to synthesize acetylcholine. Later on, the enzymes necessary for the synthesis and destruction of this transmitter substance were found in the CNS, and it was shown that the actual concentration of acetylcholine is directly proportional to the concentration of choline acetylase and not to the concentration of acetylcholine esterase.

The lowest concentrations of choline acetylase and of acetylcholine were found in the cerebellum, cerebellar peduncles, dorsal roots and optic nerves, while the highest concentrations were found in the cerebral motor cortex, caudate nucleus, thalamus, medial and lateral geniculate bodies, anterior spinal roots and brain stem (Robson and Stacey, 1962).

The acetylcholine concentration of the CNS is not constant. It decreases (for not longer than 10 seconds) during excitement and convulsions (Richter and Crossland, 1949), while it increases during ether- or barbiturate-induced general anesthesia and in sleep (Crossland and Merrick, 1954). Similarly, the stimulation of the afferent nerves, asphyxia (increase in CO_2 concentration) and the injection of adrenaline all cause an increase in free acetylcholine and a consequent elevation of acetylcholine levels in the brain. However, when acetylcholine was injected directly into the cerebral ventricles (Dikshit, 1935), it produced marked autonomic effects and behavioral changes in the direction of sleep or a stupor-like state not unlike a cataleptogenic state. This suggested that acetylcholine exerted an inhibitory rather than an excitatory action. Similar reactions were observed by Feldberg and Sherwood (1959).

There are several hypotheses on the relationship between cerebral acetylcholine concentration and psychopathology, but none has yet been fully established. For example, some investigators suggest that an excess of acetylcholine concentration may be causally related to neuroses and that a deficiency may be causally related to psychoses. It has also been suggested that chemicals which produce an increase in acetylcholine concentration in the brain, either through an increase in production or through a decrease in breakdown, may have a beneficial effect in schizophrenic patients and that drugs which have the opposite effect may be therapeutic for depressive cases.

In fact, very little is definitely known about the role of the acetylcholine in the CNS. Indeed, its effect as a synaptic transmitter in general has been firmly established in only four instances. These are at the neuromuscular junctions of the longitudinal muscle of *Hirudo medicinalis* and of the retractor muscle of *Strichopus regalis;* at the synapse between the cardio-inhibitory fibers and the heart of *Venus mercenaria;* and at some inhibitory synapses in the abdominal ganglia of *Aplysia depilans* (Tauc and Gerschenfeld 1960, 1961).

Experimental findings on the effect of pharmacological agents on acetylcholine synthesis and destruction are relatively few. It had been shown that the synthesis of acetylcholine by choline acetylase is dependent on the continuous supply of choline and glucose. This synthesis can be depressed, and consequently brain acetylcholine concentration can be decreased, by hemicholinium, a substance without any evident psychopharmacological effect. More rewarding experiments were those designed to study the effects of acetylcholine accumulation. This was first achieved by the administration of diisopropylfluorophosphate, a substance which led to electroencephalographic changes without any kind of overt behavioral effects. On the other hand, atropine and hyoscyamine, concomitantly with the increase of acetylcholine levels, also produced both electroencephalographic and behavioral alterations (Elkes, 1958). Nevertheless, when eserine was injected there was a dissociation between the electroencephalogram (alertness) and manifest behavior (drowsiness) (Bradley and Elkes, 1957). This was interpreted to mean that activation of the cortical functions occurred while the RAS of the brain stem remained unaffected. However, when connections between the thalamus and the cerebral cortex were severed, there was no longer any electroencephalographic activation (Rinaldi and Himwich, 1955).

With psychotherapeutic agents, the following effects on acetylcholine concentration were found: antipsychotic phenothiazines seemed to interfere with the cortical release of acetylcholine (Beckman, 1961); tricyclic antidepressants have been shown to be antagonistic to some of the acetylcholine actions; while sedative barbiturates have been implicated to play a role in some peripheral antiacetylcholine effects.

ii. Serotonin. Serotonin, or 5-hydroxytryptamine (5-HT), is the decarboxylation product of 5-hydroxytryptophane. The enzyme catalyzing the formation of serotonin is 5-hydroxytryptophane decarboxylase, a pyridoxal enzyme. It is well recognized that in animals only a fraction of 5HT is present in free form. Most of it is protein bound and under normal circumstances is released slowly and in small amounts. The released serotonin is destroyed by oxidation and methylation. These reactions are catalyzed by the monoamine oxidase (MAO) and catechol-*o*-methyltransferase (COMT) enzymes.

5HT is known to be present in enterochromaffin cells, platelets and mast cells (Amin *et al.*, 1954). Its distribution in the CNS was found to be distinctly different from that of acetylcholine.

Systematic investigations revealed relatively low serotonin concentration in the cerebral cortex and relatively high concentration in the brain stem, amygdala, mesencephalon and medial thalamic nuclei. There is a particularly high serotonin concentration in the hypothalamus, where the enzyme systems responsible for its synthesis and destruction are also found in large quantities.

That serotonin might be a CNS transmitter substance, or even more specifically *the* transmitter substance, of the central "parasympathetic" system was first suggested by Brodie and Shore (1957). Soon afterward, a hypothetical balance in the CNS between acetylcholine and serotonin was proposed. It was assumed that the former had a facilitatory effect on synaptic transmission and the latter an inhibitory effect. However, when serotonin was injected in small doses directly into the cerebral ventricles, it produced a definite depressant action, characterized by muscular weakness (Feldberg and Sherwood, 1954). When it was given in much larger amounts, a definite excitatory action was seen, with occasional convulsive components (Woolley and Shaw, 1954, 1957; Woolley, 1962).

There are several hypotheses on the relationship between cerebral serotonin concentration and psychopathology. It has been suggested that a relative excess of serotonin concentration has stimulating, euphorizing, antidepressant and possibly psychotomimetic effects. On the other hand, the opposite, *i.e.*, a relative deficiency, seems to have sedative, dysphoric, depressant and possibly antipsychotic effects.

In the course of psychopharmacological studies it has been shown that reserpine administration produces a decrease in the serotonin level in the brain with a concomitant sedative and cataleptic action in the animal (corresponding to the soporofic, dysphoric, depressant and possibly antipsychotic action in humans). It was also demonstrated that only the biologically active Rauwolfia alkaloids which have a psychopharmacological property effected a decrease of serotonin, whereas the biologically inactive derivatives did not. Mechanisms and effects similar to those of the Rauwolfia were seen with benzoquinolizines, *e.g.*, tetrabenazine, benzquinamide and other psychopharmacologically active synthetic derivatives of this group (Pletscher, 1957).

Evidence for the correlation between behavioral stimulation in the animal (corresponding to the euphorizing, antidepressant and possibly psychotomimetic effects in humans) and increased serotonin concentration in the brain resulted from studies with iproniazid and various other MAOI drugs. Thus, while the concomitant decrease of brain serotonin level after reserpine administration had an inhibitory effect, iproniazid caused a concomitant increase in brain serotonin concentration and had an excitatory effect on the animals' behavior.

Brodie and Shore (1959), in a series of studies, gave reserpine and iproniazid separately or in various combinations. They found that if reserpine was given alone or even if reserpine was followed by iproniazid administration, there was a definite decrease in brain serotonin concentration associated with depressant effects. They also recognized that, if iproniazid was administered alone, there was only an increase of brain serotonin level without any stimulating effect on behavior. It was only when iproniazid was followed by reserpine administration (which produced further elevation of brain 5-HT concentration) that the stimulating effects on behavior were observed.

Among the other psychotherapeutic agents, both sedative barbiturates and stimulant amphetamines exert some 5-HT-elevating action. However, in high doses amphetamines have a blocking or inhibiting effect on serotonin activity in the brain (Brodie *et al.*, 1957). The tricyclic antidepressants like the MAOI's were found to inhibit the reserpine-induced lowering of brain 5-HT concentration. In contrast, the antipsychotic phenothiazines counteract the increase of serotonin concentration after MAOI drug administration, thus showing an effect not unlike that of reserpine.

No changes in 5-HT concentration in the brain are found with anxiolytic benzodiazepines. However, the pressor effect of intravenous serotonin is slightly potentiated by these drugs. It was noted that both lysergic acid diethylamide (LSD_{25}) and its 2-bromo derivative are potent serotonin antagonists; yet only the former substance (LSD_{25}) possesses psychotomimetic action, while the latter compound is without any manifest behavioral effects.

iii. Norepinephrine. While serotonin, a tryptophan metabolite, is the decarboxylation product of 5-hydroxytrytophan, norepinephrine, a phenylalanine metabolite, is the decarboxylation product of dopamine. The enzyme catalyzing the formation of norepinephrine (NE) is dopa decarboxylase.

It is well recognized that only a part of NE is present in the free form in animals. The rest is protein bound and under normal circumstances is released very slowly. The enzymes responsible for NE destruction are MAO and COMT.

Euler (1946) was first to demonstrate the presence of NE in the brain. This was confirmed somewhat later by Holtz *et al.* (1947). Systematic investigations revealed that, while the precursor (dopamine) and the transmitter substance could be found in approximately equal amounts in the CNS, epinephrine, the oxidative deamination product of NE, is present only in a much lower concentration. It was also recognized that, in general, the distribution of NE in the different structures of the CNS corresponds to the distribution of serotonin, *i.e.*, the highest concentrations being in the hypothalamus, brain stem reticular formation, medial thalamic nuclei and around the aqueduct in the midbrain. The highest concentrations of dopamine, however, are found in decreasing amounts in the following structures: the caudate nucleus, midbrain, hypothalamus and pons.

It has been shown for some time that NE might be the transmitter substance of the central sympathetic system. More recently, a hypothetical serotonin (parasympathetic) and norepinephrine (sympathetic) balance was proposed as a functional system which presumably regulates the activity of the central autonomic nervous system centers. This hypothetical balance of NE and 5-HT is thought to be complementary to the hypothetical acetylcholine and serotonin balance which presumably regulates synaptic transmission in the CNS.

As with serotonin, there are several hypotheses based on the relationship between cerebral NE concentration and psychopathology. Although no final proof has yet been found, there are indications that a relative excess of NE concentration corresponds with stimulant, euphorizing, antidepressant and possibly psychotomimetic effects, while a relative deficiency appears to be related to sedative, dysphoric, depressant and perhaps even antipsychotic effects. Supporting this hypothesis are the findings that after the administration of the psychoactive Rauwolfia alkaloid, reserpine, or (even more prominently) the psychoactive synthetic benzoquinolizine, tetrabenazine, there was a simultaneous decrease of serotonin levels and NE concentrations, which corresponded with the sedative, depressant and possibly antipsychotic effect of these drugs. Similar behavioral effects were seen after the administration of methyldopa, a substance with an inhibitory effect on the decarboxylation of cerebral amino acids, the precursors of cerebral monoamines. Administration of methyldopa, by interfering with NE formation, results in decreased NE levels in the brain.

However, when epinephrine was injected directly into the cerebral ventricles, it produced a stuporous condition. This finding suggested that, when epinephrine enters the ventricular fluid, behavioral depression occurs and that behavioral excitation with the same substance is observed only when it is present in the blood stream (Draskoci *et al.*, 1960). Thus, while the administration of dopa (to rabbits) resulted in an increased concentration of dopamine in the caudate nucleus, without a corresponding change in norepinephrine and epinephrine levels, and appeared to increase motor activity (Bertler and Rosengren, 1959), the administration of NE or epinephrine resulted in the development of a stuporous condition associated with desynchronization of the electroencephalogram, *i.e.*, with an alerted EEG pattern (Robson and Stacey, 1962).

In the course of psychopharmacological studies, a lowering effect on hypothalamic NE levels by ether, nicotine, picrotoxin, morphine, and insulin has been demonstrated.

Among the frequently used psychopharmacological agents, sedative barbiturates were found to release NE from its protein-bound state. It was possible to potentiate the resulting vasoconstriction by cocaine and to prevent it by reserpine or tolazoline. (Increased plasma catecholamine levels in dogs have also been detected with barbiturate administration.)

The effects of stimulant amphetamines on brain NE levels differ from barbiturates. By binding the MAO enzyme, amphetamines produce an increase in brain catecholamine concentrations. Thus, even in low doses they facilitate epinephrine effects. (However, in higher concentrations they may block epinephrine action to a marked degree.) With the anxiolytic benzodiazepines, the only effect appears to be the potentiation of the arterial pressor response to NE with a resulting increase in over-all blood flow and cardiac activity.

Tricyclic antidepressants inhibit the restorage or retard the inactivation of NE, as revealed by radioactive isotope studies in which the retardation of NE uptake was measured on the heart. This effect is sometimes offered as an explanation for the marked sensitivity to catecholamines when tricyclic antidepressants are given.

The blocking of the uptake of tritium-labeled NE is not a unique property of tricyclic antidepressant drugs. Among other substances, antipsychotic phenothiazines evoke similar effects when given in appropriate doses. For example, Axelrod *et al.* (1961) were able to demonstrate that chlorpromazine can block NE uptake by peripheral tissues, and Dengler *et al.* (1961) have shown that it can also block the NE uptake of brain slices. However, in 1965 Glowinski and Axelrod reported that tricyclic antidepressants, but not chlorpromazine, prevented the uptake of intraventricularly injected, tagged NE by rat brain neurons.

The finding that tricyclic antidepressants block NE uptake by brain neurons raised the question whether there is a selective reduction of NE uptake by noradrenergic and/or dopaminergic neurons, which, according to Hillarp *et al.* (1966), are functionally and anatomically different and independent of each other. To answer this question an experiment was designed by Neff and Costa (1967) to localize drug effects on the two types of adrenergic neurons by measuring the turnover of brain dopamine (DM) and NE after the administration of desipramine, protriptyline (tricyclic antidepressants) and chlorpromazine (phenothiazine). They found that the antidepressant drugs increased brain NE synthesis without altering brain DM synthesis, in contrast to the phenothiazine substance, which increased only DM synthesis and not NE synthesis.

Furthermore, it has also been demonstrated that, while antipsychotic Rauwolfias decrease, and antidepressant MAOI's increase, brain NE concentrations, the latter increase of brain NE level can be counteracted by antipsychotic phenothiazine drugs.

In the past, the functional roles of NE and 5-HT have been subjects of much controversy, particularly in regard to their sedative or mood-lifting effects and whether their concentrations in the brain are directly correlated to manifest patterns of behavior. To answer these questions a study was designed by Matussek *et al.* (1967) in which rats were forced to swim until they were exhausted (a test frequently used in the detection of substances with mood-lifting properties). The catalepsy produced by this procedure was tested, and the NE and 5-HT concentrations were assayed by fluorescence spectrometry. Furthermore, the NE and 5-HT uptakes were measured by radioactive isotope techniques.

This study revealed that the physiological cataleptic state resulting from this procedure (in water 15°C) lasted for about 46 minutes and correlates more closely with the binding or uptake mechanism than with the total amount of amines in the CNS (a finding similar to that of Brodie *et al.*, 1962, and Carlsson *et al.*, 1963). Immediately after swimming there was at first an inhibition, which was followed by a reduction, of NE uptake in the cataleptic animals. Later there was an increase of NE uptake and a decrease in NE concentration, which was interpreted as a deficit of NE at the receptor sites. In direct contrast, *i.e.*, opposite, to the findings with NE were the results with 5-HT. There was a higher level of 5-HT concentration in the brain after swimming (also shown by Barchas and Freedman, 1963), which was correlated with a decrease in the binding of labeled 5-HT. On the basis of this, Matussek *et al.* (1967) implied that both the adrenergic and serotonergic systems are involved during sedation and that their balance can be separately and differentially influenced.

iv. γ-Aminobutyric Acid. γ-Aminobutyric acid (GABA) is formed by the decarboxylation of l-glutamic acid, and it is removed from the brain tissues by transamination by α-ketoglutarate, yielding succinic semialdehyde. The coenzyme necessary for both the synthesis and the catabolism of GABA is pyridoxal-5-phosphate, which seems to be less tightly bound to the apoenzyme in the decarboxylase, essential for GABA production, than to the transaminase, which is responsible for its destruction.

The latter reactions were also explored in brain homogenates, through which it was possible to study the conversion of GABA into succinic semialdehyde. By this means it was also possible to study the formation of γ-amino-β-hydroxybutyric acid, a substance definitely present in the dog brain, which is about twenty times as potent in preventing convulsions as GABA. The former substance may also have a therapeutic effect in schizophrenia (Hayashi, 1966).

GABA was first identified in the mammalian brain by Roberts and Frankel (1950). After its identification it was shown that it occurs only in the CNS and is generally found in the grey matter of the cerebral cortex and particularly in the globus pallidus. It is also in these regions that the GABA-synthesizing enzyme is present in high concentrations.

It was suggested that GABA might be the inhibitory transmitter in the CNS of vertebrates because of the correlation between the excitability of certain areas of the brain and their corresponding GABA content (Curtis, 1963); because of its potent depressant action on nerve cells (Eccles, 1964); and its selective blocking action on the surface cortical elements or apical dendrites (Elliot and Jasper, 1959). There is some contradictory evidence which shows that GABA does not produce hyperpolarization of nerve cells but instead has a general depressant action on all neuronal responses and that its depressant action cannot be suppressed by strychnine (Eccles, 1964). Considering all these findings, it is the concensus that while there are some striking parallels between the actions of GABA as an inhibitory transmitter, there is as yet insufficient evidence to prove that GABA is in fact this transmitter (Robson and Stacey, 1962).

There is very little information to date on the effects of chemicals and particularly of psychoactive agents on GABA concentration. It is known, however, that hydroxylamine, a substance without overt behavioral action, raises the concentration of GABA in the brain by depressing transamination, *i.e.*, the process responsible for GABA destruction. Antidepressant MAOI's of the hydrazide type, on the other hand, lower GABA concentration. This may be related to the fact that this group of MAOI's are carbonyl-trapping agents and, by producing pyridoxal deficiency, depress GABA synthesis. GABA concentrations are also decreased by reserpine, probably by a similar mechanism of action. The lower convulsive threshold simultaneously present with reduced GABA concentrations is successfully counteracted by vitamin B_6 (pyridoxine) administration (Balzer *et al.*, 1961; Matthews and Roberts, 1961; and Utley, 1963). It is interesting to note at this point that there is a structural similarity between GABA and haloperidol, a potent antipsychotic (neuroleptic) with marked extrapyramidal effects.

v. Substance P. This substance is a polypeptide extractable from the gut and active in promoting smooth muscle contractions. Its presence was first demonstrated in the CNS by Euler and Gaddum (1931), with particularly high concentrations found in the substantia nigra, hypothalamus, area postrema and cinerea.

The notion that substance P might be a CNS transmitter was proposed by Zetler *et al.* (1960) after systematic exploration of its CNS effects. In the course of these experiments, he revealed that substance P reduced spontaneous motor activity in mice, potentiated the effects of hypnotics and antagonized the action of stimulants. Prior to the discovery of these sedative effects, he found evidence of a characteristic hyperalgesic property which interfered with morphine effects (Zetler, 1953, 1958, 1959).

Subsequent to Zetler's first experiments,

it was shown that substance P gave rise to an arousal response in both the cortex and the hippocampus, which is manifested on the electrical activity as an increase of frequency with a decrease of amplitude in the cortex and an increase of frequency and synchronization in the hippocampus.

Since the administration of a transmitter of inhibitory neurons was expected to result in CNS depression and the administration of a sensory transmitter, hyperalgesia, Zetler *et al.* (1960) proposed the idea that substance P probably fulfills both of these roles, but in different areas of the CNS. Whether substance P is a CNS transmitter still remains to be seen, and its psychopharmacological implications remain to be elucidated.

While the actions of psychopharmacological substances on CNS transmitters are far from being fully explored, an authoritative view on the effect of prototype psychoactive drugs on neurohormones was succinctly presented by Himwich (1965). According to him, sedative barbiturates moderately increase neurohormonal stores. "This increase however is secondary to central depression" (as suggested by Bonnycastle *et al.*, 1962). On the other hand, anxiolytic benzodiazepines and propanediols are without any effect on the neurohormonal depots. Among the antipsychotics, the Rauwolfia alkaloid reserpine releases brain neurohormones from their depots. The alert pattern occurs simultaneously with the increased amounts of free 5-HT and NE as the neurohormonal stores are in the process of depletion. Nevertheless, after this depletion is completed and the neurohormonal levels are lowered, the spontaneous electroencephalographic activity assumes the resting pattern, frequently a sign of sedation in animals and of tranquilization in patients. In contradistinction to reserpine effects, phenothiazine tranquilization is correlated with depression of the hypothalamus and reticular formation. These are areas which contain relatively high concentrations of the neurohormones. The actions of these hormones, as revealed by Steiner and Himwich in 1962, are inhibited by phenothiazine drugs. Finally, MAOI antidepressants increase the concentration of 5-HT and NE in the brain.

Independent of the interest and research in CNS transmitters, there is an ever increasing number of investigative studies designed to elucidate the role of nucleic acids in the CNS, particularly in regard to learning and memory. This interest was aroused by Hyden (1961) and his collaborators, who put forward the notion that base changes in ribonucleic acid (RNA) may be the chemical correlates of memory for experiential events. Although the prevailing importance of RNA in memory traces has never been generally accepted, Hyden (1955, 1961, 1964) and also Landauer (1964) still maintain that RNA is a unique factor in the course of learning.

Hyden (1964) suggests that glial RNA, during the acquisition process, enters the neural tissue and depresses DNA sites so that specific RNA and protein can be synthesized. Landauer (1964), however, thinks that glial RNA entering the neurons acts directly in such a manner as to enable new protein to be synthesized.

In favor of the RNA theory is that within a limited period RNA concentration increases during functional activity, such as sensory stimulation, motor activity and learning, while it decreases during functional inactivity, such as sleep (Gaito, 1966). Furthermore, in a controlled experiment it was indicated by Babich *et al.* (1965) that learned responses of hamsters could be transferred to rats by RNA, which was extracted from the brain of the former animal and injected intraperitoneally into the latter.

During the past 15 years the growing number of psychoactive substances, improved instrumentation and increased interest in psychopharmacology have led to the accumulation of a vast amount of pharmacodynamic information. While the integration of this material is not yet complete, findings on the pharmacodynamic action of psychotropic substances with well known effects in animals are already extensively used in screening for new psychotherapeutic agents. The relationships of the data obtained by pharmacological tests, neurochemical means, conditioning procedures and neurophysiological techniques are continuously being elucidated. Nevertheless, there are still many missing links. At the present time, however, the heuristically more meaningful neurophysiological and neurochemical data are gradually replacing the pragmatic descriptive information.

B. TOXICITY

Since drugs by definition are substances which interfere with biological processes, all drugs, including the psychopharmacological compounds, are potentially toxic. The purpose of toxicological investigations is to discover, or rather uncover, the toxic or hazardous properties of a drug and to establish the circumstances in which they become manifest (Davey, 1965). From the animal toxicity data an attempt is made to anticipate the possible adverse—undesirable—effects that may be expected from the drug in humans. To overcome the limitations of the findings in animal toxicity tests, they are complemented by metabolic investigations (Brodeur, 1968).

1. Toxicity Studies

Animal toxicity studies are carried out in four steps. These are (*a*) acute studies in which the toxic effects of single doses of the psychoactive substances are established. These are followed by (*b*) subacute and (*c*) chronic toxicity determinations, which attempt to reveal the toxic effects of the substance when administered for relatively short or long periods of time. Finally, (*d*) the specific aspects of toxicity are investigated, *e.g.*, teratogenicity, carcinogenicity, etc.

a. Acute Toxicity Tests

In the acute toxicity studies the new compound is administered in single, increasing doses by various routes to small groups of animals belonging to two or more species. They are carefully observed and repeatedly examined within the first 24 hours after the medication is given and daily thereafter for an entire week. The administration of the substance to several species is important to reveal interspecies differences of drug responsivity. The administration of the drug by various routes gives useful early information regarding the absorption of the compound. Since males are usually more resistant to the toxic effects of the drug than females of the same species, and the newborn animals are more susceptible to toxic effects than the more mature, the selection of animals for the acute toxicity tests has to follow a carefully prepared design.

It is not the purpose of the acute toxicity tests to establish an exact figure for the LD_{50} *per se*, but rather to learn something about the way in which the drug is acting as a toxic substance. Thus it is essential to establish the cause of death and verify it by autopsy (Paget and Barnes, 1964). It has been noted that with any pharmacological agent immediate death and death within 24 hours are usually due to pharmacodynamic action, while death which occurs beyond this time but within the 7-day observational period is usually due to biochemical or anatomical changes.

Thus, acute toxicity tests serve the purpose of rapidly evaluating some of the inherent biological but undesirable (toxic) properties of the potentially psychoactive substance. Careful analysis of the findings may not only supply information on the potential hazards but may also provide the first clues to the mechanisms involved in the toxic (adverse) effects. Furthermore, the establishment of the seriously toxic and also the lethally toxic (LD_{50}) doses guides the toxicologist in his choice of dosages to be used in the subsequent toxicity tests.

It is generally agreed that no drug with possible psychoactive properties should be given to humans, not even in human pharmacological studies, prior to the completion of the acute toxicity testings.

b. Subacute Toxicity Tests

In the subacute toxicity studies the compound is administered by several (at least two) routes over a 2- to 12-week period (7 days a week) in at least three dosage ranges (one of them has to be large enough to be visibly effective or even lethal) to small groups of animals belonging to two or more species. They are carefully observed and repeatedly examined (weekly in the first 4 weeks and monthly thereafter) and extensive laboratory investigations, which include biochemistry, hematology and urinalyses, are carried out during the testing period. To determine any demonstrable pathology after termination of drug administration or at any time when toxic effects occur, some of the animals are sacrificed and autopsied.

The purpose of subacute toxicity studies with potential psychopharmacological agents is to uncover responses that might not be observable after a single dose; to form a basis for long term testing by providing an indication of the likely tolerated doses; and to supply sufficient evidence of safety for the first few doses of the drug which will be given to man (Paget and Barnes, 1964). Thus, subacute toxicity studies give additional information about the possible poisonous effects of the substance. They also reveal whether the medication has a cumulative action; provide guiding doses for the toxicologist for further chronic animal toxicity testings; and guide the pharmacologist for the dosage to be used in the initial human pharmacological experiments.

The actual duration of the subacute toxicity study depends on the anticipated clinical use of the drug. For drugs which are to be given only once or twice, subacute toxicity testing does not have to last longer than 2 or 3 weeks. On the other hand, for drugs intended to be administered for a period of a week, the subacute toxicity test should last at least for 4 to 5 weeks. For drugs which may be administered over a period of one month or more, the animal studies should be carried out for the full 12-week period. In spite of the fact that with most of the chemical substances, liver and kidney toxicity in animals occurs within a few days, and nervous system reactions within 3 weeks, the duration of subacute toxicity studies cannot be shortened.

No clinical pharmacological study with a possible psychoactive substance should commence prior to the termination of subacute toxicity testings.

c. Chronic Toxicity Tests

The only difference between the subacute and the chronic toxicity testing is in the duration of the study. This is extended from 3 months to a maximum of 2 years. This prolonged administration is considered essential for substances which are likely to be administered over several months, although most of the drugs (including the psychoactive compounds) produce their toxic manifestations (with the exception of carcinogenicity) within 90 days when administered in adequate doses (Brodeur, 1968).

As in the subacute toxicity study, immediately after termination of drug administration or at any time when toxic effects occur, some of the affected animals are sacrificed for pathological evidence of injury, while some others are taken off the drug and returned for further observation. The rate of recovery in this latter group is established. At the time of full recovery some of these remaining animals are sacrificed and autopsied.

In the autopsy report, the weights of the following are usually included: brain, pituitary, thymus, adrenals, gonads, heart, lungs, liver, kidney and prostate. The various parts of the body described in detail (including microscopic examination) are: skin, brain, eye, pituitary, thyroid, thymus, adrenals, tongue, stomach, small intestine, colon, heart, lung, liver pancreas, spleen, bladder, kidney, gonads, including uterus and prostate, lymph nodes and bone marrow. Particular attention is paid to the alimentary canal when the drug is given orally and to the site of injection if administered parenterally.

While there is no general agreement on how long a chronic toxicity study should last, it is usually thought that, with substances which will be used for more than 4 weeks, *e.g.*, psychopharmacological drugs, chronic toxicity testings should be conducted for at least 6 months and that, with substances where carcinogenesis is suspected, a longer period, *i.e.*, 12 to 24 months, is necessary.

No clinical investigation should commence with a potentially psychoactive compound prior to the completion of chronic toxicity testings lasting at least 6 months. On the other hand, there is no good reason why clinical pharmacological experiments cannot be performed simultaneously with the chronic toxicity studies.

d. Special Toxicity Tests

Special toxicity procedures were devised to detect potential carcinogenicity, to reveal the effects of the new drug on reproduction, to show its possible toxicity in interacting with other drugs and to recognize whether it is dependency producing.

i. Carcinogenicity. In these studies the new drug is administered over a period of 2 years in at least three dosage ranges to small groups of animals belonging to two or more species. During this period weight measurements are taken weekly. Consistent weight loss is not infrequently the first indication of a tumor. At the end of the study (or at the time of recognition of consistent weight loss) the animals are sacrificed and examined histopathologically. On the basis of the findings, the incidence, the time of appearance and the nature of the tumors are established.

Studies for carcinogenicity are essential not only for drugs which are structurally related to carcinogens and which affect mitosis but also for drugs expected to be used clinically for 6 months or longer. The latter include the psychopharmacological compounds.

ii. Reproduction. The effect of drugs on reproduction or on fetal development is explored through a number of experimental designs. The new substance is administered during pregnancy, prior to and in the period of lactation either continuously or over only a limited period of time. Information is collected on the influence of the potentially psychoactive substance on mating behavior, fertility, implantation and embryonal development (including resorption, abortion and teratogenesis). The process of delivery, the number of live births, viability of the newborn and growth of the young, etc. are all carefully assessed.

No woman of child-bearing age should be included in human studies with the new drug prior to the termination of these studies on reproductive processes.

The thalidomide "disaster" directed attention to the necessity of studying reproductive processes in animals prior to the use of a substance in human studies. Nowadays these studies are part of the required toxicity testing. Some of the findings, in reproductive studies, with some of the long established psychoactive substances were reviewed by Wortis (1964). From this it becomes evident that some of the widely used psychotropic drugs may cause fetal damage in animals without having a similar effect in humans. For example, reserpine, chlorpromazine, and meprobamate occasionally caused fetal death and significantly affected birth weight in experimental animals. Of these three compounds it was shown that chlorpromazine can retard or alter embryonic growth in mammals and salamanders (Eyal and Eyal, 1962, 1963) and that it can depress both fetal and maternal brain oxygen in the gravid guinea pig (Misrahy *et al.*, 1963). Furthermore, it was also revealed that imipramine in doses proportionate to human dosage produced a high incidence of fetal damage in the rabbit (Robson and Sullivan, 1963). In view of the fact that these drugs have been widely used clinically with no untoward effects, findings on the effect of psychoactive drugs on reproductive processes in the animals must be interpreted with caution.

iii. Drug Interaction. Additive and potentiating effects must be considered and studied. Particular attention has to be given to those drugs likely to be administered concurrently. Thus the potential hazards of barbiturates and ethyl alcohol with anxiolytic and antipsychotic substances and amphetamines or other sympathomimetics with antidepressant drugs have to be tested.

iv. Dependency. In recent years successful attempts have been made in dogs to produce dependency and consequently to develop a procedure which enables the toxicologist to explore more fully experimentally induced dependency and withdrawal manifestations in animals. Since dependency occurs not infrequently with psychoactive substances and could represent a serious drawback in the clinical usefulness of these compounds, this aspect of toxicity testing is increasingly employed in the course of animal studies with psychotropic drugs.

2. Metabolism

The value of animal toxicity findings to predict the reactions in humans has several serious drawbacks. All of these are related to the fact that various animal species (and man) may show quantitative and qualitative individual differences to a given psychopharmacological substance.

There is growing evidence which shows that the metabolic half-life of psychoactive drugs often shows interspecies variations. More frequently, the half-life is shorter in animals than in man, *e.g.*, for hexobarbital or meperidine, indicating that the animal is less susceptible to the toxic effects of these substances. Another important factor is that the metabolic processes of one species may differ entirely from those used by another. Thus, isoniazid, a substance with euphorizing properties used in the treatment of tuberculosis, is neutralized by acetylation at the level of the amine group in humans, while in the dog it is broken down through other metabolic pathways (Brodeur, 1968).

For these reasons animal toxicity tests need to be complemented by metabolic studies, since only the latter are able to reveal interspecies differences and variations.

a. General Aspects of Metabolism

The metabolism of any drug consists of two major phases: anabolism and catabolism. Anabolism in general refers to the "absorption" and "distribution," while catabolism includes the "fate" and "excretion" of the compound. More recently, the term "distribution" has been extended to "storage," and the term "fate" is being replaced by "inactivation" or "dissimilation" and "excretion."

In this modern frame of reference, absorption is considered as a multiple process. It means the traversal of the compound through several semipermeable membranes, *e.g.*, the gut-blood barrier, blood-brain barrier, etc. Among the various factors which prominently influence absorption of a drug are route of administration, solubility and physical state. It has been shown that a psychoactive substance in a crystalloid form is absorbed faster than in a colloid state and that drugs are more readily absorbed when given in solution than if administered as a dry powder. Also, for better absorption through the gastric mucosa, it is desirable that the drug should be a weak acid. When the same substance must penetrate the brain, it is preferable that it should have a high lipid solubility, so that hydrophilic groups in the molecule should be either absent or masked (Ariëns, 1964).

As a drug crosses semipermeable membranes to "reach" the "receptors" which are responsible for its biological effect, the concentration of the substance gradually decreases. Storage, inactivation and excretion are responsible for this decrease.

Storage indicates depots where part of the psychoactive drug accumulates, *e.g.*, keratinous tissues for phenothiazines. Drugs may be deposited in these depots for certain lengths of time and then return to the circulation without any transformation. Storage may take place in lipids (for liposoluble substances), on nucleic acids (for cationic substances) or on serum albumin (for anionic substances). Storage in general is disadvantageous if it keeps most of the drug out of circulation permanently, but it can be very beneficial if it helps to maintain a constant desired blood level of the substance.

Inactivation is the second mechanism responsible for a gradual decrease in concentration. In contrast to reversible storage, inactivation involves breaking old or forming new covalent bonds and is usually an irreversible process. Basically it consists of converting the drug into more polar derivatives which, because of their reduced lipid solubility, are more readily excreted by the kidney.

According to Sourkes (1962), there are seven main mechanisms which may be involved in this detoxication process. These are oxidation by microsomal enzymes in the liver (*e.g.*, amphetamines); other oxidative reactions, for example, dehydrogenation (*e.g.*, chloral hydrate) or oxidative deamination (*e.g.*, iproniazid); reduction reactions (*e.g.*, chloral hydrate); *o*-methylation (*e.g.*, catecholamines); hydrolysis of esters (*e.g.*, acetylcholine); hydrolysis of amides (*e.g.*, procaine); and conjugation with glucuronic acid, sulfuric acid, acetic acid, etc. (*e.g.*, chlorpromazine).

Grollman (1965) lists only five principal pathways of drug metabolism: oxidation, reduction, conjugation, hydrolysis and exchange reaction. Ariëns (1964) considered only four metabolic pathways crucial for psychoactive agents: oxidation, reduction, hydrolysis and conjugation.

Of the various "crucial" metabolic pathways, it seems that oxidation is the most prominent. Most of the oxidative changes are brought about by rather nonspecific enzymes located in the endoplasmatic reticulum of the liver cells. The reactions occur on sites where alcoholic hydroxyl groups or amino groups are present, especially if they are situated on a terminal carbon or alkyl chain. Since the oxidation process often results in a decreased number of atoms in the molecule, its size is consequently reduced. While reduction occurs mainly where the oxidative enzymes fail, hydrolysis is the common metabolic process for esters and glucosides, and amides as a rule remain resistant to this catabolic interaction. During the oxidation and reduction process, the change in the psychoactive molecule is such that new polar groups suitable for conjugation are formed. By the process of hydrolysis new polar groups are liberated which are suitable for conjugation (or oxidation followed by conjugation). Conjugation is the final step of inactivation, in the course of which drug molecules are bound to each other by elimination of water and formation of ethers, amides and other substitution products.

The third and last activity responsible for the decrease of psychoactive drug concentration is excretion. Excretion takes place through the kidney (urine), bile ducts (feces) and lungs (exhaled air). While inactivation is always followed by excretion, a certain amount of the drug is often excreted in its original form.

It has been reported that with certain psychoactive drugs rapid excretion can be prevented if the substance is first prepared with a high lipid solubility or if it is given together with a similar compound which has a higher affinity for the renal transport system than the investigational preparation.

b. Metabolism of Psychoactive Drugs

There are various sophisticated techniques employed to study the metabolism of drugs. These include labeling with radioactive materials; paper, thin layer, column and gas chromatographies; and electron paramagnetic resonances and nuclear magnetic resonances. From studies with these and various other techniques the metabolism of the seven most frequently used groups of psychoactive drugs has been revealed.

In brief, it is recognized that sedative barbiturates are metabolized by four (or five) metabolic pathways, primarily in the smooth-surfaced, highest density microsomes of the liver and only to a limited extent in the kidney, brain, muscle and other tissues (Friend, 1964). These metabolic pathways are oxidation of the substituent in position 5 of the ring to a ketone, alcohol or acid; loss of the alkyl groups which are attached to nitrogen; desulfuration (in case of thiobarbiturates); hydrolytic splitting of the barbiturate ring itself; and the loss of an alkyl group at position 5 with the addition of a methyl group to the ring constituent nitrogen.

Like barbiturates, the stimulant amphetamines are also metabolized primarily in the liver, where they are oxidized by microsomal enzymes. Pathways for amphetamine metabolism are demethylation (in case of methamphetamine), deamination, parahydroxylation and acetylation. The last-named metabolic process takes place in the circulation (and during urinary excretion it may be reversed).

Of the two major antidepressant categories, *i.e.*, MAOI's and tricyclics, the metabolism of the MAOI hydrazide group was found to follow two pathways. One of these is the hydrolysis of the acylhydrazine bound and cleavage of the alkyl or aralkyl substituent. Pletscher (1965) noted that this reaction may be of major importance partly because it probably yields active biological intermediates (*e.g.*, isopropylhydrazine in the case of iproniazid). The second pathway is considered to be of minor clinical significance because the metabolic end-products appear to be biologically inactive.

In contradistinction to the MAOI's, tricyclic antidepressants are metabolized by *N*-demethylation, hydroxylation and glucuronide conjugation. Thus in the case of imipramine (and of the *N*-demethyl compound), the mono- and bis-*N*-demethyl derivatives, the 2-hydroxy derivatives, as well as their glucuronides, were all isolated from the urine. In the case of amitriptyline (and of the *N*-demethyl analogue), the mono- and bis-*N*-demethyl analogues, the 10-hydroxy derivatives and their glucuronides were identified in the urine.

In a course of systematic studies the physiological distribution of injected tagged (C^{14}) amitriptyline and imipramine was studied in mice, rats and cats by Cassano *et al.* (1965). With an autoradiographic technique, they found that both compounds rapidly left the circulation and were concentrated predominantly in the brain, lung and heart. In the brain their regional distribution was found to be uneven. Shortly after injection, radioactivity appeared to be highest in the cerebral cortex, cerebellar cortex, hippocampus and in some subcortical nuclei, while 4 hours later, the radioactivity in the grey matter decreased and the white matter showed the highest activity. Furthermore, they found that both compounds were rapidly metabolized in the body and excreted to a large extent in the bile as glucuronide conjugates. The same investigators (Hansson and Cassano, 1967), in experiments with pregnant mice, showed that both substances passed the placental barrier and were concentrated mainly in the lung, liver, intestines and urinary bladder of the fetus.

The main metabolic pathways of anxiolytic benzodiazepines recognized thus far are hydroxylation and demethylation. Even after these processes, psychoactive properties are still present, and only the opening of the seven-membered ring results in a pharmacologically inactive substance.

The attempts to reveal the metabolic pathways of antipsychotic phenothiazine substances presented considerable difficulties. It took several years to establish that oxidation of the sulfur atom in position 5 and hydroxylation in positions 3 and 7 with the subsequent conjugation (with glucuronic acid) of the hydroxylation product are the essential processes involved. Other metabolic processes recognized somewhat later were demethylation and *N*-oxidation. Both occur in the side chain substituent in position 10. On the other hand, antipsychotic Rauwolfias were found to be metabolized primarily by alkaline hydrolysis. By this process reserpine is catabolized into methyl reserpate, trimethoxybenzoate and methanol. Other reserpine metabolites which were identified are syringic acid and syringoyl methyl reserpate. Since methyl reserpate is the only breakdown product isolated in the brain, some authorities consider this substance the active metabolite of the drug.

c. Special Aspects of Metabolism

Special aspects of drug metabolism are concerned with the interspecies variation and the intraspecies, possibly genetically determined, differences (Kalow, 1962). The discovery of atropine esterase in rabbits represented the first fully documented observation in this special area of research.

The first published report showing that rabbits were able to thrive on belladonna leaves appeared in Vienna in 1852 (Ammon and Savelsberg, 1949). However, the definitive paper on atropine esterase was published approximately 60 years later by Fleischmann (1910). He made the observation that atropine was inactivated *in vitro* by the serum of rabbits. The first evidence that the inactivation was due to the enzymatic destruction of atropine was given by Metzner (1912).

In no other species has atropine esterase been detected. Since then, several interspecies differences between man and animal have been described. Among them was the finding that dogs, unlike man, do not acetylate sulfonamides and that cats have minimal facilities for conjugating drugs or their metabolities with glucuronic acid. Other interspecies differences, for example, were found in amphetamine metabolism (Leake,

1958). It has been observed that fish, frogs and salamanders excrete these stimulant compounds unchanged through their skin, while toads, whose skin is not permeable to these drugs, metabolize amphetamine compounds. It has also been shown that hydroxylation of the amphetamine is one of the metabolic pathways in dogs but not in guinea pigs or rabbits. Interspecies differences with anxiolytic benzodiazepines have been found. It was shown that in dogs urinary excretion predominates, while in rats most of the drug is eliminated in the feces.

In contradistinction to these interspecies differences there are intraspecies variations. During a laboratory catastrophe in Bar Harbor, Russell (1955) found that many stocks of mice were exposed to chloroform fumes and that many of the male animals died afterward from the toxic effects on their kidneys. All the deaths occurred in 3 male strains, while the 6 other male and female strains remained unaffected. In the same year Jay (1955) demonstrated variations in sleeping time in 12 strains of mice after the administration of a sedative barbiturate (hexobarbital) drug. Other similar intraspecies variations were revealed by Rosen (1959) and Tindal (1960). They found that when iproniazid, the prototype of MAOI antidepressants, was added to the diet of AKR mice, the animals suffered severe hepatic injury and a high mortality rate, whereas Swiss and several other strains showed no ill effects. In the same year Tindal (1960) demonstrated that reserpine, the prototype of the Rauwolfia alkaloid antipsychotics, when administered during pseudopregnancy to the New Zealand white breed rabbits, produced both lactation and a decrease in the size of the thymus. No similar changes occurred in Dutch or several other strains of rabbits under the same experimental conditions.

As seen in this chapter, there are many ways in which animal pharmacodynamic and toxicity studies can be relevant to psychiatry in general and in the prediction of psychotropic properties of a substance in particular. Probably the most important contribution of animal experiments is to make detailed and stepwise analyses of the complex effects of drugs possible. There is a great diversity of methods for assessing behavioral changes of drugs in animals, however, and the meaningfulness of the findings depends largely on the discrimination with which these methods are used (Dews, 1962; and Steinberg, 1965).

Because of the many difficulties of extrapolating information from animal to man (Evarts, 1959; Irwin, 1964; and Russell, 1961), animal pharmacological data are complemented by findings based on the various phases of human studies prior to introducing a new psychopharmacological substance into clinical practice. The latter is the subject matter of the following chapters.

REFERENCES

Amin, A. H., Crawford, T. B. B., and Gaddum, J. H.: The distribution of substance P and 5-hydroxytryptamine in the central nervous system. J. Physiol. (London), *126:* 596 (1954).

Ammon, R., and Savelsberg, W.: Die enzymatische Spaltung von Atropin, Cocain und Chemisch Verwandten Estern. Ztschr. Physiol. Chem., *284:* 135 (1949).

Ariëns, E. J. (ed.): Molecular pharmacology. (Academic Press, New York, 1964.)

Askew, B. M.: A simple screening procedure for imipramine-like antidepressant agents. Life Sci., *5:* 725 (1963).

Astrup, C.: Conditional reflex studies in psychopharmacology. (Presented at the Fifth International Congress of CINP, Washington, 1966.)

Axelrod, J.: Enzymatic formation of psychotomimetic metabolites from normally occurring compounds. Science, *134:* 343 (1961).

Axelrod, J., Whitby, L. G., and Hertting, G.: Effect of psychotropic drugs on the uptake of H^3-norepinephrine by tissues. Science, *133:* 383 (1961).

Babich, F. R., *et al.:* Transfer of the response to naive rats by injection of ribonucleic acid extracted from trained rats. Science, *149:* 656 (1965).

Balzer, H., Holtz, P., and Palm, D.: Reserpine and γ-amino butyric acid content of the brain. Naunyn Schmiedeberg. Arch. Exp. Path., *241:* 190 (1961).

Bambas, B. S., *et al.:* The mechanism of the chlorpromazine effect. Zh. Nevropat. Psikhiat. Korsakov., *56:* 121 (1956).

Ban, T. A.: Conditioning and psychiatry. (Aldine Publishing Co., Chicago, 1964.)

Barchas, J. D., and Freedman, D. X.: Brain amines: response to physiological stress. Biochem. Pharmacol., *12:* 1232 (1963).

Beckman, H.: Pharmacology: the nature, action and use of drugs. (Saunders, Philadelphia, 1961.)

Bein, H. J.: Effect of reserpine on the functional strata of the nervous system. In: Psychopharmacology frontiers (ed., Kline, N. S.). (Little, Brown, Toronto, 1959.)

Bertler, A., and Rosengren, E. G.: Occurrence and distribution of catecholamines in brain. Acta Physiol. Scand., *47:* 350 (1959).

Boissier, J. R., *et al.:* Etude pharmacodynamique d'un nouveau neuroleptique majeur: le halopéridol (R 1625). II. Action sédative au niveau du système nerveux central. Thérapie, *16:* 279 (1961).

Boissier, J. R., *et al.:* Tentative de pharmacologie prévisionnell dans le domaine des neuroleptiques, action sedative centrale adrenolytique de la *N*(dimethoxy-3,4-phénéthyl)-*N*-(chloro-2-phényl) pipérazine. Arch. Int. Pharmacodyn., *133:* 29 (1961).

Bonnycastle, D. D., Bonnycastle, M. F., and Anderson, E. G.: The effect of a number of central depressant drugs upon brain 5-hydroxytryptamine levels in the rat. J. Pharmacol. Exp. Ther., *135:* 17 (1962).

Bradley, P. B.: Microelectrode approach to the neuropharmacology of the reticular formation. In: Psychotropic drugs (eds., Garattini, S., and Ghetti, V.). (Elsevier, Amsterdam, 1958.)

Bradley, P. B.: The central action of certain drugs in relation to the reticular formation. In: Reticular formation of the brain (eds., Jasper, H. H., Proctor, L. D., Knighton, R. S., Nashay, W. C., and Costello, R. T.) (Little, Brown, Boston, 1958.)

Bradley, P. B., and Elkes, J.: The effects of some drugs on the electrical activity of the brain. Brain, *80:* 77 (1957).

Bradley, P. B., and Key, B. J.: The effect of drugs on arousal responses produced by electrical stimulation of the reticular formation of the brain. Electroenceph. Clin. Neurophysiol., *10:* 97 (1958).

Bridger, W. H., and Gantt, W. H.: The effect of mescaline on differential conditional reflexes. Amer. J. Psychiat., *113:* 352 (1956).

Brodeur, J.: The pharmacologist's viewpoint. In: Toxicity and adverse reaction studies with neuroleptics and antidepressants (eds., Lehmann, H. E., and Ban, T. A.). (Q.P.R.A., Montreal, 1968.)

Brodie, B. B., Gessa, G. L., and Costa, E.: Association between reserpine syndrome and blockade of brain serotonin storage processes. Life Sci., *2:* 551 (1962).

Brodie, B. B., and Hogben, C. A. M.: Some physiochemical factors in drug action. J. Pharm. Pharmacol., *9:* 345 (1957).

Brodie, B. B., *et al.*: Possible interrelationship between release of brain norepinephrine and serotonin by reserpine. Science, *125:* 1293 (1957).

Brodie, B. B., and Shore, P. A.: A concept for a role of serotonin and norepinephrine as chemical mediators in the brain. Ann. N.Y. Acad. Sci., *66:* 631 (1957).

Brodie, B. B., and Shore, P. A.: On a role for serotonin and norepinephrine as chemical mediators in the central autonomic nervous system. In: Hormones, brain function and behavior (ed., Hoagland, H.). (Academic Press, New York, 1957.)

Brodie, B. B., and Shore, P. A.: Mechanism of action of psychotropic drugs. In: Psychopharmacology frontiers (ed., Kline, N. S.). (Little, Brown, Toronto, 1959.)

Cameron, D. E.: The experimental method in the study of human behavior; central problems. In: Psychopharmacological methods (eds., Votava, Z., Horvath, M., and Vinar, O.). (Pergamon Press, New York, 1963.)

Cameron, D. E., *et al.:* Effect of ribonucleic acid on memory defect. Amer. J. Psychiat., *120:* 320 (1963).

Cameron, D. E., *et al.:* Effects of intravenous administration of ribonucleic acid upon failure of memory for recent events in presenile and aged individuals. In: Recent advances in biological psychiatry (ed., Wortis, J.). (Plenum Press, New York, 1963.)

Carlsson, A., Jonasson, J., and Rosengren, E.: Time correlation between the effects of reserpine on behavior and storage mechanism for arylalkylamines. Acta Physiol. Scand., *59:* 474 (1963).

Carlton, P. L.: Potentiation of the behavioral effects of amphetamine by imipramine. Psychopharmacologia (Berlin), *2:* 364 (1961).

Cassano, G. B., Sjostrand, S. E., and Hansson, E.: Distribution and fate of C^{14} amitriptyline in mice and rats. Psychopharmacologia (Berlin), *8:* 12 (1965).

Chance, M. R. A.: Factors influencing toxicity of sympathomimetic amines to solitary mice. J. Pharmacol. Exp. Ther., *89:* 289 (1947).

Chen, G.: Antidepressives, analeptics, and appetite suppressants. In: Evaluation of drug activities—Pharmacometrics (eds., Laurence, D. R., and Bacharach, A. L.). (Academic Press, London, 1964.)

Chen, G., and Bohner, B.: The antireserpine effects of certain centrally-acting agents. J. Pharmacol. Exp. Ther., *131:* 179 (1961).

Cook, L., and Catania, A. C.: Effects of drugs on avoidance and escape behavior. Fed. Proc., *23:* 818 (1964).

Corne, S. T., Pickering, R. W., and Warner, B. T.: A method for assessing the effects of drugs on the central actions of 5-hydroxytryptamine. Brit. J. Pharmacol., *20:* 106 (1963).

Corson, S. A.: Pavlovian conditioning as a method for studying the mechanisms of action of minor tranquillizers. (Presented at the Fifth International Congress of CINP, Washington, 1966.)

Corson, S. A., O'Leary, E., and England, S. J. M.: The influence of meprobamate on conditioned and unconditioned visceral and motor defense responses. In: Psychopharmacological methods (eds., Votava, Z., Horvath, M., and Vinar, O.). (Pergamon Press, New York, 1963.)

Costa, E., Garattini, S., and Valzelli, L.: Interactions between reserpine, chlorpromazine and imipramine. Experientia, *16:* 461 (1960).

Courvoisier, S.: Pharmacodynamic basis for the use of chlorpromazine in psychiatry. J. Clin. Exp. Psychopath., *17:* 25 (1956).

Crossland, J., and Merrick, A. J.: The effect of anaesthesia on the actylcholine content of the brain. J. Physiol. (London), *125:* 56 (1954).

Curtis, D. R.: The pharmacology of central and peripheral inhibition. Pharmacol. Rev., *15:* 333 (1963).

Dale, H. H., Feldberg, W., and Vogt, M.: Release of acetylcholine at voluntary motor nerve endings. J. Physiol. (London), *86:* 353 (1936).

Davey, D. G.: The study of the toxicity of a potential drug; basic principles. Vol. VI, International Congress Series, No. 97. (Excerpta Medica Foundation, Amsterdam, 1965.)

Davies, E. B. (ed.): Depression—a Cambridge postgraduate medical course. (University Press, Cambridge, 1964.)

Dengler, H. J., Spiegel, H. E., and Titus, E. O.: Uptake of tritium-labelled norepinephrine in brain and other tissues of cat in vivo. Science, *133:* 1072 (1961).

Dews, P. B.: A behavioral output enhancing effect of imipramine in pigeons. Int. J. Neuropharmacol., *1:* 265 (1962).

Dikshit, R.: Action of acetylcholine on the sleep centre. J. Physiol. (London), *83:* 42 (1935).

Domenjoz, R., and Theobald, W.: Zur Pharmakologie des Tofranil (*N*-3-dimethylaminopropyliminodibenzyl hydrochloride). Arch. Int. Pharmacodyn., *120:* 450 (1959).

Draskoci, M., Feldberg, W., and Haranath, P. S.: Passage of circulating adrenaline into perfused cerebral ventricles and subarachnoid space. J. Physiol. (London), *150:* 34 (1960).

Dureman, E. I., and Henriksson, B. G.: Effects of tricyclic antidepressive compounds on operant behavior in pigeons. In: Antidepressant drugs (eds., Garattini, S., and Dukes, M. N. G.). (Excerpta Medica Foundation, Amsterdam, 1967.)

Eccles, J. C.: The physiology of synapses. (Academic Press, New York, 1964.)

Elkes, J.: Drug effects in relation to acceptor specificity within the brain: some evidence and provisional formulation. In: Neurological basis of behavior (eds., Wolstenholme, G. E. W., and O'Connor, C. M.). (Churchill, London, 1958.)

Elliot, K. A. C., and Jasper, H. H.: Gamma-aminobutyric acid. Physiol. Rev., *39:* 383 (1959).

Euler, U. S.: A specific sympathomimetic ergone in adrenergic nerve fibres (sympathin) and its relations to adrenaline and nor-adrenaline. Acta Physiol. Scand., *12:* 73 (1946).

Euler, U. S., and Gaddum, J. H.: An unidentified depressor substance in certain tissue extracts. J. Physiol. (London), *72:* 74 (1931).

Evarts, E. V. A.: A discussion of the relevance of effects on animal behavior to the possible effects of drugs on psychopathological processes in man. In: Psychopharmacology: problems in evaluation (eds., Cole, J. D., and Gerard, R. W.). (National Academy of Sciences-National Research Council, Washington, 1959.)

Eyal, H., and Eyal, Z.: The effect of chlorpromazine on the embryonic development of the emblystoma mexicanum. J. Embryol. Exp. Morph., *10:* 357 (1962).

Eyal, Z., and Eyal, H.: Growth retarding and growth promoting effect of chlorpromazine on developing emblystoma mexicanum embryos. Exp. Cell Res., *29:* 394 (1963).

Feldberg, W., and Sherwood, S. L.: Injections of drugs into the lateral ventricle of the cat. J. Physiol. (London), *123:* 148 (1954).

Feldberg, W., and Sherwood, S. L.: Behavior of cats after intraventricular injections of eserine and D.F.P. J. Physiol. (London), *125:* 488 (1959).

Fink, G. B., and Swinyard, E. A.: Comparison of anticonvulsant and psychopharmacological drugs. J. Pharm. Sci., *51:* 548 (1962).

Fleischmann, P. (1910): In: Kalow, W.: Pharmacogenetics. (Saunders, Philadelphia, 1962.)

Friedman, S. L., and Ingalls, J. W., Jr.: A note on the tilting-plane technique for measuring the performance of rats in relation to the degree of their alcohol intoxication. Quart. J. Stud. Alcohol, *21:* 217 (1960).

Friend, D. G.: Clinical evaluation of drugs. Prevention and control of adverse reactions. J.A.M.A., *187:* 348 (1964).

Friend, D. G.: Role of synthetic drugs in the therapy of mental illness. In: Molecular modification in drug design (ed., Gould, R. F.). (American Chemical Society, Washington, 1964.)

Frommel, E., *et al.:* De la pharmacodynamie differentielle des thymoanaleptiques et des substances neuroleptiques en expérimentation animale. Thérapie, *15:* 1175 (1960).

Gabay, S.: Brain transaminases in a chemically induced behavioral abnormality. In: Recent advances in biological psychiatry (ed., Wortis, J.). (Plenum Press, New York, 1966.)

Gaito, J. (ed.): Macromolecules and behavior. (Appleton-Century-Crofts, New York, 1966.)

Gaito, J.: Macromolecules and brain function. In: Macromolecules and behavior (ed., Gaito, J.). (Appleton-Century-Crofts, New York, 1966.)

Gallant, D., and Bishop, M. P.: Informal ECDEU report from Tulane (Unpublished.) Tulane, 1967.

Gantt, W. H.: Effect of B-complex vitamin on conditional reflexes in dogs. Amer. J. Clin. Nutr., *5:* 121 (1957).

Gantt, W. H.: Normal and abnormal adaptations —homeostasis, schizokinesis and autokinesis. Dis. Nerv. Syst., *18:* 30 (1957).

GANTT, W. H.: Pavlovian principles and psychiatry. Progr. Psychother., *2:* 140 (1957).

GANTT, W. H.: Pharmacological agents in the study of higher nervous activity. Dis. Nerv. Syst., *18:* 339 (1957).

GANTT, W. H.: Application of the conditional reflex method to preventive psychiatry. Dis. Nerv. Syst., *20:* 30 (1959).

GANTT, W. H.: Factors involved in the development of pathological behavior: schizokinesis and autokinesis. Perspect. Biol. Med., *5:* 473 (1962).

GANTT, W. H.: Role of drugs in conditioning. (Presented at the Fifth International Congress of CINP, Washington, 1966.)

GARATTINI, S., *et al.:* Effect of imipramine, amitriptyline and their monomethyl derivatives on reserpine activity. J. Pharm. Pharmacol., *14:* 509 (1962).

GASTAUT, H.: Etat actuel des connaissances sur l'électroencephalographie du conditionnement. Electorenceph. Clin. Neurophysiol., *6:* 133 (1957).

GASTAUT, H.: Some aspects of the neurophysiological basis of conditioned reflexes and behavior. In: The neurological basis of behavior (eds. Wolstenholme, G. E. W. and O'Connor, C. M.). (Churchill, London 1958.)

GASTAUT, H., *et al.:* A topographical study of conditioned electroencephalographic reactions which occur independently, simultaneously or successively in different cortical regions in man. Electroenceph. Clin. Neurophysiol., *8:* 728 (1956).

GATTI, G. L.: Azione dei farmaci tranquillanti sui vari tipi di compartemento del ratto condizionato. In: Psychotropic drugs (eds., Garattini, S., and Ghetti, V.). (Elsevier, Amsterdam, 1957.)

GATTI, G. L.: The effects of psychotropic drugs on avoidance behavior. (Presented at the Fifth International Congress of CINP, Washington, 1966.)

GATTI, G. L., AND BOVET, D.: Analysis of the action of the psychotropic drugs in a "lever pressing avoidance" conditioning. In: Psychopharmacological methods (eds., Votava, Z., Horvath, M., and Vinar, O.). (Pergamon Press, New York, 1963.)

GLIEDMAN, L. H., AND GANTT, W. H.: The effects of reserpine and chlorpromazine on orienting behavior and retention of conditional reflexes. Southern Med. J., *49:* 880 (1956).

GLOWINSKI, J., AND AXELROD, J.: Inhibition of uptake of tritiated noradrenaline in the intact rat brain by imipramine and structurally related compounds. Nature (London), *204:* 1318 (1964).

GLOWINSKI, J., AND AXELROD, J.: Effects of central drugs on the disposition of H^3-norepinephrine in the rat brain. (Presented at the Second Catecholamine Symposium, Milan, 1965.)

GROLLMAN, A.: Pharmacology and therapeutics. (Lea and Febiger, Philadelphia, 1965.)

HALLIWELL, G., *et al.:* A comparison of imipramine, chlorpromazine and related drugs in various tests involving autonomic functions and antagonism of reserpine. Brit. J. Pharmacol., *23:* 330 (1964).

HANSON, H. M.: The effects of amitriptyline, imipramine, chlorpromazine and nialamide on avoidance behavior. Fed. Proc., *20:* 396 (1961).

HANSSON, E., AND CASSANO, G. B.: Distribution and metabolism of antidepressant drugs. In: Antidepressant drugs (eds., Garattini S., and Dukes, M. N. G.). (Excerpta Medica Foundation, Amsterdam, 1967.)

HASSERT, G. L., *et al.:* Pharmacologic and toxicologic studies with 2-amino-5-phenyl-1,3,4-oxadiazole hydrochloride. Toxic. Appl. Pharmacol., *3:* 726 (1961).

HAYASHI, T.: Schizophrenia from the standpoint of physiology. (Presented at the Fourth World Congress of Psychiatry, Madrid, 1966.)

HECHT, K.: Comparative investigations of some centrally acting drugs with a conditioned-reflex motoric food method and a conditioned-reflex motoric escape method. In: Psychopharmacological methods (eds., Votava, Z., Horvath, M., and Vinar, O.). (Pergamon Press, New York, 1963.)

HECHT, K., *et al.:* Der Einfluss einer kleinen Dosis Reserpin (0.1 mg/kg) auf Ausbildung und Ablauf Bedingter Reaktionen I und II Ordnung. Acta Biol. Med. German, *4:* 131 (1960).

HILLARP, N. A., FUXE, K., AND DAHLSTROM, A.: Demonstration and mopping of central neurons containing dopamine, noradrenaline and 5-hydroxytryptamine and their reactions to psychopharmaca. Pharmacol. Rev., *18:* 727 (1966).

HIMWICH, H. E.: Anatomy and physiology of the emotions and their relation to psychoactive drugs. In: The scientific basis of drug therapy in psychiatry (eds., Marks, J., and Pare, C. M. B.). (Pergamon Press, Oxford, 1965.)

HIMWICH, H. E.: Comparative clinical and basic evaluation of various groups of psychotropic drugs. Psychosomatics, *6:* 254 (1965).

HIMWICH, H. E.: Psychoactive drugs. Postgrad. Med., *37:* 35 (1965).

HOLTZ, P., CREDNER, K., AND KRÖNEBERG, G.: Über das Sympathicomimetische Pressorische Prinzip des Harns. Arch. Exp. Path. Pharmakol., *204:* 228 (1947).

HYDEN, H. (1955): In: Cameron, D. E., *et al.* RNA in psychiatric therapy. In: Current psychiatric therapies (eds., Masserman, J.). (Grune and Stratton, New York, 1964.)

HYDEN, H.: Discussion: control of the mind. (Presented at the Symposium on Man and Civilization, San Francisco, 1961.)

HYDEN, H., AND EGYHAZI, E.: Changes in RNA content and base composition in cortical neurons in rats in a learning experiment involving transfer of handedness. Proc. Nat. Acad. Sci. U.S.A., *52:* 1030, 1964.

HYDEN, H., AND HARTELIUS, H.: Stimulation of the nuclein-production in the nerve cells by malononitrile and its effect on psychic functions in mental disorders. Acta Psychiat. Neurol., *48:* 1 (1948).

Hyden, H., and Pigeon, A.: A cytophysiological study of the functional relationship between oligodendroglia cells and nerve cells of Deiter's nucleus. J. Neurochem., *6:* 57 (1960).

Irwin, S.: General philosophy and methodology of screening: a multidimensional approach. (Presented at the Gordon Research Conference on Medicinal Chemistry at Colby Junior College, New London, 1959.)

Irwin, S.: The value of animal experimentation. In: Psychopharmacology frontiers (ed., Kline, N. S.). (Little, Brown, Toronto, 1959.)

Irwin, S.: Drug screening and evaluation procedures. Science, *136:* 123 (1962).

Irwin, S.: Influence of experimental variables on the rate of tolerance development to chlorpromazine and perphenazine. Fed. Proc., *21:* 419 (1962).

Irwin, S.: Determinants of variability in drug response. Psychosomatics, *5:* 174 (1964).

Irwin, S.: Drug screening and evaluation of new compounds in animals. In: Animal and clinical pharmacological techniques in drug evaluation (eds., Nodine, H., and Siegler, P. E.). (Year Book Med., Philadelphia, 1964.)

Irwin, S.: Prediction of drug effects from animals to man. In: Animal behavior and drug action (eds., Steinberg, H., *et al.*). (Little, Brown, Boston, 1964.)

Irwin, S.: Considerations for the pre-clinical evaluation of new psychiatric drugs: a case study with phenothiazine-like tranquillizers. Psychopharmacology, *9:* 259 (1966).

Irwin, S.: Psychopharmacology and drug therapy. (Paper presented at the Postgraduate Course on Animal and Clinical Pharmacology Techniques in Drug Evaluation, Philadelphia, 1966.)

Issekutz, B.: Über der Wirkung der Tropeine und Ihrer Quaterneren Ammonium Basen. Ztschr. Exp. Path. Pharmacol., *19:* 99 (1917).

Jacob, J., and Michaud, G.: Action of various pharmacological agents on the exhaustion times and the behavior of mice swimming at 20°C. Description of the technique, action of amphetamine, cocaine, caffeine, hexobarbital and meprobamate. Arch. Int. Pharmacodyn., *133:* 101 (1961).

Jacobsen, E.: The clinical pharmacology of the hallucinogen. Clin. Pharmacol. Ther., *4:* 480 (1963).

Jacobsen, E.: Investigation into the mode of action of substances acting on the central nervous system. In: Depression—a Cambridge postgraduate medical course (ed., Davies, E. B.). (University Press, Cambridge, 1964.)

Jacobsen, E.: The theoretical basis of the chemotherapy of depression. In: Depression—a Cambridge postgraduate medical course (ed., Davies, E. B.). (University Press, Cambridge, 1964.)

Jacobsen, E.: Tranquillizers and sedatives. In: Evaluation of drug activities—Pharmacometrics (eds., Laurence, D. R., and Bacharach, A. L.). (Academic Press, London, 1964.)

Janssen, P. A. J.: The evolution of the butyrophenones haloperidol and trifluperidol from meperidine-like 4-phenylpiperidines. Int. Rev. Neurobiol., *86:* 221 (1965).

Janssen, P. A. J.: The pharmacology of neuroleptic drugs. In: Haase, H. J., and Janssen, P. A. J. The action of neuroleptic drugs. (North-Holland Publishing House, Amsterdam, 1965.)

Janssen, P. A. J., Niemegeers, C. J. E., and Schellekens, K. H. L.: Is it possible to predict the clinical effects of neuroleptic drugs from animal data? Neuroleptic activity spectra for drugs. Arzneimittelforschung, *15:* 1196 (1965).

Janssen, P. A. J., *et al.*: Is it possible to predict the clinical effects of neuroleptic drugs (major tranquillizers) from animal data? Arzneimittelforschung, *15:* 104 (1965).

Jay, G. E.: Variation in response of various mouse strains to hexobarbital (evipal). Proc. Soc. Exp. Biol. Med., *90:* 378 (1955).

Kalow, W.: Pharmacogenetics: heredity and the response to drugs. (Saunders, Philadelphia, 1962.)

Kaminsky, S. D., and Savchuk, U. J.: The effect of chlorpromazine on th e higher nervous activity of dogs. (Rus.) Zh· Nevropat. Psikhiat. Korsakov., *56:* 104 (1956).

Kielholz, P.: Diagnostik und Therapie der Erschöpfungs—depressiven Zustandsbilder. Wien. Med. Wschr., *110:* 714 (1960).

Killam, E. K., and Killam, K. F., Jr.: Neurophysiological approaches to an understanding of the action of tranquillizing drugs. In: Psychopharmacology: International psychiatry clinics (eds., Kline, N. S., and Lehmann, H. E.). (Little, Brown, Boston, 1965.)

Killam, K. F., and Killam, E. K.: Central action of chlorpromazine and reserpine. In: Neuropharmacology (ed., Abramson, H.). (Madison, New York, 1960.)

Kinnard, W. J., *et al.*: Methods of evaluation of antidepressant activity. In: Antidepressant drugs (eds., Garattini, S., and Dukes, M. N. G.). (Excerpta Medica Foundation, Amsterdam, 1967.)

Konorski, J., and Miller, S.: Further remarks on two types of conditioned reflex. J. Gen. Psychol., *17:* 405 (1937).

Konorski, J., and Miller, S.: On two types of conditional reflex. J. Gen. Psychol., *16:* 264 (1937).

Kuhn, W. L., and Van Maanen, E. F.: Central nervous system effects of thalidomide. J. Pharmacol. Exp. Ther., *134:* 60 (1961).

Landauer, T. K.: Two hypotheses concerning the biochemical basis of memory. Psychol. Rev., *71:* 167, 1964.

Laurence, D. R., and Bacharach, A. L. (eds.): Evaluation of drug activities—Pharmacometrics. (Academic Press, London, 1964.)

Leake, C.: The amphetamines, their action and uses. (Charles C Thomas, Springfield, 1958.)

MacLean, P. D.: Psychosomatic disease and the "visceral brain": recent developments bearing on the Papez theory of emotion. Psychosom. Med., *11:* 338 (1949).

Magoun, H. W., and Rhines, R.: An inhibitory mechanism in the bulbar reticular formation. J. Neurophysiol., *6:* 165 (1946).

Mason, D. J.: An apparatus and method for rigorously controlling amount of reward. Psychol. Rep., *14:* 388 (1964).

Masserman, J. H.: Behavior and neurosis. (University of Chicago Press, Chicago, 1943.)

Matthews, R. J., and Roberts, B. J.: The effect of GABA on synaptic transmission in autonomic ganglia. J. Pharmacol. Exp. Ther., *132:* 19 (1961).

Matussek, N., *et al.*: Amine-metabolism in the CNS during exhaustion after swimming, and the influence of antidepressants on this syndrome. In: Antidepressant drugs (eds., Garattini, S., and Dukes, M. N. G.). (Excerpta Medica Foundation, Amsterdam, 1967.)

Metysova, J., and Metys, J.: Pharmacological properties of the desmethyl derivatives of some antidepressants of imipramine types. Int. J. Neuropharmacol., *4:* 111 (1965).

Metzner, R.: Mitteilungen über Wirkung und Verhalten des Atropins im Organismus. Arch. Exp. Path. Pharmakol., *68:* 110 (1912).

Miller, N. E.: Analytical studies of drive and reward. Amer. Psychol., *16:* 739 (1961).

Miller, N. E.: Some recent studies of conflict behavior and drugs. Amer. Psychol., *16:* 12 (1961).

Miller, N. E.: The analysis of motivational effects illustrated by experiments on amylobarbitone sodium. In: Animal behavior and drug action (eds., Steinberg, H., deReuck, A. V. S., and Knight, J.). (Churchill, London, 1964.)

Misrahy, G. A., *et al.:* The effects of drugs used in pregnancy on availability of foetal cerebral oxygen. Anesthesiology, *24:* 198 (1963).

Monnier, M., and Krupp, P.: Electrophysiologic analysis of the effect of various neuroleptic drugs (chlorpromazine, reserpine, tofranil, meprobamate). Schweiz. Med. Wschr., *89:* 430 (1959).

Moruzzi, G., and Magoun, H. W.: Brain stem reticular formation and activation of the EEG. Electroenceph. Clin. Neurophysiol., *1:* 455 (1949).

Nachmansohn, D.: Chemical and molecular basis of nerve activity. (Academic Press, New York, 1958.)

Neff, N. H., and Costa, E.: Effect of tricyclic antidepressants and chlorpromazine on brain catecholamine synthesis. In: Antidepressant drugs (eds., Garattini, S., and Dukes, M. N. G.). (Excerpta Medica Foundation, New York, 1967.)

Newton, J. E. O.: Effects of minor tranquillizers on conditional reflexes. Discussion of Doctor S. A. Corson's paper. (Presented at the Fifth International Congress of CINP, Washington, 1966.)

Norton, S.: Behavioral patterns and technique for studying psychotropic drugs. In: Psychotropic drugs (eds., Garattini, S., and Ghetti, V.). (Elsevier, Amsterdam, 1957.)

Norton, S., and deBeer, E. J.: Effects of drugs on behavioral patterns of cats. Ann. N.Y. Acad. Sci., *65:* 249 (1956).

Olds, J., and Milner, P.: Positive reinforcement produced by electrical stimulation of septal area and other regions of rat brain. J. Comp. Physiol. Psychol., *47:* 419 (1954).

Paget, G. E., and Barnes, J. M.: Toxicity tests. In: Evaluation of drug activities—Pharmacometrics (eds., Laurence, D. R., and Bacharach, A. L.). (Academic Press, London, 1964.)

Papez, J. W.: A proposed mechanism of emotion. Arch. Neurol. Psychiat., *38:* 725 (1937).

Pavlov, I. P.: Conditioned reflexes: An investigation of the physiological activity of the cerebral cortex (translated by Anrep, G. V.). (Oxford University Press, Oxford, 1928.)

Pavlov, I. P.: Lectures on conditioned reflexes (translated by Gantt, W. H.). (International Publishers, New York, 1928.)

Penfield, W., and Jasper, H. H.: Epilepsy and the functional anatomy of the human brain. (Little, Brown, Boston, 1954.)

Petersen, P. V., and Nielsen, I. M.: Chemical configuration and pharmacological action of thymoleptic drugs with special reference to a new group of bicyclic compounds. In: Antidepressant drugs (eds., Garattini, S., and Dukes, M. N. G.). (Excerpta Medica Foundation, Amsterdam, 1967.)

Pletscher, A.: Release of 5-HT by benzoquinolizine derivatives with sedative action. Science, *126:* 507 (1957).

Pletscher, A.: Pharmacology of antidepressants. In: Psychopharmacology (eds., Kline, N. S., and Lehmann, H. E.). (Little, Brown, Boston, 1965.)

Pletscher, A., Discussion. In: The scientific basis of drug therapy in psychiatry (eds., Marks, J., and Pare, C. M. B.) (Pergamon Press, Oxford, 1965.)

Pletscher, A.: Pharmacology of monoamine oxidase inhibitors. In: The scientific basis of drug therapy in psychiatry (eds., Marks, J., and Pare, C. M. B.). (Pergamon Press, Oxford, 1965.)

Plotnikoff, N.: Effects of neurotropic drugs on non-conditioned avoidance response. Arch. Int. Pharmacodyn., *145:* 3 (1963).

Quastel, J. H., Tennenbaum, M., and Wheatley, A. H.: Choline ester formation and choline esterase activities of tissues in vitro. Biochem. J., *30:* 1668 (1936).

Quastel, J. H., and Wooldridge, W. R.: Some properties of the dehydrogenating enzymes of bacteria. Biochem. J., *22:* 689 (1928).

Quinton, R. M.: The increase in the toxicity of yohimbine induced by imipramine and other drugs in mice. Brit. J. Pharmacol., *21:* 51 (1963).

Ramon y Cajal, S.: Histologie du systeme nerveux de l'homme et des vértebrés. (Maloine, Paris, 1909).

RICHTER, D., AND CROSSLAND, J.: Variation in acetylcholine content of the brain with physiological state. Amer. J. Physiol., *159:* 247 (1949).

RINALDI, F., AND HIMWICH, H. E.: A comparison of effects of reserpine and some barbiturates on the electrical activity of cortical and subcortical structures of the brain of rabbits. In: Reserpine in the treatment of neuropsychiatric, neurological and related clinical problems (ed., Miner, R. W.). (The Academy, New York, 1955.)

ROBERTS, E., AND FRANKEL, S.: γ-Aminobutyric acid in brain: its formation from glutamic acid. J. Biol. Chem., *187:* 55 (1950).

ROBSON, J. M., AND STACEY, R. S.: Recent advances in pharmacology. (Churchill, London, 1962.)

ROBSON, J. M., AND SULLIVAN, F. M.: The production of foetal abnormalities in rabbits by imipramine. Lancet, *1:* 638 (1963).

ROSEN, F.: The relationship of certain vitamin deficiencies to the toxicity of iproniazid. Ann. N.Y. Acad. Sci., *80:* 885 (1959).

RUSSELL, E. S.: Significance of physiological pattern of animal strains in biological research. Brit. Med. J., *1:* 826 (1955).

RUSSELL, R. W.: Drugs as tools in behavioral research. In: Drugs and behavior (eds., Uhr, L., and Miller, J. G.). (Wiley, New York, 1961.)

SAVCHUK, V. I.: The action of aminazine on the different parts of the brain according to the results of an experimental study. Zh. Nevropat. Psikhiat. Korsakov., *60:* 182 (1960).

SCHALLEK, W.: Neurophysiological studies with MAOI's. Dis. Nerv. Syst., *21:* 64 (1960).

SCHALLEK, W., AND KUEHN, A.: Effects of psychotropic drugs on limbic system of cats. Proc. Soc. Exp. Biol. Med., *105:* 115 (1960).

SCHECKEL, C. L., AND BOFF, E.: Behavioral effects of interacting imipramine and other drugs with d-amphetamine, cocaine and tetrabenazine. Psychopharmacologia (Berlin), *5:* 198 (1964).

SHAY, H., *et al.:* A simple method for the uniform production of gastric ulceration in the rat. Gastroenterology, *5:* 43 (1945).

SIDMAN, M.: Avoidance conditioning with brief shock and no exteroceptive warning signal. Science, *118:* 157 (1953).

SIDMAN, M.: Drug behavior interaction. Ann. N.Y. Acad. Sci., *65:* 282 (1956).

SIDMAN, M.: Behavioral pharmacology. Psychopharmacologia (Berlin), *1:* 1 (1959).

SIDMAN, M.: Some technical problems in evaluating the behavioral effects of drugs. In: Psychopharmacological methods (eds., Votava, Z., Horvath, M., and Vinar, O.). (State Medical Publishing House, Prague, 1963.)

SIEGMUND, P., AND WOLF, M.: Eine einfache Methode der Motilitätsmessung an Mäusen. Arch. Exp. Path. Pharmakol., *216:* 323 (1952).

SKINNER, B. F.: Two types of conditioned reflex and a pseudo type. J. Gen. Psychol., *12:* 66 (1935).

SKINNER, B. F.: Two types of conditioned reflex: a reply to Konorski and Miller. J. Gen. Psychol., *16:* 272 (1937).

SKLYAROVA, M. I.: The effects of reserpine and meprobamate on conditional salivary reflexes (Rus.). Tes. 20 Sov. Probl. Vyss. Nerv. Dejat, *20:* 96 (1960).

SMYTHIES, J. R.: The neurological foundations of psychiatry. (Blackwell, Oxford, 1966.)

SOURKES, T. L.: Biochemistry of mental disease. (Harper and Row, New York, 1962.)

STEDMAN, E., AND STEDMAN, E.: Mechanism of biological synthesis of acetylcholine: isolation of acetylcholine produced by brain tissue in vitro. Biochem. J., *31:* 817 (1937).

STEIN, L.: Effects and interactions of imipramine, chlorpromazine, reserpine and amphetamine on self-stimulation: possible neurophysiological basis of depression. Recent Advances Biol. Psychiat., *4:* 288 (1961).

STEIN, L.: Psychopharmacological substrates of mental depression. In: Antidepressant drugs (eds., Garattini, S., and Dukes, M. N. G.). (Excerpta Medica Foundation, Amsterdam, 1967.)

STEINBERG, H.: Methods of assessment of psychological effects of drugs in animals. In: The scientific basis of drug therapy in psychiatry (eds., Marks, J., and Pare, C. M. B.). (Pergamon Press, Oxford, 1965.)

STEINER, W. G., AND HIMWICH, H. E.: Central cholinolytic action of chlorpromazine. Science, *136:* 873 (1962).

STEWART, C. C.: Variations in daily activity produced by alcohol and by changes in barometric pressure and diet with a description of recording methods. Amer. J. Physiol., *1:* 40 (1898).

SULSER, F., AND BICKEL, M. H.: On the role of brain catecholamines in the antireserpine action of desmethylimipramine. Pharmacologist, *4:* 178 (1962).

SULSER, F., BICKEL, M. H., AND BRODIE, B. B.: The action of desmethylimipramine in counteracting sedation and cholinergic effects of reserpine-like drugs. J. Pharmacol., *144:* 321 (1964).

SULSER, F., WATTS, J., AND BRODIE, B. B.: On the mechanism of antidepressant action of imipramine-like drugs. Ann. N.Y. Acad. Sci., *96:* 279 (1962).

TAUC, L., AND GERSCHENFELD, H.: Acetylcholine as a probable transmitter of synaptic inhibition in aplysia. C. R. Acad. Sci. (Paris), *251:* 3076 (1960).

TAUC, L., AND GERSCHENFELD, H.: Acetylcholine as a probable transmitter of synaptic inhibition in the CNS of mollusca. J. Physiol., *53:* 482 (1961).

TEDESCHI, D. H., *et al.:* Interaction of neuroleptics with serotonin in the central nervous system. Rev. Canad. Biol., *20:* 209 (1961).

THUILLIER, J.: Special pharmacology of hypothalamus stimulating substances. In: Regional neurochemistry (eds., Kety, S. S., and Elkes, J.). (Pergamon Press, Oxford, 1961.)

TINDAL, J. S.: A breed difference in the lactogenic response of the rabbit to reserpine. J. Endocr., *20:* 78 (1960).

TURNER, R. A.: Screening methods in pharmacology. (Academic Press, New York, 1965.)

URSIN, H., The lack of effect of LSD_{25} on amygdaloid and cortical attention responses. Psychopharmacologia (Berlin), *3:* 317 (1962).

UTLEY, J. D.: The effects of anthranilic hydroxamic acid on rat behavior and rat brain GABA, NE and 5HT concentrations. J. Neurochem., *10:* 423 (1963).

VAILLANT, G. E.: A comparison of chlorpromazine and imipramine on behavior of the pigeons. J. Pharmacol. Exp. Ther., *146:* 377 (1964).

VALZELLI, L., CONSOLO S., AND MORPURGO, C.: Influence of imipramine like drugs on the metabolism of amphetamine. In: Antidepressant drugs (eds., Garattini, S., and Dukes, M. N. G.). (Excerpta Medica Foundation, Amsterdam, 1967.)

VANE, J. R.: A plane for evaluating potential drugs. In: Evaluation of drug activity—Pharmacometrics (eds., Laurence, D. R., and Bacharach, A. L.). (Academic Press, London, 1964.)

VERNIER, V. G.: The pharmacology of antidepressant agents. Dis. Nerv. Syst., *22:* 7 (1961).

VERNIER, V. G.: Pharmacological evidence of mode of action of antidepressant non-MAO inhibitor drugs from behavioral and electrophysiological studies. In: Antidepressant drugs of the non-MAO type (eds., Efron, D. H., and Kety, S. S.). (U.S. Dept. of Health, Education and Welfare, Bethesda, 1966.)

VERNIER, V. G., *et al.:* Pharmacological action of amitriptyline, noramitriptyline and imipramine. Fed. Proc., *21:* 419 (1962).

VERNIER, V. G., HANSON, H. M., AND STONE, C. A.: Pharmacological actions of amitriptyline, noramitriptyline and imipramine. In: Psychosomatic medicine (eds., Nodine, J. H., and Moyer, J. H.). (Lea and Febiger, Philadelphia, 1962.)

WEISSMAN, A.: Interaction effects of imipramine and d-amphetamine on non-discriminated avoidance. Pharmacologist, *3:* 60 (1961).

WOOLLEY, D. W.: The biochemical bases of psychoses or the serotonin hypothesis about mental disease. (Wiley, New York, 1962.)

WOOLLEY, D. W., AND SHAW, E. N.: A biochemical and pharmacological suggestion about certain mental disorders. Science, *119:* 587 (1954).

WOOLLEY, D. W., AND SHAW, E. N.: Evidence for the participation of serotonin in mental processes. Ann. N.Y. Acad. Sci., *66:* 649 (1957).

WORTIS, J.: Psychopharmacology and physiological treatment. Amer. J. Psychiat., *120:* 643 (1964).

ZETLER, G.: Substance P in the central nervous system. Naturwissenschaften, *40:* 559 (1953).

ZETLER, G.: Experiments on the anticonvulsive effectiveness of the polypeptide substance P. Arch. Exp. Path. Pharmakol., *237:* 11 (1959).

ZETLER, G., *et al.:* Research towards pharmacological differentiation of cataleptic effects. Arch. Exp. Path. Pharmakol., *238:* 486 (1960).

ZETLER, G., AND MOOG, E.: Die Bulbocapnin-katatonie, ihre Synergisten und Antagonisten. Arch. Exp. Path. Pharmakol., *232:* 442 (1958).

Three

Human Pharmacology

Human pharmacology is the scientific study of the effect of drugs on the human organism. The primary interest of the human pharmacologist is the drug *per se*, and his main concern is extending the knowledge of the drug's action from animal to human. In this chapter, human pharmacology will be restricted to the methods, techniques, procedures and results most pertinent to psychoactive substances.

A preliminary step in human pharmacological investigation is to establish an effective dosage range for the new substance. This is followed by pharmacodynamic and toxicity studies.

Experiments to establish the effective dosage range are carried out on young, healthy, mentally stable, volunteer adults, who have given voluntary consent for the experiment. It is essential that they are intelligent enough to give an account of their experiences while under the influence of the investigational compound.

Initially, the dose-response curves are obtained by administering single doses of the drug, progressing from minute amounts with no detectable effect to high, slightly toxic doses. The dose-response curve is based on the subjective reports of the volunteer subject; on the careful observations of the investigator; and on recordings of objective changes, *e.g.*, blood pressure, pulse rate, respiration, temperature, skin resistance, pupil size, etc. These are noted and recorded for at least 24 hours after drug administration. To uncover any possible delayed effects of the investigational compound, the experimental subject is followed up for at least a one-week period.

The "small" starting dose in the preliminary experiments is based on the findings in the animal pharmacological studies. It is generally accepted that drug dosage requirements in man, with the exception of interspecies metabolic or sensitivity differences for certain psychopharmacological compounds, are quite similar to those in animals on a milligram per kilogram basis or on the basis of the ratio of body weight to body surface area.

For all practical purposes, the amount that produces the desired effect in a dog weighing 10 kg. (22 pounds) can be given as the first dose to a human being weighing 50 kg. (110 pounds). However, if the difference between the LD_{50} (lethal dose, which produces death in 50 per cent of the animals) and the ED_{50} (effective dose which produces the desired effect in 50 per cent of the animals) is small, and consequently the therapeutic ratio of the drug is low, the first dose should be very much less.

The starting dose is usually set at one-tenth of the anticipated effective dosage. Starting with this minute amount, the single doses are gradually increased until the smallest dose which produces any of the desired effects in at least 50 per cent of the volunteers is reached or until a dose is given which produces any undesired side-effect in 25 per cent of the experimental subjects. With this data in hand human pharmacodynamic investigations may commence.

A. PHARMACODYNAMICS

There are limitations in extrapolating from animal pharmacodynamic data to man because of interspecies metabolic differences. Therefore, pharmacodynamic studies on animals have to be followed by pharmacodynamic studies in humans.

The ultimate goal of pharmacodynamic studies in humans is to enable the investigator to predict the possible clinical usefulness of a particular drug. As in animal studies, there are four major procedures available for assessing the range of activity of a new agent. First there is the phenomenological and symptomatological appraisal which subjectively assesses psychological or psychopathological changes. This is complemented by tests which objectively measure behavioral or psychophysical changes. Third, there is the exploration of the effect of the substance on the ability to form new or maintain old stimulus-response constellations by conditioning procedures. Finally, the neurophysiological and biochemical correlates of the drug's action are investigated.

1. Phenomenological and Symptomatological Appraisal

The phenomenological approach has been used extensively in the study of the pharmacodynamic action of psychoactive drugs. The value of this information depends, however, on such factors as the veracity of the subject and the sensitivity of his bodily feelings and inner experiences. It has been noted that introverts with slightly hypochondriacal tendencies are probably the best experimental subjects for this purpose, while extroverts are usually unsatisfactory (Mayer-Gross *et al.*, 1960).

While phenomenological information contributes a great deal to the knowledge of psychic experiences under the influence of various psychoactive drugs, descriptive behavioral observations are instrumental for recognizing that the human pharmacological findings are an extension of the animal pharmacological data.

Human pharmacological investigations with the seven clinically most frequently used groups of psychopharmacological substances have revealed the following data.

Sedative barbiturates produce a biphasic effect. First there is a disinhibition characterized by an increased verbal output, relief of muscular tension and loosening of associations. This is replaced, with the increasing blood concentrations of the substance, by sedation, which culminates in sleep. (If there is a deliberate attempt to interfere with sleep, a state characterized by euphoria or confusion ensues.)

As opposed to barbiturates, stimulant amphetamines in human pharmacological experiments produce increased "wakefulness," characterized by a greater awareness of the surroundings, a quicker response to environmental stimuli and a decreased sense of fatigue. A single dose may produce psychomotor stimulation, euphoria, an elevation of mood with increased initiative, confidence and decisiveness. It may also improve concentration and facilitate motor activity and speech.

It has been noted that tricyclic antidepressants in general and imipramine in particular, when given in a single dose to normals, cause a blunting of emotions without any apparent loss of initiative. (When continuously administered, the same substances may lead to difficulty in concentration and thinking.) On the other hand, MAOI antidepressants in normals produce psychomotor stimulation and a feeling of well-being, *i.e.*, euphoria. (In higher doses or by continuous administration, a toxic psychokinetic reaction occurs in some of the subjects.)

Of the various antipsychotic substances, the Rauwolfia alkaloid reserpine induces somnolence and depression, not infrequently with suicidal ideation. In contradistinction to this, the phenothiazine chlorpromazine produces manifestations more like those of imipramine. With the former, there is a greater reduction of physical activity (and even if chronically administered it does not produce cognitive impairment).

Anxiolytic benzodiazepines in general and diazepam in particular induce somnolence, drowsiness and, in higher, toxic doses, slurring of speech and ataxia. (With continuous administration, an increasing slowness of mentation and apathy develop.)

Of the various attempts to organize and communicate the descriptive information obtained in human pharmacological studies, Irwin's (1966) functional approach is one of the best. Irwin (1966) asserts that drugs do not affect behavior directly but that as chemicals they interact with other chemicals. This interaction produces alterations in the biochemical environment of cells, which lead to changes in cellular activity. This in turn affects tissue and organ *functions*. According to him, "these then modify the behavioral state of the organism, its physiological and psychological components, and the latter determines the nature of its interaction with the environment. Drugs, therefore, successively affect the various levels of integration from the simplest to the most complex, from the chemical to the psychosocial sphere."

Irwin (1966) maintains that, since the observable effects of drugs are the result of a complex drug-tissue-individual-environment interaction, they may be best understood by the functions of the CNS activity, which reflect the temperament and behavior of the organism and determine its capacity to respond. Thus he directs attention to observations on changes in psychomotor (arousal, wakefulness, activity, responses to stimuli, memory, learning, biologic drives, endurance), neurological (posture, muscle tone, equilibrium, gait, reflexes, CNS excitation) and autonomic (body temperature, sympathetic, parasympathetic) functions. Furthermore, for psychopharmacological purposes he considers the assessment of behavioral arousal as most important of the many variables involved. To support his view he refers to the fact that directly correlated with increasing levels of arousal (*e.g.*, as induced by amphetamine drugs) are increased wakefulness and responses to stimuli, apprehension, irritability, agitation, hallucinations and delusions. With decreasing levels of arousal (*e.g.*, as induced by the chlorpromazine type of drugs), there is a decrease in responsiveness to stimuli as manifested by reduced locomotor activity, stupor and coma.

Lehmann's (1960) attempt to organize the descriptive material of human psychopharmacological experiments is more clinically oriented. He considers that the effects of psychoactive drug-induced changes can be measured on the psychological parameters of arousal, mental integration and affectivity. By this approach it was demonstrated that sedative barbiturates reduced arousal in contradistinction to stimulant amphetamines, which raised it, and that various psychotomimetic substances, *e.g.*, LSD_{25}, Ditran, etc., induced a "derangement" of mental integration which could be counteracted by antipsychotic drugs, *e.g.*, phenothiazines, butyrophenones, etc.

Ditran effected a disintegration which was manifested in a disturbed state of consciousness, while lysergic acid diethylamide produced pathological integrations, *e.g.*, hallucinations. Both the Ditran-produced toxic psychosis and the LSD_{25}-produced psychopathology were counteracted by chlorpromazine. (It should be noted that the Ditran-induced toxic psychoses may also be counteracted by chlordiazepoxide, and the LSD_{25}-induced pathological integrations by diazepam.)

With regards to the "affective" psychological parameter, a feeling of well-being with a lowered state of consciousness was seen under the influence of morphine, while a feeling of well-being with a normal level of consciousness was present with some of the MAOI-antidepressant drugs. On the other hand, the Rauwolfia alkaloid reserpine —even in one high single dose—may induce transient dysthymic mood changes.

It should be noted that the phenomenological and symptomatological assessment is based on the subjective judgment of the human observer. Nevertheless, these assessments are quite useful and practical for screening and predicting the clinical usefulness of potentially psychoactive drugs.

2. Psychometrics

Psychometrics complement the subjective phenomenological and symptomatological assessment with objective instrumental measurements. Pharmacologically induced performance changes were first systematically explored by Kraepelin and his collaborators (1896). They studied the effects of alcohol, paraldehyde, chloral, morphine and several other substances on a number of psychological tests, *e.g.*, reaction time, continuous work performance, word association, time estimation, etc. Psychometric studies continued over the years (Rivers, 1908; Hollingworth, 1912; Poffenberger, 1914, 1916, 1917, 1919; Darrow, 1927, 1929; Shock, 1939; Spragg, 1941; and Gray and Trowbridge, 1942), and recently, Trouton and Eysenck (1961), have reviewed the various procedures and findings in this area of research.

In their review Trouton and Eysenck (1961) emphasized that independent of the inherent properties of a chemical substance (and apart from the mode and rate of its administration) there are other variables which influence its general effectiveness. The subject, *i.e.*, his personality, familiarity with the situation, his placebo proneness, etc., and the environment, *i.e.*, his interaction with other subjects, external reinforcement of responses, etc., are only two of the many variables which influence drug effects.

Variables that may influence drug responses are "inner environment" and "outer environment." Factors to be considered in respect to the "inner environment" are physiological (sex, age, race, constitution, dietary habits, nutritional state, sleep, body weight, periodic changes) and psychological (motivations, personality, intellect, learned responses, compliance, attitude, knowledge of drug effect). Factors to be considered in respect to the "outer environment" are physical (altitude, climate, season), social (group membership, socio-economic circumstances, life stresses) and immediate circumstances (therapeutic or experimental setting, place, atmosphere, relationship between experimenter and experimental subject, prior drug experience).

Much information has been collected on the differential effects of psychoactive drugs on various quantifiable psychological tests. While there have been a large number of procedures used for measuring various psychological functions, all of them can be classified into three major categories. In the first category are tests which measure "afferent" or perceptual functions; the second category deals with "central" or associative processes; and the third quantifies "efferent" or psychomotor activity.

An entirely different function which has been increasingly explored in human pharmacological studies under the influence of drugs is speech, a "function" which, according to Goldman-Eisler (1958), is the meeting ground for many events and processes which are sensitive to psychotropic drug effects. The effect of psychoactive drugs on speech was recently reviewed by Waskow (1966).

a. Tests for Measuring Afferent or Perceptual Functions

Among the various tests measuring afferent or perceptual functions, the Critical Flicker Fusion Frequency (CFF), the Chromatic After-image Disappearance Limen (ADL) and the Achromatic Spiral After Effect (SPIR) have been most extensively employed in human pharmacological studies.

In the CFF test, introduced independently by Talbot (1834) and Plateau (1835), the number of flickers per second at which the subject perceives the flickerings of a light source (or when the flickering light fuses into a steady beam) is recorded. In the ADL test, introduced by Lehmann (1950)—using the principles of Bidwell (1896, 1897)—the level of illumination when the chromatic after-image (*i.e.*, the green color in the standard apparatus) disappears is measured. In the SPIR test, the facilitation or depression of the after-effect is recorded. This test is based on Plateau's (1835) demonstration that normal subjects continue to see the movement of a rotating Archimedes spiral as swelling or contracting after its movement has been stopped.

In human pharmacological studies it has been revealed that CNS stimulants, *e.g.*, amphetamines, raised both the "critical frequency of fusion" and the level of illumination in which the chromatic after-image disappeared. Furthermore, they also exerted a definite facilitating action on achromatic after-effects. In contradistinction to CNS stimulants, sedatives, *e.g.*, barbiturates, had the opposite effect on these tests (Simonson *et al.*, 1941; Lehmann, 1950; Landis and Zubin, 1951; Roback *et al.*, 1952; Simonson and Brozek, 1952; Seashore and Ivy, 1953;

Lehmann and Csank, 1957; and Holland, 1960).

An effect similar to that of stimulants was observed with tricyclic antidepressants, *e.g.*, imipramine, on the CFF test and a similar effect to the sedatives with anxiolytic propanediols, *e.g.*, meprobamate, on the SPIR test (Eysenck *et al.*, 1957; Eysenck and Easterbrook, 1960; and St. Jean *et al.*, 1965). Among the antipsychotics, all four groups, *i.e.*, phenothiazines, Rauwolfias, butyrophenones and thioxanthenes, followed the sedative pattern on the CFF test, while on the ADL test there was a dissociation between the effect of chlorpromazine (a phenothiazine) and reserpine (a Rauwolfia alkaloid). The former lowered, while the latter raised, the level of illumination in which the chromatic after-image disappeared (Lehmann and Csank, 1957; Lehmann and Knight, 1958; Burbridge, 1958; Lehmann and Knight, 1960; Ban *et al.*, 1962; Ban and Schwarz, 1963; and St. Jean *et al.*, 1964).

b. Tests for Measuring Central or Associative Functions

Of the various tests measuring central or associative functions, the Word Association Time (WAT), Time Estimation Production (TEP) and Reproduction (TER), Cancellation Time (CT) and Error (CE), Digits Forward (DF) and Backward (DB), Digit Symbol Substitution (DSS), Paired Associate Learning (PAL) and the various arithmetic tests have been most extensively used in human pharmacological studies.

In the WAT test, first introduced by Galton (1879), the time lapse between the word stimulus and the verbal response is measured. According to Trautscholdt (1882), Wreschner (1900), Jung (1906, 1910, 1919) and Ivanov-Smolensky (1953), verbal reaction time is between 1 and 2.4 seconds in normal persons. Rosanoff and Rosanoff (1913) and Mitchell *et al.* (1919) recognized age, and De (1953) revealed sex differences in performance on the WAT test.

The TEP and TER tests were developed in Wundt's laboratories and used by Münsterberg (1894) and collaborators (Wundt, 1903). In the TEP test the subject is asked to estimate a certain period of time, *e.g.*, 15 seconds, while in the TER test he is presented with a 15-second time period and asked to reproduce it.

In the CT and CE tests, first introduced by Bourdon (1895) and named by Sharp (1899), the time required to complete the task of canceling off a specified digit (usually 9) is measured (CT). The specified digit (or digits) is dispensed randomly among other digits, usually in 17 rows with 35 digits in each. The wrongly canceled digits or omissions are also counted (CE).

In the DF and DB tests, first introduced in the classical experiments of Ebbinghaus (1885), and later standardized by Wechsler (1944, 1945), the number of digits the experimental subject is able to repeat in the order as they are given (DF) or in reverse order (DB) are counted.

In the DSS test, adapted from the Wechsler-Bellevue (Wechsler, 1945), predetermined symbols are given to replace numbers. The number of digits which are substituted by symbols within a predetermined period, usually one minute, are scored, and the number of errors made are recorded.

In the PAL test introduced by Calkins (1892), pairs of words are presented in varying sequence on a memory drum. As the drum rotates the stimulus word is followed by the associated word. The number of correctly associated pairs are counted.

Of the various arithmetic tests, the simple continuous addition task, the complex multiplication test and the cancellation of incorrect answers to multiplication problems have been most frequently used.

In human pharmacological studies it has been shown that CNS stimulants, *e.g.*, amphetamines, shorten WAT; produce an underestimation of time periods in both TEP and TER tests; decrease CT; improve performance on both DSS and PAL; and increase the speed in simple continuous addition tasks, while they impair complex multiplication problems (Peoples and Guttmann, 1936; Turner and Carl, 1939; Wunderle, 1941; Flory and Gilbert, 1943; Kleemeier and Kleemeier, 1947; and Düker and Düker, 1953). In contradistinction to CNS stimulants, sedatives, *e.g.*, barbiturates, in general have the opposite effect.

They prolong the duration of time that is necessary for the association of ideas; produce an overestimation of time periods on both TEP and TER tests; increase CT; reduce DF; and impair performance on PAL and of computation (Felsinger *et al.*, 1953; Lehmann and Csank, 1957; and Klerman *et al.*, 1960).

TEP and TER as well as time awareness and time perspective were tested under the influence of the sedative amobarbital (100 mg.); the stimulant dextroamphetamine (10 mg.); and the psychotomimetic psilocybin (10 mg.) by Lehmann (1967). The only consistent finding was the increase of estimated time intervals after amobarbital. It was noted that under psilocybin subjects appeared more accurate in their time estimation.

A similar effect to CNS stimulants was seen on TEP (also TER) with some of the tricyclic antidepressant, *e.g.*, imipramine and trimipramine, drugs and on the arithmetic tests with anxiolytic propanediol, *e.g.*, meprobamate compounds. On the other hand, an effect similar to that of sedatives was seen on TEP (also TER) and on PAL with reserpine, a Rauwolfia alkaloid antipsychotic substance. Other findings with antipsychotics were significant improvement on CE and DF with the phenothiazine trifluoperazine (on the latter also with the Rauwolfia alkaloid, reserpine) and a lowered performance on the DSS with chlorpromazine, a dimethylaminopropyl side chain containing phenothiazine (Lehmann, 1967; Kornetsky *et al.*, 1957; Brown *et al.*, 1958; Lehmann and Knight, 1961; Klerman *et al.*, 1960; DiMascio *et al.*, 1963; St. Jean *et al.*, 1965; and Lehmann, 1967).

c. Tests for Measuring Efferent or Psychomotor Functions

Among the various tests measuring efferent or psychomotor functions, the Tapping Speed (TS), the Reaction Time (RT) and the Pursuit Rotor (PR) tests have been most extensively used in human pharmacological studies.

In the TS test, the rate of tapping within a predetermined time period (usually 10 seconds) is counted.

In the RT test, first used by Hirsch in 1861, (the term, reaction time, was introduced later by Exner in 1870), the time lapse between the presentation of an auditory or visual stimulus and the voluntary motor response is measured (Hirsch, 1861; and Exner, 1870).

In the PR test as used by DiMascio *et al.* (1963), visual-motor coordination and steadiness is measured by the total time of contact between the stylus and a rotating disk and the number of times the stylus was moved on and off the disk.

In human pharmacological studies it has been shown that CNS stimulants, *e.g.*, amphetamines, increase TS, shorten RT and improve performance on the PR test. In contradistinction to CNS stimulants, sedatives, *e.g.*, barbiturates have the opposite effect on these tests (Carl and Turner, 1939; Eysenck *et al.*, 1957; and Trouton and Eysenck, 1961).

A similar effect with stimulants is seen with tricyclic antidepressants, *e.g.*, imipramine and trimipramine, on TS, RT and on the PR tests. Although, at first, anxiolytic propanediols, *e.g.*, meprobamate, were shown to exert an effect which resembled that of the sedatives, in more recent studies (with more appropriate dosages) this has been disproved. It now appears that their action on these tests resembles that of the stimulants. Antipsychotic drugs were found to exert a differential effect on psychomotor functions. Thus while the Rauwolfia alkaloid reserpine and the dimethylaminopropyl side chain containing phenothiazines, *e.g.*, chlorpromazine and methotrimeprazine, were shown to have an inhibitory influence on TS, the piperazine side chain containing derivatives, *e.g.*, perphenazine and trifluoperazine, improve performance on the same test. On the other hand, PR test performance was seen to be improved under the influence of the dimethylaminopropyls and impaired by the piperazines. These findings are equivocal, however, since Lehmann and Knight (1961) found that trifluoperazine, a piperazine, reduced the rate of tapping and Kornetsky *et al.* (1957) demonstrated that chlorpromazine, a dimethylaminopropyl, decreased PR test performance. The effect of various antipsychotics, *e.g.*, reserpine, methotrimeprazine and thioproperazine, on RT followed the sedative pattern (Primac *et al.*, 1957; Kornetsky, 1958; Burbridge, 1958; Schneider and Costiloe, 1959; DiMascio *et al.*, 1963; Ban *et al.*, 1962; Ban and Schwarz, 1963; and St. Jean *et al.*, 1965).

d. Other Test Procedures

Besides the psychometric procedures described, there are numerous other tests used in human psychopharmacological studies. Among them, for example, are the "nonsense syllable learning," the "clock test" of vigilance and the "ergometer test" of working capacity. A common characteristic of all three of these tests is that they are beneficially affected by stimulant amphetamines (Hollingworth, 1912; Lemmell and Hartwig, 1940; Alles and Fergen, 1942; Knoefel, 1943; Cuthbertson and Knox, 1940; and Willet, 1958). Sedative barbiturates have a less consistent effect on these tests.

An excellent review of the effects of psychoactive drugs on psychological performance in human pharmacological experiments was published by Uhr (1960). Uhr's comprehensive review includes most of the findings in this area of research up to the date of its publication. Some of the important findings presented in this review in chronological order are the following. A differential effect between two stimulants, pipradrol (a 2-benzylpiperidine derivative) and amphetamine (a phenylethylamine), was demonstrated by Payne and Moore (1955). Thus, while pipradrol, like amphetamine, delayed the fatigue-induced decrease in performance on the "SAM Multidimensional Pursuit Rotor Test," it did not produce the early rise of proficiency seen with amphetamines.

A similar performance deficit on a "simulated driving test" was reported under the influence of secobarbital (a sedative barbiturate), meprobamate (an anxiolytic propanediol) and chlorpromazine (an antipsychotic phenothiazine) (Loomis and West, 1958). Furthermore, Miller and Uhr (1960) demonstrated some impairment in accuracy and breaking reaction time under the influence of meprobamate.

A differential effect between chlorpromazine and meprobamate was demonstrated by Holliday *et al.* (1958). Thus, in contradistinction to chlorpromazine, meprobamate improved test performance during the threat of stress periods on a repetitive tracking task. Meprobamate was found to decrease GSR responses and thus adversely affects the "lie detector test" (Kristofferson and Cormack, 1959) and to reduce basal resistance throughout a period of experimentally induced stress conditions, in simple attention tasks (Uhr *et al.*, 1960).

There are a number of practical issues which have to be considered in connection with psychometric—human psychopharmacological—studies. The two most important, which may account for some of the discrepancies, are the different dosages used by various investigators and the timing of testing after drug administration.

The systematic efforts of Lehmann (1957), Kornetsky (1958), DiMascio *et al.* (1958) and others, and the numerous articles published, point out the necessity for qualifying and quantifying some of the changes induced by psychopharmacological drugs. However, in spite of the extensive exploratory work in this area, there is still no immediate clinical applicability of the psychometric findings. This does not lessen its heuristic importance.

3. Conditioning

Symptomatological assessment and psychometric test results supply important data in human pharmacology, but information regarding the effect of the compound on the different stimulus-response constellations can only be provided by the use of various conditioning procedures.

The effect of psychoactive drugs on CR phenomena has been explored in human pharmacological studies. Various conditioning techniques have been employed, and the effects of a number of psychoactive substances on CR variables have been investigated. Important contributions have been made by numerous investigators (Alexander, 1958, 1961; Lipgart, 1958; Segal and Skuin, 1958; Jus, 1959, 1961, 1962; Traugott, 1961, 1963; Tirkeltaub, 1963; Vinar, 1964; Cazzullo *et al.*, 1966; and Saarma and Saarma, 1966). The results of their work were reviewed and summarized by Astrup (1962, 1965, 1966) and Ban (1964, 1966) and in *Psychopharmacological Methods*, a volume of collected papers edited by Votava *et al.* (1963). In the majority of these studies the human pharmacological experiment was contaminated by giving the substance to psychopathological cases instead of to normal subjects and by administering it as continuous treatment instead of only as a single dose. By these "contaminations," however, it was revealed that the effects of a psychopharmacological substance are different in normal subjects than in psychiatric patients and its effects are different when it is given in a single dose than when it is continuously administered. Thus, for example, it was recognized that meprobamate induces in normals an inhibitory state with reduction and dedifferentiation of the plethysmographic responses (simultaneously with the paradoxical hypersynchrony of the electro-cerebral alerting responses). The same drug in abnormal mental states promotes differentiation by reducing excitatory phenomena (including paradoxical hypersynchrony of the electro-cerebral alerting responses) and inhibitory generalizations (which are characteristic of neurotic depression). Another example is that antipsychotic and antidepressant drugs, when given in single doses to normals, instead of affecting the psychological parameter of mental integration or mood, respectively (as seen when the substances are chronically administered to psychopathological cases), lower the level of arousal and produce inhibitory phenomena.

In human psychopharmacological studies—within the frame of reference of the classical conditioning paradigm—the autonomic and motor components of various CR phenomena, such as the extinction of the OR, CR formation, CS generalization and differentiation, are most frequently explored. The autonomic components are usually studied by measuring the galvanic skin reflex (GSR) or vascular reactions (plethysmography), while the motor components are often studied by electromyography, eyelid closure or by the even more simple finger-withdrawal technique. In spite of the differential effects of drugs on the various systems studied, certain characteristic patterns of drugs with similar psychotropic effects appear to be consistent.

CNS stimulants in general, when administered in a single dose to normals, increase the strength and decrease the latency, *i.e.*, reaction time, of the UR. They facilitate CR formation and CS differentiation. In pharmacological doses neither the OR nor CS generalization is affected by these drugs, whereas in higher toxic doses the persistence of the OR and "pathological generalized responses" become prevalent.

In contradistinction to CNS stimulants, sedatives administered in a single dose to normals decrease the strength and increase the latency of the UR. They interfere with CR formation and CS differentiation. In pharmacological doses neither the OR nor CS generalization is affected by these drugs, whereas in higher toxic doses both the OR and CS generalization are abolished.

While no consistent effect of antidepressants in human psychopharmacological studies has been recognized as yet, some differential characteristics between anxiolytic (minor tranquilizer) and antipsychotic (major tranquilizer) drugs have been revealed. Although drugs belonging to both these categories follow, by and large, the sedative pattern, anxiolytic drugs exert a predominantly inhibitory action on the autonomic components of the CR (Astrup, 1965), in contradistinction to antipsychotics, which are found to have a mainly inhibitory action on the motor components of the CR. This was clearly demonstrated for chlorpromazine by Traugott and collaborators (1958, 1960) and for reserpine by Seredina (1960).

Another technique for differentiating anxiolytics and antipsychotics was developed on the basis of conditioning principles. Finger withdrawal from a telegraph key, in the course of tapping, is first of all conditioned to a light stimulus. Thereafter the number of taps are rewarded (by monetary reward). It was found that while under the influence of antipsychotics the conditioned finger withdrawal (or even active avoidance of the shock to the conditional light stimulus) prevails; under the influence of anxiolytics, the conditioned finger withdrawal is overridden by an increase of "tolerance of the conflict situation" (Lehmann and Ban, 1966).

A comprehensive behavioral model of drug action was presented by Eysenck (1957). According to this model, human beings differ with respect to the speed with which cortical excitation and inhibition are produced or dissipated and also with respect to the strength of this (cortical) excitation and inhibition. As a second postulate, Eysenck (1957) asserted that individuals in whom the excitatory potential (process) is weak are predisposed to develop extroverted patterns of behavior or hysterical-psychopathic disorders, while those in whom the excitatory potential (process) is strong and generated quickly are predisposed to develop introverted patterns of behavior and dysthymic disorders. Applying this to drug action, Eysenck suggested that depressant drugs produce a decrease in the rate of conditioning, increase cortical inhibition, decrease cortical excitation and produce extroverted behavioral patterns or an increase in hysterical and a decrease in dysthymic symptoms; whereas stimulant drugs produce an increase in the rate of conditioning, decrease cortical inhibition, increase cortical excitation and produce introverted behavioral patterns or an increase in dysthymic and a decrease in hysterical symptoms.

One of the important assets of conditioning procedures in human pharmacological studies is that the influence of the new substance can be investigated on the same CR variables as in the animal pharmacological experiment. With more and more information on the alterations of the normal CR profile in the various psychopathologies, it has been suggested that conditioning studies in human pharmacological experiments may be useful not only for empirical prediction but also for prediction on a higher level on which a particular pathological alteration is counteracted with a substance with a particular effect (Ban, 1965, 1966).

4. Neurophysiological and Biochemical Correlates of Drug Action

a. Neurophysiological Correlates

There have been at least three electroencephalographic techniques used to study drug effects in human pharmacological studies. The most frequently used technique is to record the effect of various psychoactive agents on the spontaneous electrical activity of the brain. The effects of psychoactive drugs on evoked responses have been explored less frequently, and the results of quantitative electroencephalographic analysis under the influence of psychopharmacological compounds have only recently been reported.

i. The Effect of Drugs on the Spontaneous Electrical Activity of the Cerebral Cortex. In studying the effect of psychoactive substances on the spontaneous electrical activity of the cerebral cortex via surface electroencephalographic recordings, Bente (1961) recognized that "any approach that considers, or measures, individual characteristics (of the electroencephalogram), independent of the structural relationships, incurs the risk of serious errors." He emphasized that the changes induced by the administration of a single dose of a psychoactive drug to normal humans can not be properly evaluated by a quantitative analysis of isolated electroencephalographic characteristics (variables) such as frequency and voltage. Furthermore, he asserted that it is inadmissible to interpret a drug-induced voltage decrease or increase in alpha frequency automatically as the expression of desynchronization and to infer from this that the drug raised the level of arousal. The low voltage activity induced by the drug may represent the electroencephalographic equivalent of a decrease in vigilance as the temporary raise in alpha frequency may reflect the sleep-inducing properties of the substance.

According to Bente (1961), psychoactive drugs can be classified on the basis of their electroencephalographic effects only if all the drug-induced changes are considered in the analysis, *i.e.*, if a morphological analysis is performed in time. Since the fundamental patterns of the various consecutive stages of falling asleep are well established and since these patterns are usually influenced by psychoactive drugs, he suggested that this could be utilized as the first step in the electroencephalographic differentiation of various psychopharmacological substances.

Jasper (1941) observed and recorded the manifest behavior, awareness, and efficacy of the subject's behavioral patterns simultaneously with the changes of spontaneous electrical activity. He distinguished seven distinctly different successive steps characterized by strong, excited emotion with restricted awareness and poor efficacy of behavioral pattern (desynchronization, low amplitude, fast rhythm); alert attentiveness with selective attention and good efficacy of behavior (partial synchronization, low amplitude, fast rhythm); relaxed wakefulness with wandering attention and good efficacy of behavior (synchronization, optimal alpha rhythm); drowsiness with partial awareness and poor efficacy of behavioral pattern (reduced alpha rhythm, low amplitude, slow waves); light sleep with reduced consciousness and absence of effective behavior (no alpha rhythm, slow waves, spindle bursts); deep sleep with loss of awareness and absence of effective behavior (large and very slow waves); and coma with loss of consciousness and absence of effective behavior (isoelectric to irregular, large, slow waves).

The action of sedative barbiturates on the surface electroencephalogram begins with a fast 15 to 35 cycle per second activity, which spreads from the frontal toward the occipital cortex. With an increase in dosage, large amplitude, slow, random 2 to 8 cycle per second waves appear. With a further increase in dosage (toxic), there is a gradual decrease in the amplitude of electrical waves with brief periods of electrical silence. Opposed to barbiturates are the effects of stimulant amphetamines, which produce acceleration and desynchronization of the electroencephalogram. Under the influence of these drugs there is a shift from the resting to higher frequencies, with a simultaneous reduction of amplitude and duration of large delta waves.

Antipsychotic phenothiazines were found to produce an early slowing in the electroencephalogram (Bente, 1963). However, Bente and Itil (1955, 1957, 1959) demonstrated that the intravenously administered chlorpromazine-induced electroencephalographic somnolence was not identical with the spontaneous process of falling asleep. The most important difference, they found, was the special tendency to formation of rhythmical protracted waves with the simultaneous abatement of rapid activity forms, *e.g.*, sleep spindles. Fink (1963) recognized a shift in dominant frequency with phenothiazine drugs. He maintained that the appearance or increase in percentage time slow-wave activity and a slowing by one cycle or more per second of alpha frequencies are the principal measurable changes with these compounds. Besides the shift in dominant frequency, Fink (1963) also demonstrated an increased electrographic abundance (synchronization) and new wave forms such as high voltage slow-wave activity in paroxysmal patterns. The electroencephalographic effects of antipsychotic Rauwolfias are similar but less marked. Reserpine was found to produce an increase in percentage time slow-wave activity (Fink, 1963, and Müller and Müller, 1965) and also a diminution in the percentage time of beta activity (Fink, 1963).

In contradistinction to the antipsychotics, anxiolytic drugs, *e.g.*, benzodiazepines and propanediols, were found to produce a shift in the dominant frequency to fast activity (Müller and Müller, 1965) and an increased synchronization.

Of the two antidepressant categories, no consistent pattern could be revealed with MAOI's. In this group, pheniprazine was found to produce persistent desynchronization, iproniazid elicited sleep spindles or seizure-like electrical discharges, and tranylcypromine resulted in both, *i.e.*, first desynchronization lasting a few hours and sleep spindles thereafter. On the other hand, tricyclic antidepressant drugs were shown to induce desynchronization with a decrease of total electroencephalographic activity together with an increase in theta rhythm. Fink (1963) described both an increase in the percentage of beta activity and an increase in slow waves under the influence of these drugs. Fink (1965) also found a reduction in the total amount of alpha frequency following imipramine administration.

ii. The Effect of Drugs on Cortical Evoked Responses. Another but much less frequently used method of investigating the effects of psychoactive drugs upon brain electrical activity is the study of specific brain responses to peripheral stimulations (Müller and Müller, 1965). For this purpose, auditory or tactile stimuli are the most commonly used. Because these responses are of small amplitude they are added electronically (and photographically), and the resulting average responses are evaluated. Shagass and his collaborators (1962) were pioneers in the study of the effects of various psychopharmacological agents on cortical evoked responses. Irradiating evoked responses are occasionally used (Krugler, 1964) in human pharmacological studies.

iii. The Effect of Drugs on the Quantitative Electroencephalogram. More recently, a quantitative electroencephalographic technique has been used in human pharmacological studies by Pfeiffer *et al.* (1963). This technique is based on the application of a Drohocki integrator, which continuously summates the electrical energy content of the electroencephalogram. The output appears on one channel of the electroencephalographic recordings as a series of pulses (and the frequency is proportional to the cumulative energy). Consequently, a burst of alpha activity or a sleep spindle causes an increase in the number of pulses per unit time, while arousal with its decreased energy content causes a decrease in pulses. For statistical analysis in psychopharmacological studies, a unit of time is chosen and the number of pulses in each successive unit of time is counted and recorded (Pfeiffer *et al.*, 1965). By this procedure it was seen, for example, that anxiolytic substances tend to decrease mean electrical energy and increase the coefficient of variation on the electroencephalogram.

On the basis of electroencephalographic studies with mescaline and morphine, Wikler (1954) proposed that increased electroencephalographic abundance (*i.e.*, synchronization) was associated with decreased excitement, sedation and tranquilization, while decreased electroencephalographic abundance (*i.e.*, desynchronization) was correlated with alertness, excitement, illusions and hallucinations. This is still basically true for most of the psychoactive drugs except the anxiolytic compounds.

b. Biochemical Correlates

Bernard's (1878) dictum, "la fixité du milieu intérieur est la condition de la vie libre," was more fully appreciated when Barcroft (1934) made the first attempt to summarize the changes which occur when body fluids are altered by either composition or temperature. According to Barcroft (1934), a decrease of blood oxygen results in headache, lassitude and poor performance on psychological tests, in contradistinction to an increase which produces convulsions; a decrease in hydrogen ion concentration leads to headache and an increase to coma; a decrease of serum glucose levels produces a change in sensory-perceptual processes and behavior, culminating in coma, while an increase has a slight narcotic action; a decrease in the amount of "body water" is reflected by weakness and reduced epileptic tendency as opposed to an increase, which results in headache, nausea, dizziness, asthenia and incoordination; a decrease of sodium (Na) or calcium (Ca) salts produces fever, nervous twitchings (Na) or convulsions (Ca), while an increase produces apathy, drowsiness (Na) or atonia and stupor (Ca); and finally, a decrease of temperature leads to inertia and an increase to delirium. Barcroft (1934) concluded that changes in the internal chemical environment have their major effects on the brain. This was elaborated, but not essentially altered, by subsequent experiments which primarily aimed to produce changes by introducing various chemical substances into the "internal chemical environment" (McIlwain, 1957).

Since Barcroft's assertion, a number of chemical (inorganic and organic) "constituents" in the blood stream and urine (occasionally in the spinal fluid and saliva) have been examined under the influence of various psychoactive agents in the course of human pharmacological studies.

From the numerous investigations of the effects of psychopharmacological substances on the inorganic elements of the organism, such as sodium, potassium, calcium, magnesium, etc., it appears that all the evidence thus far has been controversial and essentially inconclusive. On the other hand, the exploration of changes in organic elements resulted in important findings.

i. Carbohydrates. Of the carbohydrates, particular attention was focused on the effect of psychoactive drugs on blood sugar (glucose) concentrations. At first it was recognized that large doses of barbiturates produce hyperglycemia. Later it was also revealed that antipsychotic Rauwolfias and phenothiazines have a similar action. A short lasting increase of glucose (also pyruvate and lactate) concentrations in the blood stream was also found with anxiolytic benzodiazepine compounds. While tricyclic antidepressants were recognized to exert a transient slight decrease on blood sugar concentration, MAOI antidepressants were shown to enhance glycolysis, reflected by a rise in blood pyruvic and lactic acid levels.

ii. Lipids. The effects of psychoactive drugs on free fatty acid and cholesterol levels in the serum have been explored. Systematic investigations of changes in serum cholesterol levels remained essentially unrevealing. But in studies on the free fatty acid concentrations it was established that like the autonomic sympathomimetic drugs the various psychotopathic substances, *e.g.*, mescaline, psilocybin and LSD_{25}, increased the blood levels of free fatty acid (Hollister, 1962). On the other hand, small, somnolence-producing amounts of insulin and high doses of nicotinic acid were found to have the opposite effect on free fatty acid concentration.

iii. Serotonin. Recently the effects of psychoactive substances on serotonin (5-hydroxytryptamine) and catecholamine metabolism have been extensively investigated in human pharmacological studies. The action of various drugs on 5-hydroxytryptamine (5-HT) levels is measured in the blood by spectrophotofluorometric methods (Waalkes, 1959) or by paper chromatographic analysis (Dalgliesh, 1956). Urinary concentrations of excreted serotonin or its catabolic end-product 5-hydroxyindoleacetic acid (5-HIAA) are more frequently determined in human pharmacological experiments. This is done by partition chromatography or gas chromatography, respectively (Sweeley and Williams, 1961).

A summary of the effects of a great number of psychoactive drugs alone or in combination on the excretion of 5-HIAA in humans (and on the level of serotonin in various tissues in animals) was presented by Garattini and Valzelli (1965). They found that the two groups of drugs of particular interest in this respect were the "releasers" of serotonin and the "inhibitors" of the MAO enzyme.

Of the serotonin releasers, interest at first was focused on the antipsychotic Rauwolfia alkaloid reserpine, which in the first hours after administration of a sufficiently high dosage was found to produce a transient increase in the excretion of the 5-HIAA in the urine (Valcourt, 1957). In contradistinction to this, the antidepressant MAOI drugs were shown to reduce the urinary excretion of 5-HIAA (simultaneously with a rise in the excretion of 5-HT glucuronide). Like the MAOI's, but by an entirely different mechanism (*i.e.*, by the inhibition of decarboxylase), methyldopa, an antihypertensive-depressant substance, was also found to diminish the excretion of 5-HIAA in the urine. On the other hand, the findings of decreased urinary excretion of 5-HIAA in animals who had been on chlorpromazine could not be clearly shown in human pharmacological studies with normal experimental subjects (Erspamer *et al.*, 1960, and Bertler, 1961).

iv. Catecholamines. The action of various drugs on catecholamines cannot be too accurately measured in the blood and entails great difficulties. However, since the introduction of fluorometric techniques (Euler, 1954), the urinary concentration of epinephrine and norepinephrine is being more readily and more accurately assessed. Of the various epinephrine metabolites such as 4-hydroxy-3-methoxymandelic acid (VMA), metanephrine, dihydroxymandelic acid and 3-methoxy-4-hydroxyphenylglycol, the amounts of VMA and metanephrine in humans have been measured very frequently (Sandler and Ruthven, 1966), as have the various norepinephrine metabolites, *e.g.*, normetanephrine (Kopin and Gordon, 1962).

In human pharmacological studies it has been found (Kety, 1966) that both tricyclic and MAOI antidepressants have a diminishing effect upon the excretion of VMA (Studnitz, 1959, and Schopbach *et al.*, 1964). In the case of imipramine, a tricyclic antidepressant substance, there was a simultaneous increase in normetanephrine excretion (Schildkraut *et al.*, 1964). It is interesting to note that, while Weil Malherbe as early as 1955 recognized that the rate of excretion of both epinephrine and norepinephrine is lowered by barbiturates in normals, the findings with psychopharmacological substances other than those mentioned have been essentially unrevealing.

Prior to the commencement of clinical pharmacological studies, these pharmacodynamic data are complemented with toxicity (acute toxicity) and metabolic studies in humans.

B. TOXICITY

There are limitations in extrapolating from animal toxicity data to man. Besides the interspecies metabolic differences, there are also intraspecies variations in human beings. Therefore, toxicity studies in animals have to be followed by toxicity studies in humans.

The ultimate goal of toxicity studies in humans is to enable the investigator to predict the possible undesired, adverse or toxic effects of a particular drug. But unlike the animal toxicity studies which are done in three stages (acute, subacute and chronic) consecutively and for all practical purposes under the same conditions for different periods of time, in the course of preclinical human pharmacological investigations, only the acute toxicity studies are conducted (subacute human toxicity is carried out in clinical pharmacology and chronic only at the time of clinical investigation). Within the frame of reference of acute toxicity studies, the secondary attributes of the substance, the effects of overdosage and hypersensitivity reactions are carefully explored. Furthermore, the metabolism of the substance in humans is also investigated.

1. Acute Toxicity Studies

Acute toxicity studies in humans are carried out on young, healthy, mentally stable, volunteer adults who have given consent for the experiment. It is essential that they are intelligent enough to give an account of their experiences while under the influence of the investigational compound.

It is the rule that acute human toxicity studies are not started prior to the full assessment of the acute toxicity studies in animals, and usually they do not commence prior to the completion of at least 2 weeks of the subacute toxicity studies in two different animal species.

The starting dosage for any drug administered in acute toxicity studies is one-tenth of the anticipated effective dosage. Only if no significant toxic effects are revealed is the dosage gradually increased until subjective experiences or objective signs of toxic effects occur. These are carefully recorded and evaluated. The duration of an acute toxicity study in humans is 1 week. Prior to drug administration, the subject is carefully assessed both physically and psychologically. These assessments are repeated several times during the first 24 hours. Also prior to and 24 hours after the study, blood and urine samples are taken for comprehensive laboratory investigations. If any toxic findings are revealed, all physical and laboratory tests are repeated until all of the ill effects disappear.

a. Secondary Attributes

Secondary attributes (including true toxicity) are side-effects due to the secondary biological properties of the substance. Sometimes these secondary attributes are of such low order of activity that they will not be evident at therapeutic dosage levels. In other instances at least one or two secondary attributes will become manifest either as a minor or a major undesirable effect. In general, however, all psychoactive drugs have shown secondary attributes in human pharmacological studies.

Most often encountered with sedative barbiturates are sluggishness, ataxia, somnolence and sleep with a concomitant slightly decreased blood pressure and heart rate. Stimulant amphetamines occasionally produce jerky movements with the increasing motor activity. Sympathicotonia is the prevailing secondary attribute of amphetamine action, as manifested by tachycardia and hypertension, palpitation sensations, etc. A single dose of amphetamine will produce insomnia in almost all normal volunteers and loss of appetite in a high percentage. In certain predisposed subjects, anginal pain and a severe headache are occasionally seen.

Anxiolytic benzodiazepines may produce a reduction of spontaneous motor activity and drowsiness and, in higher doses, ataxia. Of the antidepressants, tricyclic drugs may induce drowsiness (or insomnia), nausea, heartburn, severe orthostatic hypotensive reactions and prevailing parasympatholytic effects, while MAOI's induce increased psychomotor activity, nausea, vomiting, hypotension (rarely hypertensive crises) and headaches.

The antipsychotic groups, both phenothiazines and Rauwolfia alkaloids, reduce spontaneous motor activity and produce drowsiness. The more important secondary attributes produced by these substances are hypotension and the particularly dangerous orthostatic hypotensive reaction. Even with the single dose used in human pharmacological tests, extrapyramidal manifestations can occasionally be seen in certain predisposed subjects. However, while the secondary attributes of the Rauwolfias are predominantly parasympathetic, those of the phenothiazines are mainly sympatholytic.

b. Overdosage

The toxic effects from overdosage result from the primary and secondary attributes of the compound produced deliberately or accidentally by either too large an amount or an unusual susceptibility to the drug. Because of the moral implications and legal consequences—in contradistinction to animal studies—overdosage is not normally encountered in the course of acute toxicity testing in man. All the manifestations of overdosage are usually revealed only at a much later stage of clinical investigation.

With sedative barbiturates, severe poisoning results from amounts ten times that of the hypnotic dosage. In coma, the initially constricted pupils and rapid and shallow breathing are replaced by pupillary dilatation and Cheyne-Stokes respiration. Rapid pulse and hypotension are also characteristic features. Death is usually due to respiratory depression or renal complications.

Symptoms of overdose with stimulant amphetamines may be seen with doses as low as three times that of the therapeutic dose. They are manifest as irritability, restlessness, tension and tremor. With higher doses these symptoms precede overt psychotic manifestations or rapid, shallow respiration, pallor and collapse (occasionally death).

Overdosage with antipsychotic phenothiazines produces drowsiness, hypotension, tachycardia, tachypnea, with extrapyramidal signs, convulsions and, very infrequently, coma. The effects of overdosage of the antipsychotic Rauwolfia alkaloid reserpine differ from this only in that both the heart rate and respirations are decreased rather than accelerated.

Of the tricyclic antidepressants, overdosage with imipramine results in hyperpyrexia, disturbance of the cardiac rhythm and conduction, clonic movements, seizures, shock, and, infrequently, respiratory depression and coma. Overdosage with amitriptyline, on the other hand, manifests itself in acceleration of pulse rate, elevation of blood pressure, decreased temperature, plantar extensor response with sluggish pupils and coma.

Overdosage with MAOI antidepressants produces insomnia, restlessness, anxiety, agitation and incoherence. In case of an excessive overdosage, drowsiness, weakness, hypertension, headache and myoclonic fibrillations lead to hyperpyrexia, rigidity and coma.

Least dangerous is overdosage with anxiolytic benzodiazepine drugs. With these, drowsiness and strong sedation with ataxia are the most prominent consequences.

Antipsychotic, antidepressant and anxiolytic drugs are very extensively used. Yet overdosage with these substances is only infrequently reported. Hollister (1966) reviewed this problem and surveyed the literature. Of the antipsychotic phenothiazines, he found only five fatal cases. These all occurred accidentally in children (Dilworth *et al.*, 1963; Haggerty, 1957; Marrubini, 1959; Merchant *et al.*, 1963; and Wallman, 1957). The lowest lethal dose was 350 mg. of chlorpromazine taken by a 4-year-old child. In all cases there was an initial stage of delirium, agitation, twitching or seizures and a relatively early hypothermia with a late but often sudden respiratory failure. Hollister (1966) also noted that none of the drugs of the other antipsychotic groups, *e.g.*, the Rauwolfia alkaloids or thioxanthenes, have yet been implicated in any fatalities.

Of the antidepressants, death has been caused by substances of both the tricyclic and the MAOI antidepressant categories. In the tricyclic category 2500 mg. of imipramine caused the death of a 30-month-old child (Noack, 1960), and 1000 mg. of amitriptyline was fatal to a 15-month-old infant (Sunshine and Yaffe, 1963). The major clinical findings with both drugs were clonic movements, seizures, shock, disturbance of cardiac rhythm and conduction, deep coma and respiratory depression. In the MAOI antidepressant category, 500 mg. of tranylcypromine was fatal to a 17-year-old girl who exhibited agitation, delirium, tremor, sweating, heart block, hyperthermia, shock and coma (Bacon, 1962), while ingestion of 350 mg. of the same drug (Matter *et al.*, 1965) or 750 mg. of phenelzine (Benbow and Super, 1961) produced ataxia, weakness, drowsiness, delirium, seizures, muscle fasciculations and hyperthermia, but not death.

Of the anxiolytics, only one fatal case has as yet been reported with 20,000 mg. of the propanediol derivative meprobamate (Hollister, 1965), while no deaths have been reported from overdosage with the benzodiazepines, either chlordiazepoxide or diazepam (Zbinden *et al.*, 1961).

Hollister (1966) also reviewed the treatment of overdosage. Treatment consisted mainly of gastric lavage, norepinephrine (NE) or dextroamphetamine to control hypotension and Na-amobarbital or Na-diphenylhydantoin to control seizures in cases of phenothiazine poisoning; gastric lavage, NE, Na-amobarbital, mannitol (to hasten excretion of the drug) and dialysis (to manage hyperpyrexia) in cases of poisoning with tricyclic antidepressant drugs; and dialysis and chlorpromazine administration in cases of poisoning with MAOI compounds.

c. Hypersensitivity

Hypersensitivity includes all allergic reactions due to sensitization of some subjects to certain drugs; however, these are usually recognized only in the course of the clinical pharmacological study. On the other hand, hyperergic and idiosyncratic reactions are constantly searched for during the human pharmacological investigation.

Hyperergic reactions show signs and symptoms qualitatively similar to those produced by overdosage. The basic difference, however, is that hyperergic reactions develop to quantities of the drug which are harmless to the majority of subjects. To date, there is no way of detecting "hyperreactors" and hyperergic reactions in advance. They may occur with any of the psychoactive substances.

In contradistinction to the hyperergic reactions is idiosyncrasy, which implies an inherent qualitatively abnormal reaction.

2. Metabolism

Interspecies differences of metabolism (*i.e.*, metabolic differences between animals and man) and intraspecies metabolic variations are explored in the course of metabolic—human pharmacological—studies. Relatively few interspecies differences with psychopharmacological significance have been recognized thus far. Among them, for example, is the feeble ability of cats, unlike humans, to conjugate drugs or their metabolites with glucuronic acid.

There are at least two well known instances where genetic polymorphism of drug metabolism is known to account for intraspecies variations of toxic effects in man.

These are the pseudocholinesterase and the acetylation polymorphism.

a. Pseudocholinesterase Polymorphism

The pseudocholinesterase polymorphism was discovered in the course of investigations with succinylcholine chloride, a muscle relaxant, used as an adjuvant in general anesthesia (and for the prevention of fractures in electroconvulsive treatment). In cases of this enzymatic defect, the succinylcholine is not hydrolyzed, which accounts for the prolonged paralysis or dangerous apnea, occasionally seen following an ECT.

b. Acetylation Polymorphism

The acetylation polymorphism is particularly important from a psychopharmacological point of view. Here a metabolic factor accounts for the different speeds of inactivation of isoniazid in two different, genetically determined, phenotypes. Subjects who developed peripheral neuropathy when treated with isoniazid—a hydrazin substance, the predecessor of MAOI antidepressants—were found to be predominantly "slow acetylators" of the drug, while subjects without this adverse effect were found to be, in general, "rapid acetylators." The relevance of this information to psychopharmacology was indicated with phenelzine, a MAOI antidepressant drug, similar to isoniazid in possessing a monosubstituent hydrazine side chain. With phenelzine it was observed that in the two different phenotypes, as classified by the isoniazid test, significantly more side effects occurred in the slow acetylators.

Human pharmacology is one of the fastest growing disciplines in preclinical investigation. It is increasingly accepted that the information it offers is essential before applying animal pharmacological data in the course of clinical pharmacological experiments. More recently, there have been indications that it is advantageous to conduct at least some of the human pharmacological experiments in stressful situations. It is interesting to note how little is the dissociation between animal and human pharmacological findings, and the discrepancy can often be found and explained on the basis of structural, including metabolic, differences.

REFERENCES

Alexander, L.: Apparatus and method for the study of conditional reflexes in man. Arch. Neurol. Psychiat., *80:* 629 (1958).

Alexander, L.: Chemotherapy of depression: use of meprobamate combined with benactyzine (2-diethylaminoethyl benzilate) hydrochloride. J.A.M.A., *166:* 1019 (1958).

Alexander, L.: Effects of psychotropic drugs on conditional responses in man. In: Neuropsychopharmacology (ed., Rothlin, E.). (Elsevier, Amsterdam, 1961.)

Alexander, L.: The effect of drugs on the conditional psychogalvanic reflex in man. J. Neuropsychiat., *2:* 5 (1961).

Alles, G. A., and Fergen, G. H.: The influence of benzedrine on work decrement and the patellar reflex. Amer. J. Physiol., *136:* 392 (1942).

Astrup, C.: Schizophrenia: conditional reflex studies. (Charles C Thomas, Springfield, 1962.)

Astrup, C.: Pavlovian psychiatry—a new synthesis. (Charles C Thomas, Springfield, 1965.)

Astrup, C.: Conditional reflex studies in psychopharmacology. (Presented at the Collegium Internationale Neuropsychopharmacologicum, Washington, 1966.)

Bacon, G. A.: Successful suicide with tranylcypromine sulfate. Amer. J. Psychiat., *119:* 585 (1962).

Ban, T. A.: Conditioning and psychiatry. (Aldine Publishing Co., Chicago, 1964.)

Ban, T. A.: Methodology and pitfalls in clinical testing of psychopharmacological drugs. Chemotherapia (Basel), *9:* 223 (1964).

Ban, T. A.: Annual report of the Research Department. (Douglas Hospital, Verdun, 1965.)

Ban, T. A.: Human pharmacology and systematic clinical studies with a new phenothiazine. In: Proceedings of the Leeds Symposium (ed., Jenner, F. A.). (May and Baker, Dagenham, 1965.)

Ban, T. A.: The possible role of conditioning in the development and treatment of delinquents and criminals. (A psychiatrist's point of view.) (Presented at the Meeting of Correctional Psychologists, Montreal, 1965.)

Ban, T. A.: Trimipramine in psychiatry. In: Trimipramine: a new anti-depressant (eds., Lehmann, H. E., Berthiaume, M., and Ban, T. A.). (Q.P.R.A., Montreal, 1965.)

Ban, T. A.: Annual report of the Research Department. (Douglas Hospital, Verdun, 1966.)

Ban, T. A.: Conditioning and psychiatry. (Unwin, London, 1966.)

Ban, T. A.: Predictors of therapeutic response to drugs. Canad. Ment. Health, *14:* 23 (1966).

Ban, T. A.: Psychophysical deficit: psychiatric diagnoses. (Proceedings of the Eighteenth International Congress of Psychology, Moscow, 1966.)

Ban, T. A.: What pre-clinical information does the clinician expect to be given prior to conducting trials with a new drug? Bull. Amer. Coll. Neuropsychopharmacol., *4:* 1 (1966).

BAN, T. A., Papthomopulos, E., and Schwarz, L.: Clinical studies with thioproperazine. Compr. Psychiat., *3:* 284 (1962).

BAN, T. A., AND SCHWARZ, L.: Systematic studies with levomepromazine. J. Neuropsychiat., *5:* 112 (1963).

BARCROFT, J.: Features in the architecture of physiological function. (University Press, Cambridge, 1934.)

BENBOW, S. H., AND SUPER, W. C.: Case report of an acute overdosage of nardil. Amer. J. Psychiat., *117:* 836 (1961).

BENTE, D.: Electroencephalographic aspects in the classification of neuroleptic and thymoleptic drugs. Neuropsychopharmacol. Med. Exp., *5:* 337 (1961).

BENTE, D.: Elektroenzephologographie und Psychiatrische Pharmacotherapie. In: Anthropologishe und Naturwissenchaftliche Grundlagen der Pharmacopsychiatrie (eds., Achelis, J. D., and Ditfurth, H.). (Thieme, Stuttgart, 1963.)

BENTE, D., AND ITIL, T.: Das Verhalten des Hirnstrombildes bei Hochdosierter Behandlung mit Reserpin (serpasil) und bei Medikamentös Erzeugten Parkinsonähnlichen Zustandsbildern. Med. Klin., *50:* 1296 (1955).

BENTE, D., AND ITIL, T.: Chlorpromazine sleep as an electroencephalographic activation method. Electroenceph. Clin. Neurophysiol., *9:* 355 (1957).

BENTE, D., AND ITIL, T.: Elektroencephalographische Befunde zur Wirkungsweise des Neuroleptischen Behandlungsverfahren. Arzneimittelforschung, *7:* 611 (1957).

BENTE, D., AND ITIL, T.: Clinico-electroencephalographic investigations. In: Psychopharmacology frontiers (ed., Kline, N. S.). (Little, Brown, Toronto, 1959.)

BERNARD, C.: Les phénoménes de la vie. (Bailliére, Paris, 1878.)

BERTLER, A.: Effect of reserpine on the storage of catecholamines in brain and other tissues. Acta Physiol. Scand., *51:* 75 (1961).

BIDWELL, S.: On subjective color phenomenon attending sudden changes of illumination. Proc. Roy. Soc. Biol., *60:* 368 (1896).

BIDWELL, S.: On negative after images following brief retinal excitation. Proc. Roy. Soc. Biol., *61:* 268 (1897).

BOURDON, C.: Observations comparatives sur la reconnaisance la discrimination et l'association. Rev. Philosophique, *40:* 153 (1895).

BROWN, J., DIMASCIO, A., AND KLERMAN, G. L.: An exploratory study of the effects of tranquillizers on competitive paired associates learning. Psychol. Rep., *4:* 583 (1958).

BURBRIDGE, T. N. (1958): In: Uhr, L.: Objectively measured behavioral effects of psychoactive drugs. In: Drugs and behavior (eds., Uhr, L., and Miller, J. G.). (Wiley, London, 1960.)

CALKINS, M. V.: A suggested classification of cases of association. Philos. Rev., *1:* 389 (1892).

CARL, E. P., AND TURNER, W. D.: The effect of benzedrine sulfate (amphetamine sulfate) on performance in a comprehensive psychometric examination. J. Psychol., *8:* 165 (1939).

CAZZULLO, C. L., GOLDWURM, G. F., AND PETRELLA, F.: Correlation between psychopathological data and higher nervous activity evaluation by four reflexological methods in neuropsychiatric patients. (Presented at the Fourth World Congress of Psychiatry, Madrid, 1966.)

CUTHBERTSON, D. P., AND KNOX, J. A. C.: The effect of benzedrine on mentally deficient children. Amer. J. Ment. Defic., *45:* 59 (1940).

DALGLIESH, C. E.: Two dimensional paperchromatography of urinary indoles and related substances. Biochem. J., *64:* 481 (1956).

DARROW, C. W.: Some physiological conditions of efficiency. Psychol. Bull., *24:* 488 (1927).

DARROW, C. W.: Differences in the physiological reaction to sensory and ideational stimuli. Psychol. Bull., *26:* 185 (1929).

DE, B.: A study of the validity of the word association technique for the differentiation of normal and abnormal persons. (Dissertation, London, 1953.)

DILWORTH, N. M., DUGDALE, A. E., AND HILTON, H. B.: Acute poisoning with chlorpromazine. Lancet, *1:* 137 (1963).

DIMASCIO, A.: Drug effects on competitive-paired associate learning: relationship to and implications for the Taylor manifest anxiety scale. J. Psychol., *56:* 89 (1963).

DIMASCIO, A., *et al.*: Psychophysiologic evaluation of phenyltoloxamine: a new phrenotropic agent. Amer. J. Psychiat., *115:* 301 (1958).

DIMASCIO, A., *et al.*: The psychopharmacology of phenothiazine compounds: a comparative study of the effects of chlorpromazine, promethazine, trifluoperazine and perphenazine in normal males. J. Nerv. Ment. Dis., *136:* 15 (1963).

DÜKER, H., AND DÜKER, E.: Über die Wirkung von Pervitin auf die Psychische Leistungsfähigkeit. Z. Exp. Angew. Psychol., *1:* 32 (1953).

EBBINGHAUS, H.: Über des Gedachtnis. Untersuchungen zur Experimentellen Psychologie. (Duncker and Humbolt, Leipzig, 1885.)

ERSPAMER, V., GLÄSSER, A., AND MANTEGAZZINI, P.: Pharmacological actions of 4-hydroxytryptamine and 4-hydroxy-tryptophan. Experientia, *16:* 505 (1960).

EULER, U. S.: Adrenaline and nor-adrenaline. Triangle (Sandoz) J. Med. Sci., *1:* 101 (1954).

EULER, U. S., AND LUFT, R.: Effect of insulin on urinary excretion of adrenaline and noradrenaline. Metabolism, *1:* 528 (1952).

EXNER, S.: Bemerkungen über Intermittierende Netzhautreizung. Pfluger. Arch. Ges. Physiol., *3:* 214 (1870).

EYSENCK, H. J.: Drugs and personality. I. Theory and methodology. J. Ment. Sci., *103:* 119 (1957).

EYSENCK, H. J., CASEY, S., AND TROUTON, D. S.: Drugs and personality. II. The effect of stimulant and depressant drugs on continuous work. J. Ment. Sci., *103:* 645 (1957).

EYSENCK, H. J., AND EASTERBROOK, J. A.: Drugs and personality. VI. The effect of stimulant and depressant drugs upon body sway (static atoxia). J. Ment. Sci., *106:* 831 (1960).

Eysenck, H. J., Holland, H., and Trouton, D. S.: Drugs and personality. III. The effects of stimulant and depressant drugs on visual aftereffects. J. Ment. Sci., *103:* 650 (1957).

Felsinger, J. N., Lasagna, L., and Beecher, H. K.: The persistence of mental impairment following a hypnotic dose of barbiturate. J. Pharmacol. Ther., *109:* 284 (1953).

Fink, M.: Quantitative EEG in human psychopharmacology drug patterns. In: EEG and behavior (ed., Glaser, G. H.). (Basic Books, New York, 1963.)

Fink, M.: Quantitative EEG and human psychopharmacology. In: Applications of electroencephalography in psychiatry (ed., Wilson, W. D.). (Duke University Press, Durham, 1965.)

Flory, D., and Gilbert, J.: The effects of benzedrine sulfate and caffeine citrate on the efficiency of college students. J. Appl. Psychol., *27:* 121 (1943).

Galton, F.: Psychometric experiments. Brain, *2:* 149 (1879).

Garattini, S., and Valzelli, L.: Serotonin, (Elsevier, Amsterdam, 1965).

Goldman-Eisler, F.: Speech production and the predictability of words in content. Quart. J. Exp. Psychol., *10:* 96 (1958).

Gray, M. G., and Trowbridge, E. B.: Methods for investigating the effects of drugs on psychological function. Psychol. Res., *5:* 127 (1942).

Haggerty, R. J.: Fatal chlorpromazine poisoning. New Eng. J. Med., *256:* 527 (1957).

Hirsch, A.: Experiences chronoscopiques sur la vitesse des différentes sensations et de la transmission nerveuse. Soc. Sci. Nat. Bull., *6:* 100 (1861).

Holland, H. C.: Drugs and personality. III. A comparison of several drugs by the flicker fusion method. J. Ment. Sci., *106:* 858 (1960).

Holliday, A. R., Duffy, M. L., and Dillie, J. M.: The effect of certain tranquillizers on a stress producing behavioral task. J. Pharmacol. Exp. Ther., *122:* 32 (1958).

Hollingworth, H. L.: Psychological aspects of drug action. Psychol. Bull., *9:* 420 (1912).

Hollingworth, H. L.: The influence of caffeine on mental and motor efficiency. Arch. Psychol., *3:* 1 (1912).

Hollister, L. E.: Current concepts in therapy: complications from psychotherapeutic drugs. I. New Eng. J. Med., *264:* 291 (1961).

Hollister, L. E.: Drug-induced psychoses and schizophrenic reactions: a critical comparison. Ann. N.Y. Acad. Sci., *96:* 80 (1962).

Hollister, L. E.: Nervous system reactions to drugs. Ann. N.Y. Acad. Sci., *123:* 342 (1965).

Hollister, L. E.: Overdoses of psychotherapeutic drugs. Clin. Pharmacol. Ther., *7:* 142 (1966).

Hollister, L. E., Motzenbecker, F. P., and Degan, R. O.: Withdrawal reactions from chlordiazepoxide (librium). Psychopharmacologia (Berlin), *2:* 63 (1961).

Irwin, S.: Pharmacology and drug therapy. (Presented at Postgraduate course on Animal and Clinical Pharmacology Techniques in Drug Evaluation, Philadelphia, 1966.)

Ivanov-Smolensky, A. G.: Investigations into the interactions of the first and second signaling systems. Zh. Vyssh. Nerv. Deiat. Pavlov., *3:* 481 (1953).

Jasper, H.: Electrical activity of the brain. Ann. Rev. Physiol., *3:* 377 (1941).

Jung, C. G.: On psychophysical relation of associative experiment. J. Abnorm. Soc. Psychol., *1:* 249 (1906).

Jung, C. G.: The association method. Amer. J. Psychol., *21:* 219 (1910).

Jung, C. G.: Studies in word association. (Moffat, New York, 1919.)

Jus, A.: Clinical and experimental investigation on the action of nialamid in certain mental disorders. J. Soc. Cienc. Med. Lisboa, *1:* 235 (1959).

Jus, A.: Influence of psychotropic agents upon conditional reflexes of animals and humans. Neurol. Neurochir. Psychiat. Pol., *11:* 479 (1961).

Jus, A.: The effects of psychoactive drugs in conditional responses in animals and man. Neuropsychopharmacol., *2:* 125 (1961).

Jus, A.: Conditional reflex experimental research in the evaluation of therapeutic mechanisms of action of some psychotropic drugs. Third Wld. Congr. Psychiat., *1:* 151 (1962).

Kety, S. S.: Catecholamines in neuropsychiatric states, Pharmacol. Rev., *18:* 787 (1966).

Kleemeier, L. B., and Kleemeier, R. W.: Effects of benzedrine sulfate (amphetamine) on psychomotor performance. Amer. J. Psychol., *60:* 89 (1947).

Klerman, G. L., *et al.:* Sedation and tranquillization: a comparison of the effects of a number of psychopharmacologic agents upon normal human subjects. Arch. Gen. Psychiat., *3:* 4 (1960).

Knoefel, P. K.: The influence of phenisopropyl amine and phenisopropyl methyl amine on work output. Fed. Proc., *2:* 83 (1943).

Kopin, I. J., and Gordon, E. K.: Metabolism of norepinephrine-H^3 released by tyramine and reserpine. J. Pharmacol., *138:* 351 (1962).

Kornetsky, C.: Effects of meprobamate, phenobarbital and dextroamphetamine on reaction time and learning in man. J. Pharmacol. Exp. Ther., *123:* 216 (1958).

Kornetsky, C., Humphries, D., and Evarts, E. V.: Comparison of psychological effects of certain centrally acting drugs in man. Arch. Neurol. Psychiat., *77:* 318 (1957).

Kraepelin, E.: Der Psycholigische Versuch in der Psychiatrie. Psychol. Arbeiten, *1:* 77 (1896).

Kristofferson, A. B., and Cormack, P. H. (1959): In: Uhr, L. Objectively measured behavioral effects of psychoactive drugs. In: Drugs and behavior (eds. Uhr, L., and Miller, J. G.). (Wiley, New York, 1960.)

Krugler, J.: Electroencephalography in hospital

and general consulting practice. (Elsevier, Amsterdam, 1964.)
LANDIS, C., AND ZUBIN, J.: The effect of thorizylanine hydrochloride and phenobarbital on certain psychological functions. J. Psychol., *31:* 181 (1951).
LEHMANN, H. E.: A new preparation for sedation in organic brain disease and senile disturbances. Canad. Med. Ass. J., *60:* 157 (1949).
LEHMANN, H. E.: Preliminary report on a devise for the objective measurement of the negative after-image phenomenon. Science, *112:* 199 (1950).
LEHMANN, H. E.: The problem of evaluating psychotic art at three levels, objective, interpretive and intuitive. (Presented at the Second World Congress of Psychiatry, Zurich, 1957.)
LEHMANN, H. E.: Measurements of changes in human behavior under the effects of psychotropic drugs. In: Neuropsychopharmacology, Vol. II. (ed., Rothlin, E.). (Elsevier, Amsterdam, 1960.)
LEHMANN, H. E.: Psychoactive drugs and their influence on the dynamics of working capacity. J. Occup. Med., *2:* 523 (1960).
LEHMANN, H. E.: The place and purpose of objective methods in psychopharmacology. In: Drugs and behavior (eds., Uhr, L., and Miller, J. G.). (Wiley, New York, 1960.)
LEHMANN, H. E.: Clinical techniques for evaluating antidepressants. In: Pharmacologic techniques in drug evaluation (eds., Siegler, P. E., and Moyer, J. H.). (Year Book Medical Publishers, Chicago, 1967.)
LEHMANN, H. E.: The psychotropic drugs: their action and applications. Hospital Practice, *2:* 74 (1967).
LEHMANN, H. E.: Time and psychopathology. Ann. N.Y. Acad. Sci., *138:* 798 (1967).
LEHMANN, H. E., AND BAN, T. A.: Comprehensive clinical studies with psychoactive drugs. (Triannual report of studies with psychoactive drugs conducted at Douglas Hospital, ECDEU Progress Report, Montreal, 1966.)
LEHMANN, H. E., AND CSANK, J.: Differential screening of phrenotropic agents in man: psychophysiologic test data. J. Clin. Exp. Psychopath., *18:* 222 (1957).
LEHMANN, H. E., AND KNIGHT, D. A.: Psychophysiologic testing with a new phrenotropic drug. In: Trifluoperazine clinical and pharmacological aspects. (Lea and Febiger, Philadelphia, 1958.)
LEHMANN, H. E., AND KNIGHT, D. A.: Measurement of changes in human behavior under the effects of psychotropic drugs. (Presented at the Proceedings of the Second International meeting of the Collegium Internationale Neuropsychopharmacologicum, Basle, 1960.)
LEHMANN, H. E., AND KNIGHT, D. A.: Measurement of changes in human behavior under the effects of psychotropic drugs. Neuropsychopharmacol., *2:* 303 (1961).
LEHMANN, H. E., AND KNIGHT, D. A.: Placeboproneness and placebo-resistance of different psychological functions. Psychiat. Quart., *34:* 505 (1960).
LEHMANN, H. E., AND KNIGHT, D. A.: The psychopharmacological profile—a systematic approach to the interaction of drug effects and personality traits. In: Extrapyramidal system and neuroleptics (ed., Bordeleau, J. M.). (L'Edition Psychiatrique, Montreal, 1961.)
LEMMELL, G., AND HARTWIG, Y.: Untersuchungen über die Wirkung von Pervitin und Benzedrin auf Psychischen Gebiet. Deutsch. Arch. Klin. Med., *185:* 626 (1940).
LIPGART, N. K.: Comparative influences of phenamine on some conditional and unconditional reflexes in schizophrenic patients. Tr. 20 Sess. Ukrain. Psikoneurol. Inst., *1:* 284 (1958).
LOOMIS, T. A., AND WEST, T. C.: Comparative sedative effects of barbiturate and some tranquillizer drugs on normal subjects. J. Pharmacol. Exp. Ther., *122:* 525 (1958).
MARRUBINI, G.: Avvelenamento mortate di clorpromazina. Minerva Med., *50:* 78 (1959).
MATTER, B. J., *et al.:* Tranylcypromine sulfate poisoning. Arch. Intern. Med., *116:* 18 (1965).
MAYER-GROSS, W., SLATER, W., AND ROTH, M.: Clinical psychiatry. (Cassell, London, 1960.)
MCILWAIN, H.: Chemotherapy and the CNS. (Churchill, London, 1957.)
MERCHANT, H. C., *et al.:* A fatal case of chlorpromazine poisoning. J. A. Physicians. India, *11:* 337 (1963).
MILLER, J. G., AND UHR, L.: Behavioral toxicity as measured by tests of simulated driving and of vision. In: Drugs and behavior (eds., Uhr, L., and Miller, J. G.). (Wiley, New York, 1960.)
MITCHELL, I., ROSANOFF, I. R., AND ROSANOFF, A. J.: A study of association in negro children. Psychol. Rev., *26:* 354 (1919).
MÜLLER, H. F., AND MÜLLER, A. K.: Effects of some psychotropic drugs upon brain electrical activity. Int. J. Neuropsychiat., *1:* 224 (1965).
MÜNSTERBERG, H.: Optimal time content. Psychol. Rev., *1:* 51, 1894.
NOACK, C. H.: A death from overdosage of tofranil. Med. J. Aust., *2:* 182 (1960).
PAYNE, R. B., AND MOORE, E. W.: The effects of some analeptic and depressant drugs upon tracking behavior. J. Pharmacol., *115:* 480 (1955).
PEOPLES, S. A., AND GUTTMANN, E.: Hypertension produced with benzedrine: its psychological accompaniments. Lancet, *1:* 107 (1936).
PFEIFFER, C. C., *et al.*: Time-series frequency analysis and electrogenesis of the EEGs of normals and psychotics before and after drugs. Amer. J. Psychiat., *121:* 1147 (1965).
PFEIFFER, C. C., *et al.:* Quantitative comparisons of the electroencephalographic stimulant effects of deanol, choline, and amphetamine. Clin. Pharmacol. Ther., *4:* 461 (1963).
PLATEAU, J.: Betrachtungen über ein von Hrr. Talbot Vorgeschlagenes Photometrisches Princip. Ann. Physik. Chem., *35:* 457 (1835).
POFFENBERGER, A. T.: Psychological effects of drugs. Psychol. Bull., *11:* 418 (1914).

Poffenberger, A. T.: Psychological effects of drugs. Psychol. Bull., *13:* 434 (1916).

Poffenberger, A. T.: Psychological effects of drugs. Psychol. Bull., *14:* 409 (1917).

Poffenberger, A. T.: Psychological effects of drugs. Psychol. Bull., *16:* 291 (1919).

Primac, D. W., Mirsky, A. F., and Rosvold, H. E.: Effects of centrally acting drugs on two tests of brain damage. Arch. Neurol. Psychiat., *77:* 328 (1957).

Rivers, W. H. R.: The influence of alcohol and other drugs on fatigue. (Arnold, London, 1908.)

Roback, G. S., *et al.:* Effect of analeptic drugs on the somnifacient effect of seconal and antihistamines as measured by flicker fusion threshold. J. Appl. Physiol., *4:* 566 (1952).

Rosanoff, I. R., and Rosanoff, A. J.: A study of association in children. Psychol. Rev., *20:* 43 (1913).

Saarma, J.: Prognosis of insulin therapy in schizophrenia based on higher nervous activity data. Int. J. Psychiat., *2:* 431 (1966).

Saarma, J., and Saarma, M.: Comparative conditioning study of neuroleptics in normals and chronic schizophrenics. (Presented at the Fifth International Congress of CINP, Washington, 1966.)

Saarma, J., and Saarma, M.: Dynamics of higher nervous activity of chronic schizophrenics under treatment with aminazine, stelazine and haloperiodol. (Presented at the Third World Congress of Psychiatry, Madrid, 1966.)

Sandler, M., and Ruthven, C. R. J.: The measurement of 4-hydroxy-3-methoxymandelic acid and homovanillic acid. In: Second symposium on catecholamines (ed., Acheson, G. H.). (Williams and Wilkins, Baltimore, 1966.)

Schildkraut, J. J., *et al.:* Excretion of 3-methoxy-4-hydroxymandelic acid (VMA) in depressed patients treated with antidepressant drugs. J. Psychiat. Res., *2:* 257 (1964).

Schneider, R. A., and Costiloe, J. P. (1959): In: Schneider, R. A.: The influence of predrug level of functioning on the effects of sedatives, tranquillizers and stimulants on central autonomic function and reaction time. In: Drugs and behavior (eds., Uhr, L., and Miller. J. G.). (Wiley, New York, 1960.)

Schopbach, R. R., Kelly, A. R., and Lukaszewski, J. S.: Effects of marplan on catecholamine serotonin metabolism in humans. In: Progress in brain research (eds., Himwich, H. E., and Himwich, W. A.). (Elsevier, Amsterdam, 1964.)

Seashore, R. H., and Ivy, A. C.: Effects of analeptic drugs in relieving fatigue. Psychol. Mongr., *15:* 1 (1953).

Segal, J. E., and Skuin, E. J.: Studies of some physiological and biochemical reactions during the action of chloropromazine. Sb. Nauk. Inst. M. Asationi Tiflis, *5:* 333 (1958).

Seredina, M. I.: The effects of different doses of reserpine on the cortical dynamics and some autonomic functions in man. Tr. Inst. Vyss. Nerv. Dejat Ser. Pato-fiziol., *7:* 245 (1960).

Shagass, C., and Schwartz, M.: Excitability of the cerebral cortex in psychiatric disorders. In: Physiological correlates of psychological disorders (eds. Roessler, R., and Greenfield, N. S.). (University of Wisconsin Press, Madison, 1962.)

Shagass, C., Schwartz, M., and Amadeo, M.: Some drug effects on evoked cerebral potentials in man. J. Neuropsychiat., *3:* 49 (1962).

Sharp, S. E.: Individual psychology: a study in psychological method. Amer. J. Psychol., *10:* 329 (1899).

Shock, N. W.: Some psychophysiological relations. Psychol. Bull., *36:* 447 (1939).

Simonson, E., and Brozek, J.: Flicker fusion frequency background and application. Physiol. Rev., *32:* 349 (1952).

Simonson, E., Enzer, W., and Blankstein, S. S.: Effect of amphetamine (benzedrine) sulfate on fatigue of the CNS. War Med., *1:* 690 (1941).

Spragg, S. D. S.: The effects of certain drugs on mental and motor efficiency. Psychol. Bull., *38:* 354 (1941).

St. Jean, A., Ban, T. A., and Noe, W.: Psychopharmacological studies with neoserp and aldomet. Int. J. Neuropsychiat., *1:* 491 (1965).

St. Jean, A., *et al.:* The psychophysical effect of the butyrophenones. In: The butyrophenones in psychiatry (eds. Lehmann, H. E., and Ban, T. A.). (Quebec Psychopharmacological Research Association, Montreal, 1964.)

Studnitz, W.: Effects of marsilid on excretion of 5-methoxy-4-hydroxymandelic acid in man. Scand. J. Clin. Lab. Invest., *11:* 224 (1959).

Sunshine, P., and Yaffe, S. J.: Amitryptiline poisoning: clinical and pathological findings in a fatal case. Amer. J. Dis. Child, *106:* 501 (1963).

Sweeley, C. C., and Williams, C. M.: Gas chromatography of urinary aromatic acids. Fed. Proc., *20:* 5 (1961).

Talbot, H. F.: Experiments on light. Phil. Mag., *13:* 321 (1834).

Tirkeltaub, J. A.: The effect of tofranil on higher nervous activity and some autonomic functions in schizophrenic patients. Zh. Nevropat. Psikhiat. Korsakov., *63:* 564 (1963).

Traugott, N. N.: The mechanism of the action of chlorpromazine on the higher nervous activity of man. Zh. Vyssh. Nerv. Deiat. Pavlov., *11:* 814 (1961).

Traugott, N. N.: Clinical physiological analysis of the effects of some psychopharmacological drugs. Third Wld. Congr. Psychiat., *3:* 105 (1963).

Traugott, N. N., and Balonov, L. J.: Neurophysiological analysis of clinical states after chlorpromazine injections. Zh. Nevropat. Psikhiat. Korsakov., *58:* 585 (1958).

Traugott, N. N., *et al.:* Characteristics of cortical activity of man under the influence of chlorpromazine. Tes. 20 Sov. Probl. Vyssh. Nerv. Deiat., *1:* 128 (1960).

Trautscholdt, M.: Experimentelle Untersuchungen über die Association der Vorstellungen. (Dissertation, Leipzig, 1882.)

TROUTON, D. S.: Placebos and their psychological effects. J. Ment. Sci., *103:* 344 (1957).

TROUTON, D., AND EYSENCK, H. J.: The effects of drugs on behavior. In: Handbook of abnormal psychology (ed., Eysenck, H. J.). (Basic Books, New York, 1961.)

TURNER, W. D., AND CARL, G. P.: A further report on benzedrine sulfate (amphetamine sulfate) on performance in a comprehensive psychometric examination. J. Psychol., *8:* 165 (1939).

UHR, L.: Objectively measured behavioral effects of psychoactive drugs. In: Drugs and behavior (eds., Uhr, L., and Miller, J. G.). (Wiley, New York, 1960.)

UHR, L., PLATZ, A., AND MILLER, J. G. (1960): In: Uhr, L. Objectively measured behavioral effects of psychoactive drugs. In: Drugs and behavior (eds., Uhr, L., and Miller, J. G.). (Wiley, New York, 1960.)

VALCOURT, A. J.: Hydroxyindoleacetic acid excretion in men. Fed. Proc., *16:* 130 (1957).

VINAR, O.: A comparison of experimental conditional reflexes in schizophrenia and LSD psychosis. (Presented at the First International Congress of Social Psychiatry, London, 1964.)

VOTAVA, Z., HORVATH, M., AND VINAR, O. (eds.): Psychopharmacological methods. (Pergamon Press, Oxford, 1963.)

WAALKES, T. P. J.: The determination of serotonin (5-HT) in human blood. Lab. Clin. Med., *53:* 824 (1959).

WALLMAN, I. S.: Death from chlorpromazine poisoning. Med. J. Aust., *1:* 903 (1957).

WASKOW, I. E.: The effects of drugs on speech: a review. Psychopharmacol. Serv. Cent. Bull., *3:* 1 (1966).

WECHSLER, D.: The measurement of adult intelligence. (Williams and Wilkins, Baltimore, 1944.)

WECHSLER, D.: A standarized memory scale for clinical use. J. Psychol., *19:* 87 (1945).

WECHSLER, D.: Manual for the Wechsler adult intelligence scale. (Psychological Corp., New York, 1945.)

WEIL-MALHERBE, H.: The effect of convulsive therapy on plasma adrenaline and noradrenaline. Journal of Ment. Sci., *101:* 156 (1955).

WIKLER, A.: Clinical and electroencephalographic studies on the effects of mescaline, N-allylnormorphine and morphine. J. Nerv. Ment. Dis., *120:* 157 (1954).

WIKLER, A., AND PESCOR, F. T.: Clinical and electroencephalographic effects of drugs on man and dog. (Wm. Bird Press, Richmond, 1954.)

WILLET, R. A.: The effect of a stimulant and a depressant drug on serial rate learning of nonsense syllables. Unpublished report. (Institute of Psychiatry, London, 1958.)

WRESCHNER, A.: Eine Experimentelle Studie über die Association in Einen Falle von Idiotie. Allg. Z. Psychiat., *57:* 241 (1900).

WUNDERLE, F.: Experimental Psychologische Untersuchungen über die Wirkung des Pervitins auf Geistige Leistungen. Arch. Psychol. Z. Neurol., *113:* 504 (1941).

WUNDT, W.: Grundzüge der physiologischen Psychologie. (Engelman, Leipzig, 1903.)

ZBINDEN, G., *et al.:* Experimental and clinical toxicity of chlordiazepoxide (librium). Toxic. Appl. Pharmacol., *3:* 619 (1961).

Four

Clinical Pharmacology

The aim of clinical pharmacological studies is to reveal the effects of psychoactive substances in various psychopathologies. Thus, according to Beaulnes (1964), the clinical pharmacological study, which follows human pharmacological studies, and precedes clinical investigation, is directed toward finding pathological conditions for which the drug is therapeutically useful.

Besides discovering those psychopathological conditions for which the new investigational substance may be therapeutic, the clinical pharmacological study is also directed toward detecting any adverse effects which may occur. The latter is particularly important since this is the first time that the new drug is being chronically administered to psychiatric patients.

A. THERAPEUTIC EFFECTS

In the course of the clinical pharmacological study, besides the (1) psychopathological symptom (syndrome) assessment, other means, such as (2) psychometrics, (3) conditioning, (4) neurophysiological and (5) biochemical procedures, are used to detect the drug-induced changes.

In the evaluation of findings it has to be recognized that organismic reactivity to chronic administration of drugs may be influenced by such variables as climate; diet and nutrition; variations in sensory and social stimulation patterns in the clinical setting; interrelationship of biological and social components in population groups designated as "social class"; ethnic groups or nationalities; and cumulative effects of previous somatic treatments, particularly psychotropic drugs (WHO, 1967).

1. Psychopathological Symptom Assessment

In spite of the numerous techniques used, the assessment of changes in manifest psychopathology still remains the core of the clinical pharmacological study. Nothing can take the place of clinical acumen, although additional techniques can be helpful. This is particularly pertinent at this stage of investigation since the possible psychotherapeutic indication of the substance has not been ascertained and its therapeutic dosage ranges are still to be established. Only an uncontrolled clinical study with free dosages (within the safe limits) in a small (preferably 10, but definitely not more than 20) number of patients, conducted for a sufficiently long period of time (preferably 12 weeks but not less than 4 weeks), is practical.

The use of standardized scales and large patient samples, thought to be so important in the more advanced steps of drug evaluation, may only serve to cover up any actual changes at this stage.

Essentially, psychopathological symptom (syndrome) assessment is based on systematic (daily) clinical observations and judgment. To facilitate communication, the results are expressed as actions on psychopathological symptoms and as effects on main psychological parameters.

a. Action on Psychopathological Symptoms and Syndromes

For this purpose, the presence, absence or change of any psychopathological symptom is recorded, prior to and during the course of drug administration. In their original check list, Lehmann and Ban (1963) formulated six groups of symptom complexes reflecting psychopathological disturbances in the following areas: (1) sensory-perceptual (sensation, perception, ideation); (2) affective-relational (emotion, mood, affect); (3) adaptive (instincts, voluntary activity, automatisms); (4) cognitive (abstraction, association of ideas, thinking); (5) connective functions (consciousness, memory, attention); and (6) personality (intellect, temperament, character).

By systematically exploring the drug-induced changes in psychopathological symptoms, possible therapeutic effects on various psychopathological syndromes were revealed. For example, it was recognized that in psychiatric patients "sensory" disturbances were mainly associated with affective psychopathology, *i.e.*, emotions, affect and mood, and that these responded best to various anxiolytic (benzodiazepine, propanediol) or antidepressant (tricyclic, MAOI) compounds. Perceptual pathology, however, was most prevalently associated with altered associations and thinking and responded most favorably to various antipsychotic drugs (phenothiazines, butyrophenones, thioxanthenes, Rauwolfia alkaloids).

The prevailing approach in the assessment of new psychoactive substances in clinical pharmacological studies is to focus attention on "target symptoms" (Freyhan, 1959). The target symptom concept is based on the evidence that most psychotropic drugs act on specific symptomatic manifestations (*e.g.*, depression or hallucination) of psychiatric disorders. These target symptoms are considered as part of a context, the larger constellation of symptoms in relation to the disorder. However, many investigators are of the opinion that contemporary pharmacotherapy does not act merely by modifying the symptoms of the disorder, but also modifies its clinical course (WHO, 1967).

b. Effects on Main Psychological Parameters

Lehmann's (1961) psychophysiologically based classification of psychotropic drugs served as the starting point in developing the main psychological parameters affected by a psychopharmacological substance. The data collected is assessed for "shifts" on the psychological parameters.

In his original proposal (Lehmann, 1961), the effects of psychoactive drugs were measured by three main psychological parameters: arousal, mood and mental integration. Later, to render it useful for clinical pharmacological studies, an affective and an organicity parameter was added (Lehmann and Ban, 1966). The changes, or the "shifts," which occur on these parameters are expressed as follows: *arousal*—behavioral stimulation, excitement as opposed to behavioral inhibition, fatigue; *mood*—dysthymia, dysphoria as opposed to hyperthymia, euphoria; *mental integration*—perceptual disturbance (with or without hallucinations), thought disorder (with or without delusions) as opposed to the lack of integrational pathology; *affective*—increased preoccupation (including somatic) with the self, surplus autonomic reactivity, anxiety as opposed to impaired relational ability, impulsive actions, apathy; *organicity*—altered states of consciousness (with or without permanent memory impairment), personality changes (with or without dementia) as opposed to the lack of organic pathology.

With this parametric assessment it was revealed that amphetamines chronically administered stimulate behavior generally as measured on the arousal parameter. In depressed patients they can produce transient euphoria leading to hyperthymia, which may be replaced by dysthymia (mood parameter). The same substance in the course of chronic administration may produce, on the parameter of mental integration, perceptual disturbances or, more often, thought disorder with delusions; on the affective parameter, anxiety; and on the organicity parameter, personality changes.

By this parametric approach the behavioral inhibition, fatigue (arousal parameter) and the mood-depressant effects of the Rauwolfia alkaloid reserpine have been shown to occur prior to its beneficial action on mental integration in schizophrenics. Thus the action of reserpine was differentiated from that of chlorprothixene (a thioxanthene drug), whose beneficial action on mental integration is preceded by a slight mood-lifting effect.

Other changes observed by this approach were that the anxiolytic effect of benzodiazepines preceded their sedative action in psychoneurotic patients; the stimulating and euphorizing action of MAOI's preceded their antidepressant effect; and the mood-lifting and slightly sedative properties of some of the dibenzoazepine and dibenzocyloheptene preparations preceded their euphorizing action.

Very recently a four-dimensional conceptual model of symptomatological differences in major psychiatric disorders accessible to changes by psychotropic drugs was developed by Overall *et al.* (1967). The model was based on factor analyses of Overall and Gorham's Brief Psychiatric Rating Scale (Overall and Gorham, 1962). This provided four major syndromes. Each of these syndromes was in one end of a bipolar continuum. The opposite pole of the thinking disturbance continuum was dispensed with as inappropriate for consideration among major psychiatric disorders, and the remaining three factor dimensions (*i.e.*, extropunitiveness *versus* intropunitiveness; withdrawal—retardation *versus* agitation—excitement; and depression *versus* elation) have bipolar counterparts. Since the four-dimensional model is suggested as appropriate for characterizing patient differences in major psychiatric disorders, it may become a useful tool in clinical pharmacological studies.

2. Psychometrics

The employment of psychometric tests in clinical pharmacological studies developed in two stages. First an attempt was made to explore the characteristic psychological performance changes effected by the chronic administration of an investigational compound in patients belonging to various diagnostic categories. For this purpose a variety of testing procedures were used which included intelligence determinations, sensory-perceptual tests, simple and complex psychomotor tasks, etc. (Uhr and Miller, 1960; Ban, 1966; and Gallant *et al.*, 1965). Characteristic of this period was that these tests remained isolated measurements of the drug-induced changes and were not integrated into a comprehensive approach to further the understanding of both the action of the drug and the psychopathological condition involved.

In the second stage of development a psychometric test battery, consisting of 12 tests measuring 16 psychological functions, was constructed by Lehmann and Ban (1963). With this it became possible to establish the psychological performance (or rather deficit) profiles of the major psychiatric diagnostic categories (Donald *et al.*, 1964; and Ban, 1966). At the same time an attempt was made to reveal drug treatment-induced changes on these psychological performance profiles.

a. Assessment Methods

Lehmann and Ban's (1963) psychometric battery was the result of careful selection of established psychological tests, which were found to be of value in measuring different psychopathological syndromes. It was designed specifically for clinical use in a wide variety of cases. It took into account the difficulties encountered with long term hospitalized cases; the unmedicated acute patients who are so often irritable, distractable or frightened by complex apparatus; the chronic patients who may be too confused, incoherent or demented to perform a complex task (which has its own significance); and the fact that many psychopathological groups are easily frustrated and fatigued. Considering all these conditions, the tasks had to be simple enough to perform with minimal practice and brief enough so that the total battery could be administered within a relatively short (approximately 60 minutes) period of time.

After careful consideration and systematic exploratory work in the field, Lehmann and Ban's (1963) psychometric battery consisted of the following measurements: *afferent-perceptual tests*—Critical Flicker Fusion Frequency (CFF), Chromatic After Image Disappearance Limen (ADL) and Achromatic Spiral After Effect (SPIR); *central-associative tests*—Word Association Time (WAT), Digits Forward (DF) and Backward (DB), Time Estimation Production (TEP) and Reproduction (TER), Paired Associate Learning (PAL), Ideational Recall (IR) and Cancellation Time (CT) and Error (CE); and *efferent-psychomotor tests*—Auditory Reactions Time (RT), Tapping Speed (TS) and Track Tracer Time (TTT) and Error (TTE).

b. *Psychopathological Profiles*

Test performance (deficit) profiles on this battery were established for the following psychiatric diagnostic categories: behavior disorders (without psychosis); psychoneurotic reactions; manic-depressive psychosis (manic); psychotic depressions (acute and chronic); acute schizophrenic reactions (paranoid and undifferentiated); chronic schizophrenia (simple, paranoid and hebephrenic); and organic brain syndromes (chronic).

The most significant differential performance tendencies for the 11 diagnostic categories are as follows: *behavioral disorders* (without psychosis) showed less over-all psychological performance deficit than any of the other clinical groups. The manifest deficit was seen in the increase of TTE (with good TTT), indicating a loss of control with a maintenance of speed. *Psychoneurotics* manifested more performance deficit than patients with behavior disorders. Besides the increased TTE, they also had a prolonged RT and decreased DF and DB.

In *manic-depressive manics* there was a prominent dissociation among the psychomotor tests. Thus, RT was slightly delayed and TTT was considerably slowed as opposed to the exceptionally fast TS. This dissociation sharply distinguished these patients from *acute psychotic depressives,* who showed a consistent, impaired functioning, *i.e.*, increased RT and decreased TS. In contradistinction to the acute cases, *chronic psychotic depressives* were less impaired in RT and TS but more impaired in TTT, CT and CE. Furthermore, they also showed an increase on WAT, a decrease on PAL and IR, and a significant overestimation of time as reflected in TEP and TER.

Acute undifferentiated schizophrenics were characterized by a slight delay in WAT and RT. TS decreased and TTT and TTE increased simultaneously with impairment of IR. On the other hand, *acute paranoid schizophrenics* showed a slightly raised CFF with a slight increase of WAT, CT and RT and an impairment of PAL.

Chronic paranoid schizophrenics presented a similar psychological performance profile as their acute counterparts. They also had a lower performance on both DF and DB tests. *Chronic simple schizophrenics* differed from the chronic paranoid cases by their higher ADL, lower IR, more delayed RT, fast but inaccurate TTT and TTE and a tendency to overestimate time as reflected in TEP and TER. *Chronic catatonic schizophrenics* differed from the chronic paranoid patients by their slightly impaired SPIR and their tendency to underestimate time (TEP and TER).

In *chronic hebephrenic schizophrenics,* a greater and more generalized disturbance was revealed than in any of the other schizophrenic categories. An extremely high CFF and ADL was coupled with an impairment of SPIR. On the psychomotor tests (RT, TS and TTT), a considerable slowing was seen with relatively few errors on TTE (which resembled the performance of chronic psychotic depressives). Their overestimation of time (TEP and TER) was also similar to this latter group.

In contradistinction to hebephrenics, patients with a *chronic organic brain syndrome* showed low CFF and ADL as well as underestimation of time periods (TEP). WAT, CT and RT were increased; digit span (DF and DB) shortened; and TS, PAL and IR were reduced in this group.

The investigators pointed out the need for further modifications and adjustments of their psychometric battery to sharpen its sensitivity and discriminating power. Their differential findings must be substantiated by further studies before any definite conclusions can be established. Nevertheless, this still remains one of the first systematic attempts to express clinical psychopathology in terms of psychological performances (deficit) and to describe nosological entities in psychometric patterns. The importance of this approach is that it renders subjectively perceived psychopathological manifestations accessible for objective psychological testing. It is perhaps of equal importance that it provides an objective method for clinical psychopharmacological studies. This method may allow for an evaluation of drug effects independent of any particular theoretical frame of reference.

c. Drug-Induced Changes

There are indications that certain psychological performance deficits characteristically present in manics, chronic depressives or in chronic schizophrenics are counteracted by thioproperazine, methotrimeprazine (both phenothiazines) and thiothixene (a thioxanthene derivative), respectively. This has yet to be substantiated by further investigation. There is also some preliminary evidence that the psychological performance deficits present in behavior disorders are counteracted by propericiazine, a piperidylalkylphenothiazine compound.

3. Conditioning

Like the psychometric tests, the use of conditioning procedures in clinical pharmacological studies progressed in two stages. At first an attempt was made to explore the characteristic changes effected by the chronic administration of an investigational compound on various stimulus-response constellations. Findings at this stage were not integrated into a comprehensive approach to further the understanding of both the action of the new drug and the psychopathological condition for which the substance was useful. In the second stage of development, when conditional reflex (CR) test batteries were constructed, it became possible not only to establish the CR test profiles of various psychiatric diagnostic categories but also to reveal the drug treatment-induced changes.

a. Assessment Methods

With the use of comprehensive conditioning procedures, the differential profiles of clinical psychopathological categories have been best shown as differences in the various aspects of orienting behavior, first signal system activity, and second signal system activity.

i. Orienting Behavior. The orienting reflex (OR) was conceived by Razran (1961) as the organism's usual first reaction to any adequate stimulation and has been measured in humans by simultaneous recordings of various autonomic and skeletomuscular variables with plethysmography, electromyography, etc. The OR was originally conceptualized and described, as discussed above, by Pavlov (1928) as an innate investigatory or attitudinal reflex to indifferent stimuli.

Since Pavlov's first description, OR behavior has been extensively studied in behavioral and neurophysiological experiments in both animals and humans. The results of these investigations have been reviewed by Sokolov (1963).

ii. First Signal System Activity. By definition, first signal system activity can be initiated by any external stimulus (excluding verbal or symbolic stimuli) which elicits an unconditional (UR) or conditional reflex (CR).

The ontogenetic development of the CR formation was summarized by Peiper (1963) and Luriia *et al.* (1964). Conditional connections were found to develop in successive stages after birth. The order of their development was explored by Kasatkin (1948, 1955), who established that the CR's to auditory stimuli develop first, followed by the development of conditioned connections to vestibular and thereafter to optic stimuli. Finally, conditioned tactile reflexes are formed. The potential for these conditioned connections is already present in the first half of the second month (Kasatkin, 1955).

As a further stage in the ontogenetic development is conditional stimulus (CS) discrimination. In contradistinction to CR formation, where the CR to an auditory signal precedes the development of the CR to an optical signal, CS discrimination in the visual area (*i.e.*, the differentiation of forms and movements of objects) was found to be present earlier than differentiation in the auditory area.

First signal system activity in general and CR formation (and CS discrimination) in particular are explored via autonomic (salivary secretion), semivoluntary (eye lid closure) and voluntary (finger withdrawal) conditioning techniques.

iii. Second Signal System Activity. In the ontogenesis of man, Pavlov (1927) recognized that signals of a second order were "created, developed and perfected" in the form of spoken, heard or visible words. These new signals (or symbols) marked everything that was immediately observed and noted in the external and internal environment.

Transmission from the first to the second signal system, the relationship between the activity of the first and the second signal system and second signal system activity proper have been extensively studied.

Transmissions from the first (nonverbal) to the second (verbal) signal system was first investigated by Ivanov-Smolensky (1934, 1935), who replaced the primary auditory signal (ringing of a bell) in an established CR with the spoken or the written word "bell" or by the picture of a "bell."

In studying the relationship between first and second signal systems activity, the procedure developed by Krasnogorski (1909, 1925, 1952, 1956) was frequently used. In this procedure, the effects of conflict between the effective first signal system stimulus and the verbal second signal system stimulus was systematically explored.

Second signal system activity proper has been explored by the various semantic conditioning and word-association techniques.

The term semantic conditioning was introduced by Razran (1939), who found that college students conditioned to secrete a well defined amount of saliva at the sight of the words style, urn and surf transferred (generalized) their conditioning more toward fashion, vase and wave than to stile, earn, and serf. Razran's findings were confirmed by Reiss (1946).

Ivanov-Smolensky (1951, 1953) was among the first to use word association techniques in the frame of reference of conditioning and Astrup (1962) used word-association techniques extensively in clinical psychopathology.

b. Psychopathological Profiles

By use of the procedures described, differential "conditioning" profiles have been suggested for the following clinical psychopathological categories: psychoneuroses, manic-depressive psychosis, schizophrenias and organic brain syndromes.

i. Psychoneuroses. Orienting behavior: Among the various diagnostic groups it was demonstrated that psychoneurotics with a high level of anxiety responded more frequently than normals to indifferent stimuli (on the GSR); *i.e.*, their OR was more persistent to extinction.

First signal system activity: Independent of the clinical type in any psychoneuroses (of recent origin), an impairment of the phylogenetically and ontogenetically later developed, internal inhibitory mechanisms was found, *i.e.*, difficulty in extinguishing already established CR's and discriminating between CS's. On the other hand, in chronic psychoneurotic conditions, an inhibition more or less protective in character, *i.e.*, sleep inhibition, was demonstrated.

Second signal system activity: In hysteria disturbance of second signal system activity (with the dominance of the first signal system) was recognized to prevail in contradistinction to obsessive-compulsive neurosis and psychasthenia, in which the first signal system appeared to be more impaired (and consequently the second signal system dominated) (Ivanov-Smolensky, 1927, 1928, 1954; Seredina, 1955; Aleksandrova, 1952; Bokin, 1954; Zachepitsky, 1954; Baranov, 1955; Bokser, 1957; Harzstein, 1957; Monakhov, 1957; Khira, 1958; and Sokolova, 1958).

ii. Manic-Depressive Psychosis. Orienting behavior: The OR was found persistent in manic conditions and absent (or easily extinguished) in depressive states.

First signal system activity: CR formation was revealed to be altered in both phases of this illness. CR formation was found to be slowed in depressives, unlike manics, in whom CR's were seen to be rapidly formed. However, CS discrimination was recognized to be impaired again in both phases and sometimes even during the periods of remission.

Second signal system activity: Transmission from the first to the second signal system was found to be facilitated (or beyond a certain point became impossible) in manic conditions and decreased in depressions. Similarly, word-association time was seen to be decreased in manics and increased in depressives. While the total number of responses decreased in depressions, in manics echolalic, tautological, vague, meaningless responses as well as "clang" associations were increased (Faddeyeva, 1941, 1945, 1947; Ivanov-Smolensky, 1954; Protopopov, 1948, 1952; Moravcsik, 1911; Birnbaum, 1912; Aschaffenburg, 1896, 1904; Astrup, 1962, 1965; and Ban, 1964).

iii. Schizophrenias. Orienting behavior: Like the psychoneurotics, acute schizophrenics responded more frequently than normals to indifferent stimuli (on the GSR), while chronic schizophrenics responded significantly less often (and in a considerable percentage of these cases the OR was absent).

First signal system activity: In a comprehensive study, Astrup (1962) indicated that the absence of some of the UR's and the presence of "dissociative phenomena" are general characteristics of schizophrenic patients. Other characteristics were impaired internal inhibitory mechanisms and inertia (absence of mobility) of the basic nervous processes (*i.e.*, the excitatory and the inhibitory process). Astrup (1962) asserted that the disturbances of the higher nervous activity in schizophrenics can be explained by the principles of autokinesis and schizokinesis, as postulated by Gantt (1953, 1957, 1960). Schizokinesis implies the inherent conflict between emotional and adaptive responses (as reflected in dissociative phenomena), while autokinesis means the ability of the organism to form new patterns of behavior without external stimulation. Protective inhibition (sleep), characteristically present in some schizophrenics, was considered by him to be related to the principle of autokinesis. Other findings in chronic schizophrenics were significantly lower conditionability and CS discrimination (on the GSR) compared with normals.

Second signal system activity: While there is an interference with the transmission from the first to the second signal system, a dominant but pathologically functioning second signal system is a common characteristic of schizophrenics. In semantic conditioning a larger number of phonetographic transfers were found than in normals. It was also revealed that, while word-association time in general was increased, in catatonics the number of verbal responses and in hebephrenics the number of higher (abstract) responses were decreased. In paranoid cases the reply "no" or rejecting responses were more frequent together with egocentric and delusional responses. In simple schizophrenics "yes" replies and tautological and multiword responses were increased. In the acute forms of the illness there were a considerable number of higher reactions, while in chronic cases there was a progressive change from the general abstract to the general concrete. Then there was an increase in individual concrete responses and finally a cessation of higher responses (Ivanov-Smolensky, 1934, 1935, 1951, 1953; Peters and Murphree, 1954; Sinkevich, 1955; Zurabashvilli, 1958; Ban *et al.*, 1964; Astrup, 1962, 1965; Hattengadi *et al.*, 1966; and Cuculic *et al.*, 1967).

iv. Organic Brain Syndromes. Orienting behavior: Absence (or easily extinguishable) OR was characteristic of patients with a chronic organic brain syndrome.

First signal system activity: Both CR formation and CS discrimination were found to be decreased.

Second signal system activity: The transmission from the first to the second signal system was interfered with, and there was a dominance of first signal system activity with prevailing phonetographic transfers in semantic conditioning (Gantt and Muncie, 1942; Apter, 1955; Seredina, 1955; Gasanov, 1955; Lazarova, 1955; Linsky, 1955; Dmitriev, 1957; Astrup, 1962, 1965; and Ban, 1964, 1966).

c. Drug-Induced Changes

Extensive clinical pharmacological studies in which conditioning was used as a measurement of changes were conducted by Astrup (1962, 1965). The first important observation he made was that in cases of manifest psychopathology there were only slight differences in CR activity regardless of whether patients were under the influence of a psychoactive drug; *i.e.*, the changes in CR activity were primarily dependent on the psychiatric condition of the patient and not on the drug he was taking.

This did not mean that psychoactive substances *per se* had no effect whatsoever on CR variables in psychiatric patients. Thus, for example, schizophrenics treated with the Rauwolfia alkaloid reserpine, an antipsychotic substance, showed a stronger inhibition of UR's and gave less adequate responses on the word-association test than their untreated counterparts; or schizophrenics treated with chlorpromazine, a phenothiazine antipsychotic drug, had a stronger inhibition of UR's (while their motor CR's and associative responses were less inhibited) than similar cases not receiving the same drug. However, whatever immediate changes were effected by these substances, they always remained within the actual pathological profile.

In 311 schizophrenic patients treated with chlorpromazine, prochlorperazine, reserpine and other antipsychotic drugs, Astrup (1962) revealed that the decrease in the disturbance of the higher nervous activity and in particular of dissociative pathology paralleled clinical improvement. The best therapeutic results were obtained in the "nonsystematic cases," characterized by a comparatively acute onset but recurrent course of the illness and with only a slight degree of deterioration. On the other hand, the hebephrenic group showed the least therapeutic response. Similar findings were reported by Choi *et al.* (1966), who also noted that the relative maintenance of conditionability in schizophrenics is of predictive value for successful treatment.

In another study, Tirkeltaub (1963) explored the action of the tricyclic antidepressant imipramine on schizophrenic patients. He found "more intense and prolonged" UR's and CR's in the initial period, which were gradually replaced by inhibitory phenomena (together with the clinical worsening).

In contradistinction to this study, Alexander (1961) explored the changes in CR activity in a group of depressed patients under the influence of various MAOI (iproniazid, nialamid, isocarboxazide) and tricyclic antidepressant (imipramine) drugs. He revealed a "decrease" of CR's in cases of therapeutic success and an "increase" in CR's in the therapeutic failures.

More recently, a systematic study has been undertaken in which the conditioning profile of prototype psychoactive substances and the conditioning profiles of various clinical psychopathologies are explored by the same procedures and the same conditioning techniques. Whether comparing the drug-effect profiles with the psychopathological profiles will lead to practical implications and theoretical importance still remains to be answered (Ban, 1966).

4. Neurophysiology

The use of electrophysiological procedures in clinical pharmacological studies progressed in two stages. At first electroencephalographic changes effected by the chronic administration of the investigational compound were explored, while later the specific changes on the characteristic electroencephalographic "profiles" in the various clinical psychopathologies were studied under the influence of therapeutic administration of psychoactive drugs.

a. Assessment Methods

Differential characteristics among the various clinical psychopathological categories have been established by surface electroencephalographic (EEG) recordings, sedation threshold measurements and on the basis of changes in cerebral responsiveness to sensory stimulation (as reflected in evoked potentials).

i. Surface EEG. Surface EEG recordings of spontaneous electrical activity in the study of the variations in different psychopathologies have been extended by "activation" procedures. These include the production of alkalosis (by the administration of alkaline salts or by hyperventilation); hypoglycemia (by giving insulin); hydration (by forcing fluids or vasopressin injection); pharmacological sleep (via secobarbital Na or pentobarbital Na in combination with chloral hydrate); pharmacological excitation (by intravenous administration of pentetrazol or bemegride or by applying stroboscopy, *i.e.*, exposing the eyes to light flashes of variable frequency). In stroboscopy, within a certain range the frequency of the alpha activity in the occipital region adjusts itself to the flash rate (Walter *et al.*, 1946). This is frequently referred to as "driving" of the EEG.

ii. Sedation Threshold. Another technique frequently used in the differentiation of clinical psychopathological categories is the sedation threshold (Shagass, 1954). This is based on the administration of sodium amobarbital (0.5 mg./kg. every 40 seconds) until well past the point at which speech becomes slurred. Simultaneously the "amount" of 17 to 25 cycles per second activity recorded from the frontal areas on the electroencephalogram is measured. The curve obtained is "S" shaped and shows an "inflection point" corresponding roughly with the onset of slurred speech, beyond which the additional "amount" of fast activity produced by further increments of the drug is sharply diminished. The sedation threshold is defined as the amount of amobarbital sodium in milligrams per kilogram of body weight required to reach this "inflection point."

iii. Cerebral Responsiveness. In the past few years, Shagass *et al.*, (1961, 1964) have attempted to differentiate between the various clinical psychopathological categories on the basis of changes in cerebral responsiveness to sensory stimulation (as reflected in evoked potentials on the EEG). They used a photographic averager (built by Shipton, 1960), which was later replaced by a Memotron Computer of Average Transients (CAT). This sophisticated instrumentation made it possible to compare the beginning and the recovery, *i.e.*, the reactivity cycle of somatosensory responses in normals and psychiatric patients (Shagass and Schwartz, 1961, 1962). More recently, the "intensity-response gradient," another measure of cerebral responsiveness, has been investigated (Shagass and Schwartz, 1963). This was conceived as the curve which described the increase in response amplitude as a function of stimulus intensity.

b. *Psychopathological Profiles*

With the use of the procedures described, differential profiles for the following clinical psychopathological categories have been suggested: psychoneuroses, personality disorders, manic-depressive psychosis, schizophrenias and organic brain syndromes.

i. Psychoneuroses. Neurotics frequently show a generalized theta rhythm and fast activity (more than 13 c/s) with an amplitude rarely as high as that of the alpha rhythm. In anxiety states a relatively high incidence of low voltage fast, or beta activity and a lesser incidence of well organized alpha activity, *i.e.*, a decreased alpha index, was seen. Photic stimulation showed less "driving" than in normals within the 8 to 10 c/s range but more driving with slower than 8 c/s and higher than 10 c/s frequencies (Ulett, 1957). A stable alpha rhythm was described as characteristic of hysterical patients, and high (4.78 mg./kg.) sedation threshold was found to be characteristic of neurotic depressive cases.

ii. Personality Disorders. In some children with behavior disorders, an excess of slow activity is not an infrequent finding. This is either diffuse, or predominant in the temporal region, sometimes asymmetrically present. In the latter cases, the slow theta or delta activities are seen mainly on the left side. Similarly, in adults with personality disorders, an excess of bilateral rhythmical theta activity with an amplitude usually equal to, but sometimes greater than, that of the alpha rhythm is the commonest single finding. This theta activity is usually predominant in the temporal and the central areas, shows no blocking response to visual stimulation and is accentuated by overbreathing. In aggressive psychopathy an asymmetrical slow (3.5 c/s) activity in the posterior temporal region, more on the right than on the left side, can often be observed.

On the basis of electroencephalographic findings, Hill (1952) differentiated among three types of personality disorders. In one group there was an excess of bilateral theta activity. Another group consisted of patients with alpha rhythm variants with harmonic, particularly subharmonic, components; and in a third group episodic posterior temporal slow wave focal discharges were characteristic. It was also revealed that all of these abnormalities have a tendency not only to diminish but even to disappear with advancing age, often concomitantly with a behavioral improvement.

In studies of somatosensory cortical reactivity, patients with personality disorders and schizophrenics were clearly distinguishable from psychoneurotics and normals, but indistinguishable from one another. That is, whereas peak ratios of 1.0 or more were attained within the first 20 milliseconds by 80 per cent of normals and 74 per cent of psychoneurotics, this recovery level was reached only in 19 per cent of the patients with personality disorders and 10 per cent of schizophrenics (Shagass and Schwartz, 1962).

iii. Manic-Depressive Psychosis. A common characteristic of many manic-depressive patients is their low alpha index when compared with normals. On the other hand, beta activity in these cases is more prominent than in normals. In manics, mixed alpha and fast activity patterns with an alpha frequency of 10 c/s or faster is seen, while in depressives there is usually a mixed alpha and slow activity pattern with alpha frequencies of 10 c/s or slower.

In sedation threshold (Shagass, 1954) determination, it was recognized that, while normals had a sedation threshold of 3 mg./kg., and neurotics (including neurotic depressives) had 4.8 mg./kg., the sedation threshold of endogenous depressives was 2.8 mg./kg., and of manics, 3.5 mg./kg.

iv. Schizophrenias. According to Kennard *et al.* (1955), the EEG of schizophrenics is different from that of normals. The essential difference is the relative excess of fast activity. The average frequency of the alpha rhythm was found near the upper limit, and low voltage alpha waves were seen to be "overlaid" by increased beta activity. Furthermore, a record dominated by low voltage irregular fast activity, described by Davis (1941) as "choppy activity," is frequently reported in schizophrenics. Of the different schizophrenic conditions, in catatonic stupor the normal electroencephalographic rhythm is often replaced by generalized low amplitude 2 to 6 c/s activity. Walter (1942) revealed diffuse delta activity during catatonic episodes, and in periodic catatonia, during the acute phase, he found a high incidence of slow wave discharges in the theta and delta ranges.

It was found that schizophrenics sometimes respond to environmental stimulation only "electroencephalographically" without behavioral changes, while on other occasions their EEG response to visual stimuli, emotional disturbances or mental tasks is absent.

The use of intravenous pentetrazole combined with photic stimulation to elicit the photoconvulsive response was developed by Gastaut (1950). This photometrazol threshold was found to be low in schizophrenics (Leffman and Perlo, 1955), particularly in catatonics (Bickford, 1951; Ulett *et al.* 1953; and Leiberman *et al.*, 1954). Other findings in schizophrenics are bilateral synchronous beta and/or theta activity after intravenous thiopental administration (Goldman, 1960); a relatively low (2.7 mg./kg.) sedation threshold in the acute and a relatively high (4.27 mg./kg.) sedation threshold in the chronic stage of the illness (Shagass, 1954); and altered recovery functions of primary somatosensory responses as revealed by evoked potential techniques (Shagass and Schwartz, 1963).

v. Organic Brain Syndromes. Differential effects in acute and in chronic brain syndromes are seen. In acute brain syndromes with delirium, disorganization of the existing electroencephalographic pattern and reorganization at a lower energy level are the characteristic features. In chronic brain syndromes with prevailing dementia, on the other hand, irregularities in the background activity and interrupted or low voltage alpha rhythms are dominating. Thus, in senile dementia to a lesser extent and in arteriosclerotic dementia more prominently, the frequency, amplitude and percentage time of the alpha rhythm were found to be reduced and the amount of fast activity increased. In Pick's and Alzheimer's disease, generalized low to medium amplitude, irregular theta frequencies with little or no alpha rhythm are characteristic.

The sedation threshold in organic psychoses was found to be (1.9 mg./kg.), the lowest among all the various clinical categories tested.

c. Drug-Induced Changes

The characteristic EEG changes in the course of chronic administration of various psychopharmacological substances were summarized by Müller and Müller (1965). Various antipsychotic substances, *e.g.*, Rauwolfias, phenothiazines and butyrophenones, produce slowing of the EEG in contrast to the fast activity seen with anxiolytic drugs, *e.g.*, propanediols or benzodiazepines. Antidepressive drugs, both the tricyclic and MAOI types, were described as having a slowing effect, although at times they can produce mild accelerations. These drug-induced changes were considered to be independent of the psychopathological symptoms (or electrophysiological manifestations) present prior to treatment with the substance.

However, Bente (1963) revealed that the effect of drugs on the EEG is dependent upon the pretreatment EEG pattern. Thus, for example, he recognized a decrease of phenothiazine-induced EEG changes whenever a manic syndrome manifests itself clinically.

Of the few studies where EEG indices were used in parallel with the clinical assessment, those of Goldman (1960) and Shagass and Schwartz (1962) are of utmost importance. In Goldman's study (1960), the characteristic changes induced in schizophrenics by intravenous thiopental administration became less marked in the course of successful treatment with antipsychotic phenothiazine drugs, but reoccurred with full intensity during a relapse. These findings were confirmed by Mowrer *et al.* (1961). In the investigations of Shagass and Schwartz (1962), the tricyclic antidepressant imipramine changed the recovery function of the cortex and the amplitude of the evoked responses in the direction toward the normal in depressed (also in some paranoid) patients. This normalization corresponded with clinical improvement.

The importance of the pretreatment EEG pattern in clinical pharmacological studies cannot be sufficiently emphasized. It has been noted, for example, that the tricyclic antidepressant imipramine increased the amplitude of cortical evoked responses to sciatic nerve stimulation in the rabbit (Van Meter *et al.*, 1959) as well as in normal subjects (at least at high stimulus intensities). On the other hand, in depressions, in which the amplitude of evoked potentials is usually high, the improvement of symptoms affected by the same substance is accompanied by reduced—instead of increased—amplitude of evoked potentials. This led Shagass *et al.* (1962) to conclude that the "neurophysiological situation" in a depressed human is not the same as in one who is not depressed. The same may also apply to the biochemical or "neurochemical situation." On the basis of this, one may infer that the distinctly different neurophysiological effects of psychoactive substances in psychiatric patients (or in the various clinical psychopathologies) are the result of these differentially altered "neurophysiological" and "neurochemical situations."

5. Biochemistry

One of the first indications that the etiology of certain psychiatric disorders may be due to a biochemical disturbance was the identification of the antipellagra vitamin, nicotinamide. Rapid and dramatic improvement of both the physical and psychopathological manifestations of pellagra patients treated with nicotinamide indicated that psychiatric symptoms can result from a relative deficiency of a chemical substance (nicotinamide) in the organism and also that at least certain psychopathological manifestations can be adequately treated psychopharmacologically (Woolley, 1962).

Since this early work in the nineteen thirties, considerable progress has been made. In the past 10 years particular interest has been paid to the functional psychopathologies, and as a result some interesting data and working hypotheses have been elaborated on the biochemical mechanisms involved in schizophrenia and manic-depressive conditions.

Kety (1967) defined a good hypothesis as one which is plausible, capable of explaining the phenomena parsimoniously and heuristic; has predictive value and remains compatible with the new data that becomes available; and which can be modified in line with the new information without losing its parsimonious qualities (Himwich *et al.*, 1967).

While the biochemical basis of functional psychoses is not yet completely understood, biochemical indices measurable in the blood and in the urine (occasionally in the spinal fluid) are being increasingly investigated. Among these indices, neurohormone determinations, electrolyte assessments and several other biochemical measurements are frequently studied.

a. Neurohormones

The catecholamines (particularly dopamine and norepinephrine) and serotonin are important in this category from a clinical pharmacological point of view.

i. Catecholamines. *α. Psychopathological Basic Data.* The role of catecholamines in various clinical psychopathologies was recently reviewed by Bergsman (1959) and by Kety (1966). Kety summarized the early work of Euler (1931, 1946, 1952, 1954), in whose laboratories the fluorometric technique was developed, enabling him to measure the excretion of epinephrine (E) and norepinephrine (NE). Euler (1956) was among the first to demonstrate a significant increase in excretion of these substances under a variety of stresses, including gravitational change and muscular work. Correlations between NE excretion and aggressive states were revealed by Elmadjian *et al.* (1957) and later confirmed by Silverman and Cohen (1960). Finally the E release in uncertain and unpredictable situations was recognized by Euler (1964).

While Manger *et al.* (1957) could not find any difference in plasma catecholamine levels between patients with various psychopathology and normals, Pscheidt *et al.* (1964) reported elevated urinary excretions of both E, NE and vanilmandelic acid (VMA) in schizophrenics during acute psychotic exacerbation of their illness. Similar findings were obtained by Gjessing (1964), who in periodic catatonic patients recognized a marked elevation in urinary excretion of VMA, metanephrine and normetanephrine during their psychotic episodes, reversing to normal in the symptom-free interval.

In affective psychoses a higher excretion of E and NE was demonstrated in the manic than in the retarded depressive phase of manic-depressive psychosis by Ström-Olsen and Weil-Malherbe (1958). These findings were supported by Bergsman (1959) and Shinfuku *et al.* (1961). On the other hand, in senile psychosis a significant decrease in the urinary excretion of E was revealed.

β. Psychopathological Hypotheses. There are two catecholamine hypotheses relevant to psychopathology: the so-called catecholamine hypothesis of schizophrenia and the catecholamine hypothesis of affective disorders.

The catecholamine hypothesis of schizophrenia was put forward by Harley-Mason *et al.* (1952). It is based on the chemical relationship between mescaline and NE, which suggested that schizophrenia might be associated with an abnormality of *o*-methylation of NE, with the consequent production of some psychotoxic metabolites, such as dimethoxyphenylethanolamine, in the body (Smythies, 1967).

The catecholamine hypothesis of affective disorders was formulated by Schildkraut (1965). It is based on the recognition that those drugs which cause depletion and inactivation of NE centrally produce sedation or depression, while drugs which increase or potentiate NE are associated with behavioral stimulation or excitement and generally have an antidepressant effect in man. These findings suggested that some, if not all, depressions may be associated with a relative deficiency of NE at functionally important adrenergic receptor sites in the brain, whereas elevated mood may be associated with an excess of such amines (Schildkraut and Kety, 1967).

γ. Supporting Data. Supporting data for the catecholamine hypothesis of schizophrenia was provided by Kety (1967). He elaborated upon the notion that an alteration in biological transmethylation results in the production of abnormal methylated products (as mescaline itself is a threefold methylated congener of the normal metabolite, dopamine, which plays a crucial role in some forms of schizophrenia). The catecholamine hypothesis of schizophrenia predicted a methylation of catecholamines (which has only recently been demonstrated by Axelrod *et al.*, 1961) and the importance of 3,4-dimethoxyphenylethylamine (DMPEA) in schizophrenia. It was only 10 years later that the latter substance, which is the result of the methylation of both phenolic hydroxyl groups of catecholamines, was detected in the urine of schizophrenics (Friedhoff and Van Winkle, 1962). More recently, Faurbye and Pind (1966) reported that the compound found by Friedhoff and Van Winkle (1962) is not identical with 3,4-dimethoxyphenylethylamine but is identical with the compound demonstrated by Takessada *et al.* (1963), which is found in the urine of both schizophrenics and normals. The basis of Faurbye and Pind's (1966) assertion was that the spot of the Friedhoff and Van Winkle compound did not coincide with the spot of added authentic 3,4-dimethoxyphenylethylamine when the urine was applied to thin layer chromatography. Furthermore, Perry *et al.* (1967) have not found DMPEA in the urine of either normals or schizophrenic patients on plant-free diets. However, Friedhoff and Van Winkle's (1962) assertion was confirmed by Kuehl (1964, 1967) and Bourdillon and Ridges (1967).

Supporting data for the catecholamine hypothesis of affective disorder are primarily based on the psychopharmacological studies which demonstrated changes in serotonin levels and have shown a consistent relationship between the effects of drugs on catecholamines, particularly NE, and affective states (Schildkraut, 1965). Tetrabenazine and reserpine both produce sedation and sometimes clinical depression. They also cause depletion of both brain indoleamines (serotonin) and catecholamines. However, it was shown that administration of the catecholamine precursor dihydroxyphenylalanine will reverse reserpine sedation and restore normal behavior in animals, while administration of the indoleamine precursor 5-hydroxytryptophan does not (Carlsson *et al.*, 1957). Other evidence in favor of the catecholamine hypothesis is that the behavioral excitation following administration of MAOI drugs bears a better temporal relationship to the rise in brain NE than to the increase in brain serotonin (Spector *et al.*, 1963); that tricyclic antidepressants, *e.g.*, imipramine, inhibit the uptake of NE in the brain (Glowinski and Axelrod, 1964); and that in animals partially depleted of catecholamines by α-methylmetatyrosine, imipramine will not prevent reserpine sedation (Sulser *et al.*, 1964). Against the catecholamine hypothesis is the observation that the only effect produced by microinjection of amines into various sites in the brain is inhibition. Kety (1967), however, maintains that "it is not impossible that selective inhibition could result in stimulation." Furthermore, according to him, microinjection does not constitute a crucial test, since it may not exactly simulate the manner by which these substances are actually released nor act at the same sites in the nervous system.

δ. Psychopharmacological Implications. Psychopharmacological experimental and clinical data are in favor of the catecholamine-transmethylation hypothesis of schizophrenia and of the catecholamine hypothesis of affective disorder. An important aspect of the experimental data is the finding of

Pollin *et al.* (1961) that feeding a methyl donor, *e.g.*, methionine to schizophrenics, aggravated their clinical symptoms. This was confirmed by Alexander *et al.* (1963) and further developed by Brune and Himwich (1962), who were able to aggravate schizophrenic psychopathology by the administration of betaine, another methyl donor of a different chemical family. On the other hand, Hoffer *et al.* (1957) suggested the beneficial effect of the methyl acceptor niacin and niacinamide in the treatment of schizophrenics. Both of these substances may reduce the occurrence of 3,4-dimethoxyphenylethylamine excretion in these patients.

The psychopharmacological implications of the catecholamine hypothesis of affective disorders can be inferred from a number of pharmacological experiments. For example, both MAOI and tricyclic antidepressants have been found to decrease the urinary excretion of VMA (Studnitz, 1959; and Schildkraut *et al.*, 1964) in clinical pharmacological studies. Schildkraut (1967) was also able to demonstrate that with the decrease of VMA there is an increase in normetanephrine excretion in the course of imipramine treatment. This increase of normetanephrine excretion in patients treated with imipramine paralleled clinical improvement.

Since most VMA is derived from NE (intracellular deamination by mitochondrial MAO), the decrease of VMA in patients treated with MAOI drugs (Schildkraut, 1967) may be attributed to the chemical inhibition of the enzyme. Furthermore, Schildkraut (1967) hypothesized that the decrease of VMA in the course of imipramine treatment is the result of the decreased membrane permeability produced by this substance which might limit the access of NE to mitochondrial MAO. The gradual rise in normetanephrine during the period of clinical improvement was considered to be the result of the inhibition (produced by imipramine) of the cellular re-uptake of NE, which consequently results in a larger fraction of NE metabolized to normetanephrine.

ii. Serotonin. *α. Psychopathological Basic Data.* The role of hydroxyindoles in general and serotonin (5-HT) in particular in the various clinical psychopathologies was summarized by Benda (1959), Smythies (1960), Sprince (1961) and more recently by Garattini and Valzelli (1965). In these reviews differential values of plasma 5-HT levels (Paasonen *et al.*, 1957, 1962; Jus *et al.*, 1958; and Feldstein *et al.*, 1959) and differential values of urinary hydroxyindole concentrations (Kety, 1959; Price *et al.*, 1957; and Tissot, 1961) were given for schizophrenic and manic-depressive patients.

While serotonin levels in the majority of schizophrenic patients are within normal limits, there is at least one subgroup in which high values of serotonin (in the platelets) have been observed (Pare *et al.*, 1958). Similarly high values have been detected by Schain and Freedman (1961) in autistic children, in contradistinction to phenylketonuric and other mentally subnormal children (Berendes *et al.*, 1958; and Baldridge *et al.*, 1959). With regards to the urinary concentration, this remains unchanged in the majority of schizophrenics (Rodnight, 1956). However, there is at least one subgroup of patients that is characterized by decreased urinary 5-HT excretion (Fischer *et al.*, 1961). A similar reduction in urinary 5-HT excretion was recognized by Perry *et al.* (1964) in phenylketonuric children. On the other hand, in the study of the urinary excretion of 5-hydroxyindoleacetic acid (5-HIAA), the end product of serotonin catabolism, three groups of schizophrenics could be clearly differentiated on the basis of normal, decreased or increased urinary elimination of this substance. These three groups did not correspond to the traditional schizophrenic subcategories, although a consistently increased excretion was demonstrated in a group of catatonic schizophrenic patients by Buscaino and Stefanachi (1958). (A reduced 5-HIAA excretion was found in various mental subnormalities, including mongoloid and phenylketonuric children, by Jerome *et al.*, 1960.) Other alterations in the urinary excretion of hydroxyindoles in schizophrenics are that in general more indoles, and particularly hydroxyindoles, are detected in the urine of these patients than in normal control groups and that they may excrete 6-hydroxyskatole.

A possible relationship between tryptophan metabolism and depression was suggested by Aschcroft and Sharman (1960). They found a lowered concentration of 5-hydroxyindoles in the cerebrospinal fluid of depressed patients than in normal controls. Rodnight (1961) was first to recognize that the excretion of tryptamine was significantly reduced in these cases. This was recently confirmed by Coppen *et al.* (1965). Simultaneously with the reduced excretion of tryptamine, the excretion of xanthurenic acid was found to be increased (Cazzullo, 1966), which suggests that during depression tryptophan is metabolized to a greater extent along the kynurenine pathway. Furthermore, a decreased excretion of 5-HIAA in depressed patients was demonstrated by Pare and Sandler (1959) and, more recently, by Praag and Leijnse (1963) (Richter, 1967).

β. Psychopathological Hypotheses. There are two serotonin hypotheses relevant to psychopathology: the serotonin hypothesis of schizophrenia and the serotonin hypothesis of affective disorders.

The serotonin hypothesis of schizophrenia was put forward by Gaddum (1954) and by Woolley and Shaw (1954). It is based on the pharmacological antagonism between LSD and 5-HT, which suggested that schizophrenia might be associated with some abnormality of serotonin metabolism (Smythies, 1967).

The serotonin hypothesis of affective disorders has recently been reviewed by Richter (1967). It is based on the recognition that those drugs which cause depletion and inactivation of 5-HT centrally produce sedation or depression, while drugs which increase or potentiate 5-HT are associated with behavioral stimulation or excitement and generally have an antidepressant effect in man. These findings suggested that some, if not all, depressions might be associated with a relative deficiency of 5-HT at functionally important serotonergic receptor sites in the brain, whereas elations might be associated with an excess of such amines.

γ. Supporting Data. Supporting data for the serotonin hypothesis of schizophrenia was provided by Szara (1967), who discovered the psychotomimetic properties of the *N*-methyl derivatives of tryptamine and its analogues. According to him, there might be an abnormal *N*-methylating process in schizophrenia, with the production in the body of psychotoxic metabolites such as dimethyltryptamine. Furthermore, it was suggested that a compound like serotonin can be both *N*-methylated and *O*-methylated to yield a substance like 5-methoxy-*N*,*N*-dimethyltryptamine, a very potent disrupter of conditioned avoidance behavior in the rat (Smythies, 1967). Other supporting evidence for the serotonin hypothesis in schizophrenia was provided by Brune and Himwich (1963), who were able to demonstrate that some schizophrenics showed a striking increase in excretion of tryptamine and other tryptophan metabolites "during outbursts of psychotic behavior." The large increase in the excretion of tryptamine was accompanied by a smaller increase in indolylacetic acid, 5-hydroxyindolylacetic acid and creatinine. These findings were confirmed by Berlet *et al.* (1967), who also reported an increase in tryptamine excretion with the exacerbation of schizophrenic psychopathology. This was integrated into the transmethylation hypothesis by Kety (1967).

Supporting the serotonin hypothesis of affective disorders are primarily the psychopharmacological studies, which, while indicating changes in catecholamine levels, have also shown a relationship between the effects of these drugs on brain serotonin levels and affective states. It has been suggested that the sedation, or depressant action, of reserpine in animals might be due to the release of 5-HT rather than of catecholamines since "reserpine produces neither release of serotonin nor sedation in animals that have been previously stressed" (Brodie, 1960).

δ. Psychopharmacological Implications. Important findings are those of Sprince (1967), who reported the activation of the schizophrenic process by methionine loads. This activation of psychopathology paralleled an increase in tryptamine excretion. Prior to this, Pollin *et al.* (1961) had shown that the administration of tryptophan together with a MAOI produced an apparent activation of behavior in some patients.

In therapeutic clinical studies Pare and Sandler (1959) at first failed to observe any alleviation of depressive symptoms in patients treated with 5-hydroxytryptophan and iproniazid, a MAOI antidepressant drug. Similarly, Kline *et al.* (1964) questioned the effect of this treatment in spite of the fact that they were able to produce rapid alleviation of depression by the injection of 5-hydroxytryptophan, the precursor of 5-HT alone. However, Coppen *et al.* (1963), in a carefully controlled clinical trial, found that treatment with tryptophan together with tranylcypromine, a MAOI antidepressant drug, produced a striking improvement in depressive symptoms. These findings were confirmed by Pare (1963), who also obtained alleviation of depression by administering tryptophan and iproniazid.

b. Electrolytes

i. Psychopathological Basic Data. There has been great interest in the role of minerals (particularly sodium and potassium) in the various psychopathologies since the publication of Schottstaedt *et al.*'s (1956) report, which suggested that periods of depression are accompanied by a decreased urinary excretion of Na. However, it was only after the application of isotope dilution techniques to measure exchangeable Na and K that it was possible to demonstrate a significant dimunition of Na (but not of K) in those patients who responded to treatment, in contradistinction to those who did not (Gibbons *et al.*, 1960). In view of these findings, systematic investigations commenced (Coppen, 1960). With the isotope dilution technique they were able to demonstrate that both exchangeable and residual, intracellular and bone Na levels (but not K levels) are elevated in depressed patients, falling toward the normal in the course of recovery (Coppen *et al.*, 1962). This fall was more significant with the residual than with the exchangeable Na. Similar findings, *i.e.*, elevated exchangeable Na levels, were obtained in manics with a shift (decrease) to normal values in the course of recovery. Thus it was suggested that, for Na metabolism at least, the same mechanisms are in operation in both depressive and manic states (Coppen, 1965).

ii. Psychopharmacological Implications. The clinical psychopharmacological implications of these findings have been explored in relation to lithium treatment. Lithium treatment for manics was first suggested by Cade (1949). However, it was not until 1955 that the effect of lithium on the Na transport mechanism (across frog skin) was demonstrated by Zerahn (1955). When lithium is replaced by Na in the extracellular fluid, it produces action potentials in nerve and muscle.

Lithium has been used for approximately 20 years in psychiatric treatment with questionable success. In recent reviews of the literature, Maggs (1963) and Schou (1967) restated its usefulness in manic patients, and Hartigan (1963) indicated its possible usefulness also in the treatment of depressive conditions. Lithium acts in these conditions by competing with Na in the Na transport mechanism across membranes (Coppen *et al.*, 1965). Thus the therapeutic action of lithium in both manic and depressive conditions is considered to be the result of the decrease in residual Na brought about by the interference with the exchange of Na across the cell membrane.

c. Other Biochemical Indices

Among the various other biochemical measurements used in clinical psychopharmacological studies are nitrogen, cholesterol, calcium and steroid determinations.

i. Nitrogen. The relationship between nitrogen (N) metabolism and psychopathology was first recognized by Gjessing (1932). He was first to describe and intensively explore the condition he called periodic catatonia (Gjessing, 1932, 1935, 1938, 1939, 1960, 1961, 1963, 1964), which has become a recognized subgroup of the schizophrenias.

Recently the concept of periodic catatonia was reviewed by Minde (1966). He pointed out the correlation between changes in N metabolism, autonomic disturbances and the occurrence of varied psychopathological manifestations. All the patients diagnosed as periodic catatonics given a constant diet containing 8,000 to 11,000 mg. of N per day stored approximately 10 per cent of their daily N intake (positive N balance) until they had a reservoir of 15,000 to 30,000 mg. of N. This excess of N was then suddenly excreted (negative N balance) within a few days. On the basis of the relationship between maximum N excretion and psychic disturbances, Gjessing (1963) subdivided periodic catatonia into three subtypes. Type A showed a positive N balance during the interval between the psychic disturbance phase and was characteristic of the stuporous patient; type C had a positive N balance during the active psychic disturbance reaction phase and was characteristic of the excited patients; and type B remained in between the two in respect to the timing of the positive N balance, although it also included excited cases.

It is of psychopharmacological significance that N retention and excretion can be successfully interfered with by forcefully depleting the body of its stored N by the administration of thyroid hormone. Furthermore, thyroxine administration instituted at the proper time during the cycle stops all further periods of disturbances. On the other hand, discontinuation of thyroxine treatment brings about exacerbation of the illness.

ii. Cholesterol. Cholesterol was one of the first lipids to be measured and has been considered of special interest as an index of metabolic activity (Sourkes, 1962). Wertlake *et al.* (1958) recognized that in university students serum cholesterol levels were elevated at examination time. Furthermore, Friedman and Rosenman (1959) demonstrated that the mean serum cholesterol level was distinctly higher in subjects with intense ambition, competitive drive, constant preoccupation with occupational deadlines and a sense of time urgency than in subjects without these character traits. This was confirmed by Sloane *et al.* (1961).

Serum cholesterol levels in various psychopathologies were reviewed by Bloor (1943), Sperry (1954) and Richter (1957). Characteristically high cholesterol levels were suggested in manic-depressive psychosis and low cholesterol levels in schizophrenics (Eaton and Muntz, 1947). On the basis of their cholesterol concentration, schizophrenics with elevated, reduced or normal cholesterol values could be differentiated (McFarland and Goldstein, 1939; and Peters and Van Slyke, 1946).

The variations of free and total serum cholesterol in patients treated with psychoactive drugs (including prochlorperazine, chlorpromazine, fluphenazine, trifluoperazine, thiopropazate, methocarbamol, promazine and methoxypromazine) were reported by Denber and Teller (1966). They found the following pattern in a considerable percentage of patients: a period of little variation for 3 to 6 weeks, followed by a second period, 2 to 6 weeks, of extreme variations usually above the initial levels with changes of more than 30 mg. per cent and often over 100 mg. per cent within 1 week; finally in the third period, 6 to 12 weeks, there was little or decreasing variation. Denber and Teller (1966) revealed that in a considerable percentage of cases there was an increase of both free and total serum cholesterol levels under treatment (they excluded liver damage). Whether the changes in serum cholesterol levels under the influence of psychoactive, particularly of antipsychotic, drugs are correlated with changes in clinical psychopathology still remains to be seen.

iii. Calcium. Changes in calcium (Ca) metabolism in various clinical psychopathologies attracted interest since Flach *et al.* (1960) in a preliminary study suggested that recovery from depression, either as a result of imipramine or electroconvulsive therapy, is associated with a decrease of urinary Ca levels. Prior to this, Gour and Chaudhry (1957) had studied Ca metabolism in various clinical psychopathologies, and Coirault *et al.*, (1959) suggested variations in blood Ca concentrations (and also in 24 hours urinary Ca excretion) in the course of electroshock therapy or treatment with antidepressants.

In a systematic study with 57 patients,

Flach (1964) demonstrated a significant decrease in urinary Ca excretion in those depressed or paranoid schizophrenics who responded to imipramine or ECT treatment. On the other hand, no change in urinary Ca excretion was detected in other diagnostic groups, *e.g.*, psychoneurotics, or even within the depressives and paranoid schizophrenics who are therapeutic failures. Other common features between paranoid schizophrenics and depressives had been suggested by Böszörményi-Nagy and Gerty (1955) on the basis of "phosphorylation mechanisms."

iv. Sterolds. The psychic concomitants of changes in the 17-hydroxycorticoid supply were first recognized in the course of endocrinological disorders such as Cushing's syndrome, which is associated with an increased secretion of adrenal corticoids (especially 17-hydroxycorticoids), and Addison's disease, which is associated with a deficiency of adrenal cortical hormones (Rome and Robinson, 1959). In spite of the fact that in the former condition there is an overabundance and in the latter a deficiency of adrenal cortical hormones, Bleuler (1954) and Reiss (1958) asserted that there is no difference in the various psychiatric syndromes encountered in these two illnesses. However, Cleghorn (1957, 1965) believes that careful psychopathological appraisal and psychological testing would reveal differential characteristics. In contradistinction to the studies in which the psychological concomitants of altered adrenal cortical activity were explored, a superb review on adrenal cortical activity in pathological emotional states was presented by Rubin and Mandell (1966).

Adrenal cortical activity has been systematically investigated in psychoneurotic conditions, in the schizophrenias and in affective disorders. In *psychoneurotic* reactions a directly proportionate relationship was found between plasma (and also urinary) 17-hydroxycorticoid concentrations and anxiety levels by Persky *et al.* (1956, 1958, 1959, 1962), which was confirmed by Curtis *et al.* (1960) and Fiorica and Muehl (1962).

While plasma and urinary corticoid concentrations did not differ significantly in normals and schizophrenics (Altschule 1953; Bliss *et al.*, 1955; Smith *et al.*, 1956; Romanoff *et al.*, 1957; and Coppen *et al.*, 1967), in longitudinal investigations Rey *et al.*, (1961) and Sachar *et al.* (1963) discovered that during the exacerbation of schizophrenic psychopathology there is an increase in glucocorticoid and 17-hydroxycorticoid excretion.

Studies in affective disorders (depressions and manic-depressive reactions) generally revealed increased corticoid production and excretion in depression and a reduction of the production and excretion during mania (Rubin and Mandell, 1966). Thus, increased corticoid levels were seen in depressive cases by Bryson and Martin (1954), Board *et al.* (1956, 1957), Gibbons and McHugh (1963), Kurland (1964) and Bunney and Fawcett (1965); and decreased corticoid levels in manics, by Rizzo *et al.* (1954), Bryson and Martin (1954) and Bunney and Fawcett (1965). However, Bliss *et al.* (1956) reported on one manic patient whose 17-hydroxycorticoid level was elevated.

In psychopharmacological studies it has been shown that an intravenously administered test dose of hydrocortisone was cleared significantly faster in anxious patients than in normals (Persky *et al.*, 1956) and that during the period of lowered steroid output in manics ACTH challenge raised output to normal levels, indicating a normal adrenal responsivity in these patients (Rizzo *et al.*, 1954). More recently, the therapeutic value of cortisone, a substance with definite psychotomimetic properties, was recognized in Addison's disease. When plasma 11-hydroxycorticosteroid levels were used as indices for therapeutic changes under the influence of psychoactive drugs (or convulsive treatment), it was demonstrated that only the evening (but not the morning) plasma levels corresponded with the clinical state of the patients (Brooksbank and Coppen, 1967).

There are a number of other biochemical indices with clinical psychopharmacological significance. Among them are magnesium (Mg), free fatty acid, and ribonucleic acid (RNA). Magnesium plasma concentration has been seen to increase in the course of lithium treatment (Nielsen, 1964); free fatty acid levels were shown to correspond with psychological changes (Cleghorn *et al.*, 1967); and brain RNA concentrations (of which there is no direct measurement as yet in humans) are suggested to be inversely related to memory disturbances (Cameron *et al.*, 1964). It has been recognized that RNA concentration of cells in humans increases up to the age of 40 and decreases thereafter, paralleling the functional abilities of learning and memory in man. Cameron *et al.* (1966) have been treating patients with memory disturbances by giving RNA itself or magnesium pemoline, a substance which supposedly facilitates RNA formation, with questionable success.

B. ADVERSE EFFECTS

Besides the recognition of therapeutic actions, the detection of adverse effects and of contraindications is the other major task of the clinical pharmacological investigation.

1. Adverse Reactions

According to Hollister (1964), both drug-specific and person-specific factors may play a role in the production of adverse effects. He lists chemical structure, route of administration, dosage and duration of treatment and use of adjuvants as drug-related factors and considers age, heredity, atopic history, race, sex and other concurrent illness or treatment as person-specific factors.

Adverse effects with psychoactive substances were succinctly summarized by Caffey *et al.* (1966). They described the adverse reactions to antipsychotic, anti-anxiety (anxiolytic) and antidepressant drugs under the following headings: behavioral, central or autonomic nervous system, allergic or toxic and miscellaneous.

a. Behavioral

Adverse behavioral effects to psychoactive drugs are of particular psychopharmacological significance. Hollister (1965) further subdivided them into five different types of characteristic reactions.

Schizophrenia-like reactions can be produced with large doses of stimulants such as amphetamines or amphetamine-like drugs, *e.g.*, methylphenidate, and also with phenacemide and corticosteroids.

Depressive reactions have been described with Rauwolfia alkaloids, phenothiazines and butyrophenones and with various antihypertensive substances, such as hydralazine, guanethidine and methyldopa.

Delirium has been seen in the course of treatment with various anticholinergic drugs. These include compounds used in the treatment of paralysis agitans (*e.g.*, procyclidine, biperiden and benztropine methanesulfonate) or those prescribed as antidepressants (*e.g.*, imipramine, amitriptyline). Furthermore, isoniazid, cycloserine, procaine, bemegride, barbiturates and opiates can induce excitement in susceptible patients, while digitalis, disulfiram, mepacrine, nitrogen mustard, sulfonamides, antihistamines and penicillin have resulted in unclassifiable mental states.

Withdrawal reactions are characteristic of sedatives. Withdrawal reactions to barbiturates are the most common, but similar reactions to ethchlorvynol, glutethimide, ethinamate, meprobamate, chlordiazepoxide and diazepam have also been described.

CNS depression or oversedation is seen with the abuse of barbiturates, naphtholazine solution and antihistaminic substances.

Among the adverse behavioral effects to the three most important groups of psychoactive substances, *i.e.*, antipsychotics, anxiolytics and antidepressants, impaired psychomotor functioning and oversedation are the most frequent with antipsychotics. Toxic confusional states are rare with these drugs. Paradoxical restlessness (excitement, insomnia, bizarre dreams) have been reported. On the other hand, the most important adverse behavioral effects with anxiolytic drugs are psychomotor impairment and withdrawal reactions; and antidepressants have not infrequently been implicated in producing excitement and aggravating psychotic symptoms (Caffey *et al.*, 1966).

b. CNS and ANS

Adverse CNS reactions to psychoactive drugs were further subdivided into encephalomyelopathic reactions, convulsive, extrapyramidal and cerebrovascular reactions by Hollister (1965).

Encephalomyelopathic reactions may occur in the course of treatment with organic arsenicals, gold salts, antibacterial agents, vaccines and antisera. Cerebellar syndromes (manifested in ataxia, nystagmus and diplopia) were attributed to anticonvulsant hydantoins, excessive dosage of sedative barbiturates, anxiolytic drugs, *e.g.*, meprobamate or chlordiazepoxide, antidepressants, *e.g.*, imipramine or amitriptyline, antipsychotic compounds, *e.g.*, reserpine and various phenothiazines, and primidone.

Convulsive reactions have been encountered with analeptic and stimulant drugs, particularly with pentetrazole, picrotoxin, amphetamines, methylphenidate and bemegride, with various antidepressants (particularly the hydrazide MAOI's) and with antipsychotics (phenothiazines, Rauwolfia alkaloids).

Extrapyramidal reactions are frequent with antipsychotic drugs. Phenothiazines, Rauwolfia alkaloids, thioxanthenes, benzoquinolizines, butyrophenones and phenylpiperazine all share this common characteristic.

Cerebrovascular reactions are manifested in hypertensive encephalopathy induced by pressor amines (*e.g.*, epinephrine) or MAOI antidepressant drugs; and cerebral hypotensive reactions have been reported with antihypertensive drugs and phenothiazines.

Adverse CNS reactions to antipsychotics are body temperature changes and various neurological syndromes (including EPS and convulsions). Important and frequent autonomic (adverse) reactions with the same drugs are hypotension and tachycardia (or bradycardia), while blurred vision, aggravation of glaucoma (or peptic ulcer), fecal impaction, paralytic ileus (or diarrhea), bladder paralysis, inhibition of ejaculation and cutaneous flushing relatively rarely occur.

Adverse CNS effects to antidepressants are hyperreflexia, increased muscle tone and tremor, while those with the most serious consequences are hyperpyrexia, hypertensive crisis and intracerebral hemorrhage (particularly with MAOI's). Among the adverse ANS effects are orthostatic hypotension, constipation, delayed micturition or ejaculation, impotence and anticholinergic symptoms. In the course of treatment with these drugs, bladder and bowel paralysis and aggravation of glaucoma (particularly tricyclic drugs) are not uncommon (Caffey *et al.*, 1966).

Adverse CNS and ANS reactions to anxiolytic drugs are relatively rare. Ataxia—mainly a result of overdosage—is the most important.

c. Allergic and Toxic

Allergic or toxic reactions have been described with all three major groups of psychoactive drugs.

With *antipsychotic* compounds, harmless eosinophilia, various allergic skin manifestations, *e.g.*, dermatitis, contact dermatitis and photosensitivity reactions may occur often at an early stage of treatment. During the same period the incidence of cholestatic jaundice (with phenothiazines or thioxanthenes) is 0.5 per cent. This occasionally may lead to xanthomatous biliary cirrhosis. Cases of agranulocytosis are rare and are usually discovered in the first 12 weeks of treatment. Other infrequent adverse effects are thrombocytopenic or nonthrombocytopenic purpura, hemolytic anemias and pancytopenia. These are unrelated to the duration of treatment.

Anaphylactoid reactions, drug eruptions and mucocutaneous reactions have been reported in the course of treatment with *anxiolytic* drugs. Blood dyscrasias have been seen with both meprobamate and chlordiazepoxide.

Of the *antidepressant* drugs, agranulocytosis or cholestatic jaundice may occur with the tricyclic compounds, while cases of hepatocellular jaundice have been reported with hydrazide MAOI's.

d. Miscellaneous

Increased libido, menstrual irregularities, false pregnancy tests, lactation and gynecomastia in women; impotence in men; and weight gain and edema in both sexes may occur in the course of treatment with antipsychotic drugs. The edema (also described with antidepressants) has been attributed to an increase in antidiuretic hormone secretion.

i. Ophthalmological. In recent years, attention has been focused on the ophthalmological changes produced by antipsychotic drugs. While corneal and lens opacities are not infrequent complications with chronic high doses of chlorpromazine, these do not appear to interfere seriously with vision. On the other hand, the rather rare pigmentary retinopathy induced by thioridazine is a serious, blinding complication. Similarly, the aggravation of glaucoma by tricyclic antidepressants may have severe consequences.

ii. Electrocardiographic. ECG abnormalities, vagotonic and/or quinidine-like effects are rather rare adverse reactions of antipsychotic drugs and occur mainly with thioridazine. They are more frequent with tricyclic antidepressant compounds.

iii. Driving Skill. The high incidence of death and injury from car accidents is a major public health problem. Because of this, the effect of drugs on driving has been recently reviewed by Perry and Morgenstern (1966). The increase in reaction time, and consequently the predisposition to automobile accidents even after the consumption of only two or three drinks of whisky, is quite marked. Driving ability is usually considered to be impaired after two (12 ounces) bottles of beer or 2 ounces of whisky. It is essential to know that it takes about 2 hours to eliminate this amount of alcohol.

Sedatives also increase the hazards of driving. Hypnotic doses of barbiturates, chloral hydrate, paraldehyde, glutethimide and ethchlorvynol impair over-all efficiency, which may last for a period of 14 hours. On the other hand, the driving skill of a tense person may improve with a small dose of barbiturate drug, *e.g.*, 15 mg. of phenobarbital. While a single dose of the *stimulant* amphetamine is not incompatible with driving, prolonged use of this drug to combat fatigue may have dangerous consequences.

Although *antipsychotic* drugs have never been linked directly to accident statistics, the adverse effects of these drugs as well as of various *antidepressant* substances may be incompatible with safe driving. There is accumulating evidence that the imprecision of movements seen with some of the *anxolytic* drugs interferes with driving skill. These drugs are being increasingly implicated in automobile accidents. Whether this is due to a specific alteration produced by these drugs, their indiscriminate use or the lack of obligatory warning to patients to be careful on the road under the influence of these extensively used substances still remains unanswered.

2. Contraindications

The various contraindications of the investigational substance are intimately related to its adverse effects. There are four major areas to be explored: pregnancy, concurrent medical problems, concurrent treatment and concurrent diet.

a. Pregnancy

The whole topic of placental transfer was well reviewed by Villee (1965), who asserted that all but the largest molecules can trespass the placental membranes. The rate of transfer is primarily dependent upon the lipid solubility of the substance but is influenced also by maternal diseases such as diabetes or toxemia, which change placental permeability.

Systematic exploratory work with psychoactive drugs in this area has revealed the following.

General anesthetics (chloroform, diethylether, nitrous oxide, etc.) traverse the placenta rapidly. Since they pass into the fetal circulation swiftly, they may cause respiratory depression in the newborn. The incidence of this serious complication increases with the duration and depth of anesthesia.

Narcotic analgesics (*e.g.*, morphine, heroin) cross the placenta easily and have "depressant" effects on the fetus. As a consequence of maternal addiction, Goodfriend *et al.* (1956) have reported withdrawal symptoms, while others have described clinical depression in the newborn.

Sedatives and hypnotics achieve rapid equilibrium between the maternal and fetal blood streams. Barbital, for example, attains this equilibrium within 4 minutes. It has been noted that the mother is relatively more affected by barbiturates than the fetus. The same applies to paraldehyde. With chloral hydrate, the absence of detoxifying mechanisms in the fetus may lead to serious consequences in the newborn. Thalidomide is another example of a drug which is innocuous to the adult yet harmful to the fetus. If given between the 28th and 42nd day after conception (Cassels, 1966), even a single dose of 100 mg. may produce phocomelia, *i.e.*, short, flipper-like limbs (Taussig, 1962).

Most psychotherapeutic drugs, although they cross the placenta rather swiftly, are generally considered not to have any ill effects on the fetus. This applies to anxiolytic, antidepressant and antipsychotic compounds. While none of the anxiolytic drugs has been teratogenically implicated, the possibility of teratogenicity in animals was raised—although it could not be supported—with opipramol, a tricyclic antidepressant, and trifluoperazine, a phenothiazine antipsychotic drug.

b. Medical Problems

Of the seven most extensively used groups of psychoactive drugs, *sedative barbiturates* are absolutely contraindicated in comatose states and in acute intermittent porphyria. Impaired liver function, which delays their metabolic degradation, and impaired renal function, which decreases their elimination, may dangerously prolong the action of barbiturates and are therefore considered relative contraindications. Furthermore, barbiturates should be prescribed with caution for patients suffering from bronchopulmonary conditions and allergies. Caution should also be exercised in prescribing barbiturates for long term schizophrenics, geriatric patients and lactating mothers.

Stimulant amphetamines should not be given to patients with heart or bronchopulmonary disease and should be prescribed only with caution for hyperthyroid and hypertensive patients. They are contraindicated in manics and in the schizophrenias.

There are relatively few absolute or relative contraindications for *antipsychotic drug* administration. However, phenothiazines should not be given to patients with a history of agranulocytosis or jaundice and in acute alcoholic intoxication. Rauwolfia alkaloids are also contraindicated in depressions and in cases of peptic ulcer.

Of the two major groups of *antidepressant drugs*, tricyclic substances are absolutely contraindicated for patients with a history of agranulocytosis or severe liver impairment. They should be given with caution in cases with increased intraocular pressure (*e.g.*, glaucoma), prostatic hypertrophy, and chronic constipation. Among the absolute contraindications for MAOI antidepressants are manic conditions, liver impairment, renal disease and pheochromocytoma.

The only two absolute contraindications for *anxiolytic drugs* are shock and coma. However, it is usually agreed that diazepam should not be prescribed for cases suffering from myasthenia gravis and that oxazepam should be avoided in glaucoma.

c. Concurrent Treatment

i. Other Drugs. The combination of sedative barbiturates with antidepressant MAOI's should be given only with great caution. The same applies to the combinations of stimulant amphetamines and MAOI drugs. Furthermore, since simultaneous administration of cyclopropane or halogenated hydrocarbon anesthetics with amphetamine drugs may result in ventricular arrhythmias, tachycardia or even fatal ventricular fibrillation, combined administration of these substances is contraindicated.

While antipsychotic phenothiazines may be combined with almost any available medication, antipsychotic Rauwolfia alkaloids should be combined with cardiac drugs, *e.g.*, digitalis and quinidine, only after careful consideration. Similarly, while tricyclic antidepressants may be given together with any other drugs, MAOI antidepressants should not be used in conjunction with ether, procaine, chlorothiazide, phenylephrine and/or antiparkinson agents. On the other hand, anxiolytic drugs may be prescribed in combination with any other drug treatment. However, alcohol consumption may have dangerous consequences in the course of treatment with most psychoactive drugs.

ii. Physical Therapies. The only absolute contraindication to combining physical therapies and drugs is the simultaneous administration of antipsychotic Rauwolfia alkaloids with electroconvulsive treatment. It has been noted that the hypotensive action of ECT is intensified by antipsychotic phenothiazines and that complications are more common when insulin therapy is combined with phenothiazine treatment than when insulin is given alone.

iii. Surgery. Sedative barbiturates, antipsychotic phenothiazines and anxiolytic drugs in general can be used at any time, but tricyclic antidepressants have to be discontinued at least two days prior to surgical intervention. Amphetamines and MAOI antidepressants should be discontinued for an even longer time before any general anesthetic is administered.

d. Diet

Dietary restrictions are necessary only with the MAOI antidepressants. Since 1963 there have been a number of alarming reports of hypertensive crisis occurring in patients taking MAOI preparations. Various substances, particularly cheese, have been implicated in this serious reaction. It was suspected and later confirmed that tyramine, which was first isolated from cheese, was the chemical responsible for these reactions. The concentration of tyramine is considered to be directly proportional to the duration of aging of cheese and inversely proportional to its acidity. Therefore cheshire cheese is safer than cheddar because of its higher acid content. There is no tyramine in either cottage or cream cheeses.

Besides cheese, meat or yeast extracts may also precipitate hypertensive episodes, as was seen with Marmite, a British product prepared from brewers' yeast. The same problem can occur with chicken liver or snails. Beer and wine, particularly Chianti, contain small amounts of tyramine, but whether this is sufficient to produce a hypertensive crisis is still questionable.

In the foregoing, the measurable psychometric, conditioning, neurophysiological and biochemical correlates of clinical psychopathology have been outlined, and the therapeutic action of drugs have been screened via these indicators. With the increasing number of new psychoactive chemicals and the accumulating knowledge on their mode of action, it may not be too long before a psychopharmacologically based psychopathology will be developed in which the pathological psychiatric symptoms will be related to a particular neurochemical, neurophysiological, etc., alteration, instead of the neurochemical, neurophysiological, etc., change being viewed as part of a psychiatric syndrome. This is not an unreasonable expectation if one considers that drug effects are primarily the results of a chemical interaction which triggers off neurophysiological and neurochemical changes and, only at the end of a chain of actions, also psychological changes. Only at such time will clinical psychopharmacology progress from the present empirical to its next experimental stage of development. Until such time one must be satisfied in both psychopathological and psychopharmacological investigations with correlations which are based on statistical analysis of observations.

REFERENCES

ALEKSANDROVA, L. I.: Clinical physiologic analysis of the neurotic syndrome in the initial phase of hypertension and significance of therapeutic sleep. Zh. Nevropat. Psikhiat. Korsakov., *52:* 42 (1952)

ALEXANDER, F., *et al.:* L-methionine and *l*-tryptophan feeding in nonpsychotic and schizophrenic patients with and without tranylcypromine. J. Nerv. Ment. Dis., *137:* 135 (1963).

ALEXANDER, L.: Objective evaluation of antidepressant drug therapy by conditional reflex technique. Dis. Nerv. Syst., *22:* 14 (1961).

ALTSCHULE, M. D.: Bodily physiology in mental and emotional disorders. (Grune and Stratton, New York, 1953.)

APTER, I. M.: The characteristics of higher nervous activity in patients with epilepsy. Zh. Nevropat. Psikhiat. Korsakov., *55:* 321 (1955).

ASCHAFFENBURG, G.: Experimentelle Studien über Associationen. Die Associationen im Normalen. Z. Psychol. Arb., *1:* 209 (1896).

ASCHAFFENBURG, G.: Experimentelle Studien über Associationen. Die Ideenflucht. Z. Psychol. Arb., *4:* 235 (1904).

ASCHCROFT, G. W., AND SHARMAN, D. F.: 5-Hydroxyindoles in human cerebrospinal fluid. Nature, Lond., *186:* 1050 (1960).

ASTRUP, C.: Schizophrenia: conditional reflex studies. (Charles C Thomas, Springfield, 1962.)

ASTRUP, C.: Pavlovian psychiatry. A new synthesis. (Charles C Thomas, Springfield, 1965.)

ASTRUP, C., AND GANTT, W. H.: Effects of muscular exertion and verbal stimuli on heart rate and blood pressure in the human. Recent Advances Biol. Psychiat., *4:* 39 (1962).

ASTRUP, C., AND NOREIKY, K.: Functional psychoses: diagnostic and prognostic models. (Charles C Thomas, Springfield, 1965.)

AXELROD, J.: *O*-Methylation of epinephrine and other catechols *in vitro* and *in vivo*. Science, *126:* 400 (1957).

AXELROD, J.: The uptake and release of catecholamines and the effect of drugs. In: Progress in brain research (eds., Himwich, H. E., and Himwich, W. A. Vol. III). (Elsevier, Amsterdam, 1964.)

AXELROD, J., WHITBY, L. G., AND HERTTING, G.: Effect of psychotropic drugs on the uptake of H^3 norepinephrine by tissues. Science, *133:* 383 (1961).

AXELROD, J., *et al.*: The distribution and metabolism of lysergic acid diethylamide. Ann. N.Y. Acad. Sci., *66:* 435 (1957).

BALDRIDGE, R. C., *et al.* (1959): In: Garattini, S., and Valzelli, L. Serotonin. (Elsevier, Amsterdam, 1965.)

BAN, T. A.: Annual report of the research department. Verdun Protestant Hospital, Verdun, 1963.

BAN, T. A.: Annual report of the Research department. Douglas Hospital, Verdun, 1964.

BAN, T. A.: Conditioning and psychiatry. (Aldine Publishing Co., Chicago, 1964.)

BAN, T. A.: Annual report of the research department. Douglas Hospital, Verdun, 1966.

BAN, T. A.: Clinical pharmacology of psychotropic drugs. Appl. Ther., *8:* 145 (1966).

BAN, T. A.: Clinical pharmacology of the phenothiazines. Appl. Ther., *8:* 423 (1966).

BAN, T. A.: Clinical pharmacology of tricyclic antidepressants. Appl. Ther., *8:* 779 (1966).

BAN, T. A.: Phenothiazines alone and in combination. Appl. Ther., *8:* 530 (1966).

BAN, T. A.: Predictors of therapeutic response to drugs. Canad. Ment. Health, *14:* 23 (1966).

BAN, T. A.: Psychophysical deficit: psychiatric diagnoses. (Proceedings of the Eighteenth International Congress of Psychology, Moscow, 1966.)

BAN, T. A.: What pre-clinical information the clinician would like to have prior to the commencement of a clinical study. Bull. Amer. Coll. Neuropsychopharmacol., *4:* 1 (1966).

BAN, T. A., CHOI, S. M., AND LEE, H.: Differential conditioning in functional and organic psychoses. (Presented at the First International Congress of Social Psychiatry, London, 1964.)

BARANOV, V. G.: Data about the higher nervous activity in thyreotoxicosis and hypothyreosis. Zh. Vyssh. Nerv. Deiat. Pavlov., *5:* 336 (1955).

BEAULNES, A.: The place of clinical pharmacology in academic medicine. In: Conference on human pharmacology (eds., Murphy, C. W., and Parker, J. M.). (The Canadian Foundation for the Advancement of Therapeutics, Ste. Adele-en-Haut, 1964.)

BENDA, P. (1959): In: Garattini, S., and Valzelli, L. Serotonin. (Elsevier, Amsterdam, 1965.)

BENTE, D.: Elektroenzephalographie und Psychiatrische Pharmacotherapie. In: Anthropologische und Naturwissenschaftliche Grundlagen der Pharmacopsychiatrie (eds., Achelis, T. D., and Ditfurth, H.). (Thieme, Stuttgart, 1963.)

BERENDES, H., *et al.* (1958): In: Garattini, S., and Valzelli, L. Serotonin. (Elsevier, Amsterdam, 1965.)

BERGSMAN, A.: The urinary excretion of adrenaline and nor-adrenaline in some mental diseases. Acta Psychiat. Neurol. Scand., *133:* 33 (1959).

BERLET, H. H., *et al.*: Studies on the association of urinary tryptamine with the excretion of amino acids and 17-ketosteroid hormones in schizophrenic patients. In: Amines and schizophrenia (eds., Himwich, H. E., Kety, S. S., and Smythies, J. R.). (Pergamon Press, New York, 1967.)

BICKFORD, R. G.: Use of frequency discrimination in automatic electroencephalographic control of anesthesia. Electroenceph. Clin. Neurophysiol., *3:* 83 (1951).

BIRNBAUM, K.: Über den Einfluss von Befühlsfaktoren auf die Assoziationen. Mschr. Psychiat. Neurol., *32:* 194 (1912).

BLEULER, M.: Endocrinologische Psychiatrie. (Thieme, Stuttgart, 1954.)

BLISS, E. L., *et al*: Adrenocortical function in schizophrenia. Amer. J. Psychiat., *112:* 358 (1955).

BLISS, E. L., *et al.*: Reaction of the adrenal cortex to emotional stress. Psychosom. Med., *18:* 56 (1956).

BLOOR, W. R.: Biochemistry of the fatty acids and their compounds the lipids. (Reinhold Publishing Corp., New York, 1943.)

BOARD, F. A., PERSKY, H., AND HAMBURG, D. A.: Psychological stress and endocrine functions. Psychosom. Med., *18:* 324 (1956).

BOARD, F. A., WADESON, R., AND PERKOY, H.: Depressive affect and endocrine functions. Arch. Neurol. Psychiat., *78:* 612 (1957).

BOKIN, I. V.: Characteristics of the higher nervous activity in patients with hypertensive psychosis. Zh. Vyssh. Nerv. Deiat. Pavlov., *4:* 339 (1954).

BOKSER, O. J.: Studies of the interactions of the first and second signaling systems in Parkinsonism and chorea. Nauch. Konf. Dejat. Sign. Sist. Norm. i. Patol., *1:* 14 (1957).

BÖSZÖRMÉNYI-NAGY, I., AND GERTY, F. J.: Diagnostic aspects of study of intracellular phosphorylations in schizophrenia. Amer. J. Psychiat., *112:* 11 (1955).

Bourdillon, R. E., and Ridges, A. P.: 3,4-Dimethyoxyphenylethylamine in schizophrenia. In: Amines and schizophrenia (eds., Himwich, H. E., Kety, S. S., and Smythies, J. R.). (Pergamon Press, New York, 1967.)

Brodie, B. B.: Biochemical sites of action of psychotropic drugs. In: Neuropharmacology (ed., Abramson, H. A.). (Madison, New York, 1960.)

Brooksbank, B. W. L., and Coppen, A.: Plasma 11-hydroxycorticosteroids in affective disorders. Brit. J. Psychiat., *113:* 395 (1967).

Brune, G. G., and Himwich, H. E.: Effects of methionine loading on the behavior of schizophrenic patients. J. Nerv. Ment. Dis., *134:* 447 (1962).

Brune, G. G., and Himwich, H. E.: Biogenic amines and behavior in schizophrenic patients. In: Recent advances in biological psychiatry (ed., Wortis, J.). (Plenum Press, New York, 1963.)

Bryson, R. W., and Martin, D. F.: 17-Ketosteroid excretion in a case of manic-depressive psychosis. Lancet, *2:* 365 (1954).

Bunney, W. E., and Fawcett, J. A.: Possibility of a biochemical test for suicidal potential: an analysis of endocrine findings prior to three suicides. Arch. Gen. Psychiat., *13:* 232 (1965).

Buscaino, G. A., and Stefanachi, L.: Urinary excretion of 5-hydroxyindole-acetic acid in psychotic and normal subjects: excretion after parenteral administration of serotonin. Arch. Neurol. Psychiat., *80:* 78 (1958).

Cade, J. F. J.: Lithium salts in treatment of psychotic excitement. Med. J. Aust., *2:* 349 (1949).

Caffey, E. M., Jr., *et al.:* Antipsychotic, antianxiety and antidepressant drugs. Med. Bull., *1:* 1 (1966).

Cameron, D. E., *et al.:* Ribonucleic acid in psychiatric therapy. In: Current psychiatric therapies (ed., Masserman, J. H.). (Grune and Stratton, New York, 1964.)

Cameron, D. E., *et al.:* RNA and memory. In: Macromolecules and behavior (ed., Gaito, J.). (Appleton-Century-Crofts, New York, 1966.)

Carlsson, A., Lindquist, M., and Magnusson, T.: 3,4-Dihydroxyphenylalanine and 5-hydroxytryptophan as reserpine antagonists. Nature (London), *180:* 1200 (1957).

Cassels, D.: Placental transfer rate decides drug effect on fetus. The Medical Post, *1:* 3 (1966).

Cazzullo, C. F.: Some aspects of tryptophan metabolism in affective psychoses. Brit. J. Psychiat., *112:* 157 (1966).

Choi, S. M., *et al.:* Conditional reflex studies on the effect of psychoactive drugs in schizophrenics. Laval Méd., *37:* 122 (1966).

Cleghorn, R. A.: Steroid hormones in relation to neuropsychiatric disorders. In: Hormones, brain function and behavior (ed., Hoagland, H.). (Academic Press, New York, 1957.)

Cleghorn, R. A.: Hormones and humors. In: Proceedings of the first international congress on hormonal steroids (eds., Martini, L., and Pecile, A.). (Academic Press, New York, 1965.)

Cleghorn, J. M., *et al.:* Studies on the autonomic psychophysiology of lipid mobilization. Canad. Psychiat. Ass. J., *12:* 539 (1967).

Coirault, R., *et al.:* A new therapeutic concept in psychiatry: chemo-shock without loss of consciousness using RP 7843 (initial data). Ann. Médico Psychol. (Paris), *1:* 160 (1959).

Coirault, R., *et al.:* Chemical shock caused by RP 7843, 2-dimethylsulfonyl-10-[3-(1-methyl-4-piperazine)propyl] phenothiazine. Ann. Médico Psychol. (Paris), *2:* 45 (1959).

Coirault, R.: Introductory lessons to the study of stress. Anesth. Analg. (Paris), *16:* 1 (1959).

Coppen, A. J.: Abnormality of the blood-cerebrospinal fluid barrier of patients suffering from a depressive illness. J. Neurol. Neurosurg. Psychiat., *23:* 156 (1960).

Coppen, A. J.: Mineral metabolism in affective disorders. Brit. J. Psychiat., *111:* 1133 (1965).

Coppen, A. J., Julian, T., and Marks, V.: Body build and urinary steroid excretion in mental illness. Brit. J. Psychiat., *113:* 269 (1967).

Coppen, A. J., Malleson, A., and Shaw, D. M.: Effect of lithium carbonate on electrolyte metabolism in man. Lancet, *1:* 682 (1965).

Coppen, A. J., and Shaw, D. M.: Mineral metabolism in melancholia. Brit. Med. J., *2:* 1439 (1963).

Coppen, A. J., Shaw, D. M., and Farrell, J. P.: Potentiation of the antidepressive effect of a monoamine oxidase inhibitor by tryptophan. Lancet, *1:* 79 (1963).

Coppen, A. J., Shaw, D. M., and Mangoni, A.: Total exchangeable sodium in depressive illness. Brit. Med. J., *2:* 295 (1962).

Coppen, A. J., *et al.:* Tryptamine metabolism in depression. Brit. J. Psychiat., *111:* 993 (1965).

Coppen, A. J., *et al.:* Mineral metabolism in mania. Brit. Med. J., *1:* 71 (1966).

Cuculic, Z., *et al.:* Conditional reflex formation in different diagnostic categories. Conditional Reflex, *2:* 64 (1967).

Curtis, G. C., Cleghorn, R. A., and Sourkes, T. L.: The relationship between affect and the excretion of adrenaline, norepinephrine, and 17-hydroxycorticosteroids. J. Psychosom. Res., *4:* 176 (1960).

Davis, H., and Wallace, W. M.: Factors affecting changes produced in EEG by standardized hyperventilation. Arch. Neurol. Psychiat., *47:* 606 (1942).

Davis, P. A.: Electroencephalograms in manic-depressive patients. Amer. J. Psychiat., *98:* 430 (1941).

Denber, H. C. B., and Teller, D. N.: Variations of free and total serum cholesterol in psychiatric patients treated with psychotropic drugs (a preliminary report). In: Drugs affecting lipid metabolism (eds., Garattini, S., and Paoletti, R.). (Elsevier, Amsterdam, 1966.)

Dmitriev, L. I.: Characteristics of the combined

activity of the first and second signaling system in patients with Korsakoff's psychosis. Nauch. Konf. Dejat Syn. Sist. Norm. Patol., *1:* 34 (1957).

Donald, M. E., Ban, T. A., and Lehmann, H. E.: Psychophysical deficit and mental disorder. (Unpublished monograph, Montreal, 1964.)

Eaton, M. T., and Muntz, H. M.: Laboratory findings in affective and schizophrenic psychosis. Amer. J. Psychiat., *104:* 315 (1947).

Elmadjian, F., Hope, J. M., and Lamson, E. T.: Excretion of epinephrine and norepinephrine in various emotional states. J. Clin. Endocr., *17:* 608 (1957).

Elmadjian, F., Hope, J. M., and Pincus, G.: The action of mono-ammonium glycyrrhizinate on adrenalectomized subjects and its synergism with hydrocortisone. J. Clin. Endocr., *16:* 338 (1956).

Euler, U. S.: A specific sympathomimetic ergone in adrenergic nerve fibers (sympathin) and its relation to adrenalin and nor-adrenaline. Acta Physiol. Scand., *12:* 73 (1946).

Euler, U. S.: Adrenalin and nor-adrenalin. Triangle, *1:* 101 (1954).

Euler, U. S.: Nor-adrenalin: chemistry, physiology, pharmacology and clinical aspects. (Charles C Thomas, Springfield, 1956.)

Euler, U. S.: Quantitation of stress by catecholamine analysis. Clin. Pharmacol. Ther., *5:* 398 (1964).

Euler, U. S., and Domeij, B.: Nicotine-like action of arecoline. Acta Pharmacol. (Kobenhavn), *1:* 263 (1945).

Euler, U. S., and Gaddum, J. H.: An unidentified depressor substance in certain tissue extracts. J. Physiol. (London), *72:* 74 (1931).

Euler, U. S. and Luft, R.: Effect of insulin on urinary excretion of adrenaline and noradrenaline. Metabolism, *1:* 528 (1952).

Faddeyeva, V. K.: Changes in the higher nervous and autonomic activity in depressive states. Tes. Dokl. 9 Sov. Fiziol Posv. I.P. Pavlov, *1:* 92 (1941).

Faddeyeva, V. K.: An attempt to study experimentally the cortical dynamics of manic and depressive phases of circular psychosis. (Dissertation, Leningrad, 1945.)

Faddeyeva, V. K.: An experimental investigation of the cortical dynamics during the manic and depressive phases of circular psychosis. Ref. Nauch. Issl. Lab. Med. Biol. Nauk. SSSR, *80:* 447 (1947).

Faurbye, A., and Pind, K.: Failure to detect 3,4-dimethoxyphenylethylamine in the urine of psychotic children. Acta Psychiat. Scand., *188:* 136 (1966).

Feldstein, A., *et al.:* Blood and urinary serotonin and 5-hydroxyindole-acetic acid levels in schizophrenic patients and normal subjects. J. Nerv. Ment. Dis., *129:* 62 (1959).

Fiorica, V., and Muehl, S.: Relationship between plasma levels of 17-hydroxycorticosteroids (17-OH-CS) and a psychological measure of manifest anxiety. Psychosom. Med., *24:* 596 (1962).

Fischer, E., *et al.*: A bufotenin-like substance in the urine of schizophrenics. J. Nerv. Ment. Dis., *133:* 441 (1961).

Flach, F. F.: Metabolism in states of depression. Brit. J. Psychiat., *110:* 588 (1964).

Flach, F. F., *et al.:* The effects of electric convulsive treatments on nitrogen, calcium and phosphorus metabolism in psychiatric patients. J. Ment. Sci., *106:* 68 (1960).

Freyhan, F. A.: The clinical effectiveness of tofranil in the treatment of depressive psychoses. Canad. Psychiat. Ass. J., *4:* 86 (1959).

Freyhan, F. A.: Therapeutic implications of differential effects of new phenothiazine compounds. Amer. J. Psychiat., *115:* 577 (1959).

Friedhoff, A. F., and Van Winkle, E.: The characteristics of an amine found in the urine of schizophrenic patients. J. Nerv. Ment. Dis., *135:* 550 (1962).

Friedman, M., and Rosenman, R. H.: Association of specific overt behavior pattern with blood and cardiovascular finding; blood cholesterol level, blood clotting time, incidence of arcus senilis, and clinical coronary artery diseases. J.A.M.A., *169:* 1286 (1959).

Gaddum, J. H. (1954): In: Smythies, J. R. Introduction. Amines and schizophrenia (eds., Himwich, H. E., Kety, S. S., and Smythies, J. R.). (Pergamon Press, London, 1967.)

Gaddum, J. H., and Hameed, K. A.: Drugs which antagonize 5-hydroxytryptamine. Brit. J. Pharmacol., *9:* 240 (1954).

Gaddum, J. H., and Picarelli, Z. P.: Two kinds of tryptamine receptor. Brit. J. Pharmacol., *12:* 323 (1957).

Gaddum, J. H., and Vogt, M.: Some central actions of 5-hydroxytryptamine and various antagonists. Brit. J. Pharmacol., *11:* 175 (1956).

Gallant, D. M.: Experience with thiothixene. (Presented at the thiothixene symposium—Pfizer Medical Research Laboratories, Groton, 1965.)

Gallant, D. M., *et al.:* Further observations on trifluperidol: a butyrophenone derivative. Psychopharmacologia (Berlin), *7:* 37 (1965).

Gallant, D. M., Bishop, M. P., and Shelton, W.: SKF-10,812: a thioxanthene derivative. Curr. Ther. Res., *7:* 415 (1965).

Gallant, D. M., Bishop, M. P., and Sprehe, D.: TPS_{23}: a new thioridazine derivative. Curr. Ther. Res., *7:* 102 (1965).

Gantt, W. H.: Principles of nervous breakdown—schizokinesis and autokinesis. Ann. N.Y. Acad. Sci., *56:* 143 (1953).

Gantt, W. H.: Normal and abnormal adaptations: homeostasis, schizokinesis and autokinesis. Dis. Nerv. Syst., *18:* 7 (1957).

Gantt, W. H., and Muncie, W.: Analysis of the mental defect in chronic Korsakoff's psychosis by means of the conditional reflex method. Bull. Hopkins Hosp., *70:* 467 (1942).

Gantt, W. H., and Newton, J. E. O.: Meprobamate on acquired cardio-vascular responses and experimental catatonia. Pharmacologist, *2:* 2 (1960).

GARATTINI, S., AND VALZELLI, L.: Serotonin. (Elsevier, Amsterdam, 1965.)

GASANOV, K. A.: The neurodynamic disturbances in Korsakoff's psychosis. Tr. Nauch. Konf. Posv. 100 Let. S.S. Korsakoff, *60:* 453 (1955).

GASTAUT, H.: Combined photic and metrazol activation of the brain. Electroenceph. Clin. Neurophysiol., *2:* 249 (1950).

GIBBONS, J. L., AND MCHUGH, P. R.: Plasma cortisol in depressive illness. J. Psychiat. Res., *1:* 162 (1963).

GIBBONS, J. L., *et al.:* An endocrine study of depressive illness. J. Psychosom. Res., *5:* 32 (1960).

GJESSING, L. R.: Studies of periodic catatonia: blood levels of protein-bound iodine and urinary excretion of vanillylmandelic acid in relation to clinical course. J. Psychiat. Res., *2:* 123 (1964).

GJESSING, L. R.: Studies of periodic catatonia. II. The urinary excretion of phenolic-amines and acids with and without loads of different drugs. J. Psychiat. Res., *2:* 149 (1964).

GJESSING, R.: Beitrage zur Kenntnis der Pathophysiologie der Katatonen Stupors. Arch. Psychiat. Nervenkr., *96:* 319 (1932).

GJESSING, R.: Beitrage zur Kenntnis der Pathophysiologie der Katatonen Stupors. II. Mitteilung. Über Periodisch Rezidivierend Verlaufenden Katatonen Stupor mit Lytischem Beginn und Abschluss. Arch. Psychiat. Nervenkr., *96:* 392 (1932).

GJESSING, R.: Beitrage zur Kenntnis der Pathophysiologie der Katatonen Erregung. III. Mitteilung. Über Periodisch Rezidivierende Katatonen Erregung, mit Kritischem Beginn und Abschluss. Arch. Psychiat. Nervenkr., *104:* 355 (1935).

GJESSING, R.: Beitrage zur Kenntnis der Pathophysiologie der Katatonen Erregung. III. Mitteilung. Über Periodisch Rezidivierende Katatonen Erregung, mit Kritischem Beginn und Abschluss. Arch. Psychiat. Nervenkr., *104:* 355 (1935).

GJESSING, R.: Disturbances of somatic functions in catatonia with a periodic course and their compensation. J. Ment. Sci., *84:* 608 (1938).

GJESSING, R.: Beitrage zur Kenntnis der Pathophysiologie der Periodisch Katatonen Zustande. IV. Mitteilung. Versuch einer Ausgleichung der Funktionsstörung. Arch. Psychiat. Nervenkr., *109:* 525 (1939).

GJESSING, R.: Beitrage zur Somatologie der Periodischen Katatonie. X. Mitteilung. Pathogenetische Erwägungen. Arch. Psychiat. Nervenkr., *200:* 366 (1960).

GJESSING, R., AND GJESSING, L.: Some main trends in the clinical aspects of periodic catatonia. Acta Psychiat. Scand., *37:* 1 (1961).

GJESSING, R.: Beitrage zur Somatologie der Periodischen Katatonie. VI. Mitteilung. Umweltfaktoren, die Sich Nicht Beseitigen lassen. Arch. Psychiat. Nervenkr., *191:* 220 (1963).

GLOWINSKI, J., AND AXELROD, J.: Inhibition of uptake of tritiated-nor-adrenaline in the intact rat brain by imipramine and structurally related compounds. Nature (London), *204:* 1318 (1964).

GOLDMAN, D.: Clinical experience with trifluoperazine: treatment of psychotic states. In: Trifluoperazine. (Lea and Febiger, Philadelphia, 1958.)

GOLDMAN, D.: Effect of prochlorperazine (compazine) on psychotic states. Psychiat. Research Rep. of the American Psychiatric Association, *9:* 23 (1958).

GOLDMAN, D.: The results of treatment of psychotic states with newer phenothiazine compounds effective in small doses. Amer. J. Med. Sci., *235:* 67 (1958).

GOLDMAN, D.: Differential response to drugs useful in treatment of psychosis revealed by pentothal activated EEG. In: Recent advances in biological psychiatry (ed., Wortis, J. W.). (Grune and Stratton, New York, 1960.)

GOODFRIEND, M. J., *et al.:* Effects of maternal narcotic addiction on the new born. Amer. J. Obstet. Gynec., *71:* 29 (1956).

GOUR, K. N., AND CHAUDHRY, H. M.: Study of calcium metabolism in electric convulsive therapy (E.C.T.) in certain mental diseases. J. Ment. Sci. (London) *103:* 275 (1957).

HARLEY-MASON, J., LAIRD, A. H., AND SMYTHIES, J. R.: I. The metabolism of mescalin in the human. II. Delayed clinical reactions to mescalin. Confin. Neurol., *18:* 152 (1958).

HARLEY-MASON, J., *et al.* (1952): In: Smythies, J. R.: Introduction. In: Amines and schizophrenia (eds., Himwich, H. E., *et al.* (Pergamon Press, Oxford, 1967.)

HARTIGAN, G. F.: The use of lithium salts in affective disorders. Brit. J. Psychiat., *109:* 810 (1963).

HARZSTEIN, N. G.: The influence of psychotherapy on the higher and autonomic nervous activity in anancastic neuroses and reactive depression. Nauch. Konf. Dejat. Sign. Sist. Norm. i. Patol., *1:* 25 (1957).

HATTENGADI, S., *et al.:* The orienting response in psychiatric patients. Conditional Reflex, *1:* 214 (1966).

HILL, D.: EEG in episodic psychotic and psychopathic behavior: a classification of data. Electroenceph. Clin. Neurophysiol., *4:* 419 (1952).

HIMWICH, H. E., KETY, S. S., AND SMYTHIES, J. R. (eds.): Amines and schizophrenia. (Pergamon Press, Oxford, 1967.)

HOFFER, A.: Epinephrine derivatives as potential schizophrenic factors. J. Clin. Exp. Psychopath., *18:* 27 (1957).

HOFFER, A., *et al.:* Treatment of schizophrenia with nicotinic acid and nicotinamide. J. Clin. Exp. Psychopath., *18:* 131 (1957).

HOLLISTER, L. E.: Complications from psychotherapeutic drugs. Clin. Pharmacol. Ther., *5:* 322 (1964).

HOLLISTER, L. E.: Toxicity of psychotherapeutic drugs. Practitioner, *194:* 72 (1965).

IVANOV-SMOLENSKY, A. G.: On the methods of examining the conditional food reflexes in children and in mental disorders. Brain, *50:* 138 (1927).

IVANOV-SMOLENSKY, A. G.: Pathology of conditional reflexes and so called psychogenic depression. J. Nerv. Ment. Dis., *67:* 346 (1928).

IVANOV-SMOLENSKY, A. G.: An attempt at pathophysiological investigation of speech incoherence in schizophrenia. Ark. Biol. Nauk. Ser. B., *36:* 127 (1934).

IVANOV-SMOLENSKY, A. G.: An attempt at pathophysiological study of autism in schizophrenia. Ark. Biol. Nauk., *36:* 107 (1934).

IVANOV-SMOLENSKY, A. G.: Concerning different forms and neurodynamics of catatonic stupor. Ark. Biol. Nauk., *36:* 85 (1935).

IVANOV-SMOLENSKY, A. G.: Concerning the study of the joint activity of first and second signaling system. Zh. Vyssh. Nerv. Deiat. Pavlov., *1:* 55 (1951).

IVANOV-SMOLENSKY, A. G.: Investigation into the interaction of the first and second signaling systems. Zh. Vyssh. Nerv. Deiat. Pavlov., *3:* 481 (1953).

IVANOV-SMOLENSKY, A. G.: Essays on the pathophysiology of the higher nervous activity according to I. P. Pavlov and his school. (Foreign Languages Publishing House, Moscow, 1954.)

JEROME, H., *et al.* (1960): In: Garattini, S., and Valzelli, L. Serotonin. (Elsevier, Amsterdam, 1965.)

JUS, A., *et al.* (1958): In: Garattini, S., and Valzelli, L. Serotonin. (Elsevier, Amsterdam, 1965.)

KASATKIN, N.: Conditioned reflexes in infants. (Medicine, Moscow, 1948.)

KASATKIN, N.: Grundriss der Entwicklung der Höheren Nerventätigkeit des Kindes im Ersten Lebensjahr. (Volk und Gesundheit, Berlin, 1955.)

KENNARD, M. A., RABINOVITCH, M. S., AND FISTER, W. P.: The use of frequency analysis in the interpretation of the EEG's of patients with psychological disorders. Electroencephalograph, *7:* 29 (1955).

KETY, S. S.: Biochemical theories of schizophrenia. Science, *29:* 1529 (1959).

KETY, S. S.: Catecholamines in neuropsychiatric states. Pharmacol. Rev., *18:* 787 (1966).

KETY, S. S.: The hypothetical relationships between amines and mental illness: a critical synthesis. In: Amines and schizophrenia (eds., Himwich, H. E., Kety, S. S., and Smythies, J. R.) (Pergamon Press, Oxford, 1967.)

KHIRA, K. A.: Experimental studies of the higher nervous activity in patients with anancastic neurosis. Z. Neuropat. Vopr. Patofiziol. Vyss. nerv. Dejat., *1:* 146 (1958).

KLINE, N., SACKS, W., AND SIMPSON, G. S.: Further studies on one-day treatment of depression with 5 HTP. Amer. J. Psychiat., *121:* 379 (1964).

KRASNOGORSKI, N. I.: Über die Bedingungsreflexe in Kindesalter. Jb. Kinderheilk, *69:* 1 (1909).

KRASNOGORSKI, N. I.: The conditioned reflexes and children's neuroses. Amer. J. Dis. Child., *30:* 753 (1925).

KRASNOGORSKI, N. I.: The physiology of speech development in children. Zh. Vyssh. Nerv. Deiat. Pavlov. *2:* 474 (1952).

KRASNOGORSKI, N. I.: New data on the physiology of speech activity. Zh. Vyssh. Nerv. Deiat. Pavlov. 6*:* 513 (1956).

KUEHL, F. A.: Para-*o*-methylation of dopamine in schizophrenic and normal individuals. In: Amines and schizophrenia (eds., Himwich, H. E., *et al.*). (Pergamon Press, Oxford, 1967.)

KUEHL, F. A., *et al.:* Para-*o*-methylation of dopamine in schizophrenia. Nature (London), *203:* 154 (1964).

KURLAND, H. D.: Steroid excretion in depressive disorders. Arch. Gen. Psychiat., *10:* 554 (1964).

LAZAROVA, A. K.: Experimental studies of the disturbances of the higher nervous activity in Korsakoff's amnestic syndrome. Tr. Nauch. Konf. Posv. 100 Let. SS Korsakoff, *1:* 73 (1955).

LEFFMAN, H., AND PERLO, V. P.: Metrazol and combined photic-metrazol activated EEG in epileptic, schizophrenic, psychoneurotic and psychopathic patients. Electroenceph. Clin. Neurophysiol., *7:* 61 (1955).

LEHMANN, H. E.: Contributions to Pavlovian Conference on higher nervous activity. I. Discussion of paper presented by N. S. Kline. II. Discussion of paper presented by A. V. Snezhnevsky. Ann N.Y. Acad. Sci., *92:* 1038 (1961).

LEHMANN, H. E.: Measurement of changes in human behavior under the effects of psychotropic drugs. Neuropsychopharmacol., *2:* 291 (1961).

LEHMANN, H. E.: New drugs in psychiatric therapy. Canad. Med. Ass. J., *85:* 1145 (1961).

LEHMANN, H. E.: Selection, screening and testing of new psychiatric drugs. Proc. Third World Congr. Psychiat., *3:* 437 (1961).

LEHMANN, H. E.: The new orientation in modern nursing. Canad. Nurse, *57:* 435 (1961).

LEHMANN, H. E.: The psychopharmacological profile: a systematic approach to the interaction of drug effects and personality traits. In: Extrapyramidal System and Neuroleptics. (ed., Bordeleau, J. M.). (L'Edition Psychiatriques, Montreal, 1961.)

LEHMANN, H. E., AND BAN, T. A.: Comprehensive clinical studies with psychoactive drugs. (Bi-Annual Report of studies with phychoactive drugs, conducted at the Verdun Protestant Hospital, Montreal, 1963.)

LEHMANN, H. E., AND BAN, T. A.: Testing new psychoactive drugs. Image (Roche 14), *3:* 13 (1965).

LEHMANN, H. E., AND BAN, T. A.: Comprehensive

clinical studies with psychoactive drugs. (Tri-Annual Report of studies with psychoactive drugs, conducted at Douglas Hospital, Montreal, 1966.)

Leiberman, D. M., *et al.:* The metrazol flicker threshold in neuropsychiatric patients. Electroenceph. Clin. Neurophysiol., *6:* 9 (1954).

Linsky, V. P.: The pathophysiology of Korsakoff's syndrome. Tr. Nauch. Konf. Posv. 100 Let. SS Korsakoff, *1:* 56 (1955).

Luriia, A. R., *et al.:* O mnogoznachmosti simptomov v topicheskoi diagnostike mozgovych porazhenii. Vop. Neirokhir., *28:* 6 (1964).

Maggs, R.: Treatment of manic illness with lithium carbonate. Brit. J. Psychiat. *109:* 56 (1963).

Manger, W. M., *et al.:* Epinephrine and arterenol (norepinephrine) in mental disease. Arch. Neurol. Psychiat. (Chicago), *78:* 396 (1957).

McFarland, R. A., and Goldstein, H.: The biochemistry of manic-depressive psychosis. Amer. J. Psychiat., *96:* 21 (1939).

Minde, K.: Periodic catatonia: a review with special reference to R. Gjessing. Canad. Psychol. Ass. J., *2:* 5 (1966).

Monakhov, K. K.: The problems of the significance of the second signaling system in the elaboration of motor conditional reflexes in anancastic neurosis with a cardiophobic syndrome. Nauch. Konf. Dejat. Sign. Sist., *1:* 82 (1957).

Moravcsik, E. E.: Diagnostische Assoziationsuntersuchungen. Allg. Z. Psychiat., *68:* 626 (1911).

Mowrer, M., *et al.* (1961): In: Müller, H. F., and Müller, A. K. Effects of some psychotropic drugs upon brain electrical activity. Int. J. Neuropsychiat., *1:* 224 (1965).

Müller, H. F., and Müller, A. K.: Effects of some psychotropic drugs upon brain electrical activity. Int. J. Neuropsychiat., *1:* 224 (1965).

Nielsen, J.: Magnesium-lithium studies. Serum and erythrocyte magnesium in patients with manic states during lithium treatment. Acta Psychiat. Scand., *40:* 190 (1964).

Overall, J. E., and Gorham, D. R.: The brief psychiatric rating scale. Psychol. Rep. *10:* 799 (1962).

Overall, J. E., Hollister, L. E., and Pichot, P.: Major psychiatric disorders: a four dimensional model. Arch. Gen. Psychiat., *16:* 146 (1967).

Paasonen, M. K., and Kivalo, E. (1962): In: Garattini, S., and Valzelli, L. Serotonin. (Elsevier, Amsterdam, 1965.)

Paasonen, M. K., *et al.:* 5-Hydroxytryptamine content of structures of the limbic system. J. Neurochem., *1:* 326 (1957).

Pare, C. M. B.: Potentiation of MAO inhibitors by tryptophan. Lancet, *2:* 527 (1963).

Pare, C. M. B., and Sandler, M.: A clinical and biochemical study of a trial of iproniazid in the treatment of depression. J. Neurol. Neurosurg. Psychiat., *22:* 247 (1959).

Pare, C. M. B., Sandler, M., and Stacey, R. S. (1958): In: Garattini, S., and Valzelli, L. Serotonin. (Elsevier, Amsterdam, 1965.)

Pavlov, I. P.: Conditioned reflexes. (Oxford University Press, Oxford, 1927.)

Pavlov, I. P.: Conditioned reflexes: an investigation of the physiological activity of the cerebral cortex. (Oxford University Press, Oxford, 1928.)

Peiper, A.: Cerebral function in infancy and childhood. (International Behavioral Sciences, Series No. 61265, New York, 1963.)

Perry, C. J., and Morgenstern, A. L.: Drugs and driving. J. A.M.A., *195:* 376 (1966).

Perry, T. L., *et al.:* Failure to detect 3,4-dimethoxyphenylethylamine in urine of schizophrenics. Nature (London), *202:* 519 (1964).

Perry, T. L., *et al.:* Studies of amines in normal and schizophrenic subjects. In: Amines and schizophrenia (eds., Himwich, H. E., *et al.*). (Pergamon Press, Oxford, 1967.)

Persky, H.: Adrenocortical function during anxiety. In: Physiological correlates of psychological disorders (eds., Roessler, R., and Greenfield, N. S.). (University of Wisconsin Press, Wisconsin, 1962.)

Persky, H., *et al.:* Adrenal cortical function in anxious human subjects: plasma level and urinary excretion of hydrocortisone. Arch. Neurol. Psychiat., *76:* 549 (1956).

Persky, H., *et al.:* Relation of emotional responses and changes in plasma hydrocortisone level after stressful interview. Arch. Neurol Psychiat., *79:* 434 (1958).

Persky, H., *et al.:* Effect of hypnotically-induced anxiety on the plasma hydrocortisone level of normal subjects. J. Clin. Endocr., *19:* 700 (1959).

Peters, H. N., and Murphree, O. D.: The conditional reflex in the chronic schizophrenic. J. Clin. Psychol., *10:* 126 (1954).

Peters, J. P., and Van Slyke, D. P.: Qualitative clinical chemistry interpretations. Vol. I, 2nd ed. (Williams and Wilkins, Baltimore, 1946.)

Pollin, W., Cardon, P. V., and Kety, S. S.: Effects of amino acid feedings in schizophrenic patients treated with iproniazid. Science, *133:* 104 (1961).

Praag, H. M., and Leijnse, B.: Die Bedeutung der Monoaminoxydase-hemmung als antidepressives Princip. Psychopharmacologia (Berlin), *4:* 1 (1963).

Price, J. M., *et al.:* Quantitative studies on human urinary metabolites of tryptophan as affected by isoniazid and deoxypyridoxine. J. Clin. Invest., *36:* 1600 (1957).

Protopopov, V. P.: The somatic characteristics of manic-depressive psychoses. Zh. Nevropat. Psikhiat. Korsakov., *17:* 57 (1948).

Protopopov, V. P.: Problems of the manic-depressive psychosis. Zh. Nevropat. Psikhiat. Korsakov., *57:* 1355 (1957).

Pscheidt, G. R., *et al.:* Excretion of catecholamines and exacerbation of symptoms in schizophrenic patients. J. Psychiat. Res., *2:* 163 (1964).

RAZRAN, G.: The law of effect or the law of qualitative conditioning. Psychol. Rev., *46:* 445 (1939).

RAZRAN, G.: The observable unconscious and the inferable conscious in current Soviet psychophysiology: interoceptive conditioning, semantic conditioning, and the orienting reflex. Psychol. Rev., *68:* 100 (1961).

REISS, B. F.: Genetic changes in semantic conditioning. J. Exp. Psychol., *36:* 143 (1946).

REISS, M.: Psychoendocrinology. (Grune and Stratton, London, 1958.)

REY, J. H., *et al.:* Serial biochemical and endocrine investigations in recurrent mental illness. J. Psychosom. Res., *5:* 155 (1961).

RICHTER, D.: Biochemical aspects of schizophrenia. In: Schizophrenia: somatic aspects (ed., Richter. D.). (Pergamon Press, London, 1957.)

RICHTER, D.: Tryptophan metabolism in mental illness. In: Amines and schizophrenia (eds., Himwich, H. E., *et al.*). (Pergamon Press, London, 1967.)

RIZZO, N. D., *et al.:* Concurrent observation of behavior changes and of adrenocortical variations in a cyclothymic patient during a period of 12 months. Ann. Intern. Med., *41:* 798 (1954).

RODNIGHT, R.: Separation and characterization of urinary indoles resembling 5-hydroxytryptamine and tryptamine. Biochem. J., *64:* 621 (1956).

RODNIGHT, R.: Body fluid indoles in mental illness. Int. Rev. Neurobiol., *3:* 251 (1961).

ROMANOFF, L. P., *et al.:* Determination of tetrahydrocortisol and tetrahydrocortisone in the urine of normal and schizophrenic men. J. Clin. Endocr., *17:* 777 (1957).

ROME, H. P., AND ROBINSON, D. B.: Psychiatric conditions associated with metabolic, endocrine and nutritional disorders. In: American handbook of psychiatry (ed., Arieti, S.). (Basic Books, New York, 1959.)

RUBIN, R. T., AND MANDELL, A. J.: Adrenal cortical activity in pathological emotional states. Amer. J. Psychiat., *123:* 387 (1966).

RUBIN, R. T., MANDELL, A. J., AND CRANDALL, P. H.: Corticosteroid responses to limbic stimulation in man: localisation of stimulus sites. Science, *153:* 767 (1966).

SACHAR, E. J., *et al.:* Psychoendocrine aspects of acute schizophrenic reactions. Psychosom. Res., *25:* 510 (1963).

SCHAIN, R. J., AND FREEDMAN, D. X. (1961): In: Garattini, S., and Valzelli, L. Serotonin. (Elsevier, Amsterdam, 1965.)

SCHILDKRAUT, J. J.: The catecholamine hypothesis of affective disorders: a review of supporting evidence. Amer. J. Psychiat., *122:* 509 (1965).

SCHILDKRAUT, J. J.: Norepinephrine metabolism in depressed patients treated with imipramine. In: Antidepressant drugs (eds., Garattini, S., and Dukes, M. N. G.). (Excerpta Medica Foundation, Amsterdam, 1967.)

SCHILDKRAUT, J. J., AND KETY, S. S.: Biogenic amines and emotion. Science, *156:* 21 (1967).

SCHILDKRAUT, J. J., *et al.:* Excretion of 3-methoxy-4-hydroxy mandelic acid (VMA) in depressed patients treated with antidepressant drugs. J. Psychiat. Res., *2:* 257 (1964).

SCHOTTSTAEDT, W. W., Grace, W. J., AND WOLFF, H. G.: Life situations, behavior attitudes, emotions and renal excretion of fluid and electrolytes I, II, III and IV. J. Psychosom. Res., *1:* 75 (1956).

SCHOU, M.: The metabolism and biochemistry of lithium. In: Antidepressant drugs (eds., Garattini, S., and Dukes, M. N. G.). (Excerpta Medica Foundation, Amsterdam, 1967.)

SEREDINA, M. I.: Disturbances of the higher nervous activity in general paresis. Tr. Inst. Vyssh. Nerv. Deiat. Ser. Patofiziol., *1:* 137 (1955).

SEREDINA, M. I.: Disturbance of the neurodynamics in an anancastic neuroses. Tr. Inst. Vyssh. Nerv. Deiat. Ser. Patofiziol., *1:* 150 (1955).

SHAGASS, C.: The sedation threshold: a method for investigating tension in psychiatric patients. Electroenceph. Clin. Neurophysiol., *6:* 221 (1954).

SHAGASS, C., AND SCHWARTZ, M.: Evoked cortical potentials and sensation in man. J. Neuropsychiat., *2:* 262 (1961).

SHAGASS, C., AND SCHWARTZ, M.: Reactivity cycle of somatosensory cortex in humans with and without psychiatric disorders. Science, *134:* 1757 (1961).

SHAGASS, C., AND SCHWARTZ, M.: Excitability of the cerebral cortex in psychiatric disorders. In: Physiological correlates of psychological disorders (eds., Roessler, R., and Greenfield, N. S.). (University of Wisconsin Press, Madison, 1962.)

SHAGASS, C., AND SCHWARTZ, M.: Observations on somatosensory cortical reactivity in personality disorders. J. Nerv. Ment. Dis., *135:* 44 (1962).

SHAGASS, C., AND SCHWARTZ, M.: Cerebral responsiveness in psychiatric patients. Arch. Gen. Psychiat. (Chicago), *8:* 177 (1963).

SHAGASS, C., AND SCHWARTZ, M.: Evoked potential studies in psychiatric patients. Ann N.Y. Acad. Sci., *112:* 526 (1964).

SHAGASS, C., AND SCHWARTZ, M.: Recovery functions of somatic sensory peripheral nerve and cerebral evoked responses in man. Electroenceph. Clin. Neurophysiol., *17:* 126 (1964).

SHAGASS, C., SCHWARTZ, M., AND AMADEO, M.: Some drug effects on evoked cerebral potentials in man. J. Neuropsychiat., *3:* 49 (1962).

SHINFUKU, N., *et al.:* Catecholamine excretion in manic-depressive psychosis. Yonago Acta Med., *5:* 109 (1961).

SHIPTON, H. W.: Photographic averaging for the study of evoked cortical potentials in man. In: Medical electronics (ed., Smyth, C. W.). (Olliffe and Sons, London, 1960.)

SILVERMAN, A. J., AND COHEN, S. L.: Affect and

vascular correlates to catecholamines. Psychiat. Res. Rep. Amer. Psychiat. Ass., *12:* 16 (1960).

SINKEVICH, Z.: An attempt to investigate conditional inhibition in schizophrenics. Tr. Inst. Vyss. Nerv. Dejat Ser. Patofiziol. *1:* 13 (1955).

SLOANE, R. B., *et al.:* Some behavioral and other correlates of cholesterol metabolism. J. Psychosom. Res., *5:* 183 (1961).

SMITH, F. L., SIMON, A., AND LINGOES, J. C.: Excretion of urinary corticoids in mental patients. J. Nerv. Ment. Dis., *124:* 381 (1956).

SMYTHIES, J. R. (1960): In: Garattini, S., and Valzelli, L. Serotonin. (Elsevier, Amsterdam, 1965.)

SMYTHIES, J. R.: Introduction. In: Amines and schizophrenia (ed., Himwich, H. E., Kety, S. S., and Smythies, J. R.). (Pergamon Press, New York, 1967.)

SOKOLOV, E. N.: Orienting reflex as a cybernetic system. (Rus.) Zh. Vyssh. Nerv. Deiat Pavlov., *13:* 816 (1963).

SOKOLOVA, G. S.: Conditional traced eyelid reflexes in neurotics with depressive syndromes. Tez. 18 Sov. Probl. Vyss. Nerv. Dejat., *3:* 136 (1958).

SOURKES, T. L.: Biochemistry of mental disease. (Harper and Row, New York, 1962.)

SPECTOR, S., *et al.:* Association of behavioral effects of pargyline, a non-hydrazid MAO inhibitor with increase in brain norepinephrine. Int. J. Neuropharmacol., *2:* 81 (1963).

SPERRY, W. M.: The biochemistry of depressions. In: Depression (eds., Hoch, P. H., and Zubin, J.). (Grune and Stratton, New York, 1954.)

SPRINCE, H.: Indole metabolism in mental illness. Clin. Chem., *7:* 203 (1961).

SPRINCE, H.: Metabolic interrelationships of tryptophan and methionine in relation to mental illness. In: Amines and schizophrenia (ed., Himwich, H. E., Kety, S. S., and Smythies, J. R.). (Pergamon Press, New York, 1967.)

STRÖM-OLSEN, R., AND WEIL-MALHERBE, H.: Humoral changes in manic-depressive psychosis with particular reference to excretion of catecholamines in urine. J. Ment. Sci., *104:* 696 (1958).

STUDNITZ, W.: Effect of marsilid on excretion of 5-methoxy-4-hydroxymandelic acid in man. Scand. J. Clin. Lab. Invest., *11:* 224 (1959).

SULSER, F., BICKEL, M. H., AND BRODIE, B. B.: The action of desmethylimipramine in counteracting sedation and cholinergic effects of reserpine-like drugs. J. Pharmacol., *144:* 321 (1964).

SZARA, S.: Hallucinogenic amines and schizophrenia. In: Amines and schizophrenia (eds., Himwich, H. E., *et al.*). (Pergamon Press, Oxford, 1967.)

SZARA, S., FAILLACE, L. A., AND SPECK, L. B.: Metabolic and physiological correlates of the psychological reaction to three short-acting tryptamine derivatives. (Presented at the Fifth International Congress of the Collegium Internationale Neuro-Psychopharmacologicum, Washington, 1966.)

TAKESSADA, M., *et al.:* 3,4-Dimethoxyphenylethylamine and other amines in the urine of schizophrenic patients. Nature (London), *199:* 203 (1963).

TAUSSIG, H. B. A study of the german outbreak of phocomelia. The thalidomide syndrome. J.A.M.A., *180:* 1106 (1962).

TIRKELTAUB, J. A.: The effect of tofranil on higher nervous activity and some autonomic functions in schizophrenic patients. Zh. Nevropat. Psikhiat. Korsakov., *63:* 564 (1963).

TISSOT, R. (1961): In: Garattini, S., and Valzelli, L: Serotonin. (Elsevier, Amsterdam, 1965.)

UHR, L., AND MILLER, G. J. (eds.): Drugs and behavior. (Wiley, New York, 1960.)

ULETT, G. A.: Experience with photic stimulation in psychiatric research. Amer. J. Psychiat., *114:* 127 (1957).

ULETT, G. A., *et al.:* The EEG and reaction to photic stimulation as an index of anxiety-proneness. Electroenceph. Clin. Neurophysiol., *5:* 23 (1953).

VAN METER, W. G., OWENS, H. F., AND HIMWICH, H. E. (1959): In: Shagass, C., and Schwartz, M.: Some drug effects on evoked cerebral potentials in man. J. Neuropsychiat., *3:* 49 (1962).

VILLEE, C. A.: Placental transfer of drugs. In: Evaluation and mechanism of drug toxicity (ed., Wipple, H. E.). (Academy of Science, New York, 1965.)

WALTER, W. G.: Electroencephalography in cases of mental disorder. J. Ment. Sci., *88:* 110 (1942).

WALTER, W. G., DOVEY, V. J., AND SHIPTON, H.: Analysis of electrical response of human cortex to photic stimulation. Nature (London), *58:* 540 (1946).

WERTLAKE, P. T., *et al.:* Relationship of mental and emotional stress to serum cholesterol levels. Proc. Soc. Exp. Biol. Med., *97:* 163 (1958).

WHO, scientific group on psychopharmacology: Research in psychopharmacology. (World Health Organization Technical Report Series No. 371, World Health Organization, Geneva, 1967.)

WOOLLEY, D. W.: The biochemical bases of psychoses. (Wiley, New York, 1962.)

WOOLLEY, D. W., AND SHAW, E.: A biochemical and pharmacological suggestion about certain mental disorders. Science, *119:* 587 (1954).

ZACHEPITSKY, R. A.: Combination of sleep and psychotherapy in the treatment of neurosis. Zh. Nevropat. Psikhiat. Korsakov., *54:* 431 (1954).

ZERAHN, K.: Studies on active transport of lithium in isolated frog skin. Acta Physiol. Scand., *33:* 347 (1955).

ZURABASHVILLI, A. D. (1958): In: Astrup, C. Pavlovian psychiatry. (Charles C Thomas, Springfield, 1965.)

Five

Clinical Investigation

Clinical investigation is the last step prior to introducing a new substance for widespread use by the practicing physician. While both human and clinical pharmacology are basically "drug oriented," *i.e.*, to reveal the characteristics of a particular substance under normal and pathological conditions, clinical investigation is primarily "disease oriented," *i.e.*, to find "better" means of treating the particular psychopathological condition of a particular patient.

Some conceptualize the aim of clinical investigation as that of finding a substance with a more favorable ratio between the possible "adverse effects" of treatment and the definite "adverse effects" of the untreated disease (Marks, 1965).

During the clinical investigation the effectiveness and the safety (on long-term administration) of the new drug are assessed and compared with known drugs with established therapeutic efficacy and toxicity. Consequently, these studies are carried out on psychiatric patients who are in actual need of treatment; they are conducted in a therapeutic setting.

In this chapter some of the methodological considerations of clinical investigation will be discussed. In addition, the practical application and clinical problems encountered with psychoactive drugs will be reviewed.

A. METHODOLOGICAL CONSIDERATIONS

1. General Principles

The "design and conduct of experiments" on the psychological effects of drugs were reviewed by Nash (1959, 1960). He discussed the basic principles of a "good" design (elimination of bias, reduction of experimental error, careful selection of subjects) and gave consideration to psychological (suggestion, confounding, learning) and pharmacological (secondary drug effects, short-term *versus* long-term effects, control of effective drug concentration) effects which may influence "experimental out-comes."

Inherent in any research activity is the aim of discovering new and unknown data. Similar to other research activities, psychopharmacological clinical research proceeds through three distinctly different stages: *discovery*, *i.e.*, the recognition of the psychoactive properties of the drug; *verification*, *i.e.*, the experimental confirmation of the hypothesis which was based on uncontrolled observations; and *communication*, *i.e.*, the conveying of the information that was obtained (Bigelow and Sainz, 1962). The possible pitfalls in clinical testing in relation to these three stages have been discussed in detail by Ban (1964).

a. *Discovery*

According to Webster's Dictionary (1962), "discovery" means "to be the first," "to find out, see, know about" or "learn of the existence of something." A scientific discovery is usually based on impartial, unbiased and accurate data recorded in a particular setting. The discovery of the psychotherapeutic properties of a drug is a clinical discovery—since it is made in a clinical setting—which, however, is preceded by chemical and pharmacological research.

Thus, for example, in the case of chlorpromazine it was a French anesthesiologist (Laborit, 1951) who first recognized that those patients who were given chlorpromazine as preoperative medication became indifferent to their approaching surgical operation. He also observed that the same substance prevented postoperative restlessness. This discovery of the psychoactive properties of chlorpromazine was based on unbiased, accurate but accidental observations which were preceded, however, by extensive chemical, pharmacological and toxicological research. The therapeutic potential of the drug in psychiatry was soon recognized by Hamon *et al.* (1952) when they observed that chlorpromazine in association with pethidine resulted in transitory sedation in a case of manic agitation. About the same time, Delay *et al.* (1952) obtained symptomatic control with chlorpromazine alone in several cases of manic excitement. Thus, while in the discovery of the psychoactive properties of the drug serendipity played an important role, its actual therapeutic potential was discovered by deliberate search.

Since the discovery of the psychoactive antipsychotic properties of chlorpromazine, a great number of psychoactive drugs have been developed. Once the chemical characteristics and the pharmacological properties of these substances were known, a point was reached where it could be decided from preliminary animal pharmacological screening whether further human pharmacological or clinical pharmacological testing was indicated. Since the pharmacological psychotropic parameters are derived primarily from the activity of known psychoactive drugs, there is a danger that this may delay or even prevent further *novel discoveries* in psychopharmacology (Ban, 1964).

b. Verification

The observation of Hamon *et al.* (1952) in one single instance, and Delay and his collaborators (1952) in several manic cases, of the dramatic therapeutic effectiveness of chlorpromazine was not the end but rather the beginning of experiments with this phenothiazine drug. These experiments were intended to verify whether the discovery, *i.e.*, the strong therapeutic potential of chlorpromazine in certain psychiatric cases, could be supported.

In the stage of verification, *i.e.*, in clinical investigation, a sound knowledge of experimental methodology plays an important role. The experimental methodology of clinical investigation was succinctly presented by Hamilton (1961) in a series of lectures. He discussed the following consecutive steps in clinical investigation: observation, hypothesis, experimentation and induction.

i. Observation and Hypothesis. It is during the period of "observation" that the investigator becomes familiar with the experimental substance. This is usually achieved throughout an uncontrolled pilot study in which the drug is given in free dosages for different lengths of time to a limited number of patients of different age, sex and diagnosis with various psychopathological symptom profiles. In this step an unbiased and flexible approach is required because rigid focusing on the basis of a preconceived idea limits the scope of the available information. The experimental hypothesis is usually based on these observations.

While formulating the experimental hypothesis in the case of psychotherapeutic drugs, special emphasis must be placed on the criteria of selecting the experimental population; on the criteria of treatment, *i.e.*, what drug, what dosage and length of administration; and on the criteria of how changes ("better" or "worse") will be expressed. Failing to include at least these criteria in the experimental design leads to the danger that "if we don't know what we are talking about we can still talk and most likely talk volubly but there is small chance that we are talking to a definite point" (Wilson, 1932).

ii. Experimentation and Induction. After a hypothesis has been formulated, it is the aim of the investigator to obtain the data as quickly as possible, using the minimum number of patients for a minimum period of time to obtain the maximum amount of information. This is fully justified since no one wants to withhold a good treatment any longer than is necessary, bearing in mind the dangers of disseminating unproven or useless treatments. This goal can be achieved by an appropriate experimental design relevant to the nature of the criteria (Hamilton, 1961).

The two most important questions in the clinical investigation of psychoactive drugs are: "Does the compound have any therapeutic effect if administered in a certain dosage for a limited period to a well defined group of patients?" and "Is the compound superior, therapeutically, to other drugs already reliably established for the same purpose?"

It is at this point that the problem of controlling the experiment becomes important. Although most clinical investigators agree that a controlled design is essential, there are differences of opinion as to what constitutes a good "control procedure."

One of the best reviews on this question is that of Lehmann (1964, 1966). He reviewed the various aspects of the clinical investigation (practical, ethical, psychological and methodological) and discussed the difficulties of clinical experiments. According to Lehmann, studying the effect of an independent variable on a stable physical system requires no controls; studying the same effect on an unstable system requires controls. In the case of a physical system, the comparison of the system subjected to the effect of the independent variable with another similar system not exposed to this effect is sufficient control. If the system, however, is more complex and possesses the property of responding to stimuli with varied behavior, then a control is needed as an unspecific stimulus, *i.e.*, a single-blind placebo. Furthermore, if the system is even more complex and allows for transactional processes to develop, a double-blind control is required.

Thus, to eliminate "any effect attributable to a pill, potion, or procedure, but not to its (the drug's) pharmacodynamic or specific properties" (Wolf, 1959), a placebo is required. To eliminate the experimental error introduced by the expectations and emotional attitudes of the subjects who are receiving the drug, a single-blind procedure is essential. To eliminate not only the bias of the subject but also that of the observer, a double-blind procedure is indicated.

An exogenous placebo-controlled design with random allotment of patients to two (active-compound and placebo) treatment groups provides for a reliable answer as to whether a compound has any therapeutic effect if administered in a certain dosage for a limited period to a well defined group of patients.

However, unless an observed emergent change can be clearly linked either to the placebo, the test substance or both, then obviously administration of the placebo has been fruitless, and any consideration of the validity of the given results merely because placebo was given is unwarranted (Bigelow and Sainz, 1962). It is also stressed that whenever a placebo is used as a control it has to look exactly the same as the active compound; it has to be administered the same way; and all experimental procedures have to be alike for both substances.

To establish whether one or another drug is superior therapeutically under certain specific conditions, a double-blind controlled procedure is probably the most useful procedure at present. In contradistinction to the random design which inevitably requires a large experimental population, it is possible to derive valid conclusions from relatively small experimental groups if they are properly matched.

Theoretically, with human beings where transactional processes are present, a double-blind controlled study seems to be essential. This eliminates the bias that might be introduced through feedback mechanisms between the observed and the observer (Lehmann, 1964). Yet some investigators argue that double-blind controlled studies can obscure important and relevant findings. For example, Batterman and Grossman (1955) report on a double-blind experiment which completely obscured the therapeutic properties of the drug (which were only revealed when they switched to a single-blind placebo-controlled trial). Uhlenhuth *et al.* (1959) point out that the therapist's attitude can break through a double-blind experiment, and Hoffer and Osmond (1961) argue that when the groups under study are not homogenous the double-blind method may obscure the presence of significant differences.

The essential characteristic of a controlled experiment is that it gives a valid estimation of experimental error, which is the basis for the statistical tests of significance and makes the experiment self-contained. This enables one to form conclusions from the experimentally obtained data. It is argued that a controlled experiment is necessary since, according to the null hypothesis, any therapeutic results may have occurred by chance and there is no other way of knowing what is the frequency or rarity of this chance, *i.e.*, the probability that the findings are real (Hamilton, 1961).

In every therapeutic clinical trial with psychoactive drugs, inductive logic is used, *i.e.*, members of a class are considered and inference about the class is made on the basis of these members. The most important kind of induction is the statistical method by which general conclusions are drawn on the basis of a limited experimental sample.

In a working paper given at a Workshop of the World Health Organization, Lehmann (1966) briefly reviewed the various statistical procedures used in the clinical evaluation of psychoactive drugs (Lebedev, 1967).

According to him, simple methods of establishing statistical significance such as the "chi-square" or "t" test of the differences of the means of pretreatment and posttreatment scores or the more sensitive tests of "variance" and "covariance" are in many instances adequate. "Multiple discriminant function" analysis is indicated if the problem is to determine which of a number of factors is responsible for the observed reactions to a drug, or "factor analysis," if the problem involves the distribution of several clusters or homogenous subgroups. "Sequential analysis" is to be used when the sample size allows for statistical differences to reach significant values and is useful in experiments where subjects are gradually added to a sample group over a period of time.

Quite frequently nonparametric statistical methods are applied. These include, for example, the "Friedmann two-way analysis of variance" to detect whether there are significant differences among the treatment groups; the "Mann-Whitney U test" to compare which group responded significantly different from the other; and the "Wilcoxon matched pairs signed ranks test" to indicate significant changes in the course of treatment.

One must always bear in mind, however, that the statistical method has its own shortcomings. Among these are the type I or alpha error, namely, the finding of difference because of the choice of an inappropriate statistical technique when none actually exists, or the type II or beta error, which consists in not finding a statistically significant difference because of the insufficient size of the sample group when an actual difference does exist (Overall and Hollister, 1967). Some of the more general pitfalls of the statistical method were perhaps best expressed by Huntsman (1949), who said that "the prestige of mathematics is so great that many persons forget that even in mathematical hands, probability, chance and random mean ignorance. They come to think that, in the alembic of mathematics, chance in some way becomes certainty. They take great care to select random samples without realizing that insofar as a sample has been random, they don't know how it was selected." A more severe criticism was launched recently in the *Lancet* by Wiener (1962). He pointed out that many clinical investigators "because they are unduly sensitive or insecure regarding their lack of mathematic training and knowledge habitually hand over all their data to biometricians for analysis in order that their papers may include the appropriate chi-square tests, standard errors and so on. In that way they have come to depend more and more on mathematicians who have no knowledge or understanding of the subject to interpret their findings, instead of relying on their own experience and common sense." In essence, Wiener attempts to remind the investigator that mathematics is a poor substitute for accurate observations, reliable experimentation and common sense.

c. *Communication*

Proper communication is essential for conveying findings. It should provide information for the practitioner who is primarily interested in knowing whether the new substance can be successfully introduced in treatment. Therefore it should be formulated in simple terms and should answer the questions which are pertinent to the practicing physician, *i.e.*, under what conditions, in what dosage, for how long and with what precautions should the new drug be administered? Editorializing and presenting findings not fully supported by evidence should carefully be avoided (Bigelow and Sainz, 1962).

2. Rating Scales

The most extensively used "instruments" to measure any changes induced by an investigational compound are the rating scales. After the introduction of chlorpromazine, the growing number of new psychoactive drugs led to an increasing interest in clinical investigation and resulted in the construction of numerous rating scales. The *Handbook of Psychiatric Rating Scales* (Lyerly and Abbott, 1966) excellently reviews this particular aspect of psychiatric research, classifies the available scales and clarifies their most important theoretical and practical issues.

a. Rating Scales for Psychoneurotics

Among the various rating scales (and check lists) used to measure therapy-induced changes in psychoneurotics are the Social Ineffectiveness Scale (Parloff *et al.*, 1954), the Normative Social Ajdustment Scale (Barrabee *et al.*, 1955), the Taylor Manifest Anxiety Scale (Taylor, 1953) and the Parallel Form Anxiety Battery (Scheier and Cattell, 1958).

The *Social Ineffectiveness Scale* consists of 15 categories (of items). It reflects the degree of ineffectiveness of the relationships formed with significant people. On the other hand, in the *Normative Social Adjustment Scale* the "social adjustment" is measured in terms of effectiveness in the areas of employment, economics, family life and community. It has been shown that the *Taylor Manifest Anxiety Scale* is highly correlated with the psychasthenia and hypochondriasis scales of the Minnesota Multiphasic Personality Inventory. Consequently, it is primarily useful for clinically measuring a person's basic anxiety level. Scheier and Cattell's (1958) *Parallel Form Anxiety Battery* is more suitable for the measurement of changes, either situational or drug induced, in anxiety levels (Lehmann, 1966).

b. Rating Scales for Depressives

Among the various rating scales used to measure therapy-induced changes in depressed patients are the Feeling and Attitude Scale (Hildreth, 1964), the Clyde Mood Scale (Clyde, 1958, 1963), the Verdun Depression Scale (Lehmann *et al.*, 1958), Hamilton's Rating Scale for Depression (Hamilton, 1960), the Feelings and Concern Check List (Grinker *et al.*, 1961), the Current Behavior Check List (Grinker *et al.*, 1961), the Check List for Clinical Quantification of Depressive Reactions (Cutler and Kurland, 1961), Beck's Inventory for Measuring Depression (Beck *et al.*, 1961), the M.M.H.C. (Massachusetts Mental Health Center) Depression Rating Scale (Greenblatt *et al.*, 1962), the Psychiatric Judgment Depression Scale (Overall *et al.*, 1962), the D_{30} Scale (Dempsey, 1964) and Lubin's Adjective Check List (Lubin *et al.*, 1965).

Hildreth's (1964) *Feeling and Attitude Scale* consists of 86 items which reflect six factors: feeling state, amount of energy, outlook regarding the future, mental state, attitude toward work and attitude toward people. *Clyde's Mood Scale* (Clyde, 1963) consists of 48 items only. The six factors which these items reflect are friendly, aggressive, clear thinking, sleepy, unhappy and dizzy.

In clear distinction to the normally rather long check lists, the *Verdun Depression Rating Scale* (Lehmann *et al.*, 1958) lists only seven symptoms, *i.e.*, depressed mood, depressed facial expression, retardation, agitation, depressive ideation, insomnia and loss of weight, each of which is rated from 0 to 3. Even *Hamilton's Rating Scale for Depression* (Hamilton, 1960), one of the most widely used, is considerably longer, with its 24 items rated from 0 (absent) to 4 (severe). In an analysis of scores obtained with the first 49 patients rated on this scale, four prominent factors were revealed. The four highest loadings for each factor were as follows: Factor I—depressed mood, guilt, retardation, loss of insight; Factor II—gastrointestinal symptoms, insomnia (initial), agitation, loss of weight; Factor III—anxiety (psychic), agitation, anxiety (somatic), loss of libido; and Factor IV—insomnia (middle), general somatic symptoms, anxiety (somatic) and loss of libido.

Both the *Feelings and Concern Check List* and the *Current Behavior Check List* are described in Grinker *et al.*'s (1961) book on the *Phenomena of Depressions*. The former is a 47-item list of "feelings and concern" rated on a four-point scale by a psychiatrist, and the latter is a 139-item list of "current behavior" rated as present or absent by a nurse. The check list used by Cutler and Kurland (1961) for the *Clinical Quantification of Depressive Reactions* consists of only 27 symptoms marked as present or absent, either by a clinician or by ancillary personnel.

Beck's Inventory for Measuring Depression (*Beck et al., 1961*), constructed on the basis of observations in ambulant psychoanalytic therapy of depressed patients, consists of 94 items which are distributed over 21 symptom-attitude categories. The *M.M.H.C. Depression Rating Scale*, developed at the Massachusetts Mental Health Center by Greenblatt and associates (1962) on the basis of observations in inpatient treatment of depressive cases, consists of 28 items.

The *D_{30} Scale* was the result of reducing the 60 items of the Minnesota Multiphasic Personality Inventory depression scale to 30 by Dempsey (1964). The D_{30}, when tested for concurrent validity, showed significant correlations with *Lubin's Adjective Check List* (Lubin *et al.*, 1965).

c. Rating Scales for Schizophrenics

Among the various rating scales used to measure therapy-induced changes in schizophrenic patients, the L-M Fergus Falls Behavior Rating Scale (Lucero and Meyer, 1951), Ferguson's Hospital Ajustment Scale (Ferguson *et al.*, 1953), the Ward Behavior Rating Scale (Burdock *et al.*, 1960), Lorr's Psychotic Reaction Profile (Lorr *et al.*, 1960), the HOD test (Hoffer and Osmond, 1961), the MACC (Mobility, Affect, Cooperation and Communication) Behavioral Adjustment Scale (Ellsworth, 1962), the Central Islip Modified Malamud-Sand's Psychiatric Rating Scale (Turner *et al.*, 1962), the Inpatient Multidimensional Psychiatric Scale (Lorr *et al.*, 1963) and the Katz Adjustment Scales (Katz and Lyerly, 1963) are the ones most frequently used.

On the *L-M Fergus Falls Behavior Rating Scale* (Lucero and Meyer, 1951), eleven areas of behavior are rated by nurses on a five-point scale. (The behavioral areas scored are working behavior, eating behavior, interpersonal behavior, *i.e.*, relationship with other patients, with nonmedical and with medical personnel, acceptance of treatment, personal cleanliness, psychomotor activity, verbal behavior and toilet behavior.) Lucero and Meyer (1951) maintain that on the basis of this scale schizophrenic patients fall into different groups in accordance with the level of their behavioral adjustment. Another early rating instrument is the *Hospital Adjustment Scale* developed by Ferguson *et al.* (1953). This consists of 90 items, and its total score indicates the general level of hospital adjustment. Scores from item 1 through 42 are concerned with communication and interpersonal relations; items from 43 through 67 reflect personal cleanliness and social responsibility; and items from 68 through 90 are related to work, activities and recreation.

The *Ward Behavior Rating Scale* constructed by Burdock and collaborators (1960) was used in the National Institute of Mental Health (NIMH) Collaborative Study. This is a list of 150 behavioral items to be marked "true" or "not true" for a given patient over a specified (2 days or 1 week) time period. This was one of the first scales specifically designed to measure the severity of the illness and response to treatment. Somewhat similar to this is *Lorr's Psychotic Reaction Profile* (Lorr *et al.*, 1960), which measures ward behavior by means of 85 statements rated "true" or "not true." The Psychotic Reaction Profile consists of four scales: the withdrawal scale (which has 38 items), the thinking disorganization scale (which has 18 items), the paranoid belligerence scale (which has 24 items) and the agitated depression scale (which has 5 items).

In contradistinction to all these scales is the *HOD Test*, a simple, crude, card-sort test, which was developed by Hoffer and Osmond (1961) for entirely practical diagnostic purposes. It consists of 145 cards, each with a question on one side and a number on the other. The patient sorts the cards, depending on whether he thinks they are "true" or "false," into two separate boxes. Hoffer (1966) maintains that there is a very significant relationship between HOD scores and diagnosis, prognosis and response to treatment. Hoffer and Osmond (1961) also established a relationship between the HOD test results and an unknown factor in the urine of patients. This unknown factor, which stains mauve on paper chromatograms (at RF 0.83) was present in the majority of schizophrenic patients (Irvine, 1961; and Hoffer and Mahon, 1961), although it may also be present in about one-quarter of non-schizophrenic subjects.

A somewhat different rating instrument is the *MACC Behavioral Adjustment Scale* (Ellsworth, 1962), which consists of four behavioral clusters, mood, cooperation, communication, and social contact, each of which has four items rated on a five-point scale. The extensively used *Central Islip Modified Malamud-Sands Psychiatric Rating Scale* (Turner *et al.*, 1962) contains a 15-item list which is filled in by the ward personnel. *Lorr's Inpatient Multidimensional Psychiatric Scale* (Lorr *et al.*, 1963) is completed by trained interviewers familiar with psychiatric symptomatology. The 75 brief questions of this scale are designed to measure 10 psychotic syndromes.

Finally, the *Katz Adjustment Scales* (Katz and Lyerly, 1963) were developed to measure adjustment and social behavior of psychiatric patients in the community prior to release or during the posthospitalization period. Of the 10 scales 5 are completed by a "close" and "well informed" relative and 5 by the patient. While these scales were designed for both neurotic and psychotic patients, they have been used almost exclusively for schizophrenics.

d. Rating Scales for Various Psychopathologies

The Wittenborn Psychiatric Rating Scale (Wittenborn, 1955) and Overall and Gorham's (1962) Brief Psychiatric Rating Scale (BPRS) belong to this category.

The *Wittenborn Psychiatric Rating Scale* (Wittenborn, 1955) consists of 52 items. In spite of its length, the ratings can be completed in 15 minutes by a competent observer who knows the patient well. In its original published form it included nine symptom clusters (factors). These factors were labeled as acute anxiety (12 items); conversion hysteria (5 items); manic state (14 items); depressed state (8 items); schizophrenic excitement (23 items); paranoid condition (7 items); paranoid schizophrenia (9 items); hebephrenic schizophrenia (7 items); and phobic (4 items). However, in 1964 Wittenborn, revised his scale, which now contains 12 symptom clusters (Lehmann, 1966).

In contradistinction to the Wittenborn scale, the *BPRS* (Overall and Gorham, 1962) consists of only 16 symptom areas, which are rated on seven levels, *i.e.*, from not present, through very mild, mild, moderate, moderately severe, severe and extremely severe. The 16 items of the BPRS are somatic concern, anxiety, emotional withdrawal, conceptual disorganization, guilt feelings, tension, mannerisms and posturing, grandiosity, depressive mood, hostility, suspiciousness, hallucinatory behavior, motor retardation, uncooperativeness, unusual thought content and blunted affect. Factor analyses of this scale provided four major syndromes.

During a Workshop of the Early Clinical Drug Evaluation Units (ECDEU) held in April 1966, uniform data gathering and reporting methods were discussed. The completion of a specially devised form called Patient Record for Drug Study (PRDS) and the BPRS-18 was recommended for all patients who are given an investigational drug and was accepted by the participants. (The BPRS-18 is an extended form of the BPRS with two additional items, namely, excitement and disorientation.) In the assessment of acute and chronic schizophrenic patients in addition to the PRDS and

BPRS-18, the NOSIE-30 (Nurses Observation Scale for Inpatient Evaluation) was also recommended. The latter scale was developed by Hönigfeld and Klett (1965) and successfully used in the collaborative studies of the U.S. Veterans Administration. Furthermore, for the assessment of neurotic outpatients, the Wittenborn and Zung Scales and, for the evaluation of depressed patients, the Hamilton (or Wittenborn) and Zung rating instruments were suggested (Zung *et al.*, 1965).

Besides the selection of a particular scale for a special study, the competency of the "rater" is equally important. This was revealed in a series of six studies conducted by Lehmann *et al.* (1965). In these studies, raters of varied orientations and clinical experience but inexperienced with the particular rating scale used were asked to rate patients belonging to nine diagnostic categories on the 12 items of the Verdun Target Symptom Scale (Lehmann and Ban, 1963). The raters' accuracy was determined by comparing their ratings with those of a criterion rater and then obtaining a coefficient of congruity. This was done for each rater, each symptom item, and each patient type item.

The results indicated that psychiatrists were the most accurate raters. Since the participating psychiatrists had different theoretical backgrounds and training, the results suggested that experience was the primary factor in their agreement. It was also recognized that the scale had the highest validity on those items which were best defined and which reflected overt symptomatology. It was least valid for those items which were rather vaguely defined and which encouraged inferential reasoning. In regard to diagnosis, the scale proved to be most reliable when used on manic, depressed or general paretic patients. Finally, the results of the six experiments indicated the presence of one important factor in rater accuracy. This seems to be an unidentified personality characteristic of the rater, which may, in certain cases, either substitute for theoretical knowledge and clinical experience or, conversely, may reduce the effects of these two factors significantly.

3. Placebos

The medical use of placebos, *i.e.*, unspecific stimuli, is not new. Placebos were used therapeutically and were considered a "common place method" in the Quincy Lexicon (1787). Following this, there are only isolated references, but in the course of time the once therapeutic tool slowly became an instrument of therapeutic research.

Some of the early workers using the placebo in research were Rivers (1908) and Hollingworth (1931). The former also used double-blind procedures in evaluating the effects of alcohol on fatigue, while the latter used placebo controls in evaluating the psychological effects of caffeine.

A scholarly paper written by Pepper (1945) renewed interest in placebos, and Gold (1946) gave a new impetus to the use of placebos in therapy. However, it was only after the introduction of chlorpromazine, which was followed by an ever increasing number of new potentially psychoactive substances waiting for clinical confirmation of their therapeutic effectiveness, that the placebo-controlled design "burst into methodological and experimental prominence with the explosive brilliance of a supernova" (Lehmann, 1964). As a result, the role of placebos in clinical research became highly exaggerated (particularly by incompetent investigators who attempted to replace clinical skill and psychopathological knowledge with pseudomethodological findings). It was quite common during this period to use the term "placebo effect" for any findings which could not be attributed to any specific drug action or treatment (Hönigfeld, 1964).

Determinants of variability in drug response cannot be restricted entirely to "placebo effects." They cannot be attributed to placebo action without systematically excluding their relationship to heredity, age presence or absence of disease, constitution, temperament, baseline level of activity and environmental factors (Irwin, 1963, 1964).

Examples of hereditary influences on drug action are the well known differential sensitivity of Chinese, Whites and Negroes to alcohol, morphine or to the mydriatic effect of cocaine and ephedrine (Chen and Poth, 1929). The effect of age was clearly demonstrated with LSD_{25}. This psychotomimetic substance produced amphetamine-like stimulation without hallucination in autistic 5- to 12-year-old children. In similar but 12- to 15-year-old children, in addition to the stimulating effects, LSD_{25} also produced hallucinations (Bender *et al.*, 1962). The role of environmental factors on drug effects is seen with chlorpromazine and related drugs which are more "depressant" in an environment of 13° to 18°C than at 25° to 30°C (Berti and Cima, 1962). Another example is that in tropical countries alcoholic excess seems to be more injurious, and narcotics produce preliminary excitement and delirium more readily.

Consequently, placebo effects have to be considered within a certain framework of restrictions. According to Lehmann (1964), the "effects of a placebo while being unspecific, are not unstructured; they have meaning and their meaning is dependent on the influence of impulses coming from the cerebral cortex." Furthermore, whatever is considered to be a placebo effect must be exposed to careful experimental scrutiny.

Since the placebo is conceived as a stimulus, albeit a nonspecific stimulus, its characteristics and the influence of these characteristics on the placebo effect can be studied, as well as the characteristics of the subject who responds to placebos. Furthermore, the various effects induced by the placebo and the importance of social factors on this response can also be explored (Hönigfeld, 1964).

a. Placebo Variables

In spite of numerous studies, the relationship between the characteristics of the placebo (size, shape, color, taste, route of administration) and placebo effect remains controversial. Schindel (1962) stressed color as an important factor in placebo effect, while Glaser and Whittow (1954) found no difference in the incidence of side-effects with white-sweet compared with red-bitter placebos. The same applies to the route, the frequency of administration and the dosage. While Morison *et al.* (1961) found a greater improvement with parenteral than oral administration and Pogge and Coates (1962) revealed more side-effects when the frequency of placebo administration was increased, Goldman *et al.* (1963) and Samuels and Edison (1961) failed to demonstrate such correlations. Gruber (1956) suggested that a double dose of placebo was nearly twice as effective as a single dose, whereas Foley *et al.* (1957) asserted that placebo effects are independent of doses. All one can say at the moment is that all these various factors may be important but how they induce change in one direction or another in any given study remains uncertain.

b. Personality Variables

The existence of a particular type of personality which responds to placebos, *i.e.*, the placebo reactor, is no less controversial than the relationship between placebo characteristics and placebo effects. For a long time it was thought that clinical improvement under placebo administration depends in some important way upon suggestibility. Gliedman *et al.* (1958), using the postural Sway Test of suggestibility, could not support this assumption, *i.e.*, could not differentiate between placebo responders and nonresponders by this test. The relationship between suggestibility and the placebo response was reexamined by Steinbook, *et al.* (1965). They used the Press Test instead of the Sway Test and found that suggestibility scores were positively correlated with the decline in number and severity of psychopathological symptoms in the first 2 weeks. This correlation became much less significant toward the end of the therapy. They concluded that "something other than suggestibility must be operative in the placebo effect."

There is considerable agreement that a person might respond to a placebo one day and not on another. This was well demonstrated by Wolf (1959). Thus a placebo reactor may unpredictably turn into a nonreactor (Batterman, 1957; and Pannekoek, 1957).

In spite of this, however, Beecher (1955) was able to show that the proportion of persons who respond to placebo treatment in a wide variety of settings was a rather consistent average of 35.2 per cent. Lasagna (1954) and his collaborators went even further, and on the basis of interviews and the Rorschach test suggested that placebo reactors fall into a particular group and can be described as outward oriented, somewhat anxious and immature individuals. This was confirmed by Joyce (1959) and Gartner (1962), who used the Bernreuter Personality Inventory test and found placebo reactors less self-confident, less dominant, more sociable and more extroverted than the nonreactors. Similarly, Knowles and Lucas (1960), using the Maudsley Personality Inventory (MPI), recognized a correlation between placebo responsiveness and high scores on the MPI neuroticism scale.

In an attempt to differentiate placebo reactors from nonreactors, Klerman (1959, 1961) examined a number of criteria, such as body type, psychological, and psychomotor test responses, physiological indices and interview data. As a result, he suggested that it is possible to recognize and differentiate two types, *i.e.*, strong and weak placebo reactors. Similarly, Linton and Langs (1962), on the basis of psychological test data, suggest that strong placebo reactors are passive nonintellectual individuals with loose thinking and flattened affect, in contradistinction to the weak placebo reactors who are sensitive, introspective, and highly intellectual individuals.

The differential features of two types of placebo reactors were even further clarified by Luoto (1961, 1964) and Lehmann (1964). Luoto (1961) found that "high neurotic introverts" were positive placebo reactors, while "high neurotic extroverts" were negative placebo reactors. Lehmann (1964) showed that individuals who manifest well integrated autonomic functioning will show improved performance in certain areas under placebo conditions, in contrast to those who manifest poorly integrated autonomic functioning.

c. Placebo Effects

Both therapeutic and adverse effects have been described in the course of placebo administration. An interesting review of these was presented by Trouton (1957). Then Beecher (1960) reported on the effectiveness of placebos in a variety of pathological conditions. More recently, the multifold effects of placebos were summed up by Hönigfeld (1964) and Lehmann (1964).

i. Therapeutic Effects. Numerous symptoms, syndromes and diseases have shown favorable responses to placebo. Jellinek (1946) found placebos effective in 52 per cent of cases treated for headache, while Hillis (1952) reported that placebo was as effective as codeine in the control of coughing. Similar findings have been reported in treating hay fever, common cold, nausea, vomiting and sea sickness; and Wayne (1956) found placebo beneficial in an adrenaline-resistant asthmatic. Hamilton and Wilson (1952) had better results with a pharmacologically inert substance than with tolazoline, a vasodilator, in intermittent claudication; and Kabler (1958) was able to demonstrate in a controlled study that 62 per cent of his diabetics showed satisfactory control of blood sugar levels when treated with a placebo.

Among the various psychiatric conditions, Hampson *et al.* (1954) and Wolf (1959) independently recognized that placebo can be equal or superior to mephenesin, a muscle relaxant, for treating patients whose prevailing complaint is tension. In Hampson *et al.*'s (1954) study, while placebo was better in the first 2 weeks of treatment, the active substance and the placebo became therapeutically equal after 4 weeks. Roberts and Hamilton (1958) reported that, in neurotic anxiety reactions, patients treated with a placebo showed significant improvement in anxious mood, insomnia and tension and later on in autonomic symptoms, fears and somatic manifestations.

ii. Adverse Effects. Adverse effects of placebos were reviewed by Wolf and Pinsky (1954), Beecher (1959), Kennedy (1961) and more recently by Pogge (1963). In the last review side-effects with placebos were ranked by frequency of occurrence. Pogge (1963) found that depression of the central nervous system (drowsiness, weakness, fatigue, heaviness of limbs, motor retardation, etc.) occurred most frequently and was present in well over 6 per cent of cases. Headache ranked second, followed by stimulation of the central nervous system manifested in nervousness and insomnia. Nausea was fourth and constipation fifth. Less frequently occurring adverse effects were vertigo, dry mouth, gastrointestinal symptoms and anorexia.

In view of all the foregoing, the question arose whether placebo-prone and placebo-resistant functions could be differentiated. Lehmann and Knight (1960), in a carefully designed study, found that placebo-prone functions include autonomic reactions and psychological functions which require considerable integration. Placebo-resistant functions, on the other hand, include fundamental psychological processes which require only a minimum of integration. Furthermore, they found that the accuracy of performance is relatively placebo resistant, while the speed of performance is relatively placebo prone.

d. Social Factors

The influence of social factors on drug effects was succinctly presented by Hönigfeld (1964). He quotes Beecher (1955, 1958, 1960), who first pointed out the marked differences in pain relief produced by placebo in clinical (postoperative) *versus* experimental laboratory conditions. Other important findings in this respect were Donnelly and Zeller's (1956) and Sabshin and Ramot's (1956), who showed that more dramatic therapeutic results with major tranquilizers (antipsychotics), together with a greater enthusiasm, were seen in the "back wards" of large mental hospitals than in small psychodynamically oriented settings. Mészáros and Gallagher (1958) and Mészáros (1960), working in mental hospital settings, drew attention to the fact that improving the ward milieu by reducing staff tension has a beneficial effect on treatment; and in outpatient situations Fisher *et al.* (1962) suggested that a therapeutic orientation is more beneficial for treatment than an experimental orientation. The effect of the therapist on the outcome of treatment has also been explored (Sheard, 1963; Cohen and Struening, 1962; Gilbert and Levinson, 1963; and Klerman *et al.*, 1963).

To overcome some of the consequences of the effects of "nonspecific factors in treatment" various "blind procedures" have been introduced into therapeutic clinical trials. The nonblind experiments were replaced at first by single-blind studies, in which the experimental subject is the only one who is left "blind," *i.e.*, who is not told what drug is being given. Single-blind studies have been increasingly replaced by double-blind procedures, in which neither the experimenter nor the experimental subject knows which of the substances (active or inactive) is given to any single patient. Triple-blind procedures are also used from time to time in some of the clinical studies, in which the very nature of the substances given are not revealed. More recently, there has been a strong trend toward complementing methodological sophistication with improved clinical skill and judgment. It is becoming increasingly accepted that without the necessary clinical acumen even the best designed experiments are necessarily reduced in their value to a meaningless "clinical exercise."

B. PRACTICAL CONSIDERATIONS

1. Prediction of Therapeutic Outcome

Since psychoactive substances are usually administered over an extended period of time, it is important to find means to predict, at an early stage of treatment, whether a particular patient will respond to a particular drug. Predictive indices would render treatment more economical and would provide a more optimal therapeutic regime at an earlier stage in treatment. This in turn could help to prevent the progression of the ongoing "process" of the illness. These problems were recognized at the Workshop on Prediction of the American College of Neuropsychopharmacology (Wittenborn and May, 1966).

In his introductory presentation, Wittenborn (1966) identified at least three major classes of predictions serving somewhat different purposes in psychopharmacological studies. First there are predictive studies, which are designed to test hypotheses concerning the action of therapeutic agents. Although these studies may be relevant to the task of clinical prediction, their real purpose is to generate further understanding at a purely theoretical level. Then there are those studies which are intended to identify a therapeutic effect in a clinical context. These studies are guided by theoretical formulations concerning the nature of the therapeutic substance or by the clinical knowledge of the pathology involved. This is predictive only in the sense that some therapeutic effect is anticipated. Finally, there are studies to identify those patients who do and those who do not show the anticipated response to the therapeutic agent. These last studies can often reveal knowledge not obtainable with the other designs.

a. Prediction of Outcome of Illness

Systematic studies on prediction of therapeutic responsivity to drugs have recently been undertaken. Less sophisticated tests for predicting the outcome of a psychiatric illness to physical therapies date back at least two decades. More than 20 years ago Gottlieb and Hope (1941) pointed out the relationship between the favorable prognosis of a psychiatric illness in a particular patient and his immediate, although transient, favorable response to intravenous amobarbital.

b. Prediction of Therapeutic Response to ECT

Before Gottlieb and Hope's report (1941), Harris *et al.* (1939) and later Hoch (1946) described that the immediate response to intravenous amobarbital administration may serve as a prognostic indicator for electroshock treatment in schizophrenics. These findings were later confirmed by Frankl and Strotzka (1949) and by Cohen *et al.* (1954). Funkenstein *et al.* (1949) developed another prognostic procedure for electroconvulsive treatment (ECT) in depressed patients. The frequently quoted Funkenstein test is based on the patient's blood pressure and pulse rate responses to the intravenous injection of epinephrine and methacholine over short periods of time. Funkenstein described seven patterns of autonomic responses to these procedures, which appear to be correlated with the therapeutic response of the individual depressed patient to ECT treatment.

c. Prediction of Therapeutic Response to Pharmacotherapy

In the prediction of pharmacotherapeutic effects, much of the work has been aimed at revealing the differential therapeutic effects of various antipsychotic drugs in schizophrenic patients. Similar work has been done in investigating the differential therapeutic effects of various antidepressant drugs in depressive cases. At present there are three frequently employed approaches to this problem: the isolation of general prognostic factors, *e.g.*, age, sex, education, etc.; the systematic assessment of admission status, *e.g.*, by rating scales; and the periodic sampling of patients' behavior, feelings, etc., through standardized psychological tests (Tuma, 1966). The second approach, *i.e.*, the assessment of the patient at the time of admission by means of rating scales, has proved to be the most revealing for prognostic purposes.

i. Prediction in Schizophrenics. In schizophrenic patients Overall *et al.* (1963), using computer-derived diagnostic models, were able to demonstrate that paranoid and nonparanoid schizophrenic patients responded equally well to perphenazine, while only patients with predominantly paranoid psychopathology responded to acetophenazine. On the basis of the pretreatment scores on Lorr's (1953) multidimensional scale for rating psychiatric outpatients (in the U.S. Veterans Administration Cooperative Study), Marks (1963) was able to recognize that the responsiveness to chlorpromazine was associated with cooperativeness; to perphenazine, with sociability; to prochlorperazine, with activity level; and to trifluoperazine, with anxiety and tension.

Differential predictive indications for improvement with three phenothiazines (chlorpromazine, fluphenazine and thioridazine) were suggested by Goldberg *et al.*, (1966) in the Collaborative Multi-Hospital Study of the NIMH. While multiple correlations did not reach significance for the placebo and thioridazine patients, prediction of improvement was significant in the chlorpromazine and fluphenazine groups. By multiple regression equations it was also shown that patients who responded to chlorpromazine had been suffering from a state of high arousal manifested in irritability, agitation and confusion, in contradistinction to the fluphenazine responders, who prior to treatment had grandiose delusions and hallucinations.

Applying a typological approach to the problem of predicting response to treatment, Katz (1966) found that fluphenazine was more effective than thioridazine in reducing schizophrenic disorganization in the withdrawn suspicious group of patients, in contradistinction to thioridazine, which was significantly better in the withdrawn periodically agitated cases. On the basis of these results, Katz concluded that a given type of patient will respond better to tranquilizing drugs in general than another type; that a particular drug may be more effective in one kind of patient than another drug; and that a particular symptom complex will be differentially affected depending on the type of patient in which it occurs.

ii. Prediction in Depressives. In depressive conditions the relationship between diagnosis and outcome of treatment with a particular drug has been suggested by several authors. Kuhn (1958) reported that the proper indication for imipramine was a simple endogenous depression and that any additional complication of the depression impaired the chances for successful treatment. Kuhn's assertion was supported by Kiloh and Ball's (1961) findings. West and Dally (1959) demonstrated, on the other hand, that the MAOI antidepressant iproniazid is most specific for atypical depressions, which often resemble anxiety hysteria with depressive features.

Furthermore, Sargant and Dally (1962) differentiated among three groups of patients on the basis of their response to antidepressant treatment. The first group responded to MAOI alone; these depressed patients all had a good basic personality and a relatively stable autonomic nervous system, and their psychopathology arose only after severe stress. The patients of the second group required MAOI's in combination with chlordiazepoxide; they had a stable autonomic nervous system with prevailing anxiety, often with phobic, hysterical or obsessive coloring. The third group of patients suffered from chronic anxiety and tension states; they did not do well with combination therapy, MAOI alone increased their anxiety and they responded more favorably to short-acting barbiturates than to chloridazepoxide.

In a carefully designed methodological study, Wittenborn (1966) examined some of the pretreatment factors which qualify the effects of imipramine or iproniazid in the attempt to provide a basis for comparing these two drugs. The relative importance of various qualifying factors was assessed by means of computing first order correlations between the "qualifiers" and the criteria and then computing partial correlations between each qualifier and each criterion. As a result, he found three "qualifiers." A history of suicidal attempt had a positive implication for iproniazid and an adverse implication for imipramine treatment; a dependent, self-critical, premorbid personality had a negative implication for imipramine but was not significantly positive or negative for iproniazid treatment; and a minor degree of pretreatment paranoia had a generally adverse implication for iproniazid. The negative implications of pretreatment paranoia were not general for the imipramine group.

An entirely new approach in predicting therapeutic responsivity to drugs was recognized during the course of conditional reflex studies on the effect of psychoactive drugs in schizophrenia (Choi *et al.*, 1966). It was observed that those patients who improved clinically showed no significant changes in orienting response, unconditional reflex and disinhibitory activity while on psychoactive drugs. In those cases in which psychoactive drugs acted as suppressing agents on these variables, the patient failed in general to show any significant clinical change. In acutely disturbed patients the only predictor of psychotherapeutic drug effectiveness was dependent on whether the same level of conditional reflex activity was maintained during treatment as that recorded prior to treatment.

2. Long-Term Adverse Effects

Psychoactive drugs (particularly antipsychotic substances) are usually administered over extended periods of time. Hence, most reports on long term adverse effects to date deal almost exclusively with those effects which are attributed to the excessive and prolonged usage of antipsychotic phenothiazine drugs. Among them, irreversible extrapyramidal manifestations, skin pigmentation and ocular changes are the ones most extensively described.

a. Extrapyramidal Signs (EPS)

i. EPS in General. The appearance of dyskinesia and other extrapyramidal signs (EPS) were among the first adverse concomitant effects of treatment described with phenothiazine drugs, particularly with those which had a piperazine ring on their side chain. These EPS were assumed to be harmless and reversible. Some even considered EPS essential for the therapeutic effect of these drugs.

The whole subject of extrapyramidal side-effects was superbly reviewed by Chien and DiMascio (1967). They subdivided drug-induced extrapyramidal signs into permanent neuroleptic and paroxysmal or subacute neurodysleptic manifestations and considered the "akinetic" (hypotonia or rigidity) and "agitans" (tremor) reactions described by the European authors, which in the Anglo-American literature are referred to as "parkinsonism" or "parkinsonian-like" reactions, as permanent neuroleptic manifestations. Among the paroxysmal reactions, they distinguished between principal paroxysmal manifestations (hyperkinesia and dystonia in the European or dystonic reactions in the Anglo-American literature) and secondary subacute manifestations (psychosensory and psychomotor excitation symptoms in the European or akathisia in the Anglo-American literature).

Since extrapyramidal manifestations occur with the various antipsychotic groups of drugs such as the phenothiazines, Rauwolfias, butyrophenones and thioxanthenes, the question arose whether they are a necessary aspect of the drug's therapeutic action. The early studies of Brooks (1955), Freyhan (1955, 1959), Ayd (1955) and Goldman (1959) in North America implied that the appearance of extrapyramidal manifestations may in fact be essential for the antipsychotic action of an antipsychotic drug. (Although later on Goldman in 1961, and Freyhan in 1961, changed their position in this respect.) The relationship between extrapyramidal signs and antipsychotic potential was first questioned by Karn and Kasper (1956), but it was Hollister *et al.* (1960) and Cole and Clyde (1961) who suggested that the production of extrapyramidal signs was not essential to the clinical efficacy of antipsychotic drugs (Chien and DiMascio, 1967). This was further supported by Ban *et al.* (1962), Simpson *et al.* (1964), and Bishop *et al.* (1965).

Opposed to this is the opinion of some of the prominent European investigators such as Divry *et al.* (1960), Delay and Deniker (1961), and Sigwald *et al.* (1959), who maintain that the development of extrapyramidal signs is a prerequisite of therapeutic effects. Haase (1961) and Brune *et al.* (1962) suggest that the optimal behavioral improvement occurs when the akinetic manifestations as revealed by handwriting inhibition are noted, while Delay and Deniker (1961), supported by Morosini (1963) and Denham (1960, 1965), assert that the essential aspects of extrapyramidal manifestations are the psychic excitation and dystonic reactions, which they called the excito-motor syndrome. This is the same as Divry's (1960) neurodysleptic phenomena.

According to Denber (1961), drug-induced extrapyramidal manifestations are complex physiological-psychodynamic reactions. While Denber (1961) considers EPS as secondary elaborations of the primary central effects of the drugs, which vary from patient to patient and may have a therapeutic function, Sarwer-Foner (1960, 1961) proposes that in certain patients the pharmacological drug effect may remove or interfere chemically with activities that are used as components of ego defenses against underlying unconscious conflicts. Consequently they may cause increased anxiety, agitation and further neurotic and psychotic disturbances as well as extrapyramidal manifestations. The findings of Heninger *et al.* (1965) that physically oriented extroverts reacted negatively to the motor-inhibiting effect of chlorpromazine seems to be in favor of Sarwer-Foner's (1960, 1961) assertions.

In spite of the extensive literature on this subject, the question whether extrapyramidal manifestations in general or certain extrapyramidal signs in particular are essential for antipsychotic action still remains to be answered. At any rate, EPS are, to a greater or lesser extent, potentially present secondary attributes with all the drugs used in the treatment of psychotic patients; therefore, perhaps more important than whether EPS is present is that it points to a particular site of action.

ii. Irreversible EPS. Irreversible dyskinesias affecting the face, mouth, tongue and jaw in the course of chronic phenothiazine administration were first described by Sigwald and collaborators in 1959 and soon after by Uhrbrand and Faurbye in 1960. Renewed interest in this syndrome followed the publications of Earl and Hunter (1963) and Hunter *et al.* (1964). The last authors surveyed 450 chronic patients in a mental hospital and found irreversible dyskinesias in 13 out of 250 women (an incidence of 5 per cent). Men did not show this complication. All these cases with irreversible EPS had been on phenothiazine derivatives for 18 months to 5 years before abnormal movements were first observed. It was also recognized that the risk of developing these manifestations was greatly increased when the patient's brain was damaged or diseased.

Since treatment with antiparkinsonian drugs or even discontinuation of phenothiazine treatment (for 8 months to 3 years) remained ineffective, the dyskinesias described were considered to be irreversible extrapyramidal manifestations.

b. Skin Pigmentation

The first cases of skin pigmentation resulting from excessive phenothiazine administration were described by Ey *et al.* (1956). They reported three cases—on prolonged chlorpromazine treatment—who developed an erythematous rash with marked pigmentation of the face (which resembled a "magot chinois"). In 1962 Perrot and Bourjala published a report in a dermatological journal discussing a diagnostic problem which they called "purple face" (*visage mauve*). This discoloration was seen in a 48-year-old schizophrenic female who received chlorpromazine and later thioridazine treatment for several years.

Renewed interest in phenothiazine-induced skin pigmentation followed the work of Greiner and collaborators (1964). According to their first report, these changes occurred mainly in females (in association with amenorrhea) and were primarily seen in the sun-exposed areas of the face, neck, upper chest, dorsum of hand and lower legs after at least 3 years of intensive chlorpromazine treatment with an average daily dosage of 500 to 1000 mg. (Greiner and Berry, 1964; and Greiner and Nicolson, 1964). The work of Greiner *et al.* (1964) was followed by other studies, including Ban and Lehmann's (1965) and Satanove's (1965), and, more recently, the relevant clinical information on phenothiazine-induced skin pigmentation has been summarized by Ayd (1966).

According to Ayd (1966), some but not all phenothiazines cause a pigmentation of the light-exposed skin (face, neck, hands), and the larger the dosage and the longer the duration of administration, the greater the risk in susceptible individuals. The dermatological reaction consists of a destructive gray, violaceous discoloration of the skin causing some patients to have a purple-gray look. These changes evolve slowly and occur in less than 1 per cent of those receiving 200 mg. of chlorpromazine or more daily, and they are usually not apparent until after 2 years of continuous treatment. Ayd (1966) maintains that the fact that this phenomena had occurred most often in chlorpromazine-treated patients is more likely a reflection solely of the widespread use of this drug rather than an indication that it is more responsible for skin pigmentation than other phenothiazines.

There is no general agreement on what mechanisms are involved in the development of the pigmentary changes. One of the early hypotheses put forward by Ban and Lehmann (1965) was that phenothiazines caused a "shunting of the dopa metabolism away from the epinephrine synthesis," thereby producing increased melanin formation. Beyond a certain level (facilitated by light), the excess of melanin pigment is "dropped" from the epidermis into the dermis, where it forms a complex with the excess of chlorpromazine. The inference based on this hypothesis was that this complex—melanin and chlorpromazine—is the discoloration-producing pigment.

An even earlier hypothesis was that of Greiner (1965), who assumed that some sort of genetic defect might be present in the skin-pigmented cases. He postulated that this was caused by faulty melanin metabolism, either by a decrease of melatonin (a corpus pineal-produced hormone which reduces pigmentation) production or by an enzymatic inactivation of melatonin. According to him, in a small percentage of patients developing this side-effect the genetic defect affecting melatonin synthesis leads primarily to melanosis and only secondarily to the skin pathology seen after chlorpromazine therapy.

More recently, Forrest (1968) presented her views on this subject. She assumed that there is a chemical interaction between melanin and chlorpromazine (or other phenothiazine drugs). The most likely chemical reaction she considers is one of electron donation by chlorpromazine and of electron acceptance by melanin, so that a charge-transfer complex or some type of adduct is formed. Linking her views with Greiner's (1965) are thin layer chromatographic findings. These showed striking acquired or genetically determined differences in the metabolism of chlorpromazine between drug responders, nonresponders and patients with phenothiazine-induced skin pigmentation. Characteristic of the drug responders was a relatively large conjugate fraction in the urine and of the nonresponders, a substantially smaller conjugate fraction. Patients with skin pigmentation showed entire groups of conjugates missing.

Successful treatments of phenothiazine-induced skin pigmentation have been reported. There is some evidence that discontinuation of the drug leads to attenuation and after a considerable time to disappearance of the dermatological manifestations. Greiner and Nicolson (1965) at first suggested "dark room therapy" to facilitate melatonin production over a period of 4 weeks. Later they recommended the administration of a copper chelating agent in order to block melanin production by the inactivation of tyrosinase. For this purpose penicillamine in daily doses of 1000 mg. was given. Urinary copper excretion was significantly increased during this treatment. The therapeutic effect of penicillamine treatment in phenothiazine-induced skin pigmentation was confirmed by Gibbard and Lehmann (1966).

c. Ocular Pathology

Ocular changes in the course of thioridazine administration had been described soon after the introduction of this piperidyl side-chain containing phenothiazine substance. The pigmentary retinopathy, which causes rapid visual impairment, usually occurs within 1 to 2 months after commencement of treatment with doses above 1000 mg. a day.

A different type and less incapacitating ocular complication was described at first in skin-pigmented cases and later in a rather high percentage of patients receiving various aminopropyl or piperidyl side-chain containing phenothiazine drugs. By slit-lamp examination the occurrence of ocular changes was reported to be 37 per cent (Brill *et al.*, 1965), 33 per cent (Wetterholm *et al.*, 1965), 29 per cent (Mathalone, 1965) and 27 per cent (Barsa *et al.*, 1965) of all patients receiving phenothiazine treatment over an extended period of time. Analysis of the data suggested that the piperazine side-chain containing phenothiazines are free of this effect to date (Ayd, 1966).

Greiner and Berry (1964) were first to observe that some of their skin-pigmented cases had also developed corneal and lenticular lesions. A more detailed description of the nature of these lesions was given by Siddall (1965). Examining 78 skin-pigmented patients, he reported that 11 showed severe and 46 showed moderate corneal pigmentation. While he recognized lenticular lesions in 59 of his patients, retinal degeneration occurred only in 2. The ocular manifestations were described as a peculiar hazy-brown pigmentation of the exposed sclera and cornea. In cases in which this was found to be present, ophthalmoscopic examination revealed a dark-brown irregular, stellate or cocklebur-shaped opacity of the lenses with a dense central area and radiating branches. On slit-lamp examination, discrete yellow-white dots were seen, which were concentrated in the center with radiating arms in the anterior subcapsular pole. Under the same conditions the corneal lesions were described as yellowish-white granules—localized in the stroma—mainly in the posterior half of the cornea more centrally than peripherally.

In Ban and Lehmann's (1965) study on skin-pigmented cases, conjunctival, corneal and lens pathology were found in all but one of the experimental subjects. It was the ophthalmologist's impression (Adams, 1968) that there was a high correlation between the abnormal ocular findings and phenothiazine consumption in these cases; that the abnormal findings occurred more often in those patients with skin pigmentation and also in a higher degree of severity; that patients on chlorpromazine without skin pigmentation showed no conjunctival changes, but they were not exempt from corneal and lens pathology; and that sunlight appeared to have some relationship to the corneal and conjunctival superficial changes. The observation that the ocular changes occur in a higher incidence in the skin-pigmented cases was confirmed by Tredici *et al.* (1965) and Siddall (1965), who found eye lesions in 91 per cent and 81 per cent of their skin-pigmented cases, respectively. It was noted that in most of the cases visual acuity was not or was only slightly impaired.

Successful treatment of ocular changes was reported with dietary control of "copper" and simultaneous "penicillamine" administration. (The latter inactivates tyrosinase, the enzyme which may be responsible for the abnormal melanogenesis.) Seclusion in a dark room or melatonin injections also proved to be useful (Greiner, 1965). Replacement of the aminopropyl or piperidyl phenothiazine drug with a piperazine side-chain containing phenothiazine prevents further aggravation of eye complications, while discontinuation of phenothiazine treatment leads slowly to the reduction of eye deposits.

3. The Effects of Drug Withdrawal

a. Immediate Effects (Drug Dependence)

Over the last 15 years considerable international interest has been focused on the problems of drug dependence. Eight distinctly different types of drug dependence have now been delineated.

i. Nomenclature. Drug dependence was defined as a state of psychic or physical (or both) "dependence" on a chemical substance which develops after it is periodically or continuously administered. According to the WHO Expert Committee (1964), the characteristics of "drug dependence" vary with the agent involved in each specific case. Nevertheless, drug dependence is an all-inclusive term which encompasses drug addiction and drug habituation.

"Drug addiction" was defined (WHO Expert Committee, 1957) as a "state of periodic or chronic intoxication produced by the repeated consumption of a drug (natural or synthetic). Its characteristics include: an over-powering desire or need (compulsion) to continue taking the drug and to obtain it by any means; a tendency to increase the dose; a psychic (psychological) and generally a physical dependence on the effects of the drug; and a detrimental effect on the individual and/or society."

On the other hand, they defined "drug habituation" as a condition resulting from the repeated consumption of a drug. Its characteristics include: a desire (but not a compulsion) to continue taking the drug for the sense of improved well-being which it engenders; little or no tendency to increase the dose; some degree of psychic dependence on the effect of the drug, but absence of physical dependence, *i.e.*, of an abstinence syndrome; and possible detrimental effects on the individual.

The notion of drug tolerance has also been defined. It was described as an "adaptive state" characterized by diminished response to the same quantity of a given drug or by the fact that a larger dose is required to produce the same degree of pharmacodynamic effect (Isbell and White, 1953).

In an excellent review on drug dependence, its significance and characteristics, Eddy *et al.* (1966) explicitly emphasized the fact that both drug dependence and drug abuse may occur without the development of demonstrable tolerance.

ii. Pathomechanism. The pathomechanism of drug dependence can be discussed on the basis of several "models." The classical *cellular* model is based on the observation that to some of the dependence-producing drugs, *e.g.*, opiates, tolerance develops, followed by physical and, later on, also by psychic or emotional dependence (Isbell and White, 1953). Since, with the development of tolerance, there is a decreased response to the drug, it has been asserted that this phenomenon is the result of the "occupation" of "receptors on certain myelinated neurons" by the dependence-producing substance (which thereby exerts its pharmacologic or pathologic effects). Thus, tolerance was considered to be the consequence of either a maximal cell-receptor saturation or a change (increase) in the excitability of the cell body (or of both). In this frame of reference Seevers and Woods (1953) suggested that physical dependence is the result of "the unmasking" of this increased excitability of the cell body in the period of abstinence by the "loss" of the protecting drug. Isbell and White (1953) maintain that it is physical dependence that leads to emotional dependence, which constitutes a substitution by the use of the drug for other types of adaptive behavior.

The *neurophysiological* model of drug dependence is based on the experiments of Olds (1958), who was able artificially to induce a compulsive "pleasure seeking" behavior. In collaboration with Margules, he demonstrated (Margules and Olds, 1962) that rats, with electrodes implanted in the septal region of their brain or in the anterior part of the hypothalamus, showed a marked increase in lever pressing, *i.e.*, self-stimulation (even in preference to feeding or drinking). According to Lehmann (1963), "a model of addiction based on this observation would conceive of the addicting agent as being a suitable stimulator of the pleasure or reward centres in the brain and inducing a self-perpetuating cycle of behavior which is characterized by the continuous seeking of the special addicting agent."

The *conditioning* model, as proposed by Wikler (1948, 1953, 1963), was based on the observation that "cured" opiate addicts experienced craving and a repetition of some of the abstinence-syndrome manifestations when exposed to stimuli which were formerly strongly associated with their previous drug experiences. According to him, drug dependence can be understood as a process of conditioning in which the actual drug experience serves as the unconditional stimulus and the associated environmental factors as conditional stimuli.

Among the various *psychoanalytical* views, Rado's is one of the most frequently referred to (1933). According to him, the satisfaction obtained from the dependency-producing drug is a reactivation of the orgastic experience the infant had after breast feeding. More recently, Glover (1956) asserted that drug addiction serves to control sadism and is a protective device against paranoid psychosis. Szasz (1958) believes that it serves to deny any possible loss of primal love, while Rosenfeld (1960) maintains that ego-splitting has a prominent role in drug addiction.

iii. Classification. Whatever the mechanisms may be, drug dependency can be pragmatically classified clinically as "increment producing" or "decrement producing." Within this dichotomy (first proposed by Lehmann, 1963), drug addicts can be further subdivided into those seeking thrill producing, facilitative and derealizing, *i.e.*, increment-producing, drugs *versus* those seeking disinhibiting (pseudofacilitative), tranquilizing and stupefying, *i.e.*, decrement-producing, drugs.

The characteristic features of drug dependence on morphine, barbiturates and alcohol, cocaine, cannabis (marijuana), amphetamines, khat, and on the hallucinogen (LSD) type of drugs (Eddy *et al.*, 1966) are distinctly different. More recently, a new class of primarily physical dependence on the neuroleptic-antidepressant type of drugs was suggested by Battegay (1966), which is independent not only of tolerance but also of psychological dependence.

Morphine-type drug dependence is characterized by a strong, psychic dependence manifested as an overpowering drive to continue taking the drug. Tolerance and physical dependence develop early and increase in intensity with increasing dosage. Abstinence syndrome usually occurs a few hours after the last dose has been given and reaches its peak intensity within 24 to 48 hours. The more severe symptoms subside within 10 days. Isbell and White (1953), reporting on the symptoms of the abstinence syndrome, encountered anxiety, restlessness, body aches, insomnia, yawning, lacrimation, rhinorrhea, perspiration, mydriasis, piloerection, hot flushes, nausea, emesis, diarrhea, elevation of body temperature, respiratory rate, and systolic blood pressure, cramps, dehydration, anorexia and loss of body weight.

The most harmful aspects of this type of drug dependence arise from the constant preoccupation with the drug, which results in personal neglect, malnutrition and infections. Socially it leads to the "disruption of interpersonal relationships," to serious economic loss and not infrequently to crime.

The *barbiturate-alcohol type* of drug dependence is characterized by a psychic dependence of varying degree which may lead to periodic rather than to continuous abuse, particularly with alcohol. While there is a definite physical dependence, tolerance to these substances is irregular and incomplete. Abstinence syndrome usually begins within the first 24 hours after discontinuation and reaches peak intensity in 2 to 3 days and then subsides slowly. In the order of development the symptoms of the abstinence syndrome include: twitching of the muscles, tremor of hands and fingers, weakness, dizziness, disturbed visual perception, nausea, vomiting, weight loss, hypotension, cerebral seizure, insomnia, anxiety and delirium. Occasionally psychotic episodes, paranoid reactions, schizophrenic-like reactions, semistuporous and panicky states have been observed.

The most harmful aspects of this type of drug dependence stem from the impairment of nervous coordination and mental functions. The emotional instability leads to the deterioration of interpersonal relationships and assaultive behavior. Alcohol impairs the efficiency of thinking and psychomotor coordination, resulting in accidents and the deterioration of work performance. Excessive—and chronic—alcohol consumption predisposes the individual to such physical diseases as fatty portal cirrhosis, peripheral neuropathies, cardiomyopathies, etc., and may lead to Korsakoff's psychosis or Wernicke's encephalopathy. Consequently, the productivity of the alcoholic inevitably declines, and his family often becomes dependent on social welfare.

The *cocaine type* of drug dependence is characterized by a strong psychic—without physical—dependence and by the absence of tolerance. Digestive disorders, nausea, loss of appetite, emaciation, sleeplessness and convulsions are the common manifestations. The overestimation of capabilities, not infrequently, together with paranoid delusions and auditory, visual and tactile hallucinations, predispose the drug-dependent individual to commit dangerous, antisocial acts.

The *cannabis* (*marijuana*) *type* of drug dependence is characterized by a moderate to strong psychic—without physical—dependence and by questionable tolerance. Inertia, lethargy, self-neglect and asocial or antisocial behavior are frequently present, while the precipitation of psychosis is rather rare.

The *amphetamine type* of drug dependence is characterized by variable psychic dependence; no physical dependence (although withdrawal is usually followed by a state of mental and physical depression as the organism is freed from the persistent stimulation); and the slow development of a considerable degree of tolerance to some (but not all) of the amphetamine effects. Chronic amphetamine abuse may lead to accident proneness (due to both the excitation and the excessive fatigue, which may break through at an inopportune time) and also to dangerous antisocial acts.

The *khat type* of drug dependence resembles the amphetamine type. This is probably due to the fact that the active principle of the khat leaf is chemically and pharmacologically related to the amphetamines. Characteristics of this type of dependence are a moderate but often persistent psychic—without physical—dependence and the absence of tolerance. Besides the social and the economic there is also a physical deterioration (due to the tannin content) in khat addicts.

The *hallucinogen (LSD) type* of drug dependence is increasing in frequency. This has been reported for lysergic acid diethylamide, psilocybin and mescaline. Psychic dependence on these drugs is usually not intense, nor is there any physical dependence. On the other hand, rapidly developing and disappearing tolerance to LSD_{25} and psilocybin was revealed by Isbell *et al.* (1956) and Wolbach *et al.* (1962). This is in contradistinction to mescaline, to which tolerance develops only slowly.

The possibility of drug dependence to the *neuroleptic-antidepressant type* of drugs was explored by Battegay (1966). In the course of systematic studies he demonstrated that when antipsychotic (neuroleptic) drugs alone were withdrawn in 58 patients, 35 experienced withdrawal symptoms within the first 3 days, while 23 did not. This difference was not statistically significant. On the other hand, when antipsychotic and antiparkinsonian agents were abruptly withdrawn simultaneously in 23 patients, 20 of them experienced withdrawal symptoms and only 3 did not. This difference proved to be statistically significant. Similar results were seen for the total group of 81 patients, *i.e.*, 55 experienced withdrawal symptoms as opposed to 26 who did not.

The withdrawal symptoms after chronic administration of antipsychotic drugs were described by Battegay (1966) as subjective feeling of warmth or cold, sweating, vertigo, tachycardia, a tendency to collapse, headache, insomnia and in some cases nausea and vomiting. Other symptoms of drug withdrawal were tremor and the mouth-tongue-throat syndrome (a hyperkinesia of this whole region). Similar manifestations were observed by Kramer *et al.* (1961) following discontinuation of high dosage chronic (2 months) administration of imipramine. Thus Battegay (1966) recognized a new neuroleptic-antidepressant type of drug dependence characterized by central autonomic symptoms and central extrapyramidal signs (EPS), both of which indicate the existence of physical dependence without a demonstrable psychic dependence or tolerance.

The presence of central autonomic symptoms after the withdrawal of antipsychotic drugs had also been described by Gallant *et al.* (1964) and the exacerbation of EPS by Uhrbrand and Faurbye (1960), Ayd (1961), Delay and Deniker (1961), Haddenbrock (1964) and Degkwitz and Luxenburger (1965).

The dependence which develops with antipsychotic and antidepressant drugs is distinctly different from that which develops with anxiolytic drugs. The physical dependence on these latter substances, *e.g.*, propanediols and benzodiazepines, in addition to the autonomic manifestations may lead to muscle twitching and/or cerebral seizures in the withdrawal period. Since the dependence on anxiolytic drugs resembles that of the barbiturate-alcoholic type, physical dependence is complemented by psychic dependence and the development of tolerance.

iv. Drug Detection. The detection of dependency-producing substances in the urine in general and narcotics in particular was first studied by Mannering *et al.* (1954). He developed a method for the extraction of alkaloids from the urine and the detection of these by paper partition chromatography. One of the limitations of the Mannering method was the length of time (24 hours) it took to complete an analysis. This was overcome by Cochin and Daly (1962), who were able to demonstrate that a variety of analgesic drugs can be separated by thin layer chromatography and detected on thin layer plates with the usual alkaloid reagents. This new technique made it possible to complete an analysis of the addict's urine in 5 to 6 hours.

The Cochin-Daly (1962) technique is the one most frequently used for the detection of synthetic analgesics (Parker and Hine, 1966; and Kokoski, 1965), narcotics (Davidow, 1965; and Kokoski, 1965), amphetamines and barbiturates (Davidow, 1965; and McIsaac, 1965).

A further methodological contribution for extracting narcotics, amphetamines and barbiturates from the urine was the cation-exchange resin-loaded paper technique (Dole *et al.*, 1965). This was adapted by Jaffe (1965) for the extraction of barbiturates with an anion-exchange resin-loaded paper (Leonard, 1966).

b. Delayed Effects (Maintenance Treatment)

i. Schizophrenics and Chronic Organic Brain Syndromes. As early as 1957, Kris and Carmichael and, independently, Winkelman (1957) reported that schizophrenic patients will relapse if chlorpromazine is withheld for even a moderate period of time. These findings were supported by Caffey *et al.* (1964) and restated by Winkelman (1964). On the other hand, Good *et al.* (1958) and, independently, Diamond and Marks (1960) were able to demonstrate that chlorpromazine could be withdrawn for at least 10 to 12 weeks without any noticeable relapse, or even for a period of 5 to 6 months (Olson and Peterson, 1960; and Garfield *et al.*, 1966).

Lehmann and Ban (1966) studied the effects of discontinuation of drug therapy over a time on various psychological functions in chronic psychotic patients. They demonstrated significant changes in Reaction Time (RT) and Word Association Time (WAT). For the total group, consisting of both schizophrenic and organic patients, the salient change was the shortening of RT after the second week without medication. RT increased slowly thereafter. Even after 6 weeks without drugs, RT was still shorter than prior to drug withdrawal. Essentially there was no difference in the changes for schizophrenic and organic psychiatric patients, although patients with chronic brain syndromes did show a greater decrease in RT after the second week and weaker adaptation in the next 6 weeks. With regard to WAT, the immediate (2-week) effect of drug withdrawal for all groups was a marked blocking of associations. After the initial blocking, the long range (6-week) effect of drug withdrawal for schizophrenic patients was loosening of associations, as evidenced by a reduction in association time. In the WAT test the effect of drug withdrawal on patients with chronic brain syndrome was quite different from that of the schizophrenics. In this group blocking increased with the prolonged (6-week) duration of time.

In another study, Lehmann and Ban (1966) confirmed the finding that withdrawal of antipsychotic medication produced changes in schizophrenic and chronic brain syndrome cases. It was shown that the schizophrenic groups maintained their adjustment for approximately 1 month after the medication was discontinued. During the next 2 months they rapidly deteriorated. By the end of 6 months of no medication, compared with the psychiatric status at the time when medication was discontinued, the deterioration was significant at the 0.005 level of confidence (Wilcoxon's Matched Pairs Signed Ranks Test). The groups which were comprised of chronic brain syndrome cases showed progressive impairment with a slight rally in the sixth month. This remained still significant at the 0.01 level of confidence (Wilcoxon's Matched Pairs Signed Ranks Test) when compared with the beginning of the no-medication period.

In an after-care setting St. Laurent *et al.* (1962) indicated that discontinuation or decrease in the dosage of prochlorperazine resulted in exacerbation of symptoms, which in most cases responded promptly to resumption of maintenance therapy or to an increase of dosage. This had formerly been demonstrated by Gross (1960), who found that during the first 6 months of the after-care period those patients who were maintained on an active antipsychotic compound had only a 13 per cent relapse rate as opposed to 51 per cent for those who had been on a reduced dosage of the medication or on placebos.

On the basis of these findings, it was recommended that, after the first schizophrenic episode, medication should be continued for a period of at least 1 year after symptomatic remission; after a second episode, for not less than 4 to 5 years; after the third, for 5 to 10 years; and if there are more than three episodes the patient should be kept on medication indefinitely.

ii. Depressives. The question as to when antidepressant drug therapy can safely be discontinued has also been systematically investigated. Exacerbation of psychopathology was considered as a long term effect of discontinuation of treatment.

One of the first to provide evidence of this was Ayd (1959), who separated 20 depressive patients into five groups and discontinued the imipramine treatment of each group at different time intervals (at the end of the fourth, sixth, eighth, tenth and twelfth week). He found that within 1 to 3 days all patients in groups one and two relapsed and the same occurred within 3 to 7 days for all in group three. Within 4 to 10 days, three of four patients from group four and within 12 to 16 days two of four patients from group five again showed depressive symptoms. On the basis of these findings, Ayd (1959) suggested that depressed patients should continue on antidepressant medication for a minimum of 12 weeks after amelioration of symptoms, after which they should be gradually tapered off over a period of several months.

In a carefully designed study, a group of depressed patients were treated by a combination of electroconvulsive therapy and imipramine (or an identical placebo) during their hospitalization. On discharge the patients were switched from imipramine to placebo and vice versa. It was found that about 85 per cent of the placebo group relapsed in contrast to 20 per cent of the imipramine patients.

In a 1-year follow-up of depressed patients treated in the Cooperative Veterans Administration Study, it was demonstrated that the rate of relapse was higher in patients whose medication had been discontinued within 3 months after maximal improvement than in those who were kept on their antidepressant drugs (Hönigfeld and Lasky, 1962).

On the basis of these findings, Bennett (1966) recommended that therapy with antidepressant drugs should be continued until depressive manifestations would have ordinarily "spontaneously" remitted. In cases of reactive, neurotic depressive cases this is usually considered to be not less than 3 months; for reactive, psychotic depressive patients, at least 6 months; for endogenous, manic-depressive, depressives, from 6 to 12 months or longer; and for involutional melancholics, from 1 to 5 years.

iii. Detection of Drugs. The importance of continuous long term treatment in a variety of psychiatric conditions made it necessary to develop tests for detecting whether patients are taking their medication. The same tests can also be used in cases of overdosage with an unidentified drug and in clinical trials as a screening device to exclude the possibility of false results caused by experimental subjects who might not be taking the investigational substance.

From a practical point of view it was crucial to develop a method for the detection of phenothiazines and tricyclic antidepressants (particularly for phenothiazines, for which prolonged maintenance treatment is an essential factor in preventing relapse).

Methods for the detection of phenothiazines were developed by Forrest and Forrest (1957, 1958, 1959, 1960). At first they succeeded in developing a single procedure for the detection of chlorpromazine; subsequently they were able to extend the applicability of this procedure for the detection of promazine, trifluopromazine and finally for any piperazine side chain containing phenothiazine. In 1960 the same investigators succeeded also in developing a test for the detection of imipramine in the urine.

The Forrest test is a semiquantitative procedure which consists of adding ferric chloride, perchloric acid and nitric acid (FPN) to the urine. This gives an immediate color reaction. The shade, intensity and stability of the reaction are dependent on the chemical nature of the substance involved and the amount of the drug present in the urine. In spite of its routine use in many mental hospitals, the FPN color test in its original form gave approximately 20 per cent of false results. While some of the *false positives* were due to liver dysfunction, in the majority of cases, as demonstrated by Campbell (1965), a delayed reaction "due to possible individual patient variations" seemed to be the cause of *false negatives*. Consequently, by delaying the test readings from 1 to 10 minutes, it was possible to eliminate the false negative findings.

Other procedures for the detection and quantification of phenothiazines are those of Nadeau and Sobolewski (1959, 1960) and the bromination method of Lucas and Fabierkiewics (1963).

REFERENCES

ADAMS, K.: Ophthalmological aspects. In: Toxicity and adverse reactions studies with neuroleptics and antidepressants (eds., Lehmann, H. E., and Ban, T. A.). (Q.P.R.A., Montreal, 1968.)

AYD, F. J.: Discussion of Goldman's paper, "The effect of chlorpromazine on severe mental and emotional disturbances." In: Chlorpromazine and mental health. (Lea and Febiger, Philadelphia, 1955.)

AYD, F. J.: Chemical treatment of depression. Ann. N. Y. Acad. Sci., *80:* 734 (1959).

AYD, F. J.: Prolonged administration of chlorpromazine (thorazine) hydrochloride. J.A.M.A., *169:* 1296 (1959).

AYD, F. J.: A survey of drug-induced extrapyramidal reactions. J.A.M.A., *175:* 1054 (1961).

AYD, F. J.: Neuroleptics and extrapyramidal reactions in psychiatric patients. Rev. Canad. Biol., *20:* 451 (1961).

AYD, F. J.: Phenothiazine tranquillizers: eight years of development. Med. Clin. N. Amer., *45:* 1027 (1961).

AYD, F. J.: Phenothiazines: skin and eye complications—a further report. Int. Drug Ther. Newsletter, *1:* 2 (1966).

AYD, F. J.: Toxic somatic psychopathalogic reactions to antidepressant drugs. J. Neuropsychiat., *2:* 119 (1961).

AYD, F. J.: Prolonged pharmacotherapy and the eye. Int. Drug Ther. Newsletter, *1:* 9 (1966).

AYD, F. J.: Research and ethical directives. Int. Drug Ther. Newsletter, *1:* 7 (1966).

BAN, T. A.: Annual report of the research department. Douglas Hospital, Verdun, 1964.

BAN, T. A.: Methodology and pitfalls in clinical testing of psychopharmacological drugs. Chemotherapia (Basel), *9:* 223 (1964).

BAN, T. A., AND LEHMANN, H. E.: Skin pigmentation, a rare side effect of chlorpromazine and a hypothesis concerning one of the mechanisms of its development. Canad. Psychiat. Ass. J., *10:* 112 (1965).

BAN, T. A., *et al.:* Clinical studies with thioproperazine (Majeptil). Compr. Psychiat., *3:* 284 (1962).

BARRABEE, P., BARRABEE, E. L., AND FINESINGER, J.: A normative social adjustment scale. Amer. J. Psychiat., *112:* 252 (1955).

BARSA, J. A., NEWTON, J. C., AND SAUNDERS, J. C.: Lenticular and corneal opacities during phenothiazine therapy. J.A.M.A., *193:* 10 (1965).

BATTEGAY, R.: Drug dependence as a criterion for differentiation of psychotropic drugs. Compr. Psychiat., *7:* 6 (1966).

BATTERMAN, R. G.: Placebo and non-reactors to analgesics. Fed. Proc., *16:* 280 (1957).

BATTERMAN, R. G., AND GROSSMAN, A. J.: Effectiveness of salicylamide as analgesic and antirheumatic agent: evaluation of double blind fold technique for studying analgesic drugs. J.A.M.A., *159:* 1619 (1955).

BECK, A. J., *et al.:* An inventory for measuring depression. Arch. Gen. Psychiat. (Chicago), *4:* 561 (1961).

BEECHER, H. K.: The powerful placebo. J.A.M.A., *159:* 1602 (1955).

BEECHER, H. K.: Relation of drugs to reaction components in subjective responses. In: Psychopharmacology—pharmacologic effects on behavior (ed., Pennes, H. H.). (Hoeber, New York, 1958.)

BEECHER, H. K. (1959): In: The clinical evaluation of new drugs (eds., Waife, S. O., and Shapiro, A. P.). (Hoeber, New York, 1959.)

BEECHER, H. K.: Increased stress and effectiveness of placebos and "active" drugs. Science, *132:* 91 (1960).

BENDER, L., *et al.:* LSD-25 helps schizophrenic children. Amer. Druggist, *146:* 33 (1962).

BENNETT, I. F.: Prediction of response in the pharmacotherapy of depression. In: Prediction of response to pharmacotherapy (eds., Wittenborn, J. R., and May, P. R. A.). (Charles C Thomas, Springfield, 1966.)

BERTI, T., AND CIMA, L.: Influence of species, sex and temperature on metabolism of phenothiazines and related drugs. Psychopharmacol. Serv. Cent. Bull., *2:* 76 (1962).

BIGELOW, N., AND SAINZ, A.: Pitfalls in psychiatric research. Amer. J. Psychiat., *118:* 889 (1962).

BISHOP, M. P., GALLANT, D. M., AND SYKES, J. F.: Extrapyramidal side effects and therapeutic response. Arch. Gen. Psychiat. (Chicago), *13:* 155 (1965).

BRILL, H., SCHEIE, H. G., AND DELONG, S.: Phenothiazines, skin pigmentation and related eye findings. Amer. J. Psychiat., *122:* 326 (1965).

BROOKS, G. W. (1955): In: Chien, C., and DiMascio, A.: Drug induced extrapyramidal symptoms and their relation to clinical efficacy. Amer. J. Psychiat., *123:* 12 (1967).

BRUNE, G. G., AND HIMWICH, H. E.: Effects of methionine loading on the behavior of schizophrenic patients. J. Nerv. Ment. Dis., *134:* 447 (1962).

BRUNE, G. G., *et al.*: Relevance of drug-induced extrapyramidal reaction to behavioral changes during neuroleptic treatment. I. Treatment with trifluoperazine singly and in combination with trihexyphenidyl. Compr. Psychiat., *3:* 227 (1962).

BURDOCK, E. I., *et al.*: A word behaviour rating scale for use with mental hospital patients. J. Clin. Psychol., *16:* 246 (1960).

CAFFEY, E. M., *et al.*: Discontinuation or reduction of chemotherapy in chronic schizophrenics. J. Chronic Dis., *17:* 347 (1964).

CAMPBELL, K. N.: Phenothiazine derivatives in urine: "false negative results" with the Forrest color test (FPN) and a method for their elimination. Clin. Chem., *11:* 914 (1965).

CHEN, K. K., AND POTH, E. J.: Racial differences as illustrated by the mydriatic action of cocaine, enphthalmine and ephedrine. J. Pharmacol. Exp. Ther., *36:* 429 (1929).

CHIEN, C., AND DIMASCIO, A.: Drug-induced extrapyramidal symptoms and their relations to clinical efficacy. Amer. J. Psychiat., *123:* 12 (1967).

CHOI, S. M., *et al.*: Conditional reflex studies on the effect of psychoactive drugs in schizophrenics. Laval Méd., *37:* 122 (1966).

CLYDE, D. J.: Clyde Mood Scale. (NIMH, Bethesda, 1958.)

CLYDE, D. J.: Manual for the Clyde Mood Scale. (Biometric Laboratory, University of Miami, Coral Gables, 1963.)

COCHIN, J., AND DALY, W. J.: Rapid identification of analgesic drugs in urine with thin-layer chromatography. Experientia, *18:* 294 (1962).

COHEN, B. D., SENF, R., AND HUSTON, P. E.: Effect of amobarbital (amytal) on conceptual thinking in schizophrenia, depression and neurosis. Arch. Neurol. Psychiat., *71:* 171 (1954).

COHEN, J., AND STRUENING, E. L.: Opinions about mental illness in the personnel of two large mental hospitals. J. Abnorm. Soc. Psychol., *64:* 349 (1962).

COLE, J. O., AND CLYDE, D. J.: Extrapyramidal side effects and clinical response to the phenothiazines. Rev. Canad. Biol., *20:* 565 (1961).

CUTLER, R. P., AND KURLAND, H. D.: Clinical quantification of depressive reactions. Arch. Gen. Psychiat. (Chicago), *5:* 280 (1961).

DAVIDOW, B. (1965): In: Leonard, F.: Workshop on the detection and control of abuse of narcotics, barbiturates and amphetamines. Psychopharmacology Serv. Cent. Bull., *3:* 21 (1966).

DEGKWITZ, R., AND LUXENBURGER, O.: Das terminale extrapyramidale Insuffizienz-bzw. Defektsyndrom infolge chronischer Anwendung von Neuroleptika. Nervenarzt, *36:* 173 (1965).

DELAY, J., AND DENIKER, P.: Apport de la clinique a la connaissance de l'action des neuroleptiques. In: Extrapyramidal system and neuroleptics (ed., Bordeleau, J.). (Editions Psychiatriques, Montreal, 1961.)

DELAY, J., AND DENIKER, P.: Méthodes chimiothérapiques en psychiatrie. (Masson, Paris, 1961.)

DELAY, J., DENIKER, P., AND HARL, J. M.: Utilisation en therapeutique psychiatrique d'une phénothiazine d'action centrale elective. Ann. Medicopsychol., *2:* 112 (1952).

DELAY, J., SEGGIARO, J. A., AND DENIKER, P.: Réactions biologiques au cours des traitements par le coma hypoglycémique prolongé. Ann. Medicopsychol., *110:* 427 (1952).

DEMPSEY, P.: An unidimensional depression scale for the MMPI. J. Consult. Psychol., *28:* 364 (1964).

DENBER, H. C. B.: Psychodynamic effects of drug induced extrapyramidal reaction on ward social structure. In: Extrapyramidal system and neuroleptics (ed., Bordeleau, J. M.). (Edition Psychiatriques, Montreal, 1961.)

DENHAM, J.: Clinical use of phenothiazines. In: Marks, J., and Pare, C. M. B.: The scientific basis of drug therapy in psychiatry. (Pergamon Press, Oxford, 1965.)

DENHAM, J., AND CARRICK, D.: Therapeutic importance of extrapyramidal phenomena evoked by new phenothiazines. Amer. J. Psychiat., *116:* 927 (1960).

DEVERTEUIL, R. L., AND LEHMANN, H. E.: Therapeutic trial of iproniazid (marsilid) in depressed and apathetic patients. Canad. Med. Ass. J., *78:* 131 (1958).

DIAMOND, L. S., AND MARKS, J. B.: Discontinuance of tranquillizers among chronic schizophrenic patients receiving maintenance dosage. J. Nerv. Ment. Dis., *131:* 247 (1960).

DIVRY, P., *et al.*: Rapport sur l'activité neuropsychopharmacologique du halopéridol (R 1625). Acta Neurol. Belg., *60:* 7 (1960).

DOLE, V. P., *et al.* (1965): In: Leonard, F.: Workshop on the detection and control of abuse of narcotics, barbiturates and amphetamines. Psychopharmacol. Serv. Cent. Bull., *3:* 21 (1966).

DONNELLY, J., AND ZELLER, W.: Clinical research on chlorpromazine in state and private psychiatric hospitals. J. Clin. Exp. Psychopath., *17:* 180 (1956).

EARL, C. J., AND HUNTER, R. (1963): In: Hunter, R., *et al.* An apparently irreversible syndrome of abnormal movements following phenothiazine medication. Proc. Roy. Soc. Med., *54:* 758 (1964).

EDDY, N. B., *et al.*: Drug dependence: its significance and characteristics. Psychopharmacol. Serv. Cent. Bull., *3:* 1 (1966).

ELLSWORTH, R. B.: The MACC behavioral adjustment scale (Form II). (Western Psychological Services, Beverly Hills, 1962.)

EY, FAURE, H., AND RAPPART, P.: Les reactions d'intolerance vis-à-vis de la chlorpromazine. Encephale, *45:* 790 (1956).

FERGUSON, J. T., MCREYNOLDS, P., AND BALLACHEY, E. L.: Hospital adjustment scale.

(Consulting Psychologists Press, Palo Alto, 1953.)

Fisher, S., *et al.:* Drug-set interactions: the effect of expectations on drug response in outpatients. (Paper presented at the Congress of the CINP, Munich, 1962.)

Foley, E. F., *et al.:* Placebos: a panel on the theoretical and the practical implications on their use in experimental and clinical medicine. Illinois Med. J., *112:* 215 (1957).

Forrest, F. M., and Forrest, I. S.: A simple test for the detection of chlorpromazine in urine. Amer. J. Psychiat., *113:* 931 (1957).

Forrest, F. M., Forrest, I. S., and Mason, A. S.: A rapid urinary test for chlorpromazine, promazine and pacatal: a supplementary report. Amer. J. Psychiat., *114:* 931 (1958).

Forrest, F. M., Forrest, I. S., and Mason, A. S.: A rapid urine color test for triflupromazine (vesprin). Amer. J. Psychiat., *115:* 114 (1959).

Forrest, I. S.: Chlorpromazine metabolism. In: Toxicity and adverse reaction studies with neuroleptics and antidepressants (eds., Lehmann, H. E., and Ban, T. A.). (Q.P.R.A. Montreal, 1968.)

Forrest, I. S., and Forrest, F. M.: A rapid urine color test for imipramine (tofranil, Geigy). Amer. J. Psychiat., *116:* 840 (1960).

Frankl, V., and Strotzka, H.: Narkodiagnose. Wien. Klin. Wschr., *61:* 569 (1949).

Freyhan, F. A.: Course and outcome of schizophrenia. Amer. J. Psychiat., *121:* 161 (1955).

Freyhan, F. A.: The immediate and long range effects of chlorpormazine on the mental hospital. In: Chlorpromazine and mental health. (Lea and Febiger, Philadelphia, 1955.)

Freyhan, F. A.: Therapeutic implications of differential effects of new phenothiazine compounds. Amer. J. Psychiat., *115:* 577 (1959).

Freyhan, F. A.: Loss of ejaculation during mellaril treatment. Amer. J. Psychiat., *118:* 171 (1961).

Funkenstein, D., *et al.:* Psychophysiological study of mentally ill patients. Amer. J. Psychiat., *106:* 116 (1949).

Gallant, D. M., *et al.:* Withdrawal symptoms after abrupt cessation of antipsychotic compounds: clinical confirmation in chronic schizophrenics. Amer. J. Psychiat., *121:* 491 (1964).

Garfield, S. L., *et al.*: Withdrawal of ataractic medication in schizophrenic patients. Dis. Nerv. Syst., *27:* 321 (1966).

Gartner, K.: Experiences with the psychotropic drug N 746 (sordinol). Praxis, *51:* 774 (1962).

Gibbard, B. A., and Lehmann, H. E.: Therapy of phenothiazine-produced skin pigmentation: a preliminary report. Amer. J. Psychiat., *123:* 351 (1966).

Gilbert, D. C., and Levinson, D. J. (1963): In: Personality and social systems (eds., Smelser, N. J., and Smelser, W. T.). (Wiley, New York, 1963.)

Glaser, E. M., and Whittow, G. C.: Evidence for a non-specific mechanism of habituation. J. Physiol. (London), *122:* 43 (1953).

Glaser, E. M., and Whittow, G. C.: Experimental errors in clinical trials. Clin. Sci., *13:* 199 (1954).

Gliedman, L. H., *et al.:* Reduction of symptoms by pharmacologically inert substances and short term psychotherapy. Arch. Neurol. Psychiat., *79:* 345 (1958).

Glover, E.: On the early development of mind. (International University Press, New York, 1956.)

Gold, H. (1946): In: Lehmann, H. E.: The placebo response and the double-blind study. In: Evaluation of psychiatric treatment (eds., Hoch, P., and Zubin, J.). (Grune and Stratton, New York, 1964.)

Goldberg, S. C., Cole, J. O., and Klerman, G. L.: Differential prediction of improvement under three phenothiazines. In: Prediction of response to pharmacotherapy (eds., Wittenborn, J. R., and May, P. R. A.). (Charles C Thomas, Springfield, 1966.)

Goldman, A. R., *et al.:* Social-psychiatric determinants of placebo-reactivity in a schizophrenic population. (Eighth Annual Conference V.A. Cooperative Studies in Psychiatry, Kansas City, 1963.)

Goldman, D. (1959): In: Müller, H. F., and Müller, A. K.: Effects of some psychotropic drugs upon brain electrical activity. Int. J. Neuropsychiat., *1:* 224 (1965).

Goldman, D.: Parkinsonism and related phenomena from administration of drugs: their production and control under clinical conditions and possible relation to therapeutic effect. Rev. Canad. Biol., *20:* 549 (1961).

Goldman, H. E.: The postalcoholic syndrome. Symptomatic control with hydroxyzine. Southwest. Med., *42:* 276 (1961).

Good, W. W., Sterling, M., and Holtzman, W. H.: Termination of chlorpromazine with schizophrenic patients. Amer. J. Psychiat., *115:* 443 (1958).

Goodnow, R. E., *et al.:* Physiological performance following a hypnotic dose of barbiturate. J. Pharmacol., *102:* 55 (1951).

Gottlieb, J. S., and Hope, J. M.: Prognostic value of intravenous administration of sodium amytal in cases of schizophrenia. Arch. Neurol. Psychiat., *46:* 86 (1941).

Greenblatt, M., Grosser, G. H., and Wechsler, H.: A comparative study of selected antidepressant medications and EST. Amer. J. Psychiat., *119:* 144 (1962).

Greiner, A. C. (1965): In: Forrest, I. S.: Chlorpromazine metabolism. In: Toxicity and adverse reaction studies with neuroleptics and antidepressants (eds., Lehmann, H. E., and Ban, T. A.). (Q.P.R.A., Montreal, 1968.)

Greiner, A. C., and Berry, K.: Skin pigmentation and corneal and lens opacities with prolonged chlorpromazine therapy. Canad. Med. Ass. J., *90:* 663 (1964).

GREINER, A. C., AND NICOLSON, G. A.: Pigment deposition in viscera associated with prolonged chlorpromazine therapy. Canad. Med. Ass. J., *91:* 627 (1964).

GREINER, A. C., AND NICOLSON, G. A.: Schizophrenia melanosis. Cause or side effect? Lancet, *2:* 1165 (1965).

GREINER, A. C., NICOLSON, G. A., AND BAKER, R. A.: Therapy of chlorpromazine melanosis. Canad. Med. Ass. J., *91:* 636 (1964).

GRINKER, R. R., *et al.:* The phenomena of depressions. (Hoeber, New York, 1961.)

GROSS, M.: The impact of ataractic drugs on a mental hospital outpatient clinic. Amer. J. Psychiat., *117:* 444 (1960).

GRUBER, C. M.: Interpreting medical data. Arch. Intern. Med. (Chicago), *98:* 767 (1956).

HAASE, H. J.: Extrapyramidal modification of the fine movements—a conditio sine qua non of fundamental therapeutic action of neuroleptic drugs. Rev. Canad. Biol., *20:* 425 (1961).

HADDENBROCK, S.: Hyperkinetische Dauersyndrome nach Hochdosierter und Langstreckenbehandlung mit Neuroleptika. In: Begleitwirkungen und Misserfolge der Psychiatrischen Pharmakotherapie (eds., Kranz, H., and Heinrich, K.). (Thieme, Stuttgart 1964.)

HAMILTON, M. A.: A rating scale for depression. J. Neurol. Neurosurg. Psychiat., *23:* 56 (1960).

HAMILTON, M. A.: Lectures on the methodology of clinical research. (Livingstone, Edinburgh, 1961.)

HAMILTON, M. A., AND WILSON, G. M.: Treatment of intermittent claudication. Quart. J. Med., *21:* 169 (1952).

HAMILTON, M. A., *et al.:* A controlled trial of thiopropazate dihydrochloride (dartalan), chlorpromazine and occupational therapy in chronic schizophrenics. J. Ment. Sci., *106:* 40 (1960).

HAMON, J., PARAIRE, J., AND VELLUZ, J.: Remarques sur l'action du 4560. RP sur l'agitation maniaque. Ann. Médicopsychol., *110:* 331 (1952).

HAMPSON, J. L., *et al.:* Comparative study of the effect of mephenesin and placebo on symptomatology of mixed group of psychiatric outpatients. Bull. Hopkins Hosp., *95:* 170 (1954).

HARRIS, M. M., *et al.:* Regarding sodium amytal as a prognostic aid in insulin and metrazol therapy of mental patients. Amer. J. Psychiat., *96:* 327 (1939).

HENINGER, G., DIMASCIO, A., AND KLERMAN, G. L.: Personality factors in variability of response to phenothiazines. Amer. J. Psychiat., *121:* 1091 (1965).

HILDRETH, H.: Battery of feeling and attitude scales for clinical use. J. Clin. Psychol., *2:* 214 (1964).

HILLIS, B. R.: The assessment of cough depressing drugs. Lancet, *1:* 1230 (1952).

HIMWICH, H. E.: Prospects in psychopharmacology. J. Nerve. Ment. Dis., *122:* 413 (1955).

HIMWICH, H. E., AND RINALDI, F. A.: Analysis of the activating system including its use for screening antiparkinson drugs. Yale J. Biol. Med., *28:* 308 (1955.)

HOCH, P. H.: The present status of narcodiagnosis and therapy. J. Nerv. Ment. Dis., *103:* 248 (1946).

HOFFER, A.: Laboratory tests for following progress of schizophrenia. Dis. Nerv. Syst., *27:* 466 (1966).

HOFFER, A., AND MAHON, M.: The presence of unidentified substances in the urine of psychiatric patients. J. Neuropsychiat., *2:* 331 (1961).

HOFFER, A., AND OSMOND, H.: A card sorting test helpful in making psychiatric diagnosis. J. Neuropsychiat., *2:* 306 (1961).

HOFFER, A., AND OSMOND, H.: Double-blind clinical trials. J. Neuropsychiat., *2:* 221 (1961).

HOFFER, A., AND OSMOND, H.: The relationship between an unknown factor (UF) in urine of subjects and HOD test results. J. Neuropsychiat., *2:* 363 (1961).

HOLLINGWORTH, H. L.: The influence of caffeine on the speed and quality of performance in typewriting. Psychol. Rev., *19:* 66 (1912).

HOLLINGWORTH, H. L.: Experiments on susceptibility to drugs. Amer. J. Psychol., *43:* 139 (1931).

HOLLISTER, L. E., CAFFEY, E. M., JR., AND KLETT, C. J.: Abnormal symptoms, signs and laboratory tests during treatment with phenothiazine derivatives. Clin. Pharmacol. Ther., *1:* 284 (1960).

HÖNIGFELD, G.: Non-specific factors in treatment. I. Review of placebo reactions and placebo reactors. Dis Nerv. Syst., *25:* 145 (1964).

HÖNIGFELD, G.: Non specific factors in treatment. II. Review of social-psychological factors. Dis. Nerv. Syst., *25:* 225 (1964).

HÖNIGFELD, G., AND KLETT, C. J.: The nurses observation scale for inpatient evaluation. J. Clin. Psychol., *21:* 65 (1965).

HÖNIGFELD, G., AND LASKY, J. J.: A one year follow-up of depressed patients treated in a multi-hospital drug study. I. Social workers' evaluations. Dis. Nerv. Syst., *23:* 555 (1962).

HUNTER, R., *et al.:* A syndrome of abnormal movements and dementia in leucotomized patients treated with phenothiazines. J. Neurol. Neurosurg. Psychiat., *27:* 219 (1964).

HUNTSMAN, A. G.: Scientific research versus the theory of probabilities. Science, *110:* 566 (1949).

IRVINE, D.: Apparently non-indolic Ehrlich positive substances related to mental illnesses. J. Neuropsychiat., *2:* 292 (1961).

IRWIN, S.: Influence of external factors and arousal mechanisms on the rate of drug tolerance development. Arch. Int. Pharmacodyn., *142:* 152 (1963).

IRWIN, S.: Drug screening and evaluation of new compounds in animals. In: Animal and clinical pharmacological techniques in drug evaluation (eds., Nodine, H., and Siegler, P. E.). (Year Book Medical Publishers, Philadelphia, 1964.)

ISBELL, H., AND WHITE, W. M.: Clinical characteristics of addictions. Amer. J. Med., *14:* 558 (1953).

ISBELL, H., *et al.*: Studies on LSD-25: effects in former morphine addicts and development of tolerance during chronic administration. Arch. Neurol. Psychiat., *76:* 468 (1956).

JAFFE, G. V.: Depression in general practice. A clinical trial of a new psychomotor stimulant. Practitioner, *186:* 492 (1961).

JAFFE, J. H. (1965): In: Leonard, F.: Workshop on the detection and control of abuse of narcotics, barbiturates and amphetamines. Psychopharmacol. Serv. Cent. Bull., *3:* 21 (1966).

JELLINEK, E. M.: Clinical tests on comparative effectiveness of analgesic drugs. Biomet. Bull., *2:* 87 (1946).

JOYCE, C. R.: Consistent differences in individual reactions to drugs and dummies. Brit. J. Pharmacol., *14:* 512 (1959).

KABLER, J. D. (1958): In: Hönigfeld, G.: Non specific factors in treatment. Dis. Nerv. Syst., *25:* 145 (1964).

KARN, W. N., AND KASPER, S.: Pharmacologically induced Parkinson-like signs as index of therapeutic potential. Dis. Nerv. Syst., *20:* 119 (1956).

KATZ, M. M.: A typological approach to the problem of predicting response to treatment. In: Prediction of response to pharmacotherapy (eds. Wittenborn, J. R., and May, P. R. A.). (Charles C Thomas, Springfield, 1966.)

KATZ, M. M., AND LYERLY, S. B.: Methods for measuring adjustment and social behavior in the community. Psychol. Rep. Mono., *13:* 503 (1963).

KENNEDY, W. P.: The placebo reaction. Med. World (London), *95:* 203 (1961).

KILOH, L. G., AND BALL, J. R. B.: Depression treated with imipramine: a follow-up study. Brit. Med. J., *1:* 168 (1961).

KLERMAN, G. L.: Staff attitudes, decision-making and the use of drug therapy in the mental hospital. In: Research conference on the therapeutic community (ed., Denber, H. C. B.). (Charles C Thomas, Springfield, 1959.)

KLERMAN, G. L.: Measurement of changes in human behavior under the effects of psychotropic drugs. In: Neuropsychopharmacology (ed., Rothlin, E.). (Elsevier, New York, 1961.)

KLERMAN, G. L.: NIMH-sponsored collaborative study of phenothiazine treatment of acute schizophrenic psychoses. Psychopharmacol. Serv. Cent. Bull., *1:* 1 (1961).

KLERMAN, G. L.: The influence of personality factors on phrenotropic agent effects. Transactions of the Sixth Research Conference on Cooperative Chemotherapy Studies in Psychiatry and Broad Research Approaches to Mental Illness, *6:* 339 (1961).

KLERMAN, G. L., *et al.* (1963): In: Hönigfeld, G.: Non specific factors in treatment. Review of placebo reactions and placebo reactors. Dis. Nerv. Syst., *25:* 145 (1964).

KLINE, N. S.: Drugs in the treatment of depression: clinical studies. In: Psychiatric drugs (ed., Solomon, P.). (Grune and Stratton, New York, 1966.)

KNOWLES, J. B., AND LUCAS, C. J.: Experimental studies of the placebo response. J. Ment. Sci., *106:* 231 (1960).

KOKOSKI, R. J. (1965): In: Leonard, F.: Workshop on the detection and control of abuse of narcotics, barbiturates and amphetamines. Psychopharmacol. Serv. Cent. Bull., *3:* 21 (1966).

KRAMER, J. C., KLEIN, D. F., AND FINK, M.: Withdrawal symptoms following discontinuation of imipramine therapy. Amer. J. Psychiat., *118:* 549 (1961).

KRIS, E. B., AND CARMICHAEL, D. M.: Follow-up study on thorazine treated patients. Amer. J. Psychiat., *114:* 449 (1957).

KUHN, R.: The treatment of depressive states with G 22355 (imipramine hydrochloride). Amer. J. Psychiat., *115:* 459 (1958).

LABORIT, H.: L'hibernation artificielle. Acta Anaesth. Belg., *2:* 710 (1951).

LASAGNA, L., AND FELSINGER, J. M.: The volunteer subject in research. Science, *120:* 359 (1954).

LASAGNA, L., *et al.*: A study of the placebo response. Amer. J. Med., *16:* 770 (1954).

LEBEDEV, B. A.: Research in Psychopharmacology. (Report of W.H.O. Scientific Group, World Health Organization Technical Report Series No. 371, Geneva, 1967.)

LEHMANN, H. E.: Phenomenology and pathology of addiction. Compr. Psychiat., *4:* 168 (1963).

LEHMANN, H. E.: The placebo response and double blind study. In: The evaluation of psychiatric treatment (eds., Hoch, P. H., and Zubin, J.). (Grune and Stratton, New York, London, 1964.)

LEHMANN, H. E.: Clinical techniques for evaluating antidepressants: a review. (Presented at the Postgraduate Seminar, Animal and Clinical Pharmacologic Techniques in Drug Evaluation: American Therapeutic Society, Philadelphia, 1966.)

LEHMANN, H. E.: Individual differences in response to pharmacotherapy. In: Prediction of response to pharmacotherapy (eds., Wittenborn, J. R., and May, P. R. A.). (Charles C Thomas, Springfield, 1966.)

LEHMANN, H. E.: Methodology of clinical studies of psychotropic drugs. (Presented at the meeting of the World Health Organization Scientific Group on Research in Psychopharmacology, Geneva, 1966.)

LEHMANN, H. E.: Pharmacotherapy of schizophrenia. In: Psychopathology of schizophrenia (eds., Hoch, P. H., and Zubin, J.). (Grune and Stratton, New York, 1966.)

LEHMANN, H. E., AND BAN, T. A.: ECDEU progress report, Douglas Hospital, Verdun, 1963.

LEHMANN, H. E., AND BAN, T. A.: Comprehensive clinical studies with psychoactive drugs. (Tri-annual report of studies with psychoactive drugs, conducted at the Douglas Hospital, unpublished, Montreal, 1966.)

Lehmann, H. E., Ban, T. A., and Donald, M.: Rating the rater. Arch. Gen. Psychiat. (Chicago), *13:* 67 (1965).

Lehmann, H. E., Cahn, C. H., and DeVerteuil, R. L.: The treatment of depressive conditions with imipramine (G22355). Canad. Psychiat. Ass. J., *3:* 155 (1958).

Lehmann, H. E., and Knight, D. A.: Placebo-proneness and placebo-resistance of different psychological functions. Psychiat. Quart., *34:* 505 (1960).

Lehmann, H. E., *et al.:* Potentiation of pharmacological and therapeutic action of phenothiazines by nylidrine (arlidin). Compr. Psychiat., *5:* 36 (1964).

Lehmann, H. E., *et al.:* The effects of haloperidol on acute schizophrenic patients. A comparative study of haloperidol, chlorpromazine and chlorprothixene. In: The butyrophenones in psychiatry (eds., Lehmann, H. E., and Ban, T. A.). (Quebec Psychopharmacological Research Association, Montreal, 1964.)

Lehmann, H. E., *et al.:* The effects of trimipramine on geriatric patients. In: Trimipramine, a new antidepressant (eds., Lehmann, H. E., *et al.*). (Q.P.R.A., Montreal, 1964.)

Leonard, F.: Workshop on the detection and control of abuse of narcotics, barbiturates and amphetamines. Psychopharmacol. Serv. Cent. Bull., *3:* 21 (1966).

Linton, H. B., and Langs, R. J.: Placebo reactions in a study of LSD-25. Arch. Gen. Psychiat. (Chicago), *6:* 369 (1962).

Lorr, M.: Multidimensional scale for rating psychiatric patients. Hospital form. V.A. Tech. Bull., *43:* 10 (1953).

Lorr, M., O'Connor, J. P., and Stafford, J. W.: The psychotic reaction profile. J. Clin. Psychol., *16:* 241 (1960).

Lorr, M., *et al.:* Inpatient multidimensional psychiatric scale. (Consulting Psychologists Press, Palo Alto, 1963.)

Lubin, B., *et al.:* Adjective check lists for measurement of depression. Arch. Gen. Psychiat. (Chicago), *12:* 57 (1965).

Lucas, G. A. W., and Fabierkiewics, C.: The identification of tranquillizing drugs. J. Forensic Sci., *8:* 463 (1963).

Lucero, R. J., and Meyer, B. T.: A behavior rating scale suitable for use in mental hospitals. J. Clin. Psychol., *7:* 250 (1951).

Luoto, K.: The differential effects of personality, placebos and suggestion on timing behavior. (Unpublished Doctoral Dissertation, University of Pittsburgh, 1961.)

Luoto, K.: Personality and placebo effects upon timing behavior. J. Abnorm. Soc. Psychol., *68:* 54 (1964).

Lyerly, S. B., and Abbott, P. S.: Handbook of psychiatric rating scales. (Public Health Service Publication No. 1495, National Institutes of Mental Health, Bethesda, 1966.)

Mannering, G. J., *et al.:* Paper chromatography applied to the detection of opium alkaloids in the urine and tissues. J. Lab. Clin. Med., *49:* 292 (1954).

Margules, D. L., and Olds, J.: Identical "feeding" and "rewarding" systems in the lateral hypothalamus of rats. Science, *135:* 3501 (1962).

Marks, J.: Predrug behavior as a predictor of response to phenothiazines among schizophrenics. J. Nerv. Ment. Dis., *137:* 597 (1963).

Marks, J.: Interactions involving drugs used in psychiatry. In: The scientific basis of drug therapy in psychiatry (eds., Marks, J., and Pare, C. M. B.). (Pergamon Press, Oxford, 1965.)

Mathalone, M. B. R.: Oculocutaneous effects of chlorpromazine. Lancet, *2:* 240 (1965).

McClanahan, W. S., *et al.:* Ocular manifestations of chronic phenothiazine derivative administration. Arch. Ophthal. (Chicago), *75:* 319 (1966).

McIsaac, W. M. (1965): In: Leonard, F.: Workshop on the detection and control of abuse of narcotics, barbiturates and amphetamines. Psychopharmacol. Serv. Cent. Bull., *3:* 21 (1966).

Mészáros, A. F., and Gallagher, D. L.: Measuring indirect effects of treatment on chronic wards. Dis. Nerv. Syst., *19:* 4 (1958).

Mészáros, A. F.: Factors influencing indirect effects of tranquillizing drugs. In: Dynamics of psychiatric drug therapy (ed., Sarwer-Foner, G. J.). (Charles C Thomas, Springfield, 1960.)

Morison, R. A., *et al.:* Placebo responses in an arthritis trial. Ann. Rheum. Dis., *20:* 179 (1961).

Morosini, C.: Osservasioni sui fenomeni neurodislettici da haloperidol. Symposium internazionale sull haloperidol e triperidol. (Instituto Luso Farmaco d'Italia, Milan, 1963.)

Nadeau, G., and Sobolewski, G.: Estimation of phenothiazine derivatives (especially chlorpromazine and levomepromazine) in urine. Canad. Med. Ass. J., *80:* 826 (1959).

Nadeau, G., and Sobolewski, G.: Estimation of phenothiazine derivatives in urine. Canad. Med. Ass. J., *81:* 658 (1960).

Nash, H.: The design and conduct of experiments on the psychological effects of drugs. J. Nerv. Ment. Dis., *128:* 129 (1959).

Nash, H.: The design and conduct of experiments on the psychological effects of drugs. In: Drugs and behavior (eds., Uhr, L., and Miller, J. G.). (Wiley, New York, 1960.)

Olds, J.: Selective effects of drives and drugs on "reward" systems of the brain. In: Neurological basis of behavior (eds., Wolstenholme, G. E. W., and O'Connor, C. M.). (Little, Brown, Boston, 1958.)

Olds, J., and Olds, M. E.: Positive reinforcement produced by stimulating hypothalamus with iproniazid and other compounds. Science, *127:* 1175 (1958).

Olson, G. W., and Peterson, D. B.: Sudden removal of tranquillizing drugs from chronic psychiatric patients. J. Nerv. Ment. Dis., *131:* 252 (1960).

Overall, J. E., and Gorham, D. R.: The brief psychiatric rating scale. Psychol. Rep., *10:* 799 (1962).

Overall, J. E., and Hollister, L. E.: Psychiatric drug research sample size requirements for one versus two raters. Arch. Gen. Psychiat. (Chicago), *16:* 152 (1967).

Overall, J. E., *et al.:* Drug therapy in depression. Controlled evaluation of imipramine, isocarboxazide, dextroamphetamine-amobarbital, and placebo. Clin. Pharmacol. Ther., *3:* 16 (1962).

Overall, J. E., *et al.:* Comparison of acetophenazine with perphenazine in schizophrenics: demonstration of differential effects based on computer derived diagnostic models. Clin. Pharmacol. Ther., *4:* 200 (1963).

Pannekoek, J. H.: Critical evaluation of the efficacy of new drugs. Postgrad. Med. J., *33:* 396 (1957).

Parker, K. D., and Hine, C. H.: Manual for the determination of narcotics and dangerous drugs in the urine. Psychopharmacol. Serv. Cent. Bull., *3:* 18 (1966).

Parloff, M. B., Kelman, H. C., and Frank, J. D.: Comfort, effectiveness and self-awareness as criteria of improvement in psychotherapy. Amer. J. Psychiat., *111:* 343 (1954).

Pepper, O. H. P.: Note on placebo. Amer. J. Pharm. *117:* 409 (1945).

Perrot, P., and Bourjala, J.: Cas pour diagnostique: un visage mauve. Bull. Soc. Franc. Derm. Syph., *69:* 631 (1962).

Pogge, R. C.: The toxic placebo. I. Side and toxic effects reported during the administration of placebo medicine. Med. Times, *91:* 773 (1963).

Pogge, R. C., and Coates, E. A.: The placebo as a source of side effects in normal people: influence of gradually increasing doses. Nebraska Med. J., *47:* 337 (1962).

Quincy's Lexicon (1787): In: Lehmann, H. E.: The placebo response and the double-blind study. In: Evaluation of psychiatric treatment (eds., Hoch, P., and Zubin, J.). (Grune and Stratton, New York, 1964.)

Rado, S.: The psychoanalysis of pharmacothymia. Psychiat. Quart., *2:* 1 (1933).

Rivers, W. H. R.: The influence of alcohol and other drugs on fatigue. (Arnold, London, 1908.)

Roberts, J. M., and Hamilton, M.: Treatment of anxiety states. I. The effects of suggestion on the symptoms of anxiety states. J. Ment. Sci., *104:* 1052 (1958).

Rosenfeld, H. A.: On drug addiction. Int. J. Psychoanal., *16:* 1 (1960).

Sabshin, M., and Ramot, J.: Pharmacotherapeutic evaluation and the psychiatric setting. Arch. Neurol. Psychiat., *75:* 362 (1956).

St. Laurent, J., Cahn, C. H., and Ban, T. A.: Treatment of psychiatric patients with a phenothiazine derivative (prochlorperazine) with special reference to after care. Amer. J. Psychiat., *118:* 938 (1962).

Samuels, A. S., and Edison, C. B.: A study of the psychiatric effects of the placebo. J. Louisiana Med. Soc., *113:* 114 (1961).

Sargant, W., and Dally, P.: Treatment of anxiety states by antidepressant drugs. Brit. Med. J., *1:* 6 (1962).

Sarwer-Foner, G. J.: A methodology of testing and clinical applications of the neuroleptic drugs in psychiatry. Psychiat. Quart., *34:* 1 (1960).

Sarwer-Foner, G. J.: Recognition and management of drug-induced extrapyramidal reactions and "paradoxical" behavioral reactions in psychiatry. Canad. Med. Ass. J., *83:* 312 (1960).

Sarwer-Foner, G. J. (ed.): The dynamics of psychiatric drug therapy. (Charles C Thomas, Springfield, 1960.)

Sarwer-Foner, G. J.: Some comments with psychodynamic aspect of the extrapyramidal reactions. In: Extrapyramidal system and neuroleptics (ed., Bordeleau, J. M.). (Editions Psychiatriques, Montreal, 1961.)

Satanove, A.: Pigmentation due to phenothiazines in high and prolonged dosage. J.A.M.A., *191:* 263 (1965).

Scheier, I. H., and Cattell, R. B.: Clinical validities by analyzing the psychiatrist exemplified in relation to anxiety diagnoses. Amer. J. Orthopsychiat., *28:* 699 (1958).

Scheier, I. H., and Cattell, R. B.: The IPAT-O-A (objective anxiety battery). (IPAT, Champaign, 1959.)

Schindel, L.: Placebo in theory and practice. Antibiot. Chemother. (Basel), *10:* 398 (1962).

Seevers, M. H., and Woods, L. A.: The phenomena of tolerance. Amer. J. Med., *14:* 1 (1953).

Sheard, M.: The influence of the doctors' attitudes on the patients' response to antidepressant medication. J. Nerv. Ment. Dis., *136:* 555 (1963).

Siddall, J. R.: The ocular toxic findings with prolonged and high dosage chlorpromazine intake. Arch. Ophthal. (Chicago), *74:* 460 (1965).

Sigwald, J., *et al.:* Etude de l'action sur l'akinésie parkinsonienne de deux dérivés de l'iminodibenzyle: le chlorhydrate de *N*-(gamma-diethylaminopropyl)iminodibenzyle ou imipramine et le beta-(hydroxyethyl-4″piperazinyl)-3-propyl-5-iminodibenzyle, ou 8307 RP. Presse Med. *67:* 1698 (1959).

Simpson, G. M., *et al.:* Phenothiazine-produced extrapyramidal system disturbance. Arch. Gen. Psychiat. (Chicago), *10:* 199 (1964).

Steinbook, R. M., Jones, M. B., and Ainslie, J. D.: Suggestibility and the placebo response. J. Nerv. Ment. Dis., *140:* 87 (1965).

Szasz, T.: The role of the counterphobic mechanism in addiction. J. Amer. Psychoanal. Ass., *6:* 309 (1958).

Taylor, J. A.: A personality scale of manifest

anxiety. J. Abnorm. Soc. Psychol., *48:* 285 (1953).

Tredici, L. M., Schiele, B. C., and McClanahan, W. S.: The incidence of skin-eye syndrome. Minnesota Med., *48:* 569 (1965).

Trouton, D. S.: Placebo and their psychological effects. J. Ment. Sci., *103:* 344 (1957).

Tuma, A. H.: The prediction of response to pharmacotherapy among schizophrenics: an historical perspective. In: Prediction of response to pharmacotherapy (eds., Wittenborn, J. R., and May, P. R. A.). (Charles C Thomas, Springfield, 1966.)

Turner, W. J., Krumholz, W., and Merlis, S.: A modified Malamud-Sands rating scale for use by ward personnel. P.S.C. Bull. *2:* 17 (1962).

Uhlenhuth, E. H., *et al.:* The symptomatic relief of anxiety with meprobamate, phenobarbital and placebo. Amer. J. Psychiat., *115:* 905 (1959).

Uhrbrand, L., and Faurbye, A.: Reversible and irreversible dyskinesia after treatment with perphenazine, chlorpromazine, reserpine, and electro convulsive therapy. Psychopharmacologia (Berlin), *1:* 408 (1960).

Wayne, E. J.: Placebos. Brit. Med. J., *2:* 157 (1956).

Webster's New World Dictionary. (Nelson, Foster and Scott, Toronto, 1962.)

West, E. D., and Dally, P. J.: Effect of iproniazid in depressive syndromes. Brit. Med. J., *1:* 1491 (1959).

Wetterholm, D. H., Snow, H. L., and Winter, F. C.: A clinical study of pigmentary change in cornea and lens in chronic chlorpromazine therapy. Arch. Ophthal. (Chicago), *74:* 55 (1965).

WHO Expert Committee on mental health (alcoholism): Report on Second Session, Geneva, 1951.

WHO Expert Committee on addiction producing drugs: Seventh report. WHO Techn. Rep. Ser., *116:* 9 (1957).

WHO Expert Committee (1964): In: Eddy, N. B. *et al.:* Drug dependence: its significance and characteristics. Psychopharmacol. Serv. Cent. Bull., *3:* 1 (1966).

Wiener, A. S.: Blood groups and disease. A critical review. Lancet, *1:* 813 (1962).

Wikler, A.: Studies on conditioning of physical dependence and reinforcement of opiate drinking behavior in morphine addicted rats. (Presented at the First Annual Meeting of the American College of Neuropsychopharmacology, Washington, 1963.)

Wikler, A.: Recent progress in research on the neurophysiologic basis of morphine addiction. Amer. J. Psychiat., *105:* 329 (1948).

Wikler, A., Fraser, H. F., and Isbell, H.: *N*-Allylnormorphine: effects of single doses and precipitation of "abstinence syndromes" during addiction to morphine, methadone or heroin in man (post addicts). J. Pharmacol. Exp. Ther., *109:* 8 (1953).

Wikler, A., and Rasor, R. W.: Psychiatric aspects of drug addiction. Amer. J. Med., *14:* 566 (1953).

Wilson, A. B. (1932): In: Ban, T. A.: Methodology and pitfalls in clinical testing of psychopharmacological drugs. Chemotherapia (Basel), *9:* 223 (1964).

Winkelman, N. W.: An appraisal of chlorpromazine. Amer. J. Psychiat., *113:* 961 (1957).

Winkelman, N. W.: A clinical and socio-cultural study of 200 psychiatric patients started on chlorpromazine ten and a half years ago. Amer. J. Psychiat., *120:* 861 (1964).

Wittenborn, J. R.: Wittenborn psychiatric rating scales. (Psychological Corp., New York, 1955.)

Wittenborn, J. R.: Factors which qualify the response to iproniazid and to imipramine. In: Prediction of response to pharmacotherapy (eds., Wittenborn, J. R., and May, P. R. A.). (Charles C Thomas, Springfield, 1966.)

Wittenborn, J. R.: Introduction. In: Prediction of response to pharmacotherapy (eds., Wittenborn, J. R., and May, P. R. A.). (Charles C Thomas, Springfield, 1966.)

Wittenborn, J. R., and May, P. R. A. (eds.): Prediction of response to pharmacotherapy. (Charles C Thomas, Springfield, 1966.)

Wolbach, A. B., Isbell, H., and Miner, E. J.: Cross tolerance between mescaline and LSD-25 with a comparison of the mescaline and LSD reactions. Psychopharmacologia (Berlin), *3:* 1 (1962).

Wolf, S.: The pharmacology of placebos. Pharmacol. Rev., *11:* 689 (1959).

Wolf, S., and Pinsky, R. H.: Effects of placebo administration and occurrence of toxic reactions. J.A.M.A., *155:* 339 (1954).

Zung, W., Richards, C. B., and Short, M. J.: Self-rating depression scale in an outpatient clinic. Arch. Gen. Psychiat., *13:* 508 (1965).

Six

Recent Progress

The exploration of a new psychoactive substance is a never ending process. The various stages of the investigation from chemical synthesis to clinical application are artificially created categories. Neither the number of patients who have taken the new drug nor the length of time it has been successfully employed is an indication that the investigative work is over.

This can best be demonstrated by chloral hydrate, which was first used as a sedative-hypnotic almost 100 years ago by Liebreich (1869) and which for several decades has been considered one of the least toxic and most useful sedatives. Not until quite recently (Friend, 1964) was it revealed that the absorbed chloral hydrate is converted to trichloroethanol (which accounts for the hypnotic effects), which in turn is combined in varying amounts with glycuronic acid (in the liver) to form urochloralic acid and is excreted by the kidneys (Marshall and Owens, 1954). Individuals with an enzymatic defect which precludes elaboration of glycuronic acid, as well as the fetus and premature infants who are largely incapable of utilizing this detoxifying mechanism, can be seriously poisoned by chloral hydrate (Driscoll and Harra, 1958).

A. ADDITIONAL DATA

1. Animal Pharmacology

Some of the more recent studies in this area of research have been directed toward developing animal pharmacological tests for the detection of characteristic antipsychotic, anxiolytic and antidepressant properties of newly developed chemical substances. Perhaps the most pertinent findings are those of Guerrero-Figueroa and Gallant (1967), Berger *et al.* (1967), Spencer (1967) and Hammer and Sjöqvist (1967).

a. Antipsychotic Versus Antidepressant Effects

Guerrero-Figueroa and Gallant (1967), using the implanted electrode technique in cats, were able to demonstrate that it may be possible to predict antipsychotic and antidepressant activity by the evoked potential responses from subcortical sites. They found that antipsychotic phenothiazines, butyrophenones and dibenzoxepin compounds, despite their structural differences, all consistently facilitate the evoked potential responses in the amygdaloid complex and hippocampus and inhibit the evoked potential responses in the mesodiencephalic reticular formation. They also recognized that tricyclic antidepressants, *e.g.*, imipramine, produce the opposite effects.

b. Antipsychotic Versus Anxiolytic Effects

In the course of systematic exploratory work on the effect of various psychoactive drugs on the duration of "after discharges" (to electrical stimulation of the fornix) in the limbic system (particularly in the hippocampus), Berger *et al.* (1967) revealed a differential action between antipsychotic and anxiolytic substances. It was demonstrated by Kletzkin (1963) that under the influence of antipsychotic drugs, *i.e.*, phenothiazines, such as chlorpromazine, hippocampal stimulation produces seizures of longer duration than those recorded during control periods. Opposed to this, anxiolytic substances, *i.e.*, propanediols (meprobamate, tybamate) and benzodiazepines (chlordiazepoxide, diazepam), were seen to reduce the duration of limbic seizures (Berger *et al.*, 1967).

c. Anxiolytic and Antidepressant Effects

In the same study Berger *et al.* (1967) recognized the similarities between the action of anxiolytic and antidepressant drugs on hippocampal after-discharges. The theoretical implications of this discovery have not yet been fully explored.

The duration of hippocampal after-discharges, which usually outlast the electrical stimulation of the fornix, was consistently shortened after the administration of anxiolytic propanediols (meprobamate, tybamate), benzodiazepines (chlordiazepoxide) or tricyclic antidepressants (imipramine, amitriptyline). The same applied to the benactyzine-induced prolonged duration of hippocampal seizures, which were interfered with by anxiolytic or antidepressant drugs. On the other hand, the enhancement of after-discharges after atropine or propantheline—also central anticholinergic substances—were interfered with only by the antidepressant amitriptyline but not by the anxiolytic meprobamate or the antidepressant imipramine. While the full significance of this finding is not clearly understood as yet, it may indicate a differential action between amitriptyline on the one hand and meprobamate and imipramine on the other.

d. Antidepressant Effects

There appears to be no behavioral change in laboratory animals which can satisfactorily be described as being analogous to the state of depression in man, nor has there been any animal pharmacological test recognized as yet which adequately predicts antidepressant activity. The animal behavior which most resembles that of human depression is the reserpine-induced behavior. Concomitant with the behavioral changes, reserpine also induces hypothermia, which can be specifically prevented by antidepressant drugs but not by anticholinergic substances or sympathomimetic stimulants. In Spencer's (1967) experiment the desmethylated derivatives of the tricyclic antidepressants were found to be more active than the dimethylated compounds in this respect, and the order of activity of MAOI's reflected their relative clinical therapeutic potency.

One of the most promising leads which may enable the pharmacologist to detect potential antidepressant properties of substances in animal pharmacological studies was discovered by recognizing the antitremor properties of "imipramine-like drugs" after tremorine (or oxotremorine)—a centrally acting parasympathomimetic agent—administration (Theobald *et al.*, 1964; and Halliwell *et al.*, 1964). Since it had already been recognized that tremorine produces not only tremor but also hypothermia (Everett, 1956; and Blockus and Everett, 1957), Spencer (1965) designed an experiment to test the effect of various antidepressants on both these variables. He showed that tricyclic antidepressants and sympathomimetic stimulants were able to prevent or antagonize tremorine-induced hypothermia in a lower dosage than tremor, while MAOI's remained essentially ineffective, except when they possessed central sympathomimetic properties inherent in their structure, *e.g.*, tranylcypromine (Spencer, 1967). On the other hand, anticholinergic drugs antagonized the tremor and hypothermia at equal doses.

The biochemical basis of these findings was shown by Hammer and Sjöqvist (1967). They found that desmethylimipramine inhibits the metabolism *in vitro* and *in vivo* of tremorine in rats, thereby increasing its concentration in the visceral organs and the brain. Furthermore, they demonstrated that other tricyclic antidepressant drugs, *e.g.*, protriptyline, nortriptyline and opipramol, exert the same effect (on the metabolism *in vivo* of tremorine). On an equimolar basis desmethylimipramine was the most effective of the compounds studied.

The integration of the new information with past knowledge is an ongoing process. It seems to be that in the animal pharmacology of psychoactive substances there is an ever increasing interest in the neurochemical and neurophysiological approaches. Whether this combined approach will lead to a major breakthrough in the field remains to be seen.

2. Human Pharmacology

Human pharmacological studies are increasingly concentrating on psychophysiological measurement variables.

a. *Psychophysiological Procedures*

i. Antipsychotic Drugs. Differential effects among three of the most frequently used and potent antipsychotic substances, chlorpromazine, trifluoperazine and haloperidol, were demonstrated by Saarma and Saarma (1966) on a specially devised battery of tests. Saarma and Saarma's (1966) battery consisted of six tests. Two measured autonomic functions, *i.e.*, the functional state of the autonomic nervous system and the behavior of autonomic orienting responses; one measured first signal system activity via the "motor reflex" test; and three recorded second signal system activity by the application of word association, proofreading and learning tests.

The characteristic effects under the influence of chlorpromazine were significant impairment in the learning, proof-reading and association tasks, together with marked acceleration of heart rate and fall in blood pressure. On the other hand, trifluoperazine induced practically no changes on the learning and the word-association tests, while it produced a considerable improvement in performance in proof-reading and conditional stimulus differentiation on the motor reflex test simultaneously with a decrease in heart rate, blood pressure and weakening of the autonomic orienting responses. The effects of haloperidol, a butyrophenone substance, revealed worsening in the learning test, proof-reading and conditionability on the "motor reflex" test. CS discrimination improved under the influence of this drug, and there was a slight decrease of heart rate, blood pressure and respiration rate and a weakening of the autonomic orienting responses.

Thus chlorpromazine was found to exert a marked inhibitory action on second signal system activity simultaneously with its marked autonomic effects; trifluoperazine was seen to improve second signal system functions together with a strengthening of the (internal) inhibitory process; and haloperidol induced a slight inhibitory action on second signal system functions with a weakening of the excitory and strengthening of the inhibitory process.

ii. Anxiolytic Drugs. While no new human pharmacological procedures for detection or differentiation of antidepressants have been developed, Pishkin *et al.* (1967) have recently suggested a simple procedure for the recognition of possible anxiolytic properties of newly synthesized compounds.

In their procedure—which consisted of two phases—cognitive and physiological indices were used. In the first phase subjects were presented with a cognitive problem. They were shown a series of geometric patterns on a screen with a film projector and were asked to place these patterns in two categories by depressing one of the two response keys. The task was self-paced, and depression of the key automatically recorded the response. It also initiated a signal which provided feedback by energizing one of the two amber lights above the response keys to indicate the correctness of the response.

During problem solving subjects were administered a CS (tone) for 2 seconds immediately followed by a 2-second US (shock) at 30-second intervals for a total of 20 trials. After 5 minutes' rest a new problem-solving task was presented during which time 30 extinction trials (tone only) were administered at 1-minute intervals. There was continuous GSR recording in both phases, while samples of EMG potentials were taken initially and at 5-minute intervals throughout Phase One and at 5-minute intervals in Phase Two.

In an acute double-blind placebo-controlled study, Pishkin *et al.* (1967) showed that, under the influence of the active anxiolytic hydroxyzine, anxiety (as measured by GSR) and muscle tension (as measured by EMG) were reduced without impairment of decision making (as measured by the problem-solving task). While autonomic levels of activation decreased significantly more with hydroxyzine than with placebo, the physiological levels of activation increased with an increase in the amount of information input. Whether other anxiolytic drugs have the same effect remains to be seen.

b. Rapid Eye Movements

It has been suggested that sleep has two different phases: dreaming and nondreaming. When sleeping subjects were awakened during periods of rapid eye movements (REM) they almost always reported dreaming, while they reported very few or no dreams if awakened during the other periods of sleep. Consequently it was established that dreaming occupies about 20 per cent of the adult's night sleep and a much larger percentage of the sleep time of infants (Dement, 1960, 1963).

It has recently been demonstrated that human beings have a built-in dreaming cycle, which in a healthy adult under normal conditions results in four or five dreaming periods of increasing durations. These dreaming periods can be detected either by the fast, low voltage waves (of Stage One Sleep) on the EEG or by the REM as shown on an electro-oculogram (EOG), which is a record of the changes in electrical potential between the cornea and the retina which occur when the eyball moves (Roffwarg *et al.*, 1962; Kahn *et al.*, 1962; Antrobus, 1963; and Fisher, 1963).

The effects of various psychoactive substances on REM have been explored in human pharmacological experiments (Dement, 1963; and Fisher, 1963). It was found that small doses of lysergic acid diethylamide in normal healthy volunteers increased their REM time, while dextroamphetamine and alcohol decreased it. It was also noted that barbiturates, contrary to expectations, suppressed dreams, which might be responsible for the possible adverse behavioral effects of these drugs when given to schizophrenic patients. More recently, an attempt was made to use REM's to differentiate between various hypnotic drugs. A characteristic decrease of REM was seen with nitrazepam, a benzodiazepine preparation, and with secobarbital, while chloral hydrate did not seem to exert any particular effect on rapid eye movements. Chlorprothixene, a thioxanthene preparation, notably shortened the time of each REM period and also the duration of the "inter-dream" periods (Lehmann and Ban, 1968). The only substance to date which has been shown to increase REM sleep is γ-hydroxybutyrate, a drug related to γ-aminobutyric acid (Jouvet, 1961).

3. Clinical Pharmacology

a. Psychopathological Assessment

Besides the extension of some of the EEG work discussed above, other psychopathological indices for clinical pharmacological studies have been recognized in the spontaneous endogenous oscillating systems.

i. Electroencephalographic Indices. *α. Quantitative EEG.* The use of quantitative EEG amplitude analysis has recently been reviewed by Goldstein and Beck (1965). The most recent applications include the demonstration of the difference between EEG variability levels in chronic schizophrenics and nonpsychotic controls by Goldstein *et al.* (1963); the recognition of the relationship between changes in electrocerebral activity and changes in schizophrenic behavior by Sugerman *et al.* (1964); and the evaluation of the effects of drugs on the time-course distribution of integrated EEG values by Pfeiffer *et al.* (1965).

More recently, the work with quantitative EEG has been extended to other than schizophrenic patients by Burdick *et al.* (1967). By applying "regression analysis" they found that the slope of the regression line of standard deviation (SD) in the mean integrated area decreased from normal subjects to catatonic schizophrenics, with alcoholics and undifferentiated schizophrenics in an intermediate position. On the basis of this it was suggested that the clockwise rotation of the regression line provides a convenient measure of the level of cerebral activation or that the slope of the regression line relating SD to mean energy content may be a meaningful measure for comparing diagnostic groups with respect to their relative degrees of cerebral activation.

β. Averaged Evoked Responses. The most important characteristic of the averaged evoked response (AER) is that if conditions are kept stable a given individual will have a constant AER. In psychopathological conditions Shagass *et al.* (1964) have demonstrated that patients with schizophrenia, psychotic depressions or character disorders show an abnormally reduced AER to the second of two ulnar nerve shocks, indicating a poor "recovery" from the initial shock.

Recently Callaway and Buchsbaum (1965) revealed by AER a "segmental set" in schizophrenics. They demonstrated that only schizophrenics respond to tones of different frequencies with different AER forms, even when they have been instructed to ignore the tones. In this, schizophrenics distinctly differ from normals.

ii. Spontaneous Endogenous Oscillating Systems. The first evidence of the existence of spontaneous activity in sense organs was provided by Granit (1955), while the first demonstration of spontaneous periodic activity in the autonomic nervous system was given by Lacey and Lacey (1958).

Continuous longitudinal observations in 182 resting psychiatric patients of various diagnoses revealed spontaneous oscillations of autonomic and metabolic activity of a regularly periodic sine-wave cyclic type in the unstimulated subjects. It was the psychiatric diagnosis which was outstanding in differentiating between the group mean frequencies (Doust, 1960).

Monitoring techniques included the measurement of skin temperature, capillary blood pressure, capillary blood oxygen saturation, capillary blood flow, alveolar P CO_2, and the observation *in vivo* of changes in the intercapillary "ground substance" of the nailfold skin.

Findings pertinent to clinical pharmacological studies are that the longest cycles were found in schizophrenics and the shortest in organic patients, with affective psychoses in between the two extremes.

b. Psychopharmacological Applications

Of the numerous clinical pharmacological studies with psychoactive drugs, the following have both heuristic and practical implications.

i. Negative Findings. *α. Catecholamine Hypothesis of Schizophrenia.* α-Methylparatyrosine (AMT), a specific inhibitor of tyrosine hydroxylase, induces a reduction of norepinephrine and dopamine levels in the brain. On the basis of the catecholamine hypothesis of schizophrenia, antipsychotic properties of this substance were anticipated.

In two studies conducted independently, Gershon (1967) and Hollister (1967) failed to show any therapeutic action of AMT in schizophrenic patients. Nor did the substance produce depression or extrapyramidal adverse effects.

Attempts were made to employ coenzyme diphosphopyridine nucleotide (DPN) in the treatment of schizophrenia. This therapy was initiated on the suggested beneficial effect of long term administration of nicotinic acid or its derivative nicotinamide, which in turn was based on the transmethylation hypothesis of schizophrenia. Since nicotinamide is an integral part of the coenzyme, it was suggested (Hoffer, 1966) that its therapeutic effects were exerted by DPN and could readily be elicited by administering 1000 to 2000 mg. of this preparation orally.

In independent studies Gallant *et al.* (1966) and Kline *et al.* (1967) failed to demonstrate any therapeutic action of DPN in schizophrenic patients. Nor did the substance produce adverse effects. This whole area of research, however, is being reinvestigated and reevaluated in an international collaborative study initiated by the Canadian Mental Health Association (Ban, 1967).

β. Catecholamine Hypothesis of Affective Disorders. Dihydroxyphenylalanine (dopa) is a precursor in the synthesis of catechol amines. Dopa crosses the blood-brain barrier and reverses the behavioral and biochemical effects of reserpine in animals. Its effects were found to be enhanced by pretreatment with an MAOI. On the basis of the catecholamine hypothesis of affective disorders, antidepressant properties of this substance were anticipated.

In a clinical trial Klerman *et al.* (1963) failed to reveal any therapeutic action of dopa alone or in combination with an MAOI drug in depressed patients. A transient hypotensive effect with the combination was seen.

α-Methyldopa (AMD) is an inhibitor of

the decarboxylase enzyme system which potentiates the conversion of dopa to dopamine. On the basis of the hypothesis that in manics there is an excess of catecholamines in the CNS, an anti-manic effect of this substance was anticipated.

In a clinical trial Mosher *et al.* (1966) failed to reveal any therapeutic action of AMD in manic patients. On the other hand, some hypotensive effects were seen.

ii. Equivocal Findings. *α. RNA Hypothesis of Memory.* Magnesium pemoline (MP) is a substance with a possible facilitating effect on ribonucleic acid (RNA) synthesis. On the basis of the RNA hypothesis of memory, a beneficial effect of the substance on intelligence was anticipated.

The effects of MP on the intelligence and memory function of chronic schizophrenics were found to be equivocal in a clinical study by Gallant (1967). However, he suggested the possibility of a slight enhancement of these functions with the administration of 25 mg. daily.

iii. Positive Findings. *α. REM and Psychosis.* Chlorpromazine and trifluoperazine are phenothiazines capable of reducing the excessive REM time in sleep without discriminating the amount of eye movement which occurs in the REM stage. On the basis of the hypothesis that the reduction of REM in the REM stage is psychotogenic (while excessive REM in sleep is a characteristic of psychoses), antipsychotic properties of these substances were anticipated (Freemon *et al.*, 1965).

The antipsychotic properties of chlorpromazine and trifluoperazine are well known. The actual reduction of REM time (from 50 to 30 per cent) under the influence of trifluoperazine together with the clinical improvement was also demonstrated (Fisher, 1963).

β. Temporal Lobe Dysrhythmia and Impulsive Behavior. Diazepam is a benzodiazepine substance with an inhibitory effect on temporal lobe dysrhythmias. Since these EEG changes are characteristic of a particular kind of personality disorder, a beneficial effect of this substance in a group of patients with impulsive behavior was anticipated.

Using small doses of 5 mg. three times a day, Gallant (1967) found diazepam therapeutic for impulsive behavior disorders. He also noted that in higher doses these therapeutic neurophysiological effects seemed to be reversed.

γ. Electrolytes and Affective Disorders. Lithium is a monovalent cation which belongs to the group of alkali metals. On the basis of factual evidence that the electrolyte imbalance in both manic and depressive cases is qualitatively similar and only quantitatively different, therapeutic action of lithium in manic-depressive psychosis was anticipated.

The potent therapeutic effects of lithium in acute mania, chronic mania and hypomanic states have been described by Cade (1949), Schou (1959), Gershon and Yuwiler (1960), Maggs (1963), Strömgren and Schou (1964) and Jacobsen (1965). Its effectiveness as a prophylactic agent in recurrent manic, depressive or manic-depressive psychosis has also been demonstrated by Hartigan (1963), Baastrup (1964, 1966), Stolt (1965), Herlofsen (1965) and most recently by Baastrup and Schou (1967).

4. Clinical Investigation

While the additional clinical pharmacological information could be restricted to a factual presentation, the progress in clinical investigation is primarily concerned with singling out factors which may influence drug effects.

a. Therapeutic Effects

i. Methodological Considerations. *α. Sample Size.* The probability of obtaining significant results when true treatment differences exist in clinical investigative studies depends on the number of subjects included in the clinical trial, *i.e.*, on sample size. In a systematic study with the BPRS, Overall *et al.* (1967) indicated that in a placebo-controlled experiment with a new psychoactive substance approximately 40 to 60 patients must be included in each treatment group before it can be stated that treatment differences are significantly different. Increasing sample sizes to an acceptable level appears to them to be the only effective way at present to overcome the problem of variability in evaluating psychotherapeutic drugs.

Others are at variance with Overall *et al.* (1967). For example, Ban (1964) asserts that carefully matched groups provide grounds for reaching valid conclusions on the basis of small experimental populations. Thus a "clinical study" in which statistics are used only as a tool in the assessment does not necessarily have to be a "statistical study."

β. Reduction of Sample Size. The only means of reducing sample size—by 15 to 20 per cent—without affecting the self-sufficiency of a clinical study, according to Overall *et al.* (1967), is the use of two independent raters instead of one.

Drastic reduction of sample size was achieved by Jones and Ainslie (1966) by using a "placebo wash-out period." All patients were placed on placebo before any active medication was prescribed, which removed most of the placebo variance responsible for most of the "within-group variance" in improvement scores. In this way it was possible to demonstrate the drug effect with only a third as many patients as would otherwise have been required.

Besides the exploration of the effects of methodological changes on therapeutic outcome, systematic studies have been directed toward better understanding of the relationship between personality factors and variability in drug response on the one hand and the effect of environmental factors on treatment on the other.

ii. Personality Factors and Drug Response. *α. Psychological Factors.* In the course of a systematic study in which the effects of a number of drugs on normal male volunteers were explored, Klerman *et al.* (1959) found that extroverted athletes with a low anxiety level showed a distinctly different response to reserpine, phenyltoloxamine and a placebo than introspective introverts.

Recent experiments on the influence of personality type on drug response are those of Heninger *et al.* (1965) and Frostad *et al.* (1966). In Heninger's (1965) study it was shown that self-assertive, physically oriented extroverts experienced phenothiazine-induced sedation and psychomotor retardation as disruptive and uncomfortable and responded to it with irritability and hostility, while introspective introverts reacted with relaxation in spite of the slowing of psychomotor and cognitive functions.

Prior to this Sarwer-Foner (1960) had described the basic personality characteristic of patients in whom chlorpromazine produced an intensification of their psychopathology to the extent of causing pain, agitation, paranoid reactions, increased withdrawal or enhanced anxiety. He considered that the personalities of these patients were organized about psychomotor activity and an acting out relationship with the environment, and hypothesized that the psychomotor inhibition producing action of these drugs is ego threatening since it interferes with the activities used by the patients as major defenses against underlying conflicts. The findings of Heninger *et al.* (1965) support Sarwer-Foner's (1960) hypothesis, which was restated by him recently (1967).

Frostad *et al.*'s (1966) hypothesis on the influence of personality type on drug response was formulated in the course of studies with diazepam, a benzodiazepine anxiolytic substance. They observed that 6 out of 19 subjects responded in a paradoxical fashion to diazepam; *i.e.*, they showed a lowering of skin resistance and an increase in muscle tension. Further exploration revealed that the paradoxical reactors were more "assertive, independent, expedient, venturesome, uninhibited, imaginative and wrapped up in inner urgencies" than the other participants in the project. They characterized them arbitrarily as "action-oriented" subjects.

β. Sex and Race. Sex and race differences in improvement after 6 weeks of phenothiazine (or placebo) treatment were examined in a group of newly admitted, acutely ill schizophrenic patients by Goldberg *et al.* (1966). They found that although patients on drug treatment improved more than patients receiving placebo in both sexes the males improved on placebos markedly more than females, in contradistinction to the active drug treatment in which females improved slightly but significantly more than males.

It was also shown that more improvement

was obtained in both white and Negro patients on drug treatment than on placebo; on the active drug treatment no race differences were detected, but on placebo Negroes were found to be more therapeutically responsive than whites.

A tentative interpretation of these findings by Goldberg *et al.* (1966) is that those who have higher loading on the psychological stress factor (males and Negroes) are the placebo responders, while those who have higher loading on the genetic factor (females and whites) are the active drug responders. The possibility of environmental influences on these differential effects was previously raised by Klerman *et al.* (1964).

iii. Environmental Factors and Drug Response. Among the many consequences of the advent of modern drug therapy, Klerman (1963) considers the increasing interest in the relationship between the social environment in which the patient is treated and the effectiveness of drug treatment as one of the most important. This topic had previously been discussed by Donnelly and Zeller (1956), Sabshin and Ramot (1956), Leveton (1958), Linn (1959), Sherman (1959) and Fischer (1961). On the basis of the available evidence, Klerman (1963) elaborated on four conceptual models (which were first suggested by Fischer, 1961) on the possible relationship between the social milieu and the effects of psychopharmacological treatment.

Of the four possible relationships, in Model One, drug effects are independent of the milieu. In Model Two, an augmentation of drug effects is attributed to environmental factors. In contradistinction to these is Model Three, in which drug effects and milieu factors bear a reciprocal relationship (akin to what statisticians designate as simple or ordinal interactions). Finally, in Model Four a negative interaction between drugs and the environment is assumed (a multiplicative or disordinal interaction).

In the original exposition Klerman (1963) did not offer indicators which have helped to choose among the models presented in the actual therapeutic setting. In a more recent publication in collaboration with Goldberg *et al.* (1965), however, he was able to demonstrate that there is a group of psychiatric symptoms in schizophrenics—consisting of irritability, slow speech and movements, hebephrenic symptoms, self-care and indifference to environment—in which there is no improvement except on drug treatment.

Goldberg *et al.* (1965) also noted that these symptoms are closely related to Bleuler's (1916) fundamental symptoms in schizophrenia, in contradistinction to the placebo-prone symptoms such as auditory and non-auditory hallucinations, memory deficit and feelings of unreality, which are closely related to Bleuler's (1916) accessory symptoms. On the basis of these findings they suggested that the frequently held view that phenothiazine effects are only symptomatic and that they dampen the accessory or manifest symptoms without having an effect on the fundamental disease process is probably wrong and needs to be reevaluated.

b. Adverse Effects

i. Electrocardiographic Changes. Already in the earliest pharmacological studies with cholorpromazine (Courvoisier *et al.*, 1953) it was revealed that this drug had a powerful effect on the cardiovascular system. In a review of the literature, Kingstone (1968) divided the effects of antipsychotic drugs on the ECG into two categories: antiarrhythmic effects and the production of electrocardiographic (ECG) changes. Antiarrhythmic effects were demonstrated by Finkelstein *et al.* (1954), Dilalme and Catenacci (1955), Weinberg and Haley (1956), Melville (1958), Melville and Drapeau (1958) and Sharma and Arora (1961); and ECG changes by Moyer *et al.* (1954), Kupatz (1956), Eliakim *et al.* (1958), Royer *et al.* (1959), Teitelbaum (1963), Kelly *et al.* (1963), Graupner and Murphree (1964), Bäckman and Elosuo (1964), Desautels *et al.* (1964), Ban and St. Jean (1964), Wendkos (1964) and Ban *et al.* (1965). ECG abnormalities with antidepressants were reviewed by Lavallée (1968). He emphasized particularly the findings of Anderson and Kristiansen (1959) and Rasmussen and Kristiansen (1963) with tricyclic antidepressant drugs. This consisted of isoelectric T waves in leads I and/or

II, depression of the ST interval and frequently occurring ventricular extrasystoles (Lehman and Ban, 1968).

Interest in phenothiazine-induced ECG changes was raised after Kelly *et al.*'s (1963) report on two fatal cases in the course of thioridazine treatment. Kelly *et al.* (1963) asserted that thioridazine regularly affects the ECG and exerts a quinidine-like effect, which is the result of ventricular repolarization. They described flattened and sometimes inverted T waves and occasionally convex ST segments. In the two fatal cases—on thioridazine, 1500 and 3600 mg. a day, respectively—terminal ECG patterns were those of heart block, alternating with episodes of ventricular tachycardia. The myocardium of one of the fatal cases revealed edema, increased vascularity and some increase in connective tissue elements along with fragmentation of muscle fibers.

Further investigations were directed to reveal the characteristics and the incidence of the phenothiazine-induced ECG changes, especially to see which of the various substances are particularly implicated in the production of these alterations. In the first study by Ban and St. Jean (1964), thioridazine, chlorpromazine and trifluoperazine were administered to six patients in increasing dosages (200, 400, 800 and 1200 mg. a day for chlorpromazine and thioridazine and 8, 16, 32 and 64 mg. for trifluoperazine) for a 16-day period each in accordance to a Latin-Square design. All six patients receiving thioridazine showed ECG changes, compared with only three patients receiving chlorpromazine and one who received trifluoperazine.

In another survey in a group of 114 patients undergoing controlled drug therapy with 10 different drugs and a placebo, Ban *et al.* (1965) revealed that of the 92 patients receiving drugs other than thioridazine, 12 patients or 13 per cent yielded an abnormal ECG. In the same survey 17 or 77 per cent of all patients receiving thioridazine manifested abnormal ECG's.

In a further study by St. Jean *et al.* (1968), it was revealed that thioridazine-induced ECG changes appear at dosages above 150 mg. a day. With increasing dosage more patients were seen to be affected. At 900 mg. daily practically all ECG's were modified and a fatal case was reported. Although no tracings were taken immediately prior to the death of this patient, from the recorded evidence of a nearly fatal former experience, a period of ventricular tachycardia was assumed to have preceded death. However, by grading the ECG changes in a carefully designed experiment, Wendkos (1968) did not consider that any quantitative relationship between the magnitude of the T wave distortion and the dosage of thioridazine could be established. Nevertheless, in terms of incidence, the T wave changes occurred in 20 per cent of those receiving 200 mg. daily, in 40 per cent of those receiving 400 or 600 mg. daily and in 100 per cent of those receiving 800 mg daily in his study.

It should be noted that the thioridazine-induced ECG changes were fully reversible after ergotamine tartrate, isosorbide dinitrate or potassium mixture administration. Because of this, Wendkos (1968) considered the T wave abnormalities seen with thioridazine therapy as "expressions" of a "benign" repolarization disturbance. In variance with his views are Ballon's (1968), according to whom the fact that some of these ECG variations are modified or normalized by feeding potassium in high doses or by using drugs which are assumed to modify coronary artery circulation does not indicate that these ECG manifestations are necessarily "benign" or harmless.

On the basis of all the available evidence St. Jean (1968) asserted that psychotropic drugs which produce marked ECG alterations should be given more cautiously than heretofore in order not to expose patients to an avoidable danger.

ii. Morphological Changes in the Liver. A recent report by Bloom *et al.* (1965) restated the possibility of an asymptomatic liver disease following treatment with various antipsychotic—particularly chlorpromazine—types of drugs. After reviewing 148 autopsies in schizophrenic patients (dying between 1947 and 1959 at the Veterans Administration Hospital, Palo Alto), Hollister *et al.* (1960) asserted that morphological abnormalities of the liver are rather frequent in psychiatric patients, even in those who had never been exposed to phenothiazines. Furthermore, in cases in which the histological changes in the liver resembled those described as following chlorpromazine administration, a careful search usually revealed a plausible explanation of these abnormalities other than drug exposure (Hollister and Hall, 1966).

Prior to this, Hall and Dunlop (1955), in a placebo-controlled study designed to determine the effects of chlorpromazine, obtained liver biopsy specimens from 25 of the placebo- and from 20 of the chlorpromazine-treated patients. Identification of the slides was marked, and blind readings were made independently by a pathologist, gastroenterologist and an internist. Abnormalities were reported by the pathologist in 65 per cent of the chlorpromazine- and in 60 per cent of the placebo-treated patients; by the gastroenterologist, in 40 and 40 per cent, respectively; and by the internist, in 35 and 28 per cent, respectively. Fatty infiltration, portal fibrosis and bile duct proliferation were the most frequent changes seen appearing about equally in the two groups.

Conclusive evidence that there are no abnormal changes in the liver in patients treated with phenothiazines was given by Bengzon *et al.* (1966). In their study of the changes in certain serum enzymes during treatment with psychotropic drugs, the two liver-specific enzymes sorbitoldehydrogenase and serum glutamic pyruvic transaminase remained unaltered under the influence of the usual therapeutic doses of phenothiazines.

B. NEW APPROACHES

Probably even more important than the additional data discussed above is the development of new approaches in psychopharmacology.

1. The Functional Approach

A rational framework for the development, evaluation and use of psychoactive drugs has been systematically developed by Irwin (1967). Irwin's (1967) approach is based on the assumption of a relatedness between animal and human functioning and between the functioning of normal and disordered subjects. It commenced with a careful analysis of animal behavior and with the selection of "target functions" noticeably influenced by drug action, which were considered to be useful for predicting the therapeutic effect of psychoactive chemicals. As a further step, a corresponding assessment procedure for the patient's behavior was suggested. Finally, an adjustment was made, and the focus was directed on particular patterns of responses which rendered the measures and procedures applicable and relevant across species.

Irwin (1967) proceeded to select for the evaluation of animal behavior a number of target functions, or as he expressed it "elemental building blocks of behavior that in reality express the physiologic and psychosocial state of the organism." According to him, these are the level of wakefulness; behavioral arousal (stupor-excitability); activity; endurance; bio-social drives; set (mood), including attitudes and expectations; responsiveness to stimuli (sensory-motor and motor-affective); information processing; and physiologic (autonomic, neurologic and endocrine) functioning.

Irwin (1967) expressed the notion that these target functions are perhaps the functions which more directly arise from CNS activity and which consequently most specifically express the temperament and behavior of the organism. Alteration of any one of these by drugs, he maintains, can shift the probabilities for responding and behaving in a particular way which nevertheless is measurable in both animals and man.

For the patient assessment he devised a model in which the functions are viewed as continuously interacting with one another for establishing the changing state of the organism as it interacts with the environment. In this "schema" all subjects are defined as using "normal," "neurotic" or "psychotic" logic, the proportion of which may vary, in accordance to previous conditioning, as the environment demands. The same applies to the motor-affective behavior and the interactional responses exhibited. Mood ranges from optimistic to pessimistic and affect from euphoria, anger and anxiety to depression, each of which predisposes the subject to a particular type of behavior, *e.g.*, avoidance (to avoid punishment or denial), aggressive (offensive approach and defensive avoidance) and interactional behavior. Interactional behavior is assumed to be dynamically "moving" from "approach behavior" to "discouragement behavior," which is considered to reflect the sequence of changes from the active (extroverted) type of behavior accompanying optimism toward the passive (introverted) type of behavior associated with pessimistic expectations. This, Irwin (1967) thought, may also reflect the natural course of chronic schizophrenia toward passive avoidance behavior, apathy and depressed affect.

In Irwin's functional frame of reference the object of drug therapy was defined as modifying the functional state or disposition of the patient to reverse the direction of his responses toward normal. This, regardless of whether the patient is labeled normal, neurotic or psychotic, can be achieved by predictably modifying the target functions by drugs.

Disruptive levels of behavioral arousal, hyperactivity and avoidance responding can be counteracted by *major tranquilizers*, and disruptive sexual or aggressive bio-social drives by *narcotics*. *Minor tranquilizers* disrupt information processing in such a manner as to reduce fear-inhibited passive avoidance behavior, and *psychomotor stimulants* increase the activity, drive, vigilance and responsiveness of individuals handicapped by feelings of fatigue and low initiative.

2. The Dynamic Approach

Like Irwin's, the dynamic approach is also based on the assumption of a relatedness between animal and human functioning and between the functioning of normal and disordered subjects. But unlike the functional approach, it commences with the careful analysis of human—particularly psychopathological—behavior with the selection of dynamic stimulus-response constellations or interactions noticeably influenced by drug action and which are considered to be useful for predicting the therapeutic effect of psychoactive chemicals (Ban, 1968). As a further step, a corresponding assessment procedure for drug effects on animal behavior was suggested. Finally, an adjustment was made, and the human studies were focused on particular patterns of responses which rendered the measures and procedures applicable and relevant across species.

Ban (1968) proceeded to select for the evaluation of human behavior a number of stimulus-response constellations that he considered sufficient to express the physiological (psychological) and pathological (psychopathological) state of the organism, and which are also testable in animals. According to him, these are the startle response, *i.e.*, whether there is a response to an unexpected stimulus; the extinction of the orienting reflex (OR), *i.e.*, the ability of the CNS to inhibit the generalized response which is elicited by any indifferent stimulation; the maintenance of the unconditional reflex (UR), *i.e.*, the uninterfered with ability to respond to an unconditional stimulus; conditionability, *i.e.*, the potential for conditional reflex (CR) formation; extinction, *i.e.*, the potential to extinguish the established CR; disinhibition, *i.e.*, the ability to interfere with the function which provided for the extinction of a formerly established CR; conditional stimulus (CS) differentiation, *i.e.*, the ability to discriminate between two or more different CS's; and CS reversal, *i.e.*, the ability to turn a formerly positive CS into a negative CS and a negative into a positive one.

On the basis of these variables an attempt was made by Ban (1968) to describe both psychopathology and drug effects in these terms. Later on, the descriptive assessment was complemented with an evaluation in which—in a Pavlovian frame of reference—the state of the excitatory and the inhibitory (external and internal) processes was revealed, as well as the equilibrium and the mobility (*i.e.*, the dominance and the potential for shift in dominance) of the two basic processes and the amount of "paradoxical" responding. More recently, via the same variables, a profile of the state of arousal, affectivity and the level of mental integration have also been given.

Because of the lack of a general factor of conditioning in the human assessment it appeared to be essential to include the following conditioning techniques: galvanic skin reflex, salivary secretion (autonomic); eyelid closure (semivoluntary); and finger withdrawal (voluntary). Furthermore, Ivanov-Smolensky's (1953) procedure for testing the transmission from the first to the second signal system; a word-association technique for testing second signal system activity; and a conflict behavior procedure were also included. Consequently, in the final assessment first and second signal system activity and the relationship (dominance) between the first and the second signal system were also evaluated.

In this dynamic frame of reference the object of drug therapy was defined as that which modifies the dynamic state of the patient and reverses the direction of his pathological responses toward the physiological, *i.e.*, normal.

3. The Psychopharmacological Approach

Besides the new approaches in which the behavioral and the conditioning methods have been used in a psychopharmacological frame of reference, there is also a psychopharmacological approach slowly developing which is derived from grouping individuals on the basis of the similarity of their response patterns to various pharmacological substances. This psychopharmacological approach has already contributed observations pertinent to the analysis of clinical syndromes; to the elucidation of psychopathological mechanisms and theories; and to the delineation of concepts and nosological entities.

Some of the most pertinent knowledge derived by the application of the psychopharmacological approach was reviewed in a recent communication by the World Health Organization (WHO, 1967). It was pointed out that the newly accumulated information is in favor of the hypothesis of psychopathological diversity, gives a differential value on symptoms and opens new avenues for new symptomatological findings and groupings. It was also pointed out that the new data confirmed the concept of schizophrenia and has not invalidated the concept of manic-depressive psychosis. Furthermore, sufficient evidence has accumulated to state that contemporary pharmacotherapy does not act merely by modifying the symptoms of a disorder but that it may also modify its clinical course and evolution.

REFERENCES

Anderson, H., and Kristiansen, E. S.: Tofranil-treatment of endogenous depression. Acta Psychiat. Scand., *34:* 387 (1959).

Antrobus, J. S.: Patterns of dreaming and dream recall. Dissertation Abstract, *24:* 829, 1963.

Baastrup, P. C.: Influence of lithium ions in manic-depressive psychosis. Compr. Psychiat., *5:* 396 (1964).

Baastrup, P. C.: Lithium behandlung of manio-depressiv psykose. En psykoseforebyggende behandling smetode. (Paper read at the Seventh Scandinavian Congress of Psychopharmacology, Copenhagen, 1966.)

Baastrup, P. C., and Schou, M.: Lithium as a prophylactic agent. Arch. Gen. Psychiat. (Chicago), *16:* 162 (1967).

Bäckman, H., and Elosuo, R.: Electrocardiographic findings in connection with a clinical trial of chlorpromazine. Ann. Med. Intern. Fenn., *53:* 1 (1964).

Ballon, J.: The cardiologist's viewpoint. In: Toxicity and adverse reaction studies with neuroleptics and antidepressants (eds., Lehmann, H. E., and Ban, T. A.). (Q.P.R.A., 1968.)

Ban, T. A.: Methodology and pitfalls in clinical testing of psychopharmacological drugs. Chemotherapia (Basel), *9:* 223 (1964).

Ban, T. A.: Annual report of the research department. Douglas Hospital, Montreal, 1967.

Ban, T. A.: Prediction of therapeutic response to drugs. (Final report on Grant MA 1936 to the Medical Research Council of Canada, Montreal, 1968.)

Ban, T. A.: Psychophysical deficit and conditional reflex test variables and the classification of psychiatric patients. (Final report to the Psychiatric Services of the Province of Quebec, Montreal, 1968.)

Ban, T. A., and St. Jean, A.: The effect of phenothiazines on the electrocardiogram. Canad. Med. Ass. J., *91:* 537 (1964).

Ban, T. A., St. Jean, A., and Desautels, S.: The effects of phenothiazines on the human electrocardiogram. In: Neuropsychopharmacology. Vol. 4. (eds., Bente, D., and Bradley, P. B.). (Elsevier, Amsterdam, 1965.)

Bengzon, A., Hippius, H., and Kanig, K.: Some changes in the serum during treatment with psychotropic drugs. J. Nerv. Ment. Dis., *143:* 369 (1966).

Berger, F. M., Kletzkin, M., and Margolin, S.: The action of certain tranquilizers, antidepressants and anticholinergic drugs on hippocampal after discharges. In: Antidepressant drugs (eds., Garrattini, S., and Dukes, M. W. G.). (Excerpta Medica Foundation, New York, 1967.)

Bleuler, E. (1916): In: Bleuler, E.: Textbook of psychiatry. (MacMillan, New York, 1924.)

Blockus, L. E., and Everett, G. M.: Tremor producing drug 1,4-dipyrrolidino-2-butyne (tremorine). Fed. Proc., *16:* 283 (1957).

Bloom, J. B., Davis, N., and Wecht, C. H.: Effect on the liver of long-term tranquilizing medication. Amer. J. Psychiat., *121:* 788 (1965).

Burdick, J. A., Sugerman, A. A., and Goldstein, L.: The application of regression analysis to quantitative electroencephalography in man. Psychophysiology, *3:* 249 (1967).

Cade, J. F. J.: Lithium salts in the treatment of psychotic excitement. Med. J. Aust., *2:* 349 (1949).

Callaway, E., and Buchsbaum, M.: Effects of cardiac and respiratory cycles on averaged visual evoked responses. Electroenceph. Clin. Neurophysiol., *19:* 476 (1965).

Courvoisier, S., *et al.:* Propriétés pharmacodynamiques du chlorhydrate de chloro-3-(dimethylamino-3-propyl)-10-phenothiazine (RP 4560). Arch. Int. Pharmacodyn., *92:* 305 (1953).

Dement, W. C.: The effect of dream deprivation. Science, *131:* 1705 (1960).

Dement, W. C.: Experimental studies of dreaming. (Research Project Summaries of the National Institute of Mental Health, Bethesda, 1963.)

Desautels, S., Filteau, C., and St. Jean, A.: Ventricular tachycardia associated with administration of thioridazine hydrochloride. Canad. Med. Ass. J., *90:* 1030 (1964).

Dilalme, J. R., and Catenacci, A. J.: Chlorpromazine protection against hydrocarbon-epinephrine induced ventricular arrhythmias. Fed. Proc., *14:* 333 (1955).

Donnelly, J., and Zeller, W.: Clinical research on chlorpromazine in state and private psychiatric hospitals. J. Clin. Exp. Psychopath., *17:* 180 (1956).

Doust, J. W. L.: Spontaneous endogenous oscillating systems in autonomic and metabolic effectors: their relation to mental illness. J. Nerv. Ment. Dis., *131:* 335 (1960).

Driscoll, S. G., and Harra, D. Y. Y.: The development of enzyme systems during early infancy. Pediatrics, *22:* 785 (1958).

Eliakim, M., Isak, C., and Braun, K.: The effect of chlorpromazine on the ballistocardiogram and the electrocardiogram in man. Cardiologia (Basel), *32:* 177 (1958).

Everett, G. M.: Tremor produced by drugs. Nature (London), *177:* 1238 (1956).

Finkelstein, M. *et al.:* Effect of chlorpromazine on heart muscle and its influence on the inotropic action of three sympathomimetic amines. Fed. Proc., *13:* 354 (1954).

Fischer, S.: NIMH-PSC outpatient study of drug-set interaction. Psychopharmacol. Serv. Cent. Bull., *1:* 1 (1961).

Fisher, C.: Further experimental studies of dreaming. (Research Project Summaries, NIMH, Bethesda, 1963.)

Freemon, F. R., *et al.:* An electroencephalographic study of the effects of meprobamate on human sleep. Clin. Pharmacol. Ther., *6:* 172 (1965).

Friend, D. G.: Role of synthetic drugs in therapy of mental illness. In: Molecular modification in drug design (ed., Gould, R. F.). (American Chemical Society, Washington, 1964.)

Frostad, A. L., Forrest, T. G. L., and Bakker, C. B.: Influence of personality type on drug response. Amer. J. Psychiat., *122:* 1153 (1966).

Gallant, D. M.: Personal communication, Montreal, 1967.

Gallant, D. M., and Bishop, M. P.: The use of imipramine in high dosages: an attempt to elicit antipsychotic activity. Curr. Ther. Res., *9:* 6 (1967).

Gallant, D. M., Bishop, M. P., and Steele, C. H.: DPN(NAD-oxidized form): a preliminary evaluation in chronic schizophrenic patients. Curr. Ther. Res., *8:* 11 (1966).

Gershon, S.: Informal ECDEU report. (New York, 1967.)

Gershon, S., and Yuwiler, A.: Lithium ion: a specific psychopharmacological approach to the treatment of mania. J. Neuropsychiat., *1:* 229 (1960).

Goldberg, S. C., Klerman, G. L., and Cole, J. O.: Changes in schizophrenic psychopathology and ward behavior as a function of phenothiazine treatment. Brit. J. Psychiat., *111:* 120 (1965).

Goldberg, S. C., *et al.:* Sex and race differences in response to drug treatment among schizophrenics. Psychopharmacologia (Berlin), *9:* 31 (1966).

Goldstein, L., and Beck, R. A.: Amplitude analysis of the electroencephalogram. Review of the information obtained with the integrative method. Int. Rev. Neurobiol., *8:* 265 (1965).

Goldstein, L., *et al.:* Quantitative electroencephalographic analysis of naturally occurring (schizophrenic) and drug induced psychotic states in human males. Clin. Pharmacol. Ther., *4:* 10 (1963).

Granit, R.: Receptors and sensory perception. (Yale University Press, New Haven, 1955.)

Graupner, K. I., and Murphree, O. D.: Electrocardiographic changes associated with the use of thioridazine. J. Neuropsychiat., *5:* 344 (1964).

Guerrero-Figueroa, R., and Gallant, D. M.: Effects of pinoxepin and imipramine on the mesencephalic reticular formation and amygdaloid complex in the cat: neurophysiological and clinical correlations in human subjects. Curr. Ther. Res., *9:* 387 (1967).

GUERRERO-FIGUEROA, R., AND LESTER, B. K.: Effects of some drugs on electroencephalographic fast activity and dream time. Psychophysiology, *2:* 224 (1966).

GUERRERO-FIGUEROA, R., LESTER, B., AND HEATH, R. G.: Changes of hippocampal epileptiform activity during wakefulness and sleep. Acta Neurol. Lat. Amer., *11:* 330 (1965).

HALL, L. A., AND DUNLOP, D. J.: A study of chlorpromazine: methodology and results with chronic semi-disturbed schizophrenics. J. Nerv. Ment. Dis., *122:* 301 (1955).

HALLIWELL, G., QUINTON, R. M., AND WILLIAMS, F. E.: A comparison of imipramine, chlorpromazine and related drugs in various tests involving autonomic functions and antagonism of reserpine. Brit. J. Pharmacol., *23:* 330 (1964).

HAMMER, W., AND SJÖQVIST, F.: Inhibition of the metabolism of tremorine and oxo-tremorine in rats by antidepressants of the imipramine type. In: Antidepressant drugs (eds., Garrattini, S., and Dukes, M. N. G.). (Excerpta Medica Foundation, New York, 1967.)

HARTIGAN, G. P.: The use of lithium salts in affective disorders. Brit. J. Psychiat., *109:* 810 (1963).

HENINGER, G., DIMASCIO, A., AND KLERMAN, G. L.: Personality factors in variability of response to phenothiazines. Amer. J. Psychiat., *121:* 1091 (1965).

HERLOFSEN, H. B.: Litium behandlung ved manisk-depressiv sinnslidelse. (Paper presented at the meeting of the Norwegian Psychiatric Society, Oslo, 1965.)

HOFFER, A.: Enzymology of hallucinogens. In: Enzymes in mental health (eds., Martin, G. J., and Kisch, B.). (Lippincott, Philadelphia, 1966.)

HOFFER, A.: Laboratory tests for following progress of schizophrenia. Dis. Nerv. Syst., *27:* 466 (1966).

HOFFER, A. (1966): In: Kline, N. S., *et al.:* Controlled evaluation of nicotinamide adenine dinucleotide in the treatment of chronic schizophrenic patients. Brit. J. Psychiat., *113:* 731 (1967).

HOLLISTER, L. E.: Placebology: sense and nonsense. Curr. Ther. Res., *2:* 477 (1960).

HOLLISTER, L. E.: Personal communication, Montreal, 1967.

HOLLISTER, L. E., AND HALL, R. A.: Phenothiazine derivatives and morphologic changes in the liver. Amer. J. Psychiat., *123:* 2 (1966).

HOLLISTER, L. E., *et al.:* Causes of death in hospitalized veterans with neuropsychiatric disorders. Dis. Nerv. Syst., *21:* 315 (1960).

IRWIN, S.: A rational framework for the development, evaluation and use of psychoactive drugs. (Unpublished manuscript from the Department of Psychiatry, University of Oregon Medical School and the Oregon Regional Primate Research Center, Beaverton, 1967.)

IRWIN, S.: Psychopharmacology and drug therapy. (Oregon Regional Primate Research Center, Beaverton, 1967.)

IVANOV-SMOLENSKY, A. G.: Investigations into the interactions of the first and second signaling system. Zh. Vyssh. Nerv. Deiat. Pavlov., *3:* 481 (1953).

JACOBSEN, J. E.: The hypomanic alert: a program designed for greatest therapeutic control. Amer. J. Psychiat., *122:* 295 (1965).

JONES, M. B., AND AINSLIE, J. D.: Value of a placebo wash-out. Dis. Nerv. Syst., *27:* 393 (1966).

JOUVET, M.: Telencephalic and rhombencephalic sleep in the cat. In: The nature of sleep (eds., Wolstenholme, G. E. W., and O'Connor, M.). (Little, Brown, Boston, 1961.)

KAHN, E., *et al.:* Incidence of color on immediately recalled dreams. Science, *137:* 1054 (1962).

KELLY, H. R., FAY, J. E., AND LAVERTY, S. G.: Thioridazine hydrochloride (mellaril): its effect on the electrocardiogram and a report on two fatalities with electrocardiographic abnormalities. Canad. Med. Ass. J., *89:* 546 (1963).

KINGSTONE, E.: Electrocardiographic changes with psychoactive drugs: review of the literature—antipsychotic drugs. In: Toxicity and adverse reaction studies with neuroleptics and antidepressants (eds., Lehmann, H. E., and Ban, T. A.). (Q.P.R.A., Montreal, 1968.)

KLERMAN, G. L.: Assessing the influence of the hospital milieu upon the effectiveness of psychiatric drug therapy: problems of conceptualization and of research methodology. J. Nerv. Ment. Dis., *137:* 143 (1963).

KLERMAN, G. L., *et al.:* Clinical experience with dihydroxyphenylalanine (dopa) in depression. J. Psychiat. Res., *1:* 289 (1963).

KLERMAN, G. L., *et al.:* The influence of specific personality patterns on the reaction to phrenotropic agents. In: Biological psychiatry (ed., Masserman, J. H.). (Grune and Stratton, New York, 1959.)

KLERMAN, G. L., *et al.:* Factors influencing the clinical responses of schizophrenic patients to phenothiazine drugs and to placebo. Psychiatric Research Report, American Psychiatric Association, *19:* 97 (1964).

KLETZKIN, M.: Possible modes of action of psychotherapeutic agents in the treatment of mental disturbances. Ann. N.Y. Acad. Sci., *96:* 1 (1963).

KLINE, N. S., *et al.:* Controlled evaluation of nicotinamide adenine dinucleotide in the treatment of chronic schizophrenic patients. Brit. J. Psychiat., *113:* 731 (1967).

KUPATZ, H.: Veränderungen des Kindlichen Elektrocardiogrammes durch Megaphen. Mschr. Kinderheilk., *104:* 17 (1956).

LACEY, J. I., AND LACEY, B. C.: The relationship of resting autonomic activity to motor impulses. Res. Publ. Ass. Res. Nerv. Ment. Dis., *36:* 144 (1958).

LAVALLÉE, B.: Electrocardiographic changes

with psychoactive drugs: review of literature—antidepressant drugs. In: Toxicity and adverse reaction studies with neuroleptics and antidepressants (eds., Lehmann, H. E., and Ban, T. A.). (Q.P.R.A., Montreal, 1968.)

Lehmann, H. E.: The influence of neuroleptics and anxiolytic sedatives on conflict avoidance behavior in human subjects. (Volume dedicated to the 60th birthday of Professor Eugen Vencovsky.) (State Publishing House, Prague, 1968.)

Lehmann, H. E., and Ban, T. A.: The effect of hypnotics on rapid eye movements. (Presented at the Fourth Annual Meeting of the Canadian Society of Chemotherapy, Montreal, 1968.)

Lehmann, H. E., and Ban, T. A. (eds.): Toxicity and adverse reaction studies with neuroleptics and antidepressants. (Q.P.R.A., Montreal, 1968.)

Leveton, A. F.: The evaluation and testing of psychopharmacologic drugs. Amer. J. Psychiat., *115:* 232 (1958).

Liebreich, O. (1869): In: Sharpless, S. K.: Hypnotics and sedatives. II. Miscellaneous agents. In: The pharmacological basis of therapeutics (eds., Goodman, L. S., and Gilman, A.). (MacMillan, Toronto, 1965.)

Linn, E. C.: Drug therapy, milieu change, and release from a mental hospital. Arch. Neurol. Psychiat., *81:* 794 (1959).

Maggs, R.: Treatment of manic illness with lithium carbonate. Brit. J. Psychiat., *109:* 56 (1963).

Marshall, E. V., and Owens, A. H., Jr.: Absorption, excretion and metabolic fate of chloral hydrate and trichloroethanol. Bull. Hopkins Hosp., *95:* 1 (1954).

Melville, K. O.: Studies on the cardiovascular actions of chlorpromazine. I. Adrenergic and antifibrillatory actions. Arch. Int. Pharmacodyn., *115:* 278 (1958).

Melville, K. O., and Drapeau, I. V.: Studies on the cardiovascular action of chlorpromazine. II. Effects on cardiac output, coronary flow and heart contractions. Arch. Int. Pharmacodyn., *115:* 306 (1958).

Mosher, L. R., *et al.:* A clinical trial of alphamethyldopa in elated states. Amer. J. Psychiat., *122:* 1185 (1966).

Moyer, J. H., *et al.:* Laboratory and clinical observation on chlorpromazine: hemodynamic and toxicological studies. Amer. J. Med. Sci., *227:* 283 (1954).

Overall, J. C., Hollister, L. C., and Dellal, S. N.: Psychiatric drug research. Arch. Gen. Psychiat. (Chicago), *16:* 152 (1967).

Pfeiffer, C. C., *et al.:* Time-series frequency analysis and electrogenesis of the EEG's of normals and psychotics before and after drugs. Amer. J. Psychiat., *121:* 1147, 1965.

Pishkin, V., Shurley, J. T., and Wolfgang, A.: Stress, psychophysiological and cognitive indices in an acute double blind study with hydroxyzine in psychiatric patients. Arch. Gen. Psychiat. (Chicago), *16:* 471, 1967.

Rasmussen, E. B., and Kristiansen, P.: ECG changes during amitriptyline treatment. Amer. J. Psychiat., *119:* 781 (1963).

Roffwarg, H. P. *et al.:* Dream imagery: relationship to rapid eye movements of sleep. Arch. Gen. Psychiat. (Chicago), *7:* 235 (1962).

Royer, P., *et al.:* Les modifications de l'electrocardiogramme au cours du traitement par chlorpromazine. Ann. Medico psychol., *117:* 299 (1959).

Saarma, J., and Saarma, M.: Comparative conditioning study of neuroleptics in normals and chronic schizophrenics. (Presented at the International Congress of CINP, Washington, 1966.)

Sabshin, M., and Ramot, J.: Pharmacotherapeutic evaluation and the psychiatric setting. Arch. Neurol. Psychiat., *75:* 362 (1956).

Sarwer-Foner, G. J.: Some therapeutic aspects of the use of the neuroleptic drugs in schizophrenia, borderline states, and in the short-term psychotherapy of the neuroses. In: The dynamics of psychiatric drug therapy (ed., Sarwer-Foner, G. J.). (Charles C Thomas, Springfield, 1960.)

Sarwer-Foner, G. J. (ed.): The dynamics of psychiatric drug therapy. (Charles C Thomas, Springfield, 1960.)

Sarwer-Foner, G. J.: Discussion. (ECDEU meeting, Montreal, 1967.)

Schou, M.: Lithium in psychiatric therapy. Stock-taking after ten years. Psychopharmacologia (Berlin), *1:* 65 (1959).

Shagass, C., *et al.:* Evoked potential studies in psychiatric patients. Ann. N.Y. Acad. Sci., *112:* 526 (1964).

Sharma, P. L., and Arora, R. B.: Antiarrhythmias. II. Antiarrhythmic activity of some phenothiazine derivatives in experimental cardiac arrhythmias. Indian J. Med. Res., *49:* 1099 (1961).

Sherman, L.: The significant variables in psychopharmaceutic research. Amer. J. Psychiat., *116:* 208 (1959).

Spencer, P. S. J.: Activity of centrally acting and other drugs against tremor and hypothermia induced in mice by tremorine. Brit. J. Pharmacol., *25:* 442 (1965).

Spencer, P. S. J.: Antagonism of hypothermia in the mouse by antidepressants. In: Antidepressant drugs (eds., Garrattini, S., and Dukes, M. N. G.). (Excerpta Medica Foundation, New York, 1967.)

St. Jean, A.: General summary. In: Toxicity and adverse reaction studies with neuroleptics and antidepressants (eds., Lehmann, H. E., and Ban, T. A.). (Q.P.R.A., Montreal, 1968.)

St. Jean, A., *et al.:* Studies with thioridazine. In: Toxicity and adverse reaction studies with neuroleptics and antidepressants (eds., Lehmann, H. E., and Ban, T. A.). (Q.P.R.A., Montreal, 1968.)

Stolt, G.: Behandlung med. litium salter vid mano-depressiva stamningsstillstand. Svensk. Lakartidn., *62:* 3018 (1965).

Strömgren, E., and Schou, M.: Lithium treatment of manic states. Postgrad. Med., *35:* 83 (1964).

Sugerman, A. A., *et al.:* EEG and behavioral changes in schizophrenia. Arch. Gen. Psychiat. (Chicago), *10:* 340 (1964).

Teitelbaum, I.: Electrocardiographic changes associated with phenothiazines. Lancet, *1:* 115 (1963).

Theobald, W., *et al.:* Vergleichende Untersuchungen mit Tofranil, Pertofran und Insidon. Arch. Int. Pharmacodyn., *148:* 560 (1964).

Weinberg, S. J., and Haley, T. J.: Effect of chlorpromazine on cardiac arrhythmias induced by intra-cerebral injection of tryptamine-atrophanthidin. Arch. Int. Pharmacodyn., *105:* 209 (1956).

Wendkos, M. H.: Pharmacologic studies in a hitherto unreported benign repolarization disturbance among schizophrenics. J. New Drugs, *4:* 98 (1964).

Wendkos, M. H.: Experiments with thioridazine. In: Toxicity and adverse reaction studies with neuroleptics and antidepressants (eds., Lehmann, H. E., and Ban, T. A.). (Q.P.R.A., Montreal, 1968.)

WHO, Scientific Group on Psychopharmacology: Research in psychopharmacology. (World Health Organization Technical report Series No. 371, World Health Organization, Geneva, 1967.)

Part Two

SYSTEMATIC PSYCHOPHARMACOLOGY

Seven

Developmental Aspects

Drugs which induce behavioral changes with or without affecting psychological functions belong to nine different pharmacological groups. Substances in the first group include chemicals which have either an "inhibitory" or a "facilitating" effect on the activity of the work-performing skeletal muscles—by acting on the transmission of impulses at the site of neuromuscular junctions—and consequently on overt behavioral manifestations. Different from these are the various autonomic drugs, which act selectively on those structures which are concomitantly affected by changes in affective behavior, and the autocoids, with a distinct affinity for structures which are supposedly related to the neurochemical basis of behavior.

While the actions of these first three groups of drugs can be shown only by measuring various kinds of somatic activity, those of the remaining six groups can be inferred mainly from their effects on the various psychological functions which are involved in the reflection of the environment and the self (*i.e.*, consciousness).

In the latter groups are the classical general anesthetics whose effects are characterized by a loss of consciousness, *i.e.*, a transition in which the reflection of both the environment and the self are discontinued, and the narcotic analgesics, which only diminish the significance of conscious reflections and particularly of painful experiences.

As opposed to substances with an over-all effect on consciousness, there are other groups of drugs which have a somewhat more selective action on arousal, a basic constituent of consciousness, and consequently on attention. These are the sedatives and the stimulants, *i.e.*, drugs with a predominantly inhibitory or facilitating effect on this function.

Finally there are the psychotherapeutic drugs, with a correcting effect on pathological conscious reflections, and the psychotopathic drugs, which can induce pathological conscious experiences.

A. DRUGS WITH BEHAVIORAL EFFECTS WITH UNDECIDED PSYCHOLOGICAL ACTION

1. Drugs Acting on Skeletal Neuromuscular Junctions

These drugs are usually devoid of CNS and consequently of psychological effects. Their primary action is characterized by an interference with or facilitation of the transmission of nerve impulses at the skeletal neuromuscular junctions.

a. Neuromuscular Blocking Agents

Those substances which interrupt the transmission of nerve impulses are called neuromuscular blocking agents and in general belong to two main categories: competitive-stabilizers and depolarizing muscle-relaxants (Koelle, 1965).

i. Competitive Stabilizers. The competitive-stabilizing agents act by competing with acetylcholine, the transmitter substance, at the neuromuscular junction and thereby interfere with the performance of voluntary muscle responses. Representatives of this subgroup are curare and *d*-tubocurarine (Bernard, 1856; and Langley, 1918).

ii. Depolarizing Muscle Relaxants. The depolarizing muscle relaxants, unlike the competitive-stabilizing agents, act by depolarizing the muscle end plates and thereby interfere with the performance of voluntary muscle responses by preventing the action of acetylcholine. Representatives are decamethonium, benzoquinonium and succinylcholine. The last is extensively used as a premedication for electroconvulsive treatment in psychiatric practice.

b. Anticholinesterases

Substances which facilitate the transmission of nerve impulses at the neuromuscular junction are the cholinesterase inhibitors or anticholinesterases. The main characteristic of these drugs is that they interfere with the action of the enzyme responsible for the "destruction" of acetylcholine. Examples are physostigmine, neostigmine and edrophonium chloride (also nicotine). It has been noted that, while they interfere with the action of competitive-stabilizing agents, they leave the action of the depolarizing muscle relaxants unaffected (Koelle, 1965).

2. Autonomic Drugs

These are chemicals with a direct effect on the activity of the smooth muscles and gland cells. Their primary action is characterized by an interference with or facilitation of various autonomic nervous system functions.

Acetylcholine is the transmitter substance of the parasympathetic division of the autonomic nervous system, and norepinephrine is the transmitter substance of the sympathetic division. The only definite role of norepinephrine thus far revealed is in the transmission of impulses at the postganglionic sympathetic fiber sites, but acetylcholine seems to be important in the transmission of impulses at all preganglionic autonomic fiber sites and all postganglionic parasympathetic fiber sites.

Autonomic drugs are classified in the following subgroups: sympathomimetic substances (adrenergic drugs), sympatholytic substances (adrenergic blocking drugs), parasympathomimetic substances (cholinergic drugs) and parasympatholytic substances (cholinergic blocking drugs).

a. Adrenergic Drugs

Adrenergic drugs generally produce the following effects: mydriasis, viscid salivary gland secretion, bronchial muscle relaxation, tachycardia, coronary dilation, decreased gastrointestinal motility-tone-secretion, relaxation of the bladder detrusor muscle and contraction of the anal sphincter. Furthermore, they have a peripheral "excitatory" action which constricts the smooth muscles of the blood vessels supplying the skin and mucous membranes; a metabolic "excitatory" action manifested in an increase of glycogenolysis and liberation of free fatty acids; and a central nervous system "excitatory" action leading to wakefulness, respiratory stimulation and reduction of appetite (Innes and Nickerson, 1965).

Chemically, adrenergic drugs are subdivided into two major categories: catecholamines and noncatecholamines. Both contain naturally occurring and synthetic compounds. The parent moiety for both is the β-phenylethylamine structure, which consists of an aromatic nucleus (a benzene ring) and an aliphatic portion (ethylamine).

i. Catecholamines. Substituting the H atoms with OH groups in positions 3 and 4 of the benzene ring results in catechol; adrenergic sympathomimetic amines with these OH substitutions are called catecholamines.

Among the naturally occurring catecholamines, norepinephrine (NE), epinephrine (E) and ephedrine (Nagai, 1887) are the more important pharmacologically, while isoproterenol is the best known of the synthetic preparations. It has been noted that the last substance acts almost exclusively on the beta receptor sites, while norepinephrine acts almost exclusively on the alpha receptor sites.

Psychopharmacological Applications. In contradistinction to E, which may induce psychopathological manifestations, *e.g.*, fear, anxiety, tension, restlessness, etc., NE has been increasingly used, without any undesirable effect, as an adjuvant in behavior therapy to facilitate the extinction of old, faulty behavioral patterns and to help the establishment of new "healthy" ones. Furthermore, ephedrine is known as one of the first substances successfully used in the treatment of narcolepsy (Goodman and Gilman, 1965).

ii. Noncatecholamines. There are numerous synthetic and naturally occurring adrenergic compounds in this category. The phenylethylamines, *i.e.*, the amphetamines (Barger and Dale, 1910), are psychopharmacologically the most important (and will be discussed separately). Other drugs in this category are isoxsuprine, nylidrin (vasodilators); mephentermine, metaraminol (vasopressors); cyclopentamine, naphazoline (decongestants); and the w dely used anorexigenics such as diethylpropion, phenmetrazine, etc.

Psychopharmacological Applications. Possible potentiation of antipsychotic effects of phenothiazines by nylidrin was recognized in the laboratory by Kato and Gözsy (1964) and confirmed clinically by Lehmann and Ban (1964). Addiction to adrenergic-anorexigenic drugs has become a serious problem in recent years.

b. Adrenergic Blocking Agents

In contradistinction to adrenergic drugs are the adrenergic blocking agents. Particularly important pharmacologically are the ergot alkaloids, yohimbine and its congeners, the Rauwolfia alkaloids and methyldopa (Nickerson, 1965).

Psychopharmacological Applications. The ergot alkaloids were one of the first adrenergic blocking agents discovered. Their general pharmacological properties were explored as early as 1906 by Dale, but it took several decades before their general sedative properties, which in high doses accompany the antihypertensive effect, were shown. Both the antihypertensive and sedative effects are utilized in the preparation dihydroergotoxine, which is a mixture of equal parts of the methanesulfonates of the dihydro derivatives of the three members of the ergotoxine complex.

Yohimbine and the Rauwolfia alkaloids are closely related chemically. Yohimbine, a naturally occurring alkaloid obtained from the West African tree Yohimbèné, remains of limited clinical importance. It is occasionally used in psychiatry as an adjuvant of behavior therapy in some of the sexual neurotic cases. While the Rauwolfia alkaloids are less and less frequently used in psychiatric practice, they have become an important instrument in modern psychopharmacological research.

Methyldopa, an effective inhibitor of dopa decarboxylase, which transiently reduces 5-hydroxytryptamine formation and in a more sustained manner NE levels, was explored biochemically by Sourkes (1964) and clinically by St. Jean *et al.* (1965) and Mosher *et al.* (1966), among others. While St. Jean *et al.* (1965) have seen typical depressive manifestations in the course of treatment with this substance and suggested that it might be used as a major tranquilizer, Mosher *et al.* (1966) failed to recognize any therapeutic action (in mania).

c. Cholinergic Drugs

Cholinergic drugs are generally characterized by the following effects: miosis, watery salivary gland secretion, bradycardia, constriction of coronaries, increased gastrointestinal motility tone and secretion, contraction of the bladder detrusor muscle and relaxation of the anal sphincters. Chemicals which induce these effects are subdivided into three categories: acetylcholine and related esters, cholinesterase inhibitors, and other cholinomimetic alkaloids (Koelle, 1965). Of these, only some of the cholinomimetic alkaloids are of psychopharmacological significance.

Psychopharmacological Applications. Acetylcholine was first synthesized by Baeyer (1867), but it was Dale (1914) who recognized that the action of this substance resembles that of stimulating the parasympathetic nerves. In spite of its wide range of activity and extensive physiological and pharmacological investigations, this substance has no therapeutic value at present.

On the other hand, all three cholinomimetic alkaloids (muscarine, arecoline and pilocarpine) given by intraventricular injections have an activating effect on the paraventricular hypothalamic nuclei. It was subsequently revealed that they also evoke cortical arousal (activation of the EEG), which could be reduced or blocked by atropine and by some of the antidepressant substances.

While the clinical application of these drugs remains limited, Lehmann and Ban (1966) have reported a behavioral stimulating effect of pilocarpine in chronic psychiatric patients.

d. Cholinergic Blocking Agents

In addition to their peripheral effects, common characteristics of cholinergic blocking agents are a stimulating action on the central nervous system when given in small amounts and a depressant effect when administered in high doses (Innes and Nickerson, 1965).

The first cholinergic blocking agents were the alkaloids of the belladonna plant. Preparations of belladonna were used by the ancient Hindus, but it was not until the early nineteenth century that one of its active principles, atropine, was isolated. It took another quarter of a century before the pharmacological activity of this substance was described by Bezold and Bloebaum (1867) and Heidenhain (1872).

Psychopharmacological Applications. Atropine has been employed with questionable success in the so-called pharmacotoxic therapy of schizophrenia (Alexander, 1953); and atropine-induced psychosis has been used successfully to investigate the neurophysiological basis of hallucinatory phenomena (Giljarovskij, 1954).

Soon after the discovery of atropine, other active principles of belladonna such as hyoscyamine and hyoscine (scopolamine) were isolated, and the CNS depressant effect of the latter substance in clinical doses was noted. This depressant action of hyoscine has been utilized extensively (particularly in combination with morphine or apomorphine) to control the agitation of disturbed psychotic patients. While it is generally accepted that hyoscine induces drowsiness accompanied by a feeling of well-being (euphoria) and a pleasant fatigue that leads to dreamless sleep (the whole period covered by amnesia), it occasionally produces restlessness, excitement, hallucinations and a toxic delirious state. This condition resembles the toxic psychosis induced by atropine and is characterized by reduced electrical activity of the brain.

Procaine, a substance structurally unrelated to acetylcholine, interferes with the release of acetylcholine from the preganglionic fibers. It has been used with questionable success in attempts to improve the memory disturbance of geriatric patients (Aslan, 1960).

3. Autocoids

The third group of drugs with possible behavioral implications are the autocoids (*i.e.,* "self-medicinal agents"). This term refers to substances of intensive pharmacological activity which are present in the body under normal conditions (Goodman and Gilman, 1965). Histamine and serotonin are of paramount importance pharmacologically.

a. Histamine

Histamine, or β-imidazolylethylamine, was synthesized by Windaus and Vogt in 1907. Although it has many pharmacological actions (Douglas, 1965), it has only very limited, and mainly investigative, applications in psychiatry.

Psychopharmacological Applications. Attempts to use histamine as a diagnostic tool for schizophrenia remain unsuccessful. Histamine responses of schizophrenics were found to be equivocal (LeBlanc and Lemieux, 1961; Simpson and Kline, 1961; and Trsic *et al.*, 1967).

More important than histamine in psychopharmacology are the antihistaminic substances (Bovet and Staub, 1937; and Halpern, 1942). It was, in fact, the discovery of the potent sedative and also anxiolytic properties of promethazine (a powerful antihistaminic phenothiazine) which led to the discovery of chlorpromazine, the first synthetic antipsychotic preparation.

b. Serotonin

The other psychopharmacologically important autocoid is serotonin or (5-hydroxytryptamine) which, although known for about a century as an unidentified vasoconstrictor material of the serum, was only isolated in a crystalline complex form by Rapport *et al.* in 1948 and synthetically prepared by Hamlin and Fischer in 1951. Since then, the interest in serotonin and its functions as a central neurohumoral transmitter substance has gained increasing attention (Douglas, 1965).

Psychopharmacological Considerations. In the early nineteen fifties it was recognized that certain indole ring containing drugs with structural resemblance to serotonin, *i.e.*, bufotenine, lysergic acid diethylamide, psilocybin, etc. (Downing, 1964), exert psychotopathic effects probably through the mechanism of competitive antagonism (Twarog and Page, 1953; and Amin *et al.*, 1954). Others, *e.g.*, reserpine, which depletes serotonin storage and reduces brain serotonin levels, were shown to have sedative, tranquilizing and mood-depressing properties (Brodie *et al.*, 1955). However, other serotonin antagonists, for example, the 2-bromo derivative of lysergic acid diethylamide, lack psychotopathic effects; methysergide, a substance used in the prophylactic treatment of migraine headache, has questionable psychoactive properties; and cyproheptadine, a substance therapeutic in various allergic conditions, may produce drowsiness and exert a sedative action. Thus the role of serotonin in psychological phenomena still remains to be elucidated.

B. DRUGS WITH BEHAVIORAL EFFECTS AND PSYCHOLOGICAL ACTION

1. Substances with an Over-all Effect on Consciousness

a. General Anesthetics

Since anesthesia means the absence of sensation, the term general anesthetics refers to substances whose effects are characterized by loss of consciousness, *i.e.*, a condition in which sensorial experiencing is discontinued (Price and Dripps, 1965).

Since the middle of the nineteenth century a great number of general anesthetics have been developed. Their common characteristic is the potential to induce an "inhibitory state" of the CNS which at first extends only to the "higher" cerebral functions (consciousness) but which progresses downward to the lower centers (Grollman, 1965).

Psychopharmacological Applications. Among the various general anesthetics of particular psychopharmacological importance are carbon dioxide (Hickman, 1824), nitrous oxide (Wells, 1845) and ether (Morton, 1846). Not so long ago they were extensively used as "psycholytic" substances to facilitate the psychotherapeutic process.

The original discovery that carbon dioxide (CO_2) has a beneficial effect on abnormal mental states was made independently by Loevenhart *et al.* (1929), Solomon *et al.*, (1931) and Meduna (1950). It was considered to be particularly useful in the treatment of neurotic anxiety states and alcoholism (Wilcox, 1951). Sargant and Slater (1963) obtained good results with this treatment in posttraumatic hysterical reactions with predominantly dissociative phenomena (and the worst results in obsessional patients).

While nitrous oxide (NO_2) abreaction was found to be most useful in the presence of conversion symptoms (Alexander, 1953), ether abreaction—as introduced by Schilder and Weissmann (1927)—proved to be beneficial in cases of war neuroses (Sargant and Slater, 1963) "where one wishes to bring aggressive feelings to the fore" (Sargant and Shorvon, 1945).

b. Narcotic Analgesics

The action of narcotic analgesics on consciousness is somewhat similar to that of the general anesthetics. However, while general anesthetics induce a loss of consciousness, narcotic analgesics merely diminish the state of consciousness and, consequently, sensory experiences, motor activity and reflexes. Because of these effects, narcotic analgesics are extensively used for the relief of pain in spite of their addicting properties and other side-effects, which not infrequently include nausea, vomiting, drowsiness, dizziness, etc.

i. Categories. *α. Natural Opium Alkaloids.* Although the psychological effects of opium had been known to ancient Sumerians and its dependence-producing effects to the early Greeks, the first undisputed reference to the substance can be traced to the writings of Theophrastus, who lived in the third century B.C. Early in the nineteenth century a German pharmacist, Sertürner (1803) isolated and described the first known psychologically active opium alkaloid, which he named after Morpheus, the Greek god of dreams (morphine). Thirty years later another psychoactive alkaloid of opium, codeine, was discovered by Robiquet (1833), and in 1848, a psychologically inactive alkaloid of opium, papaverine, was reported by Merck. Since that time a great number of opium alkaloids have been isolated and found to belong to one of two chemical classes: the phenanthrenes (morphine, codeine, thebaine) and the benzyl isoquinolines (papaverine, noscapine, narceine). The former are characterized by strong psychopharmacological action; the latter class is almost entirely devoid of this quality (Jaffe, 1965).

β. Synthetic Opiates. Well known among the synthetic opium derivatives are heroin, dihydromorphine, dihyrocodeine, oxymorphone, levorphanol, ethylmorphine and apomorphine.

γ. Miscellaneous Synthetic Analgesics. Among the others, the piperidine nucleus containing compounds meperidine, methadone, alphaprodine, anileridine and piminodine are pharmacologically important.

ii. Psychopharmacological Considerations and Applications. While dependency characteristically develops in the course of administration of any of the narcotic analgesic substances, particular psychopharmacological interest has been focused on morphine. More recently, apomorphine and methadone have been increasingly applied in psychiatric treatment.

α. Morphine. Morphine is characterized by anticholinesterase activity and a distinct antiserotonin effect. It also prevents norepinephrine release from its postganglionic storage sites. The anatomical sites of action of the substance include various levels in the central nervous system. At the spinal cord level, polysynaptic reflexes are affected, *e.g.*, the ipsilateral flexor and crossed extensor reflexes are depressed; the arousal patterns produced by painful stimuli or repetitive stimulation of the brain stem reticular formation are diminished; the response of the hypothalamus to afferent stimulation is decreased; and there is also a shift in the electroencephalogram toward increased voltage and decreased frequencies. The nausea (or even vomiting) and the respiratory depression with excessive doses are attributed to the direct central medullary effects of this substance.

Simultaneously with the neurochemical and neurophysiological alterations, there are also marked psychological changes. Characteristic of these even after a single dose of morphine is the lowering of attentive and perceptual functions together with a decrease of "will power." Since during these changes the imaginative processes are usually well maintained, morphine produces in most of the exposed subjects a feeling of well-being.

In small doses it induces a definite slowing of voluntary movements and induces a "light sleep" that some described as a state of "abstraction." However, the "higher dosage"-induced sleep is deep and dreamless; and an overdosage results in coma with characteristic miotic pupils and slow respiration.

In contradistinction to single doses, chronic administration leads to permanent parasympathetic excitement with loss of ethical and moral values.

β. Morphine and Apomorphine. For a considerable time morphine was given extensively not only for the relief of pain but also for temporary behavioral control (mainly in combination with hyoscine) for acutely excited, uncontrollable, agitated psychiatric patients. Others used a hyoscine and apomorphine combination for the same purpose. The latter substance has also been extensively used in the treatment of alcoholism. In the behavior therapy of alcoholics the nausea and vomiting-producing effects of apomorphine are associated with drinking with the aim of achieving conditioned aversion to alcoholic beverages.

γ. *Methadone.* The third substance with psychopharmacological applications in this category is methadone. This drug is employed increasingly in the withdrawal treatment of morphine and related narcotic analgesic drugs. In these cases methadone, which provides for an uneventful sudden withdrawal, is substituted for the addicting drug in decreasing doses over a period of several days to one month, depending on the degree and severity of dependency.

2. Substances with a Generalized Effect on Arousal Functions

a. Sedatives

Sedatives are usually defined as substances which exert a global inhibitory effect almost equally on higher and lower cerebral structures. However, while general anesthetics and narcotic analgesics primarily affect the complex psychological function of consciousness, the action of sedatives is directed primarily toward reducing psychic arousal, *i.e.*, the psychological function of attention. Substances in this group which have been found particularly useful in facilitating sleep or to correct sleep disturbances are called hypnotics (Sharpless, 1965).

There were at least four different classes of sedatives known prior to the introduction of the barbiturates: the inorganic salts, chloral derivatives, cyclic ethers and ureides. The inorganic salts are historically the oldest. Bromides were introduced into medicine by Magendie (1821). Their sedative or, rather, central nervous system depressant effect, however, was first utilized by Lockock (1857) in the treatment of epilepsy. The rationale for this treatment was based on the belief in the relationship between epilepsy and masturbation. Since bromides, especially potassium bromide, have anaphrodisiac properties, Lockock (1857) thought they should be useful in the control of epileptic manifestations. While the rationale was wrong, the treatment proved to be successful.

Almost simultaneously with the first application of bromides, the first chloral derivative, chloral hydrate, was introduced. Although this chemical was synthesized as early as 1832 by Liebig, it was not until 1869 that Liebreich discovered its hypnotic properties.

Less than 15 years later paraldehyde was introduced into medicine by Cervello (1882), the last significant sedative prior to the discovery of ureides, the parent structure of barbiturates.

i. Categories. α. *Inorganic Salts.* While the various inorganic bromide salts were once among the most extensively used sedatives, their application today is rather limited (convulsive states in pediatric practice).

They act by replacing chlorides. Consequently, their activity depends on the amount of bromide given, the chloride intake, and on the fluid consumption and renal efficiency of the patient.

Underlying any psychological changes, there are electroencephalographic alterations, which are characterized by sustained fast wave activity at low plasma levels and diffuse slow waves at high plasma concentrations.

Psychopharmacological Considerations. Bromides are excreted very slowly by the kidneys and consequently have an accumulating property. With increasing blood concentration, undesirable side-effects occur. The earliest symptoms of bromide intoxication are fatigue and sleepiness. These are later replaced by decreased appetite, weight loss and characteristic mental dullness. A subsequent complication may be toxic delirium.

The toxic delirium induced by bromides has been of particular psychopharmacological interest. Consequently, the neurophysiological and neurochemical correlates of this artificially induced toxic psychosis have been extensively studied.

β. *Chloral Derivatives.* The first chloral derivative was chloral hydrate, an anticholinesterase which acts by transforming into trichloroethanol, a substance once widely used as a basal anesthetic.

Practical Considerations. Trichloroethanol

in varying amounts reacts (mainly in the liver) with glycuronic acid to form urochloralic acid, an inactive preparation. Individuals with an enzymatic defect precluding the formation of glycuronic acid or its conjugation with trichloroethanol may be seriously affected—poisoned in fact—by chloral hydrate. This should be taken into account when prescribing it for alcoholics with severe liver impairment. Also, since it is known that the fetus and premature infant have minimal ability to use the detoxifying mechanisms described, chloral hydrate, according to Friend (1964), should be used with caution if at all during pregnancy and the period of lactation.

Since chloral hydrate produces gastric irritation—a rather undesirable side-effect in treatment—it has been replaced more recently by chloral betaine, another chloral derivative, or by pentaerythritol chloral, one of the most stable members of this class. Other drugs in this category are butylchloral hydrate, chlorobutanol, petrichloral and chloralose.

γ. Cyclic Ethers. In this category only paraldehyde has psychopharmacological importance. Paraldehyde is a particularly rapid acting hypnotic which may be administered by various routes (oral, rectal and intramuscular). Sleep ensues within 10 to 15 minutes even after peroral usage.

Paraldehyde is a polymer of acetaldehyde without a free aldehyde group. Consequently, in high blood concentration it depresses cholinergic transmission in ganglionic and neuromuscular junctions by reducing acetylcholine liberation. It has been reported that a significant fraction of this rapidly absorbed substance is excreted unchanged in the urine.

Psychopharmacological Applications. Paraldehyde is frequently used for the control of abstinence phenomena, excitement, convulsions, intractable pain and also for night sedation. When taken as a hypnotic, a "hangover" after awakening is not infrequently seen. Even more important is that by crossing the placental barrier paraldehyde may cause a delay in respiration of the newborn which warrants cautious use of this substance in pregnancy.

δ. Ureides. The condensation of one of the amino groups of urea with a carboxyl group leads to the different monoureides, the majority of which have some hypnotic properties. Among them, carbromal, bromisoval and ectylurea are used in treatment.

More potent in their hypnotic properties are the diureides in which both of the amino groups of urea are condensed with a carboxyl group, *i.e.*, with a dicarboxylic acid. Among the diureides, most important is barbituric acid, the condensation product of urea and malonic acid, the parent compound of barbiturates.

b. Stimulants

Stimulants are usually defined as substances which exert a global excitatory effect almost equally on the higher and lower cerebral structures. While the action of sedatives is to reduce psychic arousal, the action of stimulants is in the opposite direction, which consequently improves attention (Esplin and Zablocka, 1965).

The only important stimulant drug category prior to the introduction of amphetamines were the xanthines.

i. Xanthines. The history of xanthines began with the discovery of coffee by a prior in an Arabian convent, whose shepherds complained that their goats were unable to sleep. He recognized the relationship between the insomnia and the consumption of the berries of the coffee plant growing in the nearby grazing fields.

Trimethylxanthine, the first active compound in this category, was derived from coffee arabica. It was verified as a purine derivative and named caffeine after the berry from which it was isolated.

Qualitatively similar but quantatively less stimulating are two other xanthine substances, *i.e.*, theobromine and theophylline. These are prepared from the leaves of thea chinensis and from the seeds of theobroma (cacao), respectively. All three substances have central nervous system stimulating effects, but they also show differences pharmacologically. For example, psychomotor stimulation is more pronounced with caffeine, while the greatest spasmolytic effect is attributed to theobromine. Theophylline, on the other hand, is the most effective diuretic and coronary dilator of the group.

Psychopharmacological Considerations. The stimulating effect of these drugs and particularly of caffeine is rather diffuse and extends from the cortex through the medulla to the spinal cord centers. While the medullary action of these drugs is usually considered to be responsible for the respiratory and vasomotor effects, the improvement they produce in sensory, intellectual and motor activity is attributed primarily to their cortical action.

Excessive dosage of any of these drugs, but particularly caffeine, may produce insomnia, restlessness, excitement or even delirium (and convulsions) with a characteristic tachycardia and extrasystoles. There is some evidence that chronic administration (at least of the methylxanthines) may lead to psychic dependence.

ii. Other Stimulants. Other CNS stimulants with psychopharmacological implications, extensively used in the animal pharmacological screening of psychoactive drugs, are picrotoxin, nikethamide and pentetrazol. The latter substance is used in the physical—convulsive—treatment of schizophrenics and in the pharmacological therapy of geriatric patients with equivocal results.

The most important discovery in this area of research was the synthesis of epinephrine, the vasopressor principle of the adrenal medulla, by Stolz (1904) and independently by Dakin (1905). (The parent substance of epinephrine was found to be phenylethylamine, a composite of dihydroxybenzene and ethanolamine). Following the synthesis of epinephrine, a large number of structurally related synthetic amines were studied pharmacologically by Barger and Dale (1910). Among these were the aromatic, methylated phenylethylamines, *i.e.*, amphetamines.

3. Substances with a More Specific Psychological Action

a. Psychotherapeutic Drugs

Psychotherapeutic drugs are substances primarily used in the treatment of psychiatric patients. They are usually subdivided into three major categories: antipsychotics (neuroleptics), antidepressants (thymoleptics) and anxiolytics (tranquilizers).

Apart from their therapeutic usefulness, psychotherapeutic drugs have brought about fundamental changes in the theory and practice of psychiatry. Perhaps most important is that they have provided new opportunities for investigating and reassessing neurophysiological and neurochemical concepts of psychopathology, as well as for new groupings of psychiatric patients according to their responsiveness to the various drugs.

The phenothiazines were the first among the antipsychotics to be applied therapeutically (Hamon *et al.*, 1952), soon to be followed by the Rauwolfia alkaloids (Hakim, 1953) and only much later by the butyrophenones (Divry *et al.*, 1959) and the thioxanthenes (Ravn and Rud, 1961). Of the antidepressants, both the tricyclic compounds (Kuhn, 1957) and the monoamine oxidase inhibitors (Kline *et al.*, 1957) were introduced into treatment about the same time. Of the anxiolytics, the introduction of propanediols (Osinski, 1957) preceded that of the benzodiazepines (Tobin *et al.*, 1960).

b. Psychotopathic Substances

The psychopathology-producing effects of smoking hashish, sniffing cohoba and ingesting peyotl or teonanacatl have been known for centuries. Many of these have been used during religious ceremonies in primitive societies.

Application of psychotopathic substances and consequently the study of psychopharmacologically induced psychopathology began in the first half of the nineteenth century when Moreau de Tours (1845) proposed the use of marijuana (hashish) for experimental purposes. Somewhat later, a similar suggestion was made by Kraepelin (1896), whose disciples, Knauer and Maloney (1913), were among the first to systematically study the effects of peyotl (mescaline) on humans. Since that time a great number of psychotopathic substances have been recognized and synthesized, mainly after Hofmann (1943) discovered and described the psychotopathic properties of lysergic acid diethylamide.

REFERENCES

ALEXANDER, L.: Treatment of mental disorders. (Saunders, Philadelphia, 1953.)

AMIN, A. H., CRAWFORD, T. B. B., AND GADDUM, J. H.: The distribution of substance P and 5-hydroxytryptamine in the central nervous system of the dog. J. Physiol., *126:* 596 (1954).

ASLAN, A.: Procaine therapy in old age and other disorders. Geront. Clin. (Basel), *2:* 148 (1960).

BAEYER, A.: Über das Neurin. Liebig. Ann. Chem., *142:* 322 (1867).

BAN, T. A.: Brom-Sevenal. Elme és Idegápolás, *2:* 82 (1956).

BARGER, G., AND DALE, H. H.: Chemical structure and sympathomimetic action of amines. J. Physiol., *41:* 19 (1910).

BERNARD, C.: Analyse physiologique des propriétés des systèmes musculaire et nerveux au moyer du curare. C. R. Acad. Sci. (Paris), *43:* 825 (1856).

BEZOLD, A., AND BLOEBAUM, F. (1867): In: Innes, I. R., and Nickerson, M.: Drugs inhibiting the action of acetylcholine on structures innervated by postganglionic parasympathetic nerves. In: The pharmacological basis of therapeutics (eds., Goodman, C. S., and Gilman, A.) (MacMillan, New York, 1965.)

BOVET, D., AND STAUB, A. M.: Action protectrice des éthers phénotiques au cours de l'intoxication histaminique. C. R. Soc. Biol. (Paris), *124:* 547 (1937).

BRODIE, B. B., PLETSCHER, A., AND SHORE, P. A.: Evidence that serotonin has a role in brain function. Science, *122:* 968 (1955).

BRODIE, B. B., SHORE, P. A., AND SILVER, S. L.: Potentiating action of chlorpromazine and reserpine. Nature (London) *175:* 1133 (1955).

CERVELLO, V. (1882): In: Sharpless, S. K.: Hypnotics and sedatives. II. Miscellaneous agents. In: The pharmacological basis of therapeutics (eds., Goodman, L. S., and Gilman, A.). (MacMillan, Toronto, 1965.)

DAKIN, H. D.: On the physiological activity of substances indirectly related to adrenalin. Proc. Roy. Soc. (London), *76:* 491 (1905).

DALE, H. H. (1906): In: Nickerson, M.: Drugs inhibiting adrenergic nerves and structures innervated by them. In: The pharmacological basis of therapeutics (eds., Goodman, L. S., and Gilman, A.). (MacMillan, New York, 1965.)

DALE, H. H.: The action of certain esters and ethers of choline and their relation to muscarine. J. Pharmacol. Exp. Ther., *6:* 147 (1914).

DALE, H. H.: Chemical transmission of the effects of nerve impulses. Brit. Med. J., *1:* 835 (1934).

DIVRY, P., *et al.:* Etude et expérimentation cliniques du R 1625 ou halopéridol, nouveau neuroleptique et "neurodysleptique." Acta Neurol. Belg., *59:* 377 (1959).

DOUGLAS, W. W.: Histamine and antihistamines. In: The pharmacological basis of therapeutics (eds., Goodman, L. S., and Gilman, A.). (MacMillan, New York, 1965.)

DOUGLAS, W. W.: 5-Hydroxytryptamine and antagonistic polypeptides, angiotension and kinins. In: The pharmacological basis of therapeutics (eds., Goodman, L. S., and Gilman, A.). (MacMillan, New York, 1965.)

DOWNING, D. F.: Psychotomimetic compounds. In: Psychopharmacological agents (ed., Gordon, M.). (Academic Press, New York, 1964.)

EBIN, D. (ed.): The drug experience. (Orion Press, New York, 1961.)

ESPLIN, D. W., AND ZABLOCKA, B.: Central nervous system stimulants. In: The pharmacological basis of therapeutics (eds., Goodman, L. S., and Gilman, A.). (MacMillan, Toronto, 1965.)

FRIEND, D. G.: Clinical evaluation of drugs. Prevention and control of adverse reactions. J.A.M.A., *187:* 348 (1964).

FRIEND, D. G.: Role of synthetic drugs in the therapy of mental illness. In: Molecular modifications in drug design (ed., Gould, R. F.). (American Chemical Society, Washington, 1964.)

GILJAROVSKIJ, A. W.: Psychiatry. (Medgiz, Moskow, 1954.)

GOODMAN, L. S., AND GILMAN, A. (eds.): The pharmacological basis of therapeutics. (MacMillan, New York, 1965.)

GORDON, M. (ed.): Psychopharmacological agents. (Academic Press, New York, 1964.)

GOULD, R. F. (ed.).: Molecular modification in drug design. (American Chemical Society, Washington, 1964.)

GROLLMAN, A.: Pharmacology and therapeutics. (Lea and Febiger, Philadephia, 1965.)

HAKIM, R. A.: Indigenous drugs in the treatment of mental diseases. (Presented at the Sixth Gujurat and Saurashtra Provincial Medical Conference, Baroda, 1953.)

HALPERN, B. N.: Les antihistaminiques de synthése. Essais de clinicothérapie des états allergiques. Arch. Int. Pharmacodyn., *68:* 339 (1942).

HAMLIN, K. E., AND FISCHER, F. E.: The synthesis of 5-hydroxytryptamine. J. Amer. Chem. Soc., *73:* 5007 (1951).

HAMON, J., Paraire, J., and Velluz, J.: Remarques sur l'action du 4560 RP sur l'agitation maniaque. Ann. Medico psychol., *110:* 331 (1952).

HEIDENHAIN, R. P. H. (1872): In: Innes, I. R., and Nickerson, M.: Drugs inhibiting the action of acetylcholine on structures innervated by postganglionic parasympathetic nerves. In: The pharmacological basis of therapeutics (eds., Goodman, L. S., and Gilman, A.). (MacMillan, New York, 1965.)

HICKMAN, H. H.: A letter on suspended animation containing experiments showing that it may be safely employed on animals, with the view of ascertaining its probable utility in surgical operations on the human subject. (W. Smith, Ironbridge, 1824.)

HOFMANN, A. (1943): In: Downing, D. F.: Psychotomimetic drugs. In: Psychopharmacological agents (ed., Gordon, M.). (Academic Press, New York, 1964.)

HOFMANN, A. (1943): In: Mayer-Gross, W., Slater, E., and Roth, M. Clinical Psychiatry. (Cassell, London, 1960.)

INNES, I. R., AND NICKERSON, M.: Drugs inhibiting the action of acetylcholine on structures innervated by postganglionic parasympathetic nerves (antimuscarinic or atropinic drugs). In: The pharmacological basis of therapeutics (eds., Goodman, L. S., and Gilman, A.). (MacMillan, New York, 1965.)

JAFFE, J. H.: Narcotic analgesics. In: The pharmacological basis of therapeutics (eds., Goodman, L. S., and Gilman, A.). (MacMillan, Toronto, 1965.)

KATO, L., AND GÖZSY, B.: Effect of depressants and stimulants of the central nervous system on the capillary endothelium. International symposium on neuroleptic drugs. Rev. Canad. Biol., *20:* 261 (1961).

KATO, L., AND GÖZSY, B.: Personal communication, Montreal, 1964.

KLINE, N. S.: Clinical experiences with iproniazid (marsilid). (Hoffmann-La Roche, New York, 1957.)

KLINE, N. S., LOOMER, H. P., AND SAUNDER, J. C.: Clinical and pharmacodynamic evaluation of iproniazid as psychic energizer. APA Psychiat. Res. Rep. Amer. Psychiat. Ass., *8:* 129 (1957).

KNAUER, A., AND MALONEY, W. J.: A preliminary note on the psychic action of mescaline with special reference to the mechanisms of visual hallucinations. J. Nerv. Ment. Dis., *40:* 425 (1913).

KOELLE, G. B.: Anticholinesterase agents. In: The pharmacological basis of therapeutics (eds., Goodman, L. S., and Gilman, A.). (MacMillan, Toronto, 1965.)

KOELLE, G. B.: Neuromuscular blocking agents. In: The pharmacological basis of therapeutics (eds., Goodman, L. S., and Gilman, A.). (MacMillan, Toronto, 1965.)

KOELLE, G. B.: Parasympathomimetic agents. In: The pharmacological basis of therapeutics (eds., Goodman, L. S., and Gilman, A.). (MacMillan, Toronto, 1965.)

KRAEPELIN, E.: Der Psychologische Versuch in der Psychiatrie. Psychol. Arbeiten, *1:* 77 (1896).

KUHN, R.: Über die Behandlung Depressiver Zustande mit Einem Iminodibenzylderivat (G22355). Schweiz. Med. Wschr., *87:* 1135 (1957).

LANGLEY, J. N.: On the stimulation and paralysis of nerve cells and nerve endings. Paralysis by curare, strychnine and brucine and its antagonism by nicotine. J. Physiol. (London), *52:* 247 (1918).

LEBLANC, J., AND LEMIEUX, L.: Histamine and mental disease. Med. Exp. (Basel), *4:* 217 (1961).

LEHMANN, H. E., AND BAN, T. A.: Notes from the log-book of a psychopharmacological research unit. Canad. Psychiat. Ass. J., *9:* 111 (1964).

LEHMANN, H. E., AND BAN, T. A.: Progress report —early clinical drug evaluation unit, Douglas Hospital, Montreal, 1966.

LEHMANN, H. E., *et al.*: Potentiation of pharmacological and therapeutic action of phenothiazines by nylidrin (arlidin). Compr. Psychiat., *5:* 36 (1964).

LEHMANN, H. E., BERTHIAUME, M., AND BAN, T. A. (eds): Trimipramine, a new antidepressant. (Q.P.R.A., Montreal, 1964.)

LIEBIG, J. (1832): In: Sharpless, S. K.: Hypnotics and sedatives. II. Miscellaneous agents. In: The pharmacological basis of therapeutics (eds., Goodman, L. S., and Gilman, G.). (MacMillan, Toronto, 1965.)

LIEBREICH, O. (1869): In: Friend, D. G.: Role of synthetic drugs in therapy of mental illness. In: Molecular modification in drug design (ed., Gould, R. F.). (American Chemical Society, Washington, 1964.)

LOCKOCK, C. (1857): In: Sharpless, S. K.: Hypnotics and sedatives. II. Miscellaneous agents. In: The pharmacological basis of therapeutics (eds., Goodman, L. S., and Gilman, A.). (MacMillan, Toronto, 1965.)

LOEVENHART, A. S., LORENZ, W. F., AND WATERS, R. M.: Cerebral stimulation. J.A.M.A., *92:* 880 (1929).

MAGENDIE, F. (1821): In: Friend, D. G.: Role of synthetic drugs in therapy of mental illness. In: Molecular modification in drug design (ed., Gould, R. F.). (American Chemical Society, Washington, 1964.)

MAYER-GROSS, W., SLATER, E., AND ROTH, M.: Clinical psychiatry. (Cassell, London, 1960.)

MEDUNA, L. J.: Carbon dioxide therapy: a neurophysiological treatment of nervous disorders. (Charles C Thomas, Springfield, 1950.)

MERCK, E. (1848): In: Jaffe, J. H.: Narcotic analgesics. In: The pharmacological basis of therapeutics (eds., Goodman, L. S. and Gilman, A.). (MacMillan, Toronto, 1965.)

MOREAU DE, J. J. TOURS (1845): In: The drug experience (ed., Ebin, D.). (Orion Press, New York, 1961.)

MORTON, W. T. G. (1846): In: Morton, W. J.: Memoranda relating to the discovery of surgical anesthesia and Dr. William T. G. Morton's relation to this event. Postgrad. Med. Sch., *20:* 333 (1905).

MORTON, W. J.: Memoranda relating to the discovery of surgical anesthesia and Dr. William T. G. Morton's relation to this event. Postgrad. Med. Sch., *20:* 333 (1905).

MOSHER, L. R., KLERMAN, G. L., AND GREANEY, J. F.: A clinical trial of alphamethyldopa in elated states. Amer. J. Psychiat., *122:* 1185 (1966).

NAGAI, N.: Ephedrine. Pharm. Zeitung *32:* 700 (1887).

NICKERSON, M.: Drugs inhibiting adrenergic nerves and structures innervated by them.

In: The pharmacological basis of therapeutics (eds., Goodman, L. S., and Gilman, A.). (MacMillan, New York, 1965.)

Osinski, W. A.: Treatment of anxiety states with meprobamate. Ann. N.Y. Acad. Sci., *67:* 766 (1957).

Price, H. L., and Dripps, R. D.: General anesthetics. III. Intravenous anesthetics. In: The pharmacological basis of therapeutics (eds., Goodman, L. S., and Gilman, A.). (MacMillan, Toronto, 1965.)

Rapport, M. M., Green, A. A., and Page, I. H.: Serum vasoconstrictor (serotonin). Isolation and characterization. J. Biol. Chem., *176:* 1243 (1948).

Ravn, J., and Rud, C.: Sordinol: a new psychotropic drug. Clinical trial on 95 patients. Ugeskr. Laeg., *123:* 1663 (1961).

Robiquet, J. P. (1833). In: Jaffe, J. H.: Narcotic analgesics. In: The pharmacological basis of therapeutics (eds., Goodman, L. S., and Gilman, A.). (MacMillan, Toronto, 1965.)

Sargant, W., and Shorvon, H. J.: Acute war neuroses: special reference to Pavlov's experimental observations and mechanisms of abreaction. Arch. Neurol. Psychiat., *54:* 231 (1945).

Sargant, W., and Slater, E.: An introduction to physical methods of treatment in psychiatry. (Livingstone, London, 1963.)

Schilder, P., and Weissmann, M.: Atherisierung Geisteskranker. Fortschr. Neurol. Psychiat., *11:* 779 (1927).

Schwarz, L., Ban, T. A., and Smith, R.: Clinical trial with cyclopentimine. Amer. J. Psychiat., *118:* 254 (1961).

Sertürner, F. W. (1803). In: Jaffe, J. H.: Narcotic analgesics. In: The pharmacological basis of therapeutics (eds., Goodman, L. S., and Gilman, A.). (MacMillan, Toronto, 1965.)

Sharpless, S. K.: Hypnotics and sedatives. II. Miscellaneous agents. In: The pharmacological basis of therapeutics (eds., Goodman, L. S., and Gilman, A.). (MacMillan, Toronto, 1965.)

Simpson, G. M., and Kline, N. S.: Histamine wheel formation and mental illness. J. Nerv. Ment. Dis., *133:* 19 (1961).

Solomon, H. C., *et al.:* Some effects of the inhalation of carbon dioxide and oxygen and of intravenous sodium amytal on certain neuropsychiatric conditions. Amer. J. Psychiat., *10:* 761 (1931).

Sourkes, T. L.: Inhibition of dihydroxyphenylalanin decarboxylase by derivatives of phenylalanine. Arch. Biochem., *51:* 444 (1964).

St. Jean, A., Ban, T. A., and Noe, W.: The effect of trimipramine on psychophysical test performances. In: Trimipramine, a new antidepressant (eds., Lehmann, H. E., Berthiaume, M., and Ban, T. A.). (Q.P.R.A., Montreal, 1964.)

St. Jean, A., Ban, T. A., and Noe, W.: Psychopharmacological studies with neoserp and aldomet. Int. J. Neuropsychiat., *1:* 491 (1965).

Stolz, F.: Über adrenalin and alkylaminoacetobenzcatechin. Ber. Ges. Chem., *37:* 4149 (1904).

Tobin, J. M., *et al.:* Preliminary evaluation of librium (RO-5-0690) in treatment of anxiety reactions. Dis. Nerv. Syst., *21:* 11 (1960).

Trsic, J., *et al.:* Resistance to histamine in human skin after electroconvulsive treatment. Med. Pharmacol. Exp. (Basel), *17:* 200 (1967).

Twarog, B. M., and Page, J. H.: Serotonin content of some mammalian tissues and urine and a method for its determination. Amer. J. Physiol. *175:* 157 (1953).

Wells, H. (1845): In: Keys, T. E.: The history of surgical anesthesia. (Schuman's, New York, 1945.)

Wilcox, P. H.: Psychopenetration. Dis. Nerv. Syst., *12:* 35 (1951).

Windaus, A., and Vogt, W.: Synthese des Imidazolylethylamines. Ber. Ges. Chem., *40:* 3691 (1907).

Eight

The Barbiturates

In the course of the past fifty years more than 2500 barbiturates have been synthesized, and at least 50 of them have been employed clinically. These compounds are widely used; there is hardly anyone in a civilized country in the second half of the twentieth century who has not at one time or another taken a barbiturate drug.

A. BASIC DATA

1. Historical Aspects

Barbiturates developed from the ureides, which are formed by the combination of urea and organic acids. In the monoureides only one of the amino groups of urea is condensed with a carboxyl group. Some of the monureides are weak hypnotics, *e.g.* carbromal. In the diureides both of the amino groups of urea are condensed with two carboxyl groups containing acids. One of these is malonylurea, the condensation product of urea and malonic acid, commonly called barbituric acid.

The basic constituent of barbituric acid is a six-membered ring. It is an oxybarbiturate, different from the thiobarbiturates—the condensation product of thiourea and malonic acid—in which the carbonyl oxygen in position 2 is replaced by a sulfur atom.

Malonylurea (barbituric acid) was first successfully prepared in 1864 by Adolph von Baeyer, who celebrated his now famous synthesis with his friends on St. Barbara's Day, the patron saint of artillery officers. Whether the name of the substance is the result of adding urea to the name of this saint or the name of a popular Munich waitress will never be known (Sharpless, 1965).

Although barbituric acid itself is an inactive substance, it is the carrier for active synthetic preparations. Some believe that the potential of the substance has not been sufficiently explored in spite of the numerous compounds derived from it.

Barbiturates are those derivatives of barbituric acid in which the two hydrogens on the carbon atom in position 5 of the basic ring are substituted with alkyl or aryl groups. The first barbiturate introduced into medical practice was diethylbarbituric acid or barbital, which was synthesized by Fischer and von Mering in 1903. While barbital, with its rather long duration of action and strong sleep-producing effect, was particularly effective as a hypnotic, the second oldest barbiturate, phenobarbital (introduced by Loewe *et al.* in 1912) proved to be more useful as a sedative and anticonvulsant drug.

2. Mechanism of Action

Since the early years of the century many hypotheses on the mechanism of action of these drugs have been put forward. These range from psychodynamic to physiochemical concepts.

The psychodynamic concept is based on the assumption that anxiety is the result of unconscious, instinctual impulses growing beyond the level that the ego can control without primary process defenses. The

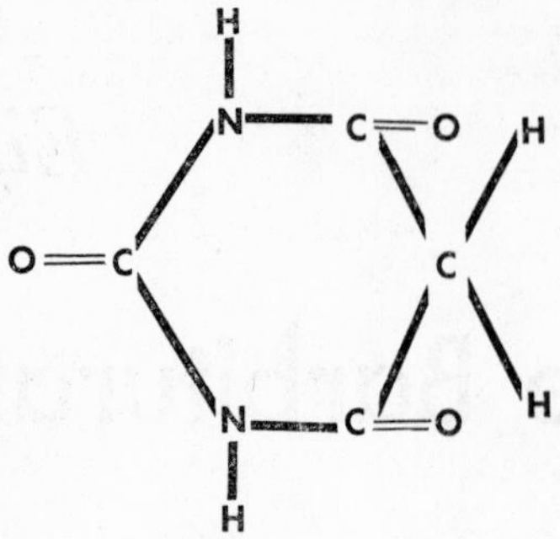

Barbituric Acid

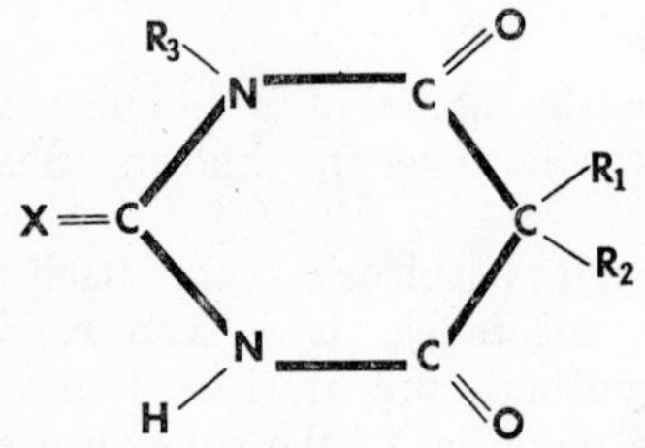

General Formula

FIG. 8. Barbituric acid and the general formula of barbiturates.

persistence of this anxiety leads to pathological symptoms. It is believed that barbiturates may abate the urgency of the situation and defer the development of psychopathological manifestations without having any effect in resolving the actual conflict. In other words, barbiturates are thought to act directly upon ego functions without influencing ego libido (Ostow, 1962).

Other theories propose that barbiturate action is the result of its interference with the oxidation of glucose or with the processes by which energy is acquired and stored by the cells or with the processes by which this stored energy is utilized.

In spite of the increasing information on the neurochemical and neurophysiological concomitants of barbiturate action, there is still no general agreement as to which of the known actions of the molecule account for its particular usefulness in different psychiatric conditions. Nevertheless, research to modify and change the therapeutic effects of barbital—the first therapeutically used member of this group—led to the synthesis of a large number of barbiturate drugs with distinctly different properties.

3. Structure and Activity

It was discovered that to obtain barbiturates with sedative or hypnotic properties the two hydrogen atoms in position 5 of the psychotherapeutically inactive barbituric acid had to be replaced by alkyl or aryl groups. Substitution of the two hydrogens by ethyl groups resulted in barbital (Fischer and von Mering, 1903), which became the first clinically used barbiturate derivative. It has sedative and hypnotic properties and a rather long duration of action. Replacement of one of the ethyl groups of barbital by a phenyl radical yielded phenobarbital (Loewe *et al.*, 1912), the second most extensively used member of this group with a similarly long duration of action. The presence of the phenyl group in the molecule potentiated the capacity of the drug to decrease cortical motor activity and added selective anticonvulsant properties to the range of activity of the compound. Thus phenobarbital is more valuable as an anticonvulsant than as a hypnotic and in certain cases controls cerebral seizures even below the sedative dose.

Further systematic exploratory work demonstrated that structural changes which result in an increased lipid solubility of the molecule in general are associated with a decreased latency period in the onset of action, more rapid metabolic degradation with a consequent decreased duration of action and quite frequently increased hypnotic activity. This can be achieved by an increase in the length of one or both of the alkyl side chains in position 5; replacement of the carbonyl oxygen by a sulfur atom in position 2; and methylation of the nitrogen atom in position 3.

It has also been recognized that barbiturate drugs with a branched side chain are usually shorter acting than those with a straight side chain and that those with unsaturated side groups are in general more active than those with saturated ones.

Thus increasing the length of one of the alkyl side-chains of barbital in position 5 by one carbon atom results in butobarbital, a shorter acting barbiturate with faster onset and decreased duration of action than barbital, while a further increase of one more carbon atom results in pentobarbital, a short acting compound with a stronger hypnotic effect than butobarbital. Extending the length of the ethyl side chain of pentobarbital by one carbon atom yields secobarbital, a short acting and potent sleep-inducing drug.

The thiobarbiturates are the outcome of the replacement of the carbonyl oxygen in position 2 by a sulfur atom. Unlike the oxybarbiturates, which maintain their carbonyl oxygen, these drugs are characterized by extremely rapid onset and ultra-short duration of action. Because of these properties, only those thiobarbiturates which have a relatively high molecular weight such as thiamylal, methitural and the most frequently used member of the group, thiopental, have a satisfactory margin of safety for clinical application. These extremely potent compounds are used either intravenously or rectally to induce general anesthesia.

Methylation of one of the nitrogen atoms in the barbituric acid nucleus, usually in position 3, increases the affinity of the molecule for lipids and decreases the duration of its action. The result of this (methylation) is the group of *N*-alkyl barbiturates. Among these are the long acting mephobarbital and metharbital, both known as potent anticonvulsant agents, and the ultra-short acting methohexital and hexobarbital.

These two ultra-short acting drugs are extensively used in general anesthesia. Methohexital has the shortest duration of action of any of the currently available barbiturates.

The increased hypnotic potency occurring with the increase in the length of one or both of the alkyl side chains in position 5 is limited to a total of 6 to 7 carbon atoms. Longer side-chains yield compounds which exhibit convulsive properties. Similarly, while methylation in position 3 leads to anticonvulsant drugs, substitution of both hydrogens in position 1 and 3 results in convulsants. It has also been shown that introduction of functional or polar groups into the alkyl side-chains (such as ether or keto groups, hydroxyl, amino or carboxyl groups) abolishes the hypnotic activity of barbiturate compounds (Friend, 1964).

4. Metabolism

The fate of the different barbiturate compounds from the time they are first administered until they are excreted from the organism can be readily followed by means of ultraviolet spectrography or chromatography or by the use of radioactive drugs (labeled with N^{15}, C^{14} or S^{35}). Their distribution in the central nervous system has been intensively studied by means of autoradiography and radioassay.

In the course of these studies it has been observed that there is no impenetrable barrier to the diffusion of barbiturates in the body. Within a limited period of time, determined by the characteristics of the individual substance, they are distributed to all tissues and fluids, including the milk of lactating mothers. They cross the placental barrier and can be detected in the blood of the fetus.

a. *Absorption*

The absorption of barbiturates is primarily dependent on their lipid solubility. This is generally expressed by the partition coefficient, which is the ratio between the lipid and water solubility of each substance. Greater lipid solubility results in a faster onset of action, an increased speed of metabolism but a shorter duration of action.

b. *Distribution and Storage*

Distribution and storage are also influenced by the protein-binding capacity of these drugs, which depends on the same structural features as the affinity to non-polar solvents. Regulated by these factors, barbiturates are readily absorbed from the sites of oral or parenteral administration. In the blood stream they are reversibly bound to plasma protein, mainly to albumin—the ultra-short acting thiopental to a much greater extent than the long acting barbital. Because the cerebrospinal fluid (CSF) is protein free, the maximum CSF level of barbiturates is always less than the plasma concentration. After passing the blood-brain barrier, barbiturates reach their highest concentration first in the cortex and geniculate bodies probably because of the good blood supply of these areas. The subcortical white matter of the cerebral hemispheres is penetrated less rapidly than the gray cortical areas. Eventually, however, these drugs are uniformly distributed in the brain. Simultaneously with passing the blood-brain barrier, barbiturates also enter the tissues of various organs, reaching maximum concentration at first in the heart, liver and kidneys, only later in the skin and finally in the lipid-containing tissues, *e.g.*, body fat. Although barbiturates have the same relative affinity to tissue proteins as to plasma proteins, their relative concentration in organ tissues is always higher than their plasma level.

c. Degradation and Excretion

The duration of action of different barbiturates depends on their physical redistribution, metabolic degradation and renal excretion.

The role of physical redistribution *in vivo* can easily be demonstrated by the ultra-short acting thiopental. Given intravenously, this drug reaches its maximum concentration within 30 seconds in the brain, liver, kidneys and heart. It exerts a central depressant action that results in sleep. The characteristically rapid emergence from sleep is due to a shift in the concentration of the substance from the brain to other tissues. In the first 15 to 20 minutes after administration the decline in brain concentration of thiopental, simultaneously with awakening, is due to the uptake of the drug by the skin; the further decline in brain concentration in 1 to 3 hours is due to the uptake of the drug by the lipid-containing tissues.

Metabolic degradation is the second process responsible for the limited duration of action of barbiturate drugs. It is generally true that the shorter acting barbiturates are metabolized faster and more completely than the longer acting ones. The longer acting oxybarbiturates are catabolized only in the liver, while the shorter acting thiobarbiturates may also be metabolized in the kidneys and the brain.

In the liver the usual metabolic change is the transformation of lipid-soluble (nonpolar) agents into more polar derivatives that can be excreted by the kidneys. Additional metabolic pathways are the loss of an alkyl group in position 5 of the barbituric acid ring, detoxication in general or the oxidation of substituents in position 5 in particular. The resulting ketone or alcohol may be excreted as free compounds or in a conjugated form with glucuronic acid. *N*-alkyl barbiturates are metabolized through *N*-dealkylation and thiobarbiturates through desulfuration. During their catabolism, some of the *N*-alkyl barbiturates are converted into active metabolites, *e.g.*, mephobarbital into phenobarbital and metharbital into barbital, while the thiobarbiturates are converted to their corresponding oxybarbiturates, *e.g.*, thiopental yields pentobarbital. Finally, the barbiturate ring is destroyed by hydrolytic splitting (Sourkes, 1962).

The site of metabolism of barbiturates in the liver is in the smooth-surfaced, lightest density microsomes. The enzyme systems involved require both triphosphopyridine nucleotide and oxygen to perform this function. These microsomal enzymes are very sensitive to external or internal influences. They may be inhibited by the metabolic changes present in diabetes mellitus, the toxic products of obstructive jaundice or by nutritional deficiencies. Among the various exogenous chemical substances, a predominantly inhibiting effect is exerted by azacyclonol, imipramine, iproniazid and various other hydrazine drugs. The inhibition of the activity of the microsomal enzymes has a potentiating effect on the action of barbiturate drugs. On the other hand, a weak inhibitory effect with a subsequent enzyme induction is exerted by glutethimide, meprobamate, chlorpromazine, pyrimidine, several monoamine oxidase inhibitor drugs and, interestingly, also by phenobarbital and barbital.

Barbiturates and their metabolites are

excreted mainly in the urine and only to a very limited extent in the feces. Renal excretion is primarily responsible for the elimination of barbiturates which are not destroyed in the body. It is also known that the long acting barbital is excreted almost entirely unchanged in the urine, while the short acting pentobarbital or ultra-short acting hexobarbital and thiopental are almost completely metabolized.

Excretion of barbiturates in general is slow and takes place over several days. For example, in normal adults 8 per cent of an orally given single hypnotic dose of barbital is eliminated in the first 12 hours and only 20 per cent in the first 24 hours. Furthermore, traces of barbital may be detected for as long as 8 to 12 days after the administration of a single dose. Elimination of these drugs through the kidneys is dependent upon the tubular reabsorption of undissociated barbiturates. Since this decreases with an increase in the pH of the urine, there is a good possibility of increasing—even tripling—the elimination of these drugs by simple measures such as the administration of alkalis (*e.g.*, sodium bicarbonate) and diuretics (Musser and Bird, 1961).

5. Chemical and Neurophysiological Correlates of Drug Action

a. Chemical Correlates

The psychoactive properties of barbiturates cannot be reduced to a single concomitant of drug action. There are a number of changes described in the central nervous system and in the periphery which are related to the effect of these compounds. Among these the most frequently discussed is the interference of barbiturates with oxidative phosphorylation in the central nervous system.

The original hypothesis that barbiturates may interfere with oxidative phosphorylation—which is one of the essential mechanisms of normal brain metabolism—was based on the correct assumption that under barbiturate anesthesia there is a decreased concentration of inorganic phosphate, along with a decreased utilization of adenosine triphosphate (ATP) in the central nervous system, as indicated by reduced cerebral oxygen uptake and by diminished lactic acid and heat production. The finding that following intracisternal injection of radioactive phosphate there is an increase in the specific activity of ATP and consequently that there is also an increase in the concentration of phosphocreatinine gave experimental evidence to support the original hypothesis. More recently, it has been shown with mitochondrial preparations that barbiturates reduce oxidative metabolism. Brody and Bain (1954) have demonstrated that the uptake of inorganic phosphate is decreased in these mitochondrial preparations which in turn reduces the oxidative metabolism (phosphorylation) both *in vitro* and *in vivo*.

Whether this uncoupling of oxidative phosphorylation is responsible for the psychotropic effects of barbiturates still remains undecided. Militating against a unitary theory is the fact that interference with oxidative phosphorylation is not a common characteristic of all barbiturates, although the majority of them exerts this effect, and that this interference has also been shown with other agents, *e.g.*, salicylates, which do not have sedative or hypnotic properties.

An antiacetylcholine effect of barbiturates was suggested by the inhibition of the increase in salivation and in intestinal activity after acetylcholine administration. It was shown that certain barbiturates, *e.g.*, thiobarbiturates, release norepinephrine from its protein-bound storage depots in or near the smooth muscles of the vascular system. The resulting vasoconstriction can be potentiated by cocaine and prevented by reserpine or tolazoline. Other findings include occasionally increased plasma catecholamine levels in dogs and hyperglycemia, which may occur with large doses.

b. Neurophysiological Correlates

Barbiturates have an over-all effect on the nervous system. The influence they exert on the various nervous tissues depends on the dosage and route of administration and also on the degree of the system's inherent and acquired sensitivity. This is further modified by the actual state of the nervous system at the time the drug is given.

The functional alterations in the nervous system induced by barbiturate compounds will now be described from the lowest level of integration to the cerebral cortex.

i. Autonomic Nervous Systems. The inhibitory effect of barbiturates on the parasympathetic ganglia can be shown by the interference with the cardiac effects (deceleration) produced by electrical stimulation of the vagus nerve. This parasympatholytic effect is usually stronger with oxybarbiturates than with thiobarbiturates. Barbiturates also exert a selective inhibition on the transmission of impulses in the sympathetic ganglia. This occurs at such low concentrations that there is no detectable effect on nerve conduction or on the neuroeffector junctions. On the other hand, since it is also present in the anesthetic dose, it may account for the hypotension occasionally seen with some of the intravenously given barbiturate compounds and in severe barbiturate intoxication.

ii. Spinal Cord. Barbiturates have an inhibitory effect on both the mono- and polysynaptic reflexes of the spinal cord. There is some evidence that polysynaptic pathways are the more susceptable. The effect of barbiturates on the transmission function in the monosynaptic spinal reflex arc has been analyzed by means of intracellular recordings from motorneurons in the anterior gray columns of the spinal cord. It was found that barbiturates depress the monosynaptic excitatory postsynaptic potentials. This effect takes place in such low doses that they effect neither resting transmembrane potentials nor the electrical properties of these membranes.

iii. Brain Stem Reticular Formation. While the vital centers in the medulla oblongata are affected only by excessive dosages of barbiturates, there are indications that the brain stem reticular activating system is particularly sensitive to the depressant effect of these drugs. This can be shown by the increased threshold to direct electrical stimulation in the reticular activating system and by the depression of the potentials evoked in this system by a variety of sensory stimuli even after small dosages of barbiturates. Simultaneously with this inhibition, barbiturates have an excitatory effect on certain areas of the hippocampus.

Some believe that the main action of barbiturates is in the areas of the diencephalon concerned with sleep (Grollman, 1958). During physiological sleep there are cyclic periodic episodes of rapid eye movements (REM), relatively high frequency electroencephalographic activity with phasic movements of the extremities (sharp diminution in tonic muscle tension) and dreams. Barbiturates, particularly oxybarbiturates (like the amphetamines) reduce the total REM time. Whether this is responsible for the deleterious effects of barbiturates on certain psychic functions is still unknown.

iv. Cortex. The cortical concomitants of barbiturate action, as seen on the electroencephalogram, begin with a fast 15 to 35 cycle per second activity which spreads from the frontal to the parietal and occipital cortex, accompanied by changes in the state of consciousness. With increase in dosage, large amplitude, slow random (2 to 8 cycle per second) waves appear, resembling those seen in physiological sleep. With further increase in dosage, there is a gradual decrease in the amplitude of electrical waves with brief periods of electrical silence. These periods become increasingly prolonged, and it is inadvisable to let them last longer than 5 to 6 seconds even under fully controlled circumstances, *e.g.*, in surgical anesthesia.

Other neurophysiological concomitants of barbiturate administration are the depression of repetitive activity, believed by some to be responsible for wakefulness and also for the spread of epileptiform activity. Repetitive activity is depressed in the spinal cord, midbrain reticular formation, thalamus, retina and in the cerebral cortex. There is also an enhancement of the recruiting response of the anterior thalamic part of the reticular formation and a raised threshold as well as a shortened duration of after-discharges in the cerebral cortex.

6. Behavioral Pharmacology

Barbiturates induce a wide range of behavioral changes in animals and man. It was recognized at an early stage of animal experimentation that barbiturates have some local anesthetic action on the sensory-perceptual side of the reflex arc. Thus direct application of pentobarbital to the peripheral nerve produces increase in the threshold to electrical stimulation; reduction of amplitude of spike potentials; prolongation of relative and absolute refractory periods; and slowing of conduction velocity. Unmyelinated fibers are more sensitive in this respect than the myelinated ones. While in small doses barbiturates may increase the reaction to painful stimuli, in higher dosages they are able to relieve the distress of pain, although less effectively than morphine. Furthermore, they enhance the analgesic action of salicylates and paraaminophenol derivatives.

a. Animal Studies

Of the various central effects of barbiturates, one of the most widely discussed and clinically used is their anticonvulsant action. They are capable of counteracting the convulsions of tetanus or status epilepticus or the convulsions artificially induced by strychnine, picrotoxin or cocaine. This anticonvulsant action is not abolished by amphetamine compounds, which antagonize the sedative effect of these drugs.

Barbiturates have a characteristic biphasic effect on behavioral tests. The disinhibition usually present with low doses gives place to a sedative and finally a hypnotic effect as the dosage is increased. When given in medium or high dosages, in the Open Field Test, which gives tridimensional information, they inhibit "voluntary" ambulation primarily, but also "emotional" defecation and "instinctual" rearing. The degree of the decrease of voluntary activity is easily determined in the Activity Cage, and it has been found to be directly proportionate to the dosage administered. In the Inclined Screen Test, in which the animal can maintain a position under normal conditions, and in the Taming Effect Test, which measures the decrease in defensive aggression of monkeys, barbiturates are effective only in sedative doses.

The same applies to unconditional and conditional reflexes, both of which become simultaneously inhibited only on a substantially high dosage. On the other hand, in somewhat lower doses they prevent or counteract conflicting stimuli-produced experimental neuroses.

The sedative effect of barbiturates is potentiated by minor or major tranquilizers and counteracted by stimulant drugs.

b. Human Studies

The biphasic effect of barbiturates already noted on animal behavioral tests can best be shown in humans, in whom disinhibition can easily be detected in the increase in verbal output and by the loosening of associations as a result of the diminishing of conscious control. With increased blood levels this disinhibitory effect is replaced by sedation and finally by sleep with characteristically fewer rapid eye movements than under physiological conditions.

If barbiturate administration cannot be followed by sleep, a state characterized by euphoria or confusion (resembling inebriation) occurs. Otherwise, sleep in not infrequently followed by a hangover (particularly with the long acting compounds) and some transient impairment of mental functioning. In patients with organic psychopathology, barbiturates, even in low doses, may have a paradoxical effect and not infrequently produce delirium instead of sedation.

In psychometric tests barbiturates have a characteristic effect on various psychological functions. They lower Critical Flicker Fusion Frequency, *i.e.*, the number of flickers per second at which the subject begins to see a previously steady light flicker. They also lower the Chromatic After-Image Disappearance Limen and inhibit the Achromatic After-Effect.

Barbiturates decrease the number of digits a subject is able to repeat forward, decrease Tapping Speed on a telegraph key and increase visual and auditory Reaction Time. Some interpret the increased scores on the Body Sway test as an indication that these drugs increase suggestibility, while others maintain that this effect may be due to the "unsteadiness" produced by the drug.

In human conditioning procedures in general barbiturates diminish the strength of unconditional reflexes; decrease the number of stimulations required to extinguish orienting reflexes; and lower conditionability (Ban, 1964).

B. CLINICAL DATA

1. Indications and Contraindications

a. Indications

Barbiturates are successfully administered in numerous pathological conditions. Besides the therapeutic indications, they are frequently given for diagnostic purposes and occasionally as prognostic indicators of treatment.

i. Diagnostic and Prognostic Applications. Intraarterially barbiturates are used in neurosurgery to identify the dominant cerebral hemisphere, and intravenously they are used in neurology to activate latent abnormalities on the electroencephalogram. Barbiturates are given intravenously by the electrophysiologist to measure the sedation threshold, which is characteristic for different psychopathologies, and by the psychiatrist for differential diagnosis of catatonic stupor and stuporous depression, conditions resembling each other in their overt behavioral manifestations. During barbiturate-induced disinhibition (most commonly induced by amobarbital, less often by pentobarbital), depressive ideation or concealed suicidal tendencies may openly appear and can be distinguished from schizophrenic psychopathology. The degree and duration of the period of disinhibition in the same conditions may also indicate the amount of benefit to be expected from convulsive treatment, since it induces, transiently, an effect (disinhibition) similar to that produced by electroshock for a longer period of time.

ii. Therapeutic Indications. There is probably no other group of drugs in the pharmacopeia with as wide a range of therapeutic indications as the barbiturates. They are extensively used by general practitioners, pediatricians, psychiatrists and other specialists.

α. Internal Medicine. Barbiturates are mainly prescribed as daytime sedatives or as hypnotics for the symptomatic treatment of insomnia. For daytime sedation, amobarbital and phenobarbital are usually favored. They are given to irritable, anxious and tense patients, to hyperthyroid cases, in essential hypertension and in cardiac failure. Among functional and organic gastrointestinal symptoms, a beneficial effect has been observed in nausea and vomiting and also in peptic ulcers and colitis because of reduced gastric secretion or reduction in the mobility of the sigmoid colon. When sleep is desired, oxybarbiturates are usually given. The faster and shorter acting secobarbital has proved to be a useful sleep inducer, and the slower but longer acting barbital, a useful sleep sustainer.

β. Pediatrics. Barbiturates are mainly used for sedation of children in stressful situations, during illness and in preparation for routine examination of the ears, nose and throat. They may be therapeutic in pylorospasm of infants and helpful in croup and whooping cough.

γ. Surgery. In surgery, or rather for surgical anesthesia, thiobarbiturates and ultra-short acting barbiturates are widely used, *e.g.*, methitural, thiamylal, thiopental, methohexital or hexobarbital. These drugs may be used for surgical anesthesia of short duration or to induce general anesthesia. Barbiturates may also be used as preanesthetic and postoperative medication in local or general anesthesia.

δ. Neurology and Psychiatry. Epilepsy remains one of the most important indications. Until the introduction of diphenylhydantoin (Merritt and Putnam, 1938), bromides and phenobarbital were for all practical purposes the only drugs used for the control of cerebral seizures. Best results with barbiturates are obtained in cases of grand mal seizures. In these conditions the administration of phenobarbital, mephobarbital or metharbital are the most effective.

The anticonvulsant properties of barbiturates may also be effective in tetanus, eclampsia, etc. Of the extrapyramidal manifestations, dramatic responses have been described with parenterally administered barbiturates in acute dystonia and in cases of choreiform movements.

Barbiturates in general are not indicated in functional psychoses, although as emergency measures they are still frequently (and successfully) used (amobarbital intramuscularly and thiopental intravenously) in the control of acutely excited or agitated patients.

Transient improvement in catatonic stupor can be produced by intravenous administration of barbiturates (amobarbital, pentobarbital, etc.). Improvement has also been described in some schizo-affective and manic-depressive psychoses—conditions which in principle are not to be treated with barbiturate compounds. Similarly catatonic stupor, stuporous depression may also respond to intravenous barbiturate administration, and in certain therapy-resistant manic patients regular addition of a small dosage of barbital often has a beneficial effect.

The major psychiatric indications for barbiturates are the different psychoneuroses. Intravenously administered barbiturates may have a dramatic effect on functional amnesia and conversion symptoms of abrupt and recent onset. Orally given barbiturates are beneficial in patients with anxiety states, phobic attacks, psychosomatic conditions and in some of the sexual neuroses. Barbiturates are indicated in all the neurotic conditions in which suppresion of excitement, nervousness and tension is desirable and also in all of those conditions in which disinhibition and recall of repressed material may be therapeutically useful (Mayer-Gross *et al.*, 1960; Gregory, 1961; Kalinowsky and Hoch, 1961; Musser and Bird, 1961; and Sargant and Slater, 1963.)

b. Contraindications

There are relatively few absolute contraindications to barbiturate treatment. These are comatose states, particularly hepatic coma and acute intermittent porphyria. By stimulating porphyrin synthesis, barbiturates can precipitate an attack which may culminate in paralysis or death.

Impaired liver function, by slowing the metabolic degradation of barbiturates, may dangerously prolong their action and hence is a relative contraindication (Meyler, 1963). This applies particularly to cirrhosis and obstructive or parenchymal jaundice. Impaired renal function, particularly uremia, nutritional deficiencies, myxedema, myasthenia, diabetes mellitus, pulmonary infections, bronchitis and allergies are also relative contraindications. Alcohol consumption in the course of barbiturate treatment may have serious consequences (Jenner, 1965).

It is generally agreed that barbiturates should not be given to the elderly and arteriosclerotic because they may cause a rather prolonged (sometimes for even 24 hours) confusional state; to the chronically depressed because they may aggravate the depression; to the chronic schizophrenic because they antagonize his appropriate drug treatment; and in general to unstable persons who are particularly predisposed to become dependent on these compounds.

Since barbiturates cross the placental barrier and can also be found in the milk of the lactating mother, they should only be given cautiously (and preferably not at all) during pregnancy or in the period of lactation.

There has been no carcinogenic effect attributed to barbiturate drugs even after prolonged administration.

2. Therapy with Barbiturate Drugs Alone and in Combination with Other Treatments

a. Barbiturate Drugs Alone

It is important to give these drugs (*i*) in adequate dosages, (*ii*) by appropriate routes, (*iii*) following well established clinical procedures, and (*iv*) for no longer a period of time than is absolutely necessary.

i. Dosage. While the therapeutic dosage range of each barbiturate drug differs slightly, it generally holds true that the single sedative dose which is repeated three or four times a day is one-third or one-fourth of the single hypnotic dose that is given once at bedtime. It also holds true that in principle all the barbiturates can be used as anticonvulsants in anesthetic dosage, but mephobarbital, metharbital and phenobarbital are effective in a considerably lower dosage.

The average adult hypnotic dose of the various barbiturates ranges from 40 mg. to 500 mg. It is 40 to 100 mg. for aprobarbital, butabarbital, pentobarbital and secobarbital; 100 to 200 mg. for amobarbital, cyclobarbital, diallylbarbituric acid, phenobarbital, talbutal, and vinbarbital; 200 to 350 mg. for heptabarbital, hexethal and probarbital; and 350 to 500 mg. for barbital.

The same compounds are given in a considerably lower dosage to infants and children. Approximately one-fifth of the average adult dose is given below 1 year of age; one-third from 1 to 2 years and one-half from 2 to 6.

In cases of severe convulsions Na pentobarbital (300 to 500 mg.), Na amobarbital (400 to 800 mg.) and Na thiopental (100 to 200 mg.) are slowly administered intravenously.

ii. Routes of Administration. Barbiturates may be obtained as powders, elixirs, syrups, drops, capsules, tablets, sustained-release capsules, delayed-release coated tablets, etc. They can also be given rectally as suppositories and injected intramuscularly or intravenously.

For oral administration the sodium salts of barbiturates are the most rapidly absorbed (although they may also cause epigastric distress somewhat more frequently). While oral administration is satisfactory in the majority of instances and for most of the adult cases, infants, small children and patients with prolonged convulsive states may require suppositories.

Intramuscularly, barbiturates are given in 10 per cent sodium salt solutions. They have to be given deep in the appropriate gluteal muscles since subcutaneous injection (particularly of thiobarbiturates) may cause necrosis and sloughing.

While hexobarbital, methitural, methohexital, thiamylal and thiopental can only be given intravenously, other barbiturates are given intravenously only in emergency situations, in general anesthesia, for convulsive patients and for neurological and psychiatric diagnostic or therapeutic purposes.

The concentration of most of the barbiturates for intravenous administration is a 5 per cent aqueous solution, but the ultra-short acting thiobarbiturates are given in a 2.5 per cent and the ultra-short acting methohexital in a 1 per cent solution. All these solutions should be given slowly (1 to 2 ml. per minute) to avoid hypotension, laryngospasm and apnea.

Intravenous barbiturates should never be given without adequate preparation for emergency measures to support respiration and counteract circulatory collapse. In this way the occurrence of fatal accidents can be almost entirely eliminated.

iii. Treatment Procedures. One of the most frequently used "clinical procedures" of barbiturate administration in psychiatry is continuous therapy. In the treatment of the neuroses (or when given as a sedative), phenobarbital, for example, is administered in 30-mg. doses, which are taken at first three times daily. Depending on individual variations, severity of the symptoms, chronicity of the condition and previous exposure to the drug, the dosage may have to be increased up to a total of 300 mg. a day. More recently, a kind of discontinuous treatment with barbiturates was reported to be successful. This consists of administering these drugs in 2- or 3-week courses with drug-free intervals of 1 or 2 weeks.

Insomnia is treated with single doses given at bedtime. In cases in which there is difficulty in falling asleep, the short acting barbiturates are indicated, *e.g.*, pentobarbital, secobarbital, etc. When sleep is disturbed by nocturnal or early morning awakening, the longer acting drugs, whose peak effect comes on later and lasts 6 to 8 hours, are more useful (Matthews *et al.*, 1964). Because of the delay in the onset of its hypnotic action, barbital is given three-quarters of an hour prior to going to bed. In certain conditions, *e.g.*, the initial period of endogenous depression, there is no good reason for not giving the barbiturate hypnotic regularly every night, while in others, *e.g.*, neurotic conditions, it is advisable to have placebo nights with increasing frequency.

One of the most common psychiatric uses of barbiturates is in the treatment of certain neuroses by abreaction. The purpose of abreaction is to "encourage" a suppressed or repressed emotional experience to be "relived." Amphetamines appear to be more effective in the "civilian" setting than the barbiturates, but the latter are superior to amphetamines in dealing with conditions that develop in combat or in the course of "crushing, threatening events," particularly in those cases "where the reaction to these experiences is a state of profound inhibition" (Sargant and Slater, 1963).

This inhibition can be successfully overcome by intravenous barbiturates, *e.g.*, amobarbital or thiopental. Intravenous amobarbital produces relaxation of tension at a dosage much lower than that which produces hypnosis, while with thiopental the point at which relaxation is achieved coincides almost with the point at which clouding of consciousness begins. Amobarbital merely produces emotionally colored verbal expression, *i.e.*, ventilation of the suppressed or repressed material, while thiopental may produce a more dramatic effect, with an intensive reliving of the traumatic experience in words and actions.

For abreaction, amobarbital is given in a 10 per cent or occasionally in a 5 per cent solution. In the majority of cases, 5 ml. of the 10 per cent or 10 ml. of the 5 per cent solution (both administered in 10 minutes) is needed for successful treatment.

After administration of between 300 and 500 mg. of amobarbital, most patients relax; tears appear; and they begin to verbalize feelings. When the desirable state of communication is reached, no further drug is given, but the needle is kept in the vein so that injection can be resumed when the stream of talk slackens or blocks and tension reappears.

Thiopental is preferred in 2.5 per cent or occasionally in 5 per cent solution for abreactive treatment. It is common practice to ask the patient to count backward during the period of injection. When the patient's speech slows down becomes slurred or if the patient becomes confused, administration of the drug is discontinued. Readiness for treatment can be recognized by the relaxed face and glassy stare of the patient. Because aggressive outbursts are frequent, some advise the administration of the injection through a rubber cannula to allow for gross motor movements.

Barbiturates are also used in narcosynthesis treatment, which is primarily indicated in those neuroses in which anxiety-produced inhibition prevail (Alexander, 1953).

Another treatment method is continuous narcosis or prolonged sleep therapy. This involves the administration of barbiturates in sufficient dosage to keep the patient asleep for 18 to 20 hours a day over a 2-week period. This treatment apparently originated in Sweden around the beginning of the century, but it was not until 1922 that Kläsi in Switzerland introduced barbiturates for this purpose. Optimal results with minimal therapeutic risks could not, however, be achieved with these drugs alone, and since the early periods of sleep therapy, barbiturates have been given in combination with other pharmacological treatments.

iv. Duration of Treatment and the Problem of Addiction. The duration of drug administration depends on the therapeutic indication and purpose, but barbiturates should never be given any longer than is absolutely necessary. Tolerance and dependence develop quickly, although true addiction is rather rare.

Jenner (1965) recommends limiting the use of barbiturates to short term treatment in hospital as a "prelude" to psychodynamic investigations or other treatments. He considers these substances very reliable if large doses can be used, and the resultant drowsiness is unimportant. He emphasizes that barbiturates can produce considerable confusion and if large doses are administered for a long time addiction may occur, with severe withdrawal phenomena, including cerebral seizures and delirium, which may lead to a state of exhaustion and even death.

Tolerance to barbiturates is at least partly the result of the activation by the drug of its own metabolizing enzyme system in the liver, which leads to more rapid detoxication. Consequently, there is a decrease in sleeping time and an increase in the dose required to maintain a specific tissue concentration.

In animals, tolerance to barbiturates develops rapidly, often after only two or three administrations of the drug. Another phenomenon, usually called "acute tolerance," occurs even more quickly. In case of acute tolerance, the plasma concentration at the time of awakening from barbiturate intoxication varies directly with the dose administered.

Addiction (of a "pernicious type") develops only when approximately four times the usual dose is given daily over a period of at least 3 months. The basis of addiction is the pharmacodynamic adaptation of the nervous tissue to the presence of the drug. Thus addicts become resistant to the hypnotic effect of barbiturates, without the lethal dose being significantly increased. They develop a psychic and physical dependence, which can be measured by the severity of the abstinence syndrome upon sudden withdrawal of the drug. Factors which influence the abstinence syndrome are the depth, duration and continuity of intoxication prior to drug withdrawal and the rate at which the drug is removed from the tissues.

The withdrawal syndrome may consist only of paroxysmal electroencephalographic abnormalities without any other manifestations. With somewhat higher dosages or longer duration of administration there may be weakness, tremulousness, anxiety and insomnia, which may subside or give place to delirium and/or grand mal seizures.

The withdrawal syndrome from large amounts of barbiturates taken over an extended period of time in untreated cases subsides in approximately 8 days. In the course of drug withdrawal there are at least five distinct stages. The first two stages with short acting barbiturates occur within the first 12 to 16 hours. During this period the blood level of the drug at first declines, concomitant with a transient clinical improvement. From this seemingly improved state the patient passes into the second stage, characterized by increasing restlessness, anxiety, tremulousness and weakness, sometimes associated with abdominal cramps, nausea, vomiting and, not infrequently, orthostatic hypotension. After 24 hours, this picture is replaced by the manifestations of the third stage: extreme weakness, coarse tremor and hyperactive tendon reflexes. This is the period when the patient pleads for the drugs.

The peak of the withdrawal syndrome—fourth stage—with short acting barbiturates is reached after 48 to 72 hours (with long acting ones on the seventh to eighth day) and is characterized by cerebral seizures. Some of the patients who have seizures improve afterward, while others become delirious, usually between the fourth and seventh day. A clouded sensorium, disorientation, visual hallucinations, frightening dreams, anxiety, agitation and hyperthermia are the pathological symptoms present which may lead to exhaustion and/or cardiovascular collapse. The fifth and last stage is a period of prolonged sleep from which the patient awakens tired, but recovered.

To prevent the withdrawal syndrome, discontinuation of barbiturate treatment should always be carried out gradually. If there is any evidence of drug dependence, pentobarbital should be substituted for the implicated drug. For this purpose, approximately 200 to 400 mg. (or even more) of pentobarbital are given every 6 hours, to the point where symptoms of mild intoxication occur. The patient is kept on a dosage which produces nystagmus, ataxia and slurred speech for a period of 24 to 36 hours. After a stabilization period, the drug is slowly tapered off at the rate of 100 mg. a day. Thus, withdrawal is completed from 10 days to 3 weeks.

More recently, the best results in the prevention of the withdrawal syndrome have been obtained with the combined administration of chlorpromazine and sodium diphenylhydantoin. The same combination is useful even if the withdrawal syndrome is already manifest.

b. Barbiturate Drugs in Combination with Other Treatments

Not infrequently barbiturate drugs are administered in conjunction with other treatments: physical, pharmacological or psychological.

i. Physical. *α. ECT*. Both electroconvulsive (ECT) and insulin therapies may be combined with barbiturate administration. Since the early nineteen-fifties it has become common practice to carry out ECT under thiopental narcosis, most of the time in combination with a curare-like compound (succinylcholine chloride). Some believe that this reduces the fear usually associated with convulsive treatment and that it also reduces the risk of possible complications. On the other hand, the hypotensive effects of barbiturates are intensified by ECT, and therefore it is necessary to maintain the patient in a recumbent position for at least 30 minutes after consciousness is regained.

β. Insulin. Occasionally insulin (modified or somnolent) therapy is combined with barbiturate administration. This reduces the infrequent cerebral seizures seen with insulin, but it predisposes the patient to confusional states. Because of the slight hyperglycemic action of barbiturates, it also alters the required insulin dosage.

ii. Pharmacological. Barbiturates are available commercially in a great number of combinations with other drugs. For example, one barbiturate substance is mixed with another, or with amphetamines, bromides, xanthines, belladonna alkaloids or nicotinic acid. There are also analgesic, tranquilizer (minor and major), sympathomimetic amine, antihistamine, spasmolytic, vitamin, antibiotic, digestive enzyme, gastric antacid and absorbent combinations manufactured by the pharmaceutical industry.

α. Other Drugs. It should be noted that administration of barbiturates with other drugs not only has an influence—positive or negative—on barbiturate metabolism and consequently barbiturate action but also possibly has a yet undetermined effect on the action of the concomitantly given substance itself. This applies to imipramine, azacyclonol, hydrazine drugs in general and iproniazid in particular, all of which have an inhibitory effect on enzymes of barbiturate metabolism, as well as to glutethimide, meprobamate, chlorpromazine, primidone, etc., which have an opposite, *i.e.*, stimulating, effect on the same enzymes. The fact that barbiturates increase the metabolism of bishydroxycoumarin and consequently increase prothrombin time cannot be emphasized enough, since the combined administration of anticoagulants and sedatives is a common and accepted practice in cardiac cases with coronary illness.

β. Sleep Treatment. The combination of barbiturates with other sedative or hypnotic drugs or, more recently, with chlorpromazine in sleep treatment is frequently used; continuous narcosis may be conducted by the daily administration of secobarbital (300 mg.), pentobarbital (300 mg.), barbital (450 mg.) and chlorpromazine (300 mg.) in three equally divided doses adjusted according to requirements. A somewhat similar combination, *i.e.*, thiopental intravenously and amobarbital and chlorpromazine intramuscularly, is employed in semi-sleep treatment, which does not require the hospitalization of the patient.

iii. Psychological. *α. Psychotherapy.* Barbiturates may be used in both psychotherapies and behavior therapies. They are administered in narcoanalysis and narcosynthesis (mainly as an abreactive agent). While the facilitating effect of intravenous barbiturates on psychotherapy by pharmacological reduction of cortical inhibition and resistance is known, this treatment is little used.

β. Behavior Therapy. Behavior therapists often utilize these drugs, particularly amobarbital. By interfering with the appearance of the autonomic response to the repeated presentation of the pathology-producing situation, barbiturates may produce deconditioning (via generalization). This has been used in the therapy of ejaculatio praecox with equivocal success.

3. Adverse Reactions and Their Treatment

a. Adverse Reactions

In the course of barbiturate administration a number of undesirable reactions may occur. These can affect any of the functional systems of the organism, causing mild discomfort or severe pathological changes that call for untimely termination of treatment. According to the nature of the undesired manifestation, adverse barbiturate reactions are classed as psychiatric, neurological, cardiovascular, respiratory, gastrointestinal, genitourinary, hepatobiliary and dermatological. Occasionally agranulocytosis and other blood dyscrasias have been described (Jenner, 1965).

i. Psychiatric. These range from an idiosyncratic hangover or excitement through symptoms resembling alcoholic inebriation to severe toxic delirium and confusional states.

Chronic excessive barbiturate usage produces a profound change in personality, starting with exaggeration of the basic personality traits. Frequently the initial symptoms are affective in nature (euphoria and elation are commonly seen, while in some cases, depression and suicidal tendencies become evident). These manifestations are cccasionally replaced by irritability and quarrelsomeness, leading to a hostile attitude and paranoid ideation. If barbiturate administration continues, a general sluggishness with poor attention (reduced vigilance and reduced tenacity), difficulty in thinking, poor memory and faulty judgment may become the predominant psychopathological features. At this stage emotional lability may be replaced by emotional incontinence, as shown by an untidiness in personal habits, and may finally culminate in a toxic confusional state. Others develop a so-called acute toxic delirium on the basis of chronic barbiturate intoxication with vivid visual (and less frequently auditory) hallucinations, leading occasionally to a chronic psychosis with marked mood swings.

ii. Neurological. The neurological changes characteristic of barbiturate intoxication are usually diffuse, pointing to no specific location in the central nervous system. Among these, thick, slurred speech and nystagmus are of crucial importance in establishing the diagnosis of barbiturate intoxication, but diplopia, strabismus and difficulty in accommodation are also rather commonly present. Vertigo, positive Romberg sign, ataxic gait and muscular hypotonia and dysmetria indicate the effect of the drug on cerebellar structures, while decreased skin reflexes or bilateral Babinski signs and ankle clonus point toward different sites of action.

iii. Cardiovascular. Adverse cardiovascular effects range from slight decrease in heart rate and blood pressure, as in normal sleep, to cardiovascular collapse. In general, with increasing dosages there is a negative inotropic effect (reversible by sympathomimetic amines), which with a further increase in dosage gives place to reduction in the contractile force of the heart and vessels. Cardiac arrhythmias are, however, rare.

It has long been recognized that there is a difference between oxybarbiturates and thiobarbiturates in their initial cardiovascular action. While oxybarbiturates tend to cause vasodilation with a fall in blood pressure—more pronounced in hypertensive patients—thiobarbiturates tend to cause vasoconstriction attributed to the release of catecholamines in the perivascular tissues. Thus, thiopental often has a slight hypertensive effect at the commencement of intravenous administration.

Other cardiovascular effects of thiopental include a decrease in cardiac output, intrathoracic blood volume, venous pressure, cerebral blood flow and cerebrospinal fluid pressure and an increase in heart rate, peripheral resistance and extremital blood flow.

iv. Respiratory. Under the influence of barbiturates, the "neurogenic drive" of respiration (brain stem reticular activating system) is reduced, and the control of respiration becomes dominated at first by the "chemical drive," *i.e.*, the direct action of CO_2 and H ions on the medullary respiratory centers, and later on by the "hypoxic drive," mediated by the chemoreceptors of the carotid and aortic bodies. With a further increase in blood concentration, the hypoxic drive also fails (Grollman, 1958).

The protective respiratory reflexes are only slightly depressed in barbiturate intoxication. The cough reflex particularly is maintained for some time. Therefore, coughing, sneezing and hiccoughing are rather common during intravenous barbiturate administration, and laryngospasms are considered to be one of the most dangerous of the respiratory complications.

It has been noted that cardiovascular collapse is rather rare. This is probably because respiratory arrest occurs first.

v. Gastrointestinal. Gastric secretion may be somewhat depressed. With oxybarbiturates there is also a decreased tone in the gastrointestinal musculature with a reduced amplitude of rhythmic contractions. Since hypnotic doses reduce the motility of the sigmoid colon, an intestinal-colonic hypermotility is frequently encountered as a rebound phenomena upon awakening from barbiturate-induced sleep.

vi. Genitourinary. It has been shown that pentobarbital interferes with the tubular reabsorption of sodium and glucose in the kidneys. Barbiturates in blood concentrations higher than the therapeutic levels depress the smooth muscles of the urinary bladder. They also produce a slight decrease in urinary flow. The severe oliguria or anuria which may occur in acute barbiturate poisoning is, however, mainly the result of hypotension and is not due to the direct effect of barbiturates on the genitourinary system.

While hypnotic doses do not affect the activity of the uterus, anesthetic doses decrease the force and frequency of contractions during labor. This is aggravated by the fact that barbiturates have a depressant effect on the fetus.

vii. Hepatobiliary. Although therapeutic doses do not impair hepatic functions, in anesthetic doses or in hypersensitive individuals liver damage may occur. There is, however, evidence that barbiturates increase the activity of liver enzyme systems, specifically, the ones responsible for their own metabolism; the biotransformation of a number of foreign organic compounds and endogenous steroids; the rate of ascorbic acid synthesis; and the synthesis of porphyrins. The effect of barbiturates on the last enzyme (see above) may lead to the precipitation of attacks of acute intermittent porphyria in prediposed subjects.

As a consequence of all the effects on the hepatobiliary system, there is an increase in the size and weight of the liver, with changes in the structure of the endoplasmic reticulum following chronic barbiturate administration.

viii. Dermatological. Skin eruptions are one of the commonest adverse reactions with barbiturates. Most frequently these are maculopapular or urticarial in nature, spreading diffusely over the trunk and extremities. Other dermatological reactions are localized swellings of the eyelids, cheeks, and lips, erythematous dermatitis, bullous cutaneous lesions and, rarely, exfoliative dermatitis and the Stevens-Johnson syndrome.

ix. Overdosage. A special aspect of adverse reactions is that of overdosage, which in the period 1957 to 1963 in New York City alone was responsible for 8469 poisonings with 1165 deaths, half of them suicidal attempts. One quarter of the suicides are cases of so-called "drug automatism," wherein the patient, if he fails to fall asleep after the second barbiturate-containing sleeping pill, may become confused and, unwittingly, gradually ingest an overdose.

Severe poisoning may be produced by barbiturates above ten times the hypnotic dose. Blood levels of poisoning are 3 mg./100 ml. to 10 mg./100 ml. One of the highest toxic doses ingested followed by recovery, reported to date, was 25 g. taken by a 37.7 kilogram woman, who had a peak blood level of 29 mg./100 ml.

In severe intoxication the patient is in coma, although deep reflexes are maintained for quite some time. Pupils are constricted at first but later become dilated; rapid and shallow breathing is replaced by Cheyne-Stokes respiration; blood pressure falls and the shock syndrome develops with rapid pulse and cold and sweaty skin. Renal failure may precede respiratory complications. If resuscitation fails, the patient will die of respiratory depression.

b. Treatment of Adverse Reactions

Most adverse reactions to barbiturates usually respond well to a decrease in dosage. In the majority of patients, however, barbiturate administration is discontinued and replaced by a nonbarbiturate hypnotic, sedative or minor tranquilizer drug. It is of great practical importance to know that the somnolence commonly produced by barbiturates can be counteracted by amphetamine preparations without interfering with the anticonvulsant effect and that the laryngospasm occurring during ECT, due to thiopental administration, promptly responds to an additional dose of succinylcholine.

In cases of barbiturate intoxication, treatment depends on the clinical manifestations. If discovered early, gastric lavage is recommended. To facilitate elimination, the administration of diuretics along with alkalination to decrease tubular reabsorption and increase urinary excretion is routinely used in most of the toxicological centers. At the same time, fluid and electrolyte balance are carefully maintained by glucose and saline infusion and antibiotics are given prophylactically to prevent secondary infections. Specific barbiturate antagonists may also be given. Among them, bemegride is somewhat stronger than amiphenazole. They stimulate respiration and reflex activity and reverse the electroencephalographic pattern of depression, but they do not increase the rate of barbiturate elimination, nor do they shorten the duration of coma.

The adverse and toxic effects of barbiturates on the cardiovascular, renal and respiratory systems are of particular concern. Cases of heart failure are treated by digitalization, and the negative inotropic effect is counteracted by sympathomimetic amines. To stimulate circulation, analeptics, *i.e.*, ephedrine, levarterenol, methoxamine, phenylephrine and amphetamines, are extensively used, but methylphenidate, nikethamide, pentetrazol and picrotoxin are probably even more frequently given. In case of shock, 2000 or 3000 ml. of dextran, concentrated albumin or blood are given, and if after the administration of 1000 ml. the shock still persists, norepinephrine is added to the infusion.

With satisfactory renal function, alkalination and forced diuresis are achieved by simultaneous administration of diuretics, 3000 to 4000 ml. of isotonic or hypotonic sodium bicarbonate solution or a solution of urea and sodium lactate. In case of renal failure, hemodialysis may be a lifesaving procedure.

Preparation for artificial respiration, intubation or tracheotomy is essential in barbiturate poisoning. Respiratory stimulants may be given. Epinephrine, dextroamphetamine, bemegride, amiphenazole, pentetrazol and picrotoxin may also be used. When respiratory paralysis supervenes, preference should be given to phthalic acid-bis-diethylamide or amphetamine, while picrotoxin and bemegride, because of their convulsant action, should be avoided (Grollman, 1958). It should be noted that bemegride may induce a toxic delirium or confusional state. This, as well as the delirium which develops from chronic barbiturate administration, can be controlled by phenothiazines, particularly chlorpromazine.

4. The Use of Barbiturates in Medical Practice

The choice of barbiturate for any individual patient depends primarily on the condition the drug is administered for, but also on the patient's physical condition and psychic disposition and on the experience of the physician. With these considerations, of the three main groups of barbiturates, oxybarbiturates are primarily used as sedatives or hypnotics, thiobarbiturates to induce general anesthesia and *N*-alkyl barbiturates to prevent or counteract convulsions.

Oxybarbiturates are most frequently prescribed in the treatment of nighttime or daytime sedation. Nighttime sedatives or hypnotics are needed for sleeping difficulties, which are manifested in three distinctly different patterns. The first type of insomnia is present in tense, agitated and overactive patients who have difficulty in relaxing and consequently in falling asleep. For this, a rapid acting, quickly metabolized sleep *inducer*, such as heptabarbital or the even more frequently used secobarbital, is useful. An entirely different kind of insomnia is present in very anxious and disturbed patients. This is characterized by fluctuations between waking and sleeping in varying frequency. This type of disturbance requires a sleep *maintainer* such as butobarbital or the extensively used pentobarbital. Finally, the third type of insomnia is characterized by early awakening, which can be controlled by a sleep *sustaining* drug, *e.g.*, barbital. It is also important to know that barbital is a useful adjuvant medication in the treatment of endogenous depression and can be helpful in cases as an adjuvant medication in an uncontrollable manic. Among the various oxybarbiturates, amobarbital and phenobarbital are probably the most frequently used for daytime sedation. Other short acting barbiturates used as sedatives or hypnotics are allylbarbituric acid, butallylonal, butethal, cyclobarbital, hexethal, probarbital, talbutal and vinbarbital; among the long acting compounds used are aprobarbital and diallylbarbituric acid. Phenobarbital, which belongs to this category is a most effective anticonvulsant barbiturate.

Among the thiobarbiturates, thiopental is probably the safest and the most extensively used to induce surgical anesthesia; thiamylal and methitural are also used for this purpose.

The *N*-alkyl barbiturate preparations are used as anticonvulsants. The long acting mephobarbital and metharbital are used in the control of grand mal seizures, and the ultra-short acting methohexital and methitural, in status epilepticus. Both of the latter drugs are used to induce surgical anesthesia, methohexital prior to electroconvulsive therapy and methitural for abreactive treatment.

In liver and renal disease the catabolism and excretion of barbiturates may be delayed, and consequently their effect may be potentiated. It also holds true that other drugs administered concurrently may potentiate or interfere with barbiturate treatment. In the elderly suffering from cerebral arteriosclerosis, oxybarbiturates may have a paradoxical effect; and barbiturates in predisposed individuals may produce dependence.

SUMMARY

The introduction of barbiturates in the early years of the century had a profound effect on psychiatric practice. A large number of formerly untreatable patients became accessible to treatment; and by improving the diagnosis in others, barbiturates facilitated the application of an appropriate therapy. The most significant results occurred in the treatment of various neurotic patients in whom the suppression or repression of emotional experiences led to the clinical syndrome or in whom the disinhibition produced by intravenous administration of these drugs broke through the manifestations of inhibitory phenomena produced by ultramaximal stimulation, *i.e.*, stimulation beyond the individual's tolerance. That barbiturates are helpful in the differential diagnosis of catatonic or depressive stupor became particularly important after the introduction of phenothiazines in the treatment of schizophrenia and monoamine oxidase inhibitors in the treatment of depression. By early differential diagnosis with the help of barbiturates it is possible to avoid giving MAO inhibitors, which may aggravate schizophrenic psychopathology in patients in a catatonic stupor; similarly, it is possible to avoid giving phenothiazines, which may aggravate depression, to patients suffering from stuporous depression.

Fifty years after their introduction, oxybarbiturates in general are still in the front rank among drugs administered for the various insomnias; phenobarbital stands among the "firsts" in the treatment of the various epilepsies. Similarly, thiobarbiturates and some of the ultra-short acting barbiturates are still extensively used in the introduction of general anesthesia. On the other hand, they are somewhat less frequently prescribed for daytime sedation.

There is increasing attention being paid to the change that various drugs produce on barbiturate action and on the effect barbiturates have on the metabolism of other therapeutically used compounds. The personality changes and toxic psychopathological reactions that may develop in the course of barbiturate treatment and the fact that acute intoxication with these drugs accounts for approximately 25 per cent of all deaths due to acute poisoning admitted to general hospitals are also increasingly stressed.

Even after 50 years of successful therapeutic application, barbiturate compounds may still have many secrets yet to be discovered.

REFERENCES

Alexander, L.: Treatment of mental disorders. (Saunders, Philadelphia, 1953.)

BAEYER, A. (1864): In: Sharpless, S. K.: Hypnotics and sedatives. I. The barbiturates. In: The pharmacological basis of therapeutics (eds., Goodman, L. S., and Gilman, A.). (MacMillan, Toronto, 1965.)

BAN, T. A.: Conditioning and psychiatry. (Aldine, Chicago, 1964.)

BRODY, T. M., AND BAIN, J. A.: Barbiturates and oxidative-phosphorylation. J. Pharmacol. Exp. Ther., *110:* 148 (1954).

FISCHER, E. AND MERING, J. (1903): In: Sharpless, S. K.: Hypnotics and sedatives. I. The barbiturates. In: The pharmacological basis of therapeutics (eds., Goodman, L. S., and Gilman, A.). (MacMillan, Toronto, 1965.)

FRIEND, D. G.: Role of synthetic drugs in therapy of mental illness. In: Molecular modification in drug design (ed., Gould, R. F.). (American Chemical Society, Washington, 1964.)

GREGORY, I.: Psychiatry. (Saunders, Philadelphia, 1961.)

GREGORY, R.: The brain as an engineering problem. In: Current problems in animal behavior (eds., Thorpe, W. H., and Zangwill, O. L.). (University Press, Cambridge, 1961.)

GROLLMAN, A.: The effect of various hypotensive agents on the arterial blood pressure of hypertensive rats and dogs. J. Pharmacol., *114:* 263 (1955).

GROLLMAN, A.: Pharmacology and therapeutics. (1st Ed.) (Lea and Febiger, Philadelphia, 1958.)

GROLLMAN, A.: Pharmacology and therapeutics. (2nd Ed.). (Lea and Febiger, Philadelphia, 1965.)

JENNER, F. A.: Use of drugs in anxiety states. In: The scientific basis of drug therapy in psychiatry (eds., Marks, J., and Pare, C. M. B.). (Pergamon Press, Oxford, 1965.)

KALINOWSKY, L. B., AND HOCH, P. H.: Somatic treatments in psychiatry. (Grune and Stratton, New York, 1961.)

KLÄSI, J.: Über Somnifen, eine Medicamentoese Therapie Schizophrener Aufregungszustaende. Schweiz. Arch. Neurol. Psychiat., *8:* 131 (1921).

KLÄSI, J.: Über die Therapeutische Anwendung der "Dauernarkose" mittels Somnifen bei Schizophrenen. Z. Ges. Neurol. Psychiat., *74:* 557 (1922).

LEHMANN, H. E., AND BAN, T. A.: Studies with new drugs in the treatment of convulsive disorders. Int. J. Clin. Pharmacol., *3:* 231 (1968).

LEHMANN, H. E., AND BAN, T. A.: The effect of hypnotics on rapid eye movements. (Presented at the Fourth Annual Meeting of the Canadian Society of Chemotherapy, Montreal, 1968.)

LEHMANN, H. E., AND BAN, T. A. (eds.): Toxicity and adverse reaction studies with psychoactive drugs. (Q.P.R.A., Montreal, 1968.)

LOEWE, S., *et al.* (1912): In: Sharpless, S. K.: Hypnotics and sedatives. I The barbiturates. In: The pharmacological basis of therapeutics (eds., Goodman, L. S., and Gilman, A.). (MacMillan, Toronto, 1965.)

MARKS, J., AND PARE, C. M. B. (eds.): The scientific basis of drug therapy in psychiatry. (Pergamon Press, Oxford, 1965).

MATTHEWS, V., LEHMANN, H. E., AND BAN, T. A.: A comparative study of thirteen hypnotic drugs. Appl. Ther., *6:* 806 (1964).

MAYER-GROSS, W., *et al.*: Clinical psychiatry. (Cassell, London, 1960.)

MERRITT, H. H., AND PUTNAM, T. J.: A new series of anticonvulsant drugs tested by experiments on animals. Arch. Neurol. Psychiat., *39:* 1003 (1938).

MEYLER, L. (ed.): Side effects of drugs. (Excerpta Medica Foundation, Amsterdam, 1960.)

MEYLER, L. (ed.): Side effects of drugs. (Excerpta Medica Foundation, Amsterdam, 1963.)

MEYLER, L. (ed.): Side effects of drugs. (Excerpta Medica Foundation, Amsterdam, 1964.)

MEYLER, L., AND PECK, H. M.: Drug-induced diseases. (Charles C Thomas, Springfield, 1962.)

MUSSER, R. D., AND BIRD, J. G.: Modern pharmacology and therapeutics. (MacMillan, New York, 1961.)

OSTOW, M.: Extrapyramidal system and neuroleptics. In: Extrapyramidal system and neuroleptics (ed., Bordeleau, J. M.). (L'Edition Psychiatriques, Montreal, 1961.)

OSTOW, M.: The clinical estimation of ego libido content. Int. J. Psychoanal., *42:* 486 (1961).

OSTOW, M.: Drugs in psychoanalysis and psychotherapy. (Basic Books, New York, 1962.)

OSTOW, M.: Meprobamate sedative or tranquilizer. J.A.M.A., *193:* 249 (1965).

SARGANT, W., AND SLATER, E.: An introduction to physical methods of treatment in psychiatry. (Livingstone, Edinburgh, 1963.)

SHARPLESS, S. K.: Hypnotics and sedatives. I. The barbiturates. In: The pharmacological basis of therapeutics (eds., Goodman, L. S., and Gilman, A.). (MacMillan, Toronto, 1965.)

SHARPLESS, S. K., AND HALPERN, L. M.: The electrical excitability of chronically isolated cortex studied by means of permanently implanted electrodes. Electroenceph. Clin. Neurophysiol., *14:* 244 (1962).

SHARPLESS, S. K., AND JASPER, H.: Habituation of the arousal reaction. Brain, *79:* 655 (1956).

SOURKES, T. L.: Biochemistry of mental disease. Harper and Row, New York, 1962.)

Nine

The Amphetamines

A. BASIC DATA

1. Historical Aspects

The parent compound of the amphetamines, a volatile phenylpropylamine, was first prepared by Edeleano in 1895. It was not until 1910 that Barger and Dale reported that this substance is not only chemically related to epinephrine but also similar in its action. More than a decade passed before Chen and his associates (1929, 1930) aroused interest in another substance of this group which was obtained from the Chinese herb Ma Huang (*Ephedra vulgaris*). This new drug, ephedrine, which proved to be particularly useful in the treatment of bronchial asthma, was the immediate predecessor of amphetamine.

In the search for a substitute for the scarce ephedrine Alles (1927) synthesized amphetamine, an alkylamine with sympathomimetic properties. The basic constituent of amphetamine (α-methylphenethylamine or phenylisopropylamine) is a benzyl ring in which an ethylamine group is attached in position 1.

Alles' (1927) hopes for the therapeutic usefulness of the substance in bronchial asthma were not fulfilled, but it was soon recognized that the new drug produced arousal and characteristic behavioral effects opposite to those of the already extensively used barbiturates. Several other amphetamines have been synthesized, *e.g.*, dextroamphetamine, methamphetamine, etc., and for a time the amphetamines became one of the most extensively used groups of drugs (Leake, 1958).

2. Action Mechanism

While all three amphetamines have definite behavioral stimulating effects, the action mechanism that leads to behavioral arousal is not yet fully understood. Theories range from psychodynamic to neurochemical concepts.

One psychodynamic formulation asserts that amphetamines are egotonics and thus their primary action is to improve ego functions. Accordingly, these substances can be utilized to strengthen the ego when its function is impaired (Ostow, 1962). A neurochemical hypothesis maintains that amphetamines may act on receptors related to the upper part of the reticular activating system by interfering with a naturally occurring catecholamine present in this area (Elkes, 1958).

In spite of the increasing information on the neurochemical and neurophysiological concomitants of the pharmacological effects of the amphetamines, there is still no general agreement as to which of the known actions of the molecule account for its psychoactive properties.

3. Structure and Activity

The parent substance of amphetamine drugs is the amphetamine base, a colorless liquid with an amine odor and an acid, burning taste, which on exposure to air rapidly changes into carbonate. Both the

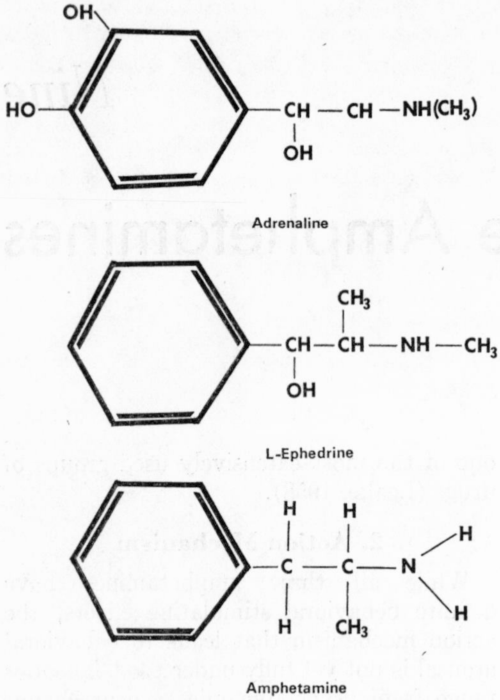

Adrenaline

L-Ephedrine

Amphetamine

FIG. 9. The evolvement of amphetamine from adrenaline.

base and the carbonate are volatile and as such evaporate slowly at room temperature. Amphetamines are most frequently available in the form of the racemic amphetamine sulfate or amphetamine phosphate, both of which are white, nonvolatile, water-soluble powders with a bitter taste.

Racemic amphetamine consists of two isomers. One is levorotatory and the other dextrorotatory to polarized light. The levoisomer has a characteristically strong "pressor action" with poor analeptic properties; the dextroisomer has less "pressor action" but is a powerful analeptic. The latter is a white, odorless, crystalline powder which is only slightly soluble in alcohol but freely soluble in water. It is usually administered in the form of dextroamphetamine sulfate, a substance with a characteristically strong alerting effect on the central nervous system with relatively weak generalized sympathomimetic action. Furthermore, the dextroisomer is twice as powerful as the racemic compound as a central nervous system stimulant and three to four times more potent in all respects than the levoisomer substance.

Another dextroisomer is methyl or methamphetamine, a water-, alcohol- and chloroform-soluble substance which lacks the characteristic fatigue-reducing effect of dextroamphetamine and has a somewhat weaker central effect, although it is more potent in this respect than the racemic compound.

While methamphetamine in small doses produces central nervous system stimulation without significant peripheral action, in somewhat larger doses this stimulant action may be complemented by a hypertensive effect.

Other less frequently used members of the amphetamine category are *N*-nicotinoylamphetamine, biphetamine and hydroxyamphetamine. The effects of *N*-nicotinoylamphetamine (Arbusov, 1952), resemble those of dextroamphetamine, although it is weaker pharmacologically and clinically. Unlike all the other amphetamine preparations, it has a mild hypotensive—rather than hypertensive—property. Biphetamine is a resin conjugate of racemic amphetamine sulfate and is given for appetite depression; and hydroxyamphetamine, which is entirely lacking in central nervous system stimulant effects, is successfully used in hypotensive states, Stokes-Adams syndrome, nasal congestion and as a mydriatic.

In the course of systematic exploratory research—first to synthesize amphetamines in general and then amphetamines with central, *i.e.*, behavioral stimulating or peripheral, *e.g.*, vasoconstricting effects—three basic principles on structure-activity relationships were recognized. The first was derived from examining the common and the differential features of epinephrine, ephedrine and the amphetamines. As a result it was suggested that the lack of hydroxyl radicals on the benzyl ring in ephedrine and in the amphetamines is responsible for the more prolonged action of these latter drugs; and it was recognized that the central stimulating effect of amphetamines can be separated from their peripheral vasoconstrictor action by saturating the benzyl ring.

Thus propylhexedrine was synthesized and used as an inhalant in the treatment of nasal congestion. This substance is entirely free from the abuses of the related phenylmethyl compound (amphetamine) which has been used extensively by "thrill seekers" for its "stimulating" effects.

Finally it was suggested that substitution on the first carbon atom of amphetamine results in compounds that tend to have increased central stimulating effects with reduced peripheral sympathomimetic action.

On the basis of these principles amphetamine drugs were placed on a hypothetical continuum. On one end of this continuum are the drugs with predominantly central (*e.g.*, dextroamphetamine sulfate) and on the other end those with mainly peripheral (*e.g.*, hydroxyamphetamine hydrobromide) actions (Grollman, 1958; Leake, 1958; and Innes and Nickerson, 1965).

4. Metabolism of Amphetamine Compounds

a. Absorption

Amphetamines are promptly absorbed, and their effects can be seen within 30 minutes after oral and 5 minutes after parenteral administration.

b. Distribution and Storage

The absorbed amphetamine can be detected in protein-bound form in both the blood and the various tissues. The largest amount is found in the liver, much less in the kidneys and only traces in the central nervous system structures.

c. Degradation and Excretion

There are interspecies variations in amphetamine metabolism. It is well known that fishes, frogs and salamanders excrete amphetamine unchanged through their skin, while toads metabolize amphetamines (an interesting phenomenon of functional adaptation) since their skin is not permeable to these drugs. Another interspecies variation was pointed out by Axelrod (1964), who showed that hydroxylation of the amphetamine ring takes place in dogs but not in guinea pigs or rabbits.

In mammals in general and humans in particular the site of the prevailing catabolic changes is the liver, where amphetamines are oxidized by the dehydrogenating microsomal enzyme system (but not by monoamine oxidase enzymes which are inhibited, at least *in vitro*, by these drugs) to phenylacetone and ammonia; and deaminated by monohydric phenols (phenoloxidase) in the presence of ascorbic acid (Sourkes, 1962). Consequently, in the case of an unsatisfactory ascorbic acid supply, the excretion of unmetabolized amphetamines increases.

Other routes of catabolism are parahydroxylation (with a resulting metabolite which is devoid of central nervous system stimulating effects) and acetylation (which takes place in the circulation).

There are great individual variations in the rate of excretion of amphetamines, although under normal circumstances a relatively large proportion of the drug ingested is excreted unchanged through the kidneys. Urinary excretion of a single dose is generally complete within 72 hours and, after discontinuation of prolonged drug administration, within 8 days.

5. Chemical and Neurophysiological Correlates of Drug Action

a. Chemical Correlates

It was surmised that amphetamines react with the MAO enzyme and thus prevent the effect of the latter in the catabolism of epinephrine, norepinephrine and serotonin. This mechanism was thought to be responsible for the reduction of aldehyde formation, which consequently allows for an improvement in brain respiration and increased central nervous system activity. Furthermore, since ergotropic functions are mediated by NE and trophotropic activities by 5-HT (Brodie *et al.*, 1956), it was considered that amphetamines in low dosages may cause their characteristic central stimulating effect by the activation of ergotropic functions, while in high dosages they block or inhibit trophotropic activity also.

Indications against the MAOI hypothesis of amphetamine action are the findings that amphetamines may still exert their action after catecholamines have been depleted by reserpine or in subjects who have previously been given a monoamine oxidase inhibitor drug; and that in low doses amphetamines increase the epinephrine effect, while in high doses they antagonize it.

b. Neurophysiological Correlates

Sympathomimetic effects and stimulation of the cerebrospinal axis are characteristics of amphetamine action. There is evidence for the direct passage of these drugs across the blood-brain barrier and indications of a decreased cerebral blood flow.

i. Autonomic Nervous System. Amphetamines exert sympathomimetic effects, which are responsible for the dilatation of pupils; constriction of blood vessels; blanching of mucous membranes; rise of blood pressure; rapid heart rate; dilatation of bronchi; increased muscle tension; elevated blood sugar level; and hastened blood coagulability. More recently, depolarization and blocking of activity in the autonomic ganglia have also been shown under the influence of these drugs.

ii. Spinal Cord. In the spinal cord there is evidence of facilitation of synaptic transmissions, which leads to quickened responses to external stimuli, manifested in both mono- and polysynaptic reflexes.

iii. Brain Stem Reticular Formation. The medullary action of amphetamines is seen in the stimulation of respiratory centers and indirectly by the interference with the depressant effect of morphine. Their effects on the brain stem reticular activating system are primarily seen in the lowering of the arousal threshold and indirectly by the reversal of barbiturate effects on these structures. Bradley and Key (1958, 1959), in animal experiments, have demonstrated that with increasing doses of amphetamines the behavioral and electroencephalographic thresholds for arousal gradually decrease. This applies to both environmental and direct stimulation of the brain stem reticular activating system structures, implying that besides the lowering of the threshold of sensory impulses to peripheral stimulation, amphetamines also possess a direct stimulating action on the brain stem. These result in increased alertness, attentiveness and awareness of the surroundings (accompanied by desynchronization of the electrocortical pattern).

There is a definite inhibition of trophotropic and activation of ergotropic functions of the mid-brain by amphetamine drugs. The slowing of the low voltage, high frequency EEG activity in rabbits after transection of the mid-brain at the posterior border of the pons (following atropine administration) is restored by dextroamphetamine, methamphetamine and ephedrine, but not by epinephrine. Similarly, the slow electroencephalographic pattern produced by transection of the anterior border of the pons is activated by dextroamphetamine, whereas the very slow electroencephalographic activity induced by rostral transection of the mid-brain is not altered by this group of drugs.

iv. Hypothalamus. The effect of amphetamines on the hypothalamus was explored by Brobeck *et al.* (1956). He was able to demonstrate that amphetamines stimulate the medial portion of the hypothalamus which contains an inhibitory center for food intake and exert an inhibitory effect on the "appetite centers" located in the lateral region of the same structure.

v. Cerebral Cortex. It was believed that the predominant effect of amphetamines on the cerebral cortex is stimulation, manifested in increased attentiveness and awareness, improved mental processes and reduction of fatigue. It had also been shown that the cortical stimulating effect of amphetamines is more marked in humans than in animals. Experimental data supporting these findings are acceleration and desynchronization of the human electroencephalogram; a shift from the resting to higher frequencies; reduction of amplitude and duration of large delta waves (present during sleep, after prolonged insomnia and in narcolepsy); counteraction of postconvulsive confusional state simultaneously present with the slow wave electroencephalogram; abolishment of both petit mal seizures and "spike and dome dysrhythmia" in children; and improvement of behavioral disorder concomitant with a rhythm of six cycles per second in children (with or without altering the electroencephalogram). More recently, it has been shown in rabbits that the amphetamine-produced desynchronization is restricted to the frontal cortex, while occipital leads depict slow waves of high voltage activity. This was further clarified by showing that the amphetamine-induced desynchronization results in inhibition of spikes produced by topical application of 0.1 per cent strychnine on the frontal cortex and that amphetamines also have an inhibitory effect on the evoked responses of the visual cortex. This line of investigation was pursued by Marazzi *et al.* (1956) and led to the conclusion that amphetamines may inhibit the passage of impulses across the neuronal ganglionic synapses in the brain with a consequent reduction of the over-all inhibitory action of the cerebral cortex. Thus, according to Marazzi, the alerting effect is a release phenomenon.

6. Behavioral Pharmacology

Amphetamines induce behavioral changes in animals and man over a wide range of functions. The initial mild sympathomimetic effects are progressively replaced by toxic manifestations. The LD_{50} of amphetamines is approximately 150 mg. per kg. Marked excitement, roughening of hair, tremor and clonic convulsions precede death. (Hemorrhages in the lungs and spleen are seen in post mortem examinations.)

a. Animal Studies

The effect of amphetamines on systems of lower complexity than the human has been extensively explored. It was shown that when amphetamines were given to spiders they induce erratic and rapid web spinning. When given to chicks—about 5 days old—they induced continuous twittering, excitement and droopy wings and when applied in a 1 per cent solution to the abdomen of fireflies, they caused a persistence of glow. Direct application to living tissues in the mammalian organism causes blanching of the mucous membranes for about 30 to 60 minutes. This local effect is responsible for the relief of nasal congestion if the drug is inhaled and may also be responsible for the reduction of gastric secretion with consequent loss of appetite.

The initial experiments with amphetamines were conducted on the gastrocnemius muscles of frogs. Where both gastrocnemius muscles were stimulated with the same electrical current, it was found that there was an increased tone and contractibility with a greater degree of relaxation between contractions on the muscle painted with a 1 per cent solution of amphetamine sulfate. When the same muscles were stimulated to produce fatigue, it was found that amphetamine sulfate significantly delayed the appearance of the characteristic fatigue curve.

In conditioning studies in animals it has been shown that these drugs decrease differentiation of conditional stimuli in dogs (classical paradigm), while they increase the rate of bar pressing for food reward in rats (operant paradigm). Amphetamines also help to restore the usual rate of bar pressing response after its extinction (by nonreinforcement), while they do not improve maze learning in rats.

In interaction with other drugs it has been shown that amphetamines enhance the analgesic effect of morphine and meperidine but decrease the sedative effect of these drugs. It has also been shown that administration of amphetamines does not protect against the anesthetic or lethal dose of pentothal, but it may be useful for counteracting its adverse effects. While ergotamine blocks amphetamine actions, amphetamines exert some reserpine antagonism effects.

b. Human Studies

In humans, 10 to 30 mg. of dextroamphetamine sulfate given in a single dose produce wakefulness, greater awareness of surroundings, a quicker response to environmental stimuli and a decreased sense of fatigue. This dose increases initiative, confidence, decisiveness and concentration; it induces euphoria, elation with increased motor activity and speech. While performance of simple mental tasks and physical activities is improved, and consequently more work is accomplished, the number of errors is not necessarily decreased.

Bleuler (1949) described the state of habitual users of these drugs as self-assured and confident with a tendency to sexual excitement easily satisfied by fantasy. Their "state of mind" swings between restlessness and motor overactivity and fatigue and exhaustion. This may result in an incapacitating condition in which the regular activities of the patient are interfered with.

Of the individual functions, increased visual and auditory acuity with increased capacity for mental processes have been shown. A systematic appraisal of drug effects on various psychophysical functions has shown that of the afferent (perceptual) tests, Critical Flicker Fusion Frequency is raised and Chromatic Spiral After-Image is facilitated; on the central (intrinsic-associative) tests, color naming on the Stroop tests is improved, Ideational Recall facilitated and Time underestimated; and on the efferent (psychomotor) tasks, auditory and visual Reaction Time and Cancellation Time and Error are decreased, Tapping Rate increased and Tracktracer Time decreased, while Tracktracer Error remains unchanged.

In Astrup's (1966) Word Association conditioning experiments, amphetamines improved conditionability and differentiation, facilitated the transmission from the first to the second signal system and improved second signal system activity.

B. CLINICAL DATA

1. Indications and Contraindications

a. Therapeutic Indications

Amphetamines are successfully administered in numerous conditions (Alexander, 1953; Leake, 1958; Grollman, 1958; Remmen *et al.*, 1962; and Sargant and Slater, 1963). Occasionally they are given to normal healthy adults, particularly when it is necessary for them to remain alert over an unusually long period, *e.g.*, war, emergencies, etc. Of the pathological conditions—besides the neuropsychiatric indications—they are frequently prescribed in obesities of various etiology, and to counteract the toxic effects (vasomotor collapse, respiratory depression) of narcotics, hypnotics and sedatives. They are less frequently used to replace ephedrine in the treatment of bronchial asthma (their original indication) and to counteract hypotension. They are used somewhat more often in colds and hay fever to relieve nasal congestion and in pregnancy and seasickness to reduce nausea and vomiting. Only rarely are they employed locally as mydriatics.

The neuropsychiatric indications of amphetamines range from functional to organic conditions, although they are now less frequently used than before.

i. Psychoneuroses. Amphetamines are used widely in various psychoneurotic conditions. There are indications that they improve the chronic fatigue of neurasthenic patients, while in neurotic depressive reactions the findings in therapeutic clinical trials remained equivocal. Favorable results are usually obtained in mildly depressed patients characterized by "morning melancholia" or slight retardation. There are no fully substantiated reports on the beneficial effect of these drugs on the depressive features of geriatric patients.

ii. Pathological Personalities. Sometimes psychopathic conditions "improve" with amphetamine medication. The periodic and recurrent aggressive outbursts of children associated with electroencephalographic changes, *i.e.*, persistent theta rhythm, have been beneficially influenced by these drugs, as have adults of immature personality with characteristic outbursts of spontaneous aggression. It has been noted that both groups have a characteristically high tolerance for amphetamine drugs.

iii. Organic Brain Syndromes. Amphetamines are used in the hyperkinetic-hyperactivity syndrome of children, characterized by poor concentration, irritability, impulsiveness and explosiveness. Another characteristic feature of this condition is the low convulsive threshold to pentetrazol. In the course of successful amphetamine treatment this convulsive threshold is raised to a normal level, and the activity of the child becomes less disjointed and more constructive and his attention span is lengthened.

In adults, amphetamine therapy was once

frequently used in alcoholism and morphine addiction. In acute alcoholic intoxication, amphetamine compounds as direct antagonists calm the excited, hyperactive, irritable patient, improving his coordination and coherence. They may also have a beneficial effect in the withdrawal period from morphine.

Among the therapeutic indications for amphetamines are various epilepsies. As early as 1935, Prinzmetal and Bloomberg introduced amphetamine treatment for narcolepsy. Later on, these drugs have also been successfully used in the treatment of pyknolepsy and in patients with other epileptic equivalents, *e.g.*, episodic mood swings or exacerbations of irritability. In grand mal or petit mal epilepsies they are used only as adjuvant medication to counteract the drowsiness and sluggishness, a common side-effect of anticonvulsant drugs. Other indications are postencephalitic parkinsonism and spasmodic torticollis, sexual tension and enuresis (Gwynne-Jones, 1960).

b. Contraindications

There are numerous conditions in which amphetamines should be taken with caution or in which they are contraindicated. It is generally accepted that in cases of heart disease or malnutrition amphetamines should be prescribed only after careful consideration and that caution should be exercised in hyperthyroid and hypertensive patients. Amphetamines are contraindicated in long standing bronchial asthma associated with a significant degree of emphysema and degenerative heart disease and also in angina pectoris.

Among the various psychopathologies, manic conditions are considered to be absolute and the schizophrenias relative contraindications of amphetamine treatment. Neurotic depression and drug dependency with prominent anxiety may become worse when treated with these drugs. Although amphetamines are therapeutic in certain psychopathic conditions, they should be prescribed with extreme caution for psychopaths, particularly those with a history of homicidal tendencies.

Amphetamines may prevent or counteract some of the adverse effects of monoamine oxidase inhibitor compounds, but they definitely aggravate others (*e.g.*, hypertensive crisis). Simultaneous administration of cyclopropane or halogenated hydrocarbon anesthetics may result in ventricular arrhythmias, tachycardia or even fatal ventricular fibrillation.

Among the different amphetamine preparations, relative contraindications of methamphetamine administration are arteriosclerosis, hypertension, coronary disease, myocardial damage, hyperthyroidism, insomnia and schizophrenia; those of amphetamine sulfate, phosphate and of dextroamphetamine sulfate are prepsychotic and hyperactive states, cardiovascular disease, including hypertension, and sensitivity to sympathomimetic drugs. The frequent use of these drugs to overcome sleepiness and to increase energy and alertness should be discouraged.

There is no evidence that these drugs should not be administered during pregnancy or in the period of lactation, nor has any carcinogenic effect been reported.

2. Therapy with Amphetamines Alone and in Combination with Other Treatments

a. Amphetamines Alone

In the therapeutic administration of amphetamines it is important to give these drugs in adequate dosage, by appropriate routes, following well established clinical procedures and for no longer than necessary.

i. Dosage. The therapeutic dosage range of each of the amphetamines differs slightly, but it generally holds true that if amphetamine sulfate is taken as a unit and prescribed in a dosage of 20 mg. a day for a patient, then the equivalent amount of dextroamphetamine sulfate is 15 mg. and of methamphetamine hydrochloride, 10 mg. The less frequently used biphetamine resinate is given in the same dosage as amphetamine sulfate, and the rarely used *N*-nicotinylamphetamine is given in a slightly (10 to 20 per cent) higher dosage. Hydroxyamphetaamine hydrobromide, an amphetamine without psychiatric indications, is applied topically in a 1 per cent solution.

Of the various therapeutic indications, the lowest dosages are used in the different psychoneurotic conditions or for weight-reducing purposes: amphetamine sulfate, 10 to 20 mg.; dextroamphetamine sulfate, 5 to 15 mg.; and methamphetamine sulfate 2.5 to 10 mg. a day. For neurological indications in general and particularly for relieving the rigidity of extrapyramidal manifestations, slightly higher dosages are needed; *e.g.*, in postencephalitic parkinsonism, 10 to 25 mg. a day of dextroamphetamine sulfate are usually given.

High dosages are required in narcolepsy and barbiturate poisoning or to obtain analeptic effects. In cases of narcolepsy, for example, it is not unusual to give 90 mg. a day of dextroamphetamine sulfate. In barbiturate poisoning 100 to 200 mg. of methamphetamine hydrochloride can be administered within a 24-hour period. Occasionally 5 to 10 mg. per kg. are needed to achieve a proper analeptic effect.

Age has less influence on the adequate dosage of these drugs than the actual therapeutic indication. Thus, for geriatric cases one may prescribe the actual adult dosage or somewhat less, while for aggressive, hyperactive children a dosage as high as 60 mg. per day is frequently needed for successful treatment.

ii. Routes of Administration. In historical sequence, the volatile amphetamine base was used at first via an inhaling device to give symptomatic relief in nasal congestion and hay fever. The instrument for this treatment—the so-called amphetamine inhaler—was introduced in 1932. A few years later hydroxyamphetamine hydrobromide was prepared in a 1 per cent aqueous solution. This, however, was applied topically. As such it has been used locally as a mydriatic or a nasal decongestant. Amphetamines are also given per os, rectally and parenterally.

The most frequent route is the oral, although the rectal route is often used, *e.g.*, by means of retention enema. Although amphetamines are promptly absorbed from the gastrointestinal tract, they have a relatively long lasting effect. The resinated combination of racemic amphetamine is very slowly released after oral ingestion, and its effects may last for 10 hours. Similarly *N*-nicotinylamphetamine is available in spansules from which the active ingredient is only gradually and slowly released.

Amphetamines may be given subcutaneously, intramuscularly or intravenously. Methamphetamine hydrochloride is most frequently and amphetamine sulfate only rarely chosen for parenteral usage.

In cases of respiratory depression or when analeptics are needed, methamphetamine hydrochloride is used intravenously first and then intramuscularly. In diagnostic or therapeutic exploration of psychiatric patients the same compound is given by the intravenous route.

iii. Treatment Procedures. Prior to commencement of treatment with any of the amphetamine drugs a test—sensitivity—dose should be given. Sensitivity is determined by the administration of 2.5 mg. of any of the preparations (orally or subcutaneously). If there is any evidence of agitation or depression, further administration of these drugs should be carefully avoided.

The course of treatment depends on the condition for which the drug is prescribed. In cases of intoxication due to alcohol or barbiturates, if the patient is in coma, treatment with these drugs may commence with intravenous administration of 40 mg. of methamphetamine hydrochloride. Half of this dosage may be repeated every 30 minutes until consciousness is fully regained. In other instances intravenous administration is followed by intramuscular treatment, in which the same dose as given intravenously is administered at hourly intervals. In some cases of light intoxication with barbiturates, 40 mg. of methamphetamine given intravenously may have a dramatic effect clinically and also electrophysiologically. Within 10 seconds the slow activity on the electroencephalogram, characteristic of deep barbiturate narcosis, is replaced by the fast activity prevalent in light barbiturate narcosis and 8 minutes later the normal waking rhythm is restored. In other instances, treatment is continued for 1 or 2 days, and some cases may receive as much as 400 mg. of the amphetamine drug within a period of 48 hours.

In contrast to the treatment of intoxication, in which amphetamines are given just for the acute period, these drugs may be given over an extended period, in narcolepsy, for example (not infrequently for the rest of the patient's life). In some of these cases the drug has to be given every 4 hours.

The treatment of hyperkinetic children extends over 6 months, during which time the drug is administered at least three times a day. For obese patients amphetamines are usually given half an hour before each meal, preferably for not longer than 2 to 3 months; for neurasthenic cases (to overcome fatigue), to reduce morning melancholia or to counteract the hangover and thus break the drinking cycle of alcoholics, the course of treatment consists of administration of a single dose which is taken after breakfast over a period of a few weeks. In the treatment of enuresis, the dosage is given at bedtime.

In most of the cases, however, these drugs should not be given before meal or at bedtime because they may interfere with both appetite and sleep.

iv. Duration of Treatment. Except in narcolepsy, amphetamines should be given only for a limited period, *i.e.*, preferably less than 3 months. During this time two distinct phases can be discerned: the first, of short duration, characterized by increasing susceptibility and the second, by some tolerance, particularly to the appetite-reducing effect.

Some patients experience the initial stimulation as euphoria or even elation. There is quite often a temptation to repeat the experience, which after a certain time period may result in habituation, with increasing doses needed to achieve the same effect. The progressively increasing doses (ingestion of 1700 mg. per day of dextroamphetamine sulfate has been reported) after a certain time may produce chronic restlessness, interference with appetite and eventually depressive symptoms with fatigue. In the majority of cases, however, there is no significant addiction with characteristic physical and psychological manifestations and thus no real craving. Amphetamine drugs may usually be withdrawn without any accompanying symptoms.

b. Amphetamines in Combination with Other Treatments

Amphetamines are not infrequently administered in conjunction with other treatments: pharmacological and psychological.

i. Pharmacological. Amphetamines are most frequently administered in conjunction with barbiturates. The drowsiness-producing effects of barbiturates are eliminated by this combination.

Commercially available amphetamine-barbiturate combinations are: Ambar I (methamphetamine hydrochloride, 10 mg., and phenobarbital, 64.8 mg.); Ambar II (methamphetamine hydrochloride, 15 mg., and phenobarbital, 64.8 mg.); Amyldex No. 1 (dextroamphetamine sulfate, 10 mg., and amobarbital, 60 mg.); Bitab 77 (dextroamphetamine sulfate, 12 mg., and phenobarbital, 48 mg.); Desbutal capsules (methamphetamine hydrochloride, 5 mg., and pentobarbital sodium, 30 mg.); Desbutal gradumets (methamphetamine hydrochloride, 10 mg., and pentobarbital sodium, 60 mg.), etc.

Other drug combinations have been used in the treatment of parkinsonism, epilepsy and neurasthenia. In parkinsonism, amphetamines had been frequently combined with belladonna alkaloids. To relieve rigidity, dextroamphetamine sulfate was commonly given together with atropine and to control oculogyric crises with low doses of scopolamine hydrobromide. More recently, amphetamines have been occasionally administered in combination with specific antiparkinsonism drugs.

While in certain epilepsies amphetamines may be therapeutically successful when given alone, in others they are administered in combination with other anticonvulsant drugs, particularly those of the hydantoin group. The fact that amphetamines counteract drowsiness is of great advantage in some of these long-term therapies.

The combination of morphine with amphetamines in the treatment of certain coronary conditions was at one time considered advantageous. Similarly, the combined administration of amphetamines with vitamins and iron (*e.g.*, Dexavite) for some neurasthenic patients was once favored. None is used any longer.

ii. Psychological. Both psychotherapies and behavior therapies are occasionally combined with amphetamine administration.

α. Psychotherapy. In the psychotherapies amphetamines are used in abreaction. In a civilian setting, amphetamine-induced abreaction is considered to be superior to that produced by barbiturate drugs, in contrast to the combat situation (Sargant and Slater, 1963).

β. Behavior Therapy. In the behavior therapy of bed wetting, amphetamines are increasingly used. Patients are fully awakened by the sound of a bell in case of bed wetting and instructed to visit the toilet (even if there is no urge to urinate). Seven uninterrupted (dry) nights with normal fluid intake and seven uninterrupted nights after one or two cups of water before retiring are considered to be signs of successful treatment. There is some evidence that amphetamine drugs given prior to retiring shorten the time required for therapeutic results (Gwynne-Jones, 1960).

3. Adverse Reactions and Their Treatment

a. Adverse Reactions

In the course of amphetamine administration a number of reactions occur which are unnecessary and undesired in the particular therapeutic situation. According to their nature, the undesired manifestations are classed as psychiatric, neurological, autonomic, endocrine, cardiovascular, respiratory, gastrointestinal, genitourinary, metabolic and hematological.

i. Psychiatric. These range from mild psychological changes to severe psychotic reactions. Increased wakefulness, talkativeness, motor activity and insomnia are commonly seen and frequently precede a state in which the patient becomes increasingly nervous, tense, apprehensive, restless and agitated. If drug administration is continued, this condition is replaced by increasing fatigue and depression (occasionally with suicidal intent). In some cases, latent delinquent behavior becomes manifest (Scott and Willcox, 1965).

Amphetamines may precipitate the onset of a schizophrenic episode, but they may also produce a psychosis that has a closer resemblance to schizophrenia than that induced by any of the presently known hallucinogenic drugs. The typical amphetamine psychosis is a well defined clinical syndrome characterized by paranoid manifestations with auditory and visual hallucinations with clear consciousness. Because of this, it resembles paranoid schizophrenia, from which it is differentiated by the prominence of visual hallucinations and the absence of a schizophrenic type of thought disorder (Bell, 1965).

Amphetamines, particularly amphetamine sulfate, occasionally induce a toxic confusional state but more often induce a transient delirium with memory disturbance. The lowest dosage which has resulted in an amphetamine psychosis is 55 mg.; the highest, 1500 mg. of amphetamine sulfate. The shortest duration of amphetamine administration prior to the psychotic manifestations has been a single dose; the longest, several years. The shortest duration of the psychosis has been 36 hours, and the most prolonged has lasted several months (Connell, 1958).

ii. Neurological. Characteristic neurological reactions of chronic amphetamine administration are headache, dizziness and vertigo. Tremor, increased reflexes and jerky and tremulous movements occur frequently, while acuity of smell and taste are only rarely changed.

iii. Autonomic. Characteristic autonomic reactions of chronic amphetamine administration are sympathicotonia in general and mydriasis, dry mouth and excessive sweating in particular.

iv. Endocrine. Adverse endocrinological effects in the course of amphetamine treatment are rare. Inhibition of the estrus cycle and inhibition of the liberation of antidiuretic hormones have been produced by massive dosage. It has been noted that, while an acute dosage may increase libido and facilitate ejaculation, chronic administration may lead to the reduction of sexual desire and performance.

v. Cardiovascular. Characteristic amphetamine effects are tachycardia and hypertension with a rapid pulse rate. Only occasionally are there paradoxical responses (bradycardia, hypotension). With higher doses, palpitations, extrasystoles, paroxysmal tachycardias, arrhythmias and anginal pains are quite common. The vessels of the skin and mucous membranes are constricted, while those of the skeletal muscles are dilated. There may also be a decrease in cerebral blood flow and a reduced oxygen consumption in the brain.

vi. Respiratory. In general, amphetamines are respiratory stimulants. They have a mild dilatory effect on the bronchial tree. In humans, overdosage may produce rapid, shallow breathing.

vii. Gastrointestinal. While these drugs reduce hunger by their CNS activity, they nevertheless have an inhibitory effect on salivary and gastric secretion and gastrointestinal motility. In cases in which enteric activity is pronounced, amphetamine preparations may counteract forceful gastrointestinal movement or even spasm, while in cases where the intestines are relaxed, high doses may cause diarrhea and abdominal cramps.

viii. Genitourinary. Amphetamines have a distinct tonic effect on the uterine musculature, but they diminish the amplitude (strength) of the contractions of this organ. The contractile effect of amphetamines on the urinary bladder sphincter may cause pain and difficulties in micturition. Occasionally, diuresis and, even less frequently, hematuria have been attributed to amphetamine administration.

ix. Metabolic. Amphetamine drug administration influences metabolism to the extent that glycogenolysis is increased in the liver and muscles. Simultaneously, there is liberation of free fatty acids from the adipose tissues. While on the one hand the metabolic effect of amphetamines may result in a slight rise in the blood sugar level, in other cases it may decrease it, especially in diabetic patients.

x. Hematological. Contraction of the spleen in the course of amphetamine treatment may produce a prompt but temporary increase in the number of circulating red blood cells and polymorphonuclear leucocytes. Another effect is hastened coagulation time, which occurs more often with racemic amphetamine than with the other preparations.

xi. Overdosage. Severe toxic reactions have been described with a single dose as low as 30 mg., survival with a single dose as high as 500 mg. and death after a rapid intravenous injection of 120 mg. of dextroamphetamine. Symptoms of overdosage are irritability, restlessness, tension and tremor, which precede, in certain cases, psychotic manifestations; other signs are rapid, shallow respiration, pallor and collapse. In cases of survival, headache, depression, arrhythmia and anginal pain are the common clinical features.

b. Treatment of Adverse Reactions

Some of the unpleasant autonomic effects can be counteracted by combining amphetamines with barbiturates. Mild adverse effects respond promptly to reduction in dosage, while in severe reactions, discontinuation of treatment is indicated. This can be carried out abruptly because there are usually no severe withdrawal symptoms even in cases of chronic intoxication with these drugs. Sedative or tranquilizer drugs alleviate the irritability present in the first days of drug withdrawal.

The treatment of overdosage is systematic sedation with barbiturate or phenothiazine drugs. A nitrate or a rapidly acting alpha receptor blocking agent is given in cases of marked hypertension. It has been noted that atropine may increase the pressor effect of amphetamine drugs, while cocaine may reverse the occasional paradoxical fall in blood pressure.

4. The Use of Amphetamines in Medical Practice

Amphetamines are extensively used and abused in everyday practice. D,L-Amphetamine sulfate was the first commercially available amphetamine. It was registered by the trade mark Benzedrine, after one of the compound's chemical names, benzyl-methyl-carbinamine. It is available in tablets and also in injectable form. D,L-Amphetamine is primarily a sympathomimetic drug. It produces definite central nervous system stimulation, fatigue reduction and mild vasoconstriction. (Racemic amphetamine is also available as its phosphate salt.)

Dextroamphetamine sulfate is stronger than D,L-amphetamine in its central nervous system stimulating property and is available in tablet form and as an elixir. It also reduces fatigue, probably more so than any of the other amphetamine compounds, with practically no peripheral concomitant effects, *e.g.*, vasoconstriction.

Methamphetamine hydrochloride is stronger than D,L-amphetamine but weaker than dextroamphetamine sulfate in its central stimulating effect, while in its sympathomimetic action it is weaker than D,L-amphetamine but stronger than dextroamphetamine. This substance is available in tablets and elixirs, but it is probably most frequently purchased in a sterile solution for parenteral use. Methamphetamine hydrochloride is prescribed for central nervous system stimulation, for diagnostic and therapeutic interviews and at one time also for the treatment of hypotension.

Of the other amphetamine preparations, biphetamine resinate, *N*-nicotinoylamphetamine and hydroxyamphetamine hydrobromide are only occasionally used. While hydroxyamphetamine hydrobromide is without any psychiatric indication and is entirely lacking in central nervous system effects, it is a good vasoconstrictor and is also given as a mydriatic or for cardiac acceleration. On the other hand, *N*-nicotinoylamphetamine has central nervous system stimulating properties, reduces fatigue without producing vasoconstriction. It is used mainly for appetite depression, as is biphetamine resinate, which has a characteristically prolonged—10 hours—effect because the active ingredient is released from the preparation rather slowly.

The central nervous system stimulating properties of the three most widely used amphetamines make them particularly useful in the treatment of certain neurotic—particularly neurasthenic—conditions, in narcolepsy or in counteracting the effect of central nervous system depressant drugs, *e.g.*, barbiturates. While the indiscriminate use of these drugs in the various depressive conditions is discouraged, their administration for hyperkinetic children and for a selected group of patients with personality disorders is suggested.

These drugs should be given after meals to avoid weight reduction and should not be given later than 4 P.M. to prevent insomnia.

SUMMARY

One end of the "amphetamine axis" consists of drugs with predominantly peripheral sympathomimetic actions, *e.g.*, hydroxyamphetamine, while the other end consists of drugs with mainly central nervous system stimulating effects, *e.g.*, dextroamphetamine. Of the three most frequently used amphetamine preparations, amphetamine sulfate has the strongest peripheral and the weakest central effects and dextroamphetamine sulfate has the strongest central and the weakest peripheral action; methamphetamine hydrochloride is intermediate in both respects.

Of the various neuropsychiatric conditions, amphetamines have proven to be beneficial in some of the epileptic disorders, particularly narcolepsy, in certain extrapyramidal manifestations, in behavior disorders of children, especially those with abnormal electroencephalograms, and in neurasthenia. Their effect in the various depressions is controversial. While they usually induce a transient period of well-being, continued administration leads to aggravation of the original condition. Tolerance develops in the course of chronic administration, and, depending on predisposition, a reversible paranoid psychotic reaction or a toxic delirious dysmnesic syndrome can occur.

Amphetamines should be prescribed only after the most careful appraisal of the patient's pathological manifestations and circumstances and preferably only for a limited period of time.

REFERENCES

ALEXANDER, L.: Treatment of mental disorders. (Saunders, Philadelphia, 1953.)

ALEXANDER, L.: Epinephrine-mecholyl test (Funkenstein test). Its value in determining the recovery potential of patients with mental disease. Arch. Neurol. Psychiat., *73:* 496 (1955).

ALLES, G. A.: Comparative physiological action of phenylethanolamines. J. Pharmacol. Exp. Ther. *32:* 121 (1927).

ARBUSOV, S.: On the pharmacology of phenatine. Farmakol. Toksik., *15:* 46 (1952).

ASTRUP, C.: Pavlovian psychiatry. (Charles C Thomas, Springfield, 1965.)

ASTRUP, C.: Conditional reflex studies in psychopharmacology. (Presented at the Fifth International Congress of CINP, Washington, 1966.)

ASTRUP, C., AND RASMUSSEN, J.: Is there an enhancing effect of neuroleptic drugs on blood coagulation and thrombosis? Thromb. Diath. Haemorrh., *13:* 418 (1965)

AXELROD, J.: The uptake and release of catecholamines and the effect of drugs. In: Progress in brain research, Vol. VIII (eds., Amine, B., Himwich, H. E., and Himwich, W. A.). (Elsevier, Amsterdam, 1964.)

BARGER, G., AND DALE, H. H.: Chemical structure and sympathomimetic action of amines. J. Physiol. (London), *41:* 19 (1910).

BELL, D. S.: Comparison of amphetamine psychosis and schizophrenia. Brit. J. Psychiat., *3:* 701 (1965).

BLEULER, M. (1949): In: Mayer-Gross, W., *et al.:* Clinical Psychiatry. (Cassell, London, 1960.)

BRADLEY, P. B., AND KEY, B. J.: The effect of drugs on arousal responses produced by electrical stimulation of the reticular formation of the brain. Electroenceph. Clin. Neurophysiol., *10:* 97 (1958).

BRADLEY, P. B., AND KEY, B. J.: A comparative study of the effects of drugs on the arousal system of the brain. Brit. J. Pharmacol., *14:* 340 (1959).

BROBECK, J. R., LARSSON, S., AND REYES, I.: A study of the electrical activity of the hypothalamic feeding mechanism. J. Physiol. (London), *132:* 358 (1956).

BRODIE, B. B., PLETSCHER, A., AND SHORE, P. A.: Possible role of serotonin in brain function and in reserpine action. J. Pharmacol., *116:* 9 (1956).

BRODIE, B. B., SHORE, P. A., AND PLETSCHER, A.: Serotonin-releasing activity limited to Rauwolfia alkaloids with tranquillizing action. Science, *123:* 992 (1956).

CHEN, K. K., AND POTH, E. J.: Racial differences as illustrated by the mydriatic action of cocaine, enphthalmine and ephedrine. J. Pharmacol. Exp. Ther., *36:* 429 (1929).

CHEN, K. K., AND SCHMIDT, C. F.: Ephedrine and related substances. Medicine (Balt.), *9:* 1 (1930).

CONNELL, P. H.: Amphetamine psychoses. (Chapman and Hall, London, 1958.)

EDELEANO, L.: Über einige Derivate der Phenylmethacrylsaure der Phenylisobuttersaure. Ber. Deutsch. Chem. Ges., *20:* 616 (1895).

ELKES, J.: Effects of psychosomimetic drugs in animal and man. In: Neuropharmacology (ed., Abramson, H. S.). (Madison, New York, 1957.)

ELKES, J.: Drug effects in relation to acceptor specificity within the brain: some evidence and provisional formulation. In: Ciba Foundation Symposium on The neurological basis of behavior (eds., Wolstenholme, G. E. W., and O'Connor, C. M.). (Churchill, London, 1958.)

ELKES, J., ELKES, C., AND BRADLEY, P. B.: The effect of some drugs on the electrical activity of the brain and on behavior. J. Ment. Sci., *100:* 125 (1954).

GOODMAN, L. S., AND GILMAN, A.: The pharmacological basis of therapeutics. (MacMillan, New York, 1955.)

GROLLMAN, A.: Pharmacology and therapeutics. (1st Ed.) (Lea and Febiger, Philadelphia, 1958.)

GROLLMAN, A.: Pharmacology and therapeutics. (2nd Ed.) (Lea and Febiger, Philadelphia, 1965.)

GWYNNE-JONES, H.: The behavioral treatment of enuresis nocturna. In: Behavior therapy and the neuroses (ed., Eysenck, H. J.). (Pergamon Press, New York, 1960.)

INNES, I. R., AND NICKERSON, M.: Drugs inhibiting the action of acetylcholine on structures innervated by postganglionic parasympathetic nerves (antimuscarinic or atropinic drugs). In: The pharmacological basis of therapeutics (eds., Goodman, L. S., and Gilman, A.). (MacMillan, Toronto, 1965.)

LEAKE, C. D.: The amphetamines: their actions and uses. (Charles C Thomas, Springfield, 1958.)

LEAKE, C. D.: The evaluation of the new drug carisoprodol. In: The pharmacology and clinical usefulness of carisoprodol (ed., Miller, J. G.). (Wayne State University Press, Detroit, 1959.)

MARAZZI, A. S., AND HART, E. R.: The possible role of inhibition at adrenergic synapses in the mechanisms of hallucinogenic and related drug action. J. Nerv. Ment. Dis., *122:* 453 (1955).

MARAZZI, A. S., HART, E. R., AND COHN, V. H.: Pharmacology of the nervous system. Progr. Neurol. Psychiat., *11:* 565 (1956).

MAYER-GROSS, W., *et al.:* Clinical psychiatry. (Cassell, London, 1960.)

OSTOW, M.: Drugs in psychoanalysis and psychotherapy. (Basic Books, New York, 1962.)

PRINZMETAL, M., AND BLOOMBERG, W.: The use of benzedrine for the treatment of narcolepsy. J.A.M.A., *105:* 2051 (1935).

REMMEN, E., *et al.:* Psychochemotherapy. (Western Medical Publications, Los Angeles, 1962.)

SARGANT, W., AND SLATER, E.: An introduction to physical methods of treatment in psychiatry. (Livingstone, Edinburgh, 1963.)

SCOTT, P. D., AND WILLCOX, D. R. C.: Delinquency and the amphetamines. Brit. J. Psychiat., *3:* 865 (1965).

SOURKES, T. L.: Biochemistry of mental disease. (Harper and Row, New York, 1962.)

Ten

The Phenothiazines

In the past decade at least fifty million patients have received chlorpromazine (CPZ) and more than ten thousand reports (Jarvik, 1965) have been published on the drug that heralded a new psychopharmacological era in psychiatry. One may safely compare the impact of the introduction of CPZ to that of penicillin.

A. BASIC DATA

1. Historical Aspects

The basic constituent of CPZ is the phenothiazine nucleus which consists of two benzol rings attached to each other by a sulfur and a nitrogen atom (Bernthsen, 1883).

The origin of this nucleus is in the benzodioxane structure. Variations of the benzodioxane structure led through ethers of the ethanolamine, ethylenediamine and finally diphenylamine types to the phenothiazine derivatives. Phenothiazine is the parent substance of the thionine dyes, of which methylene blue was used as an intestinal and urinary antiseptic (Einhorn, 1891). When the toxic effect of phenothiazine on various bacteria, insects and helminths was discovered, the drug became extensively used as an anthelminthic in the treatment of enterobiasis (Kuitunen-Ekbaum, 1941). The expectation that one of these might be effective in the treatment of protozoal infections, however, was not fulfilled. Instead, it has been found that diethazine and ethopropazine are successful antiparkinson drugs and that promethazine and pyrathiazine are potent antihistaminic agents (Gordon *et al.*, 1964).

In the course of treatment of allergic conditions with promethazine, sedation was noted to be the prominent side-effect. To enhance this sedative action a large number of modifications of promethazine were synthesized and studied. This work resulted in the synthesis of CPZ in which the two carbon—ethyl—side chain of promethazine was replaced by a three carbon—propyl—chain and in which the hydrogen atom of the phenothiazine nucleus in position 2 was substituted with a chlorine. These modifications not only greatly enhanced the sedative effect but, as was later discovered, also added tranquilizing and antipsychotic properties to the compound.

Since the antihistaminic potency of CPZ was found to be inferior to that of promethazine, the hypothesis that this antihistaminic property is responsible for the therapeutic effect of the drug in schizophrenics was not supported. Instead, another hypothesis received increasing attention. This was based on the actual application of the drug as a "stabilisateur végétatif" to bring about a condition—in surgical patients and cases in shock—that Laborit (1951) described by his concept of "artificial hibernation." Under artificial hibernation, consciousness is maintained, but an indifference to the surroundings develops. This, in turn, leads to relaxation with a simultaneous decrease of the usual adaptive responses to stress. Thus, if one accepts the theory that stress leads to mental breakdown by exhausting the body's

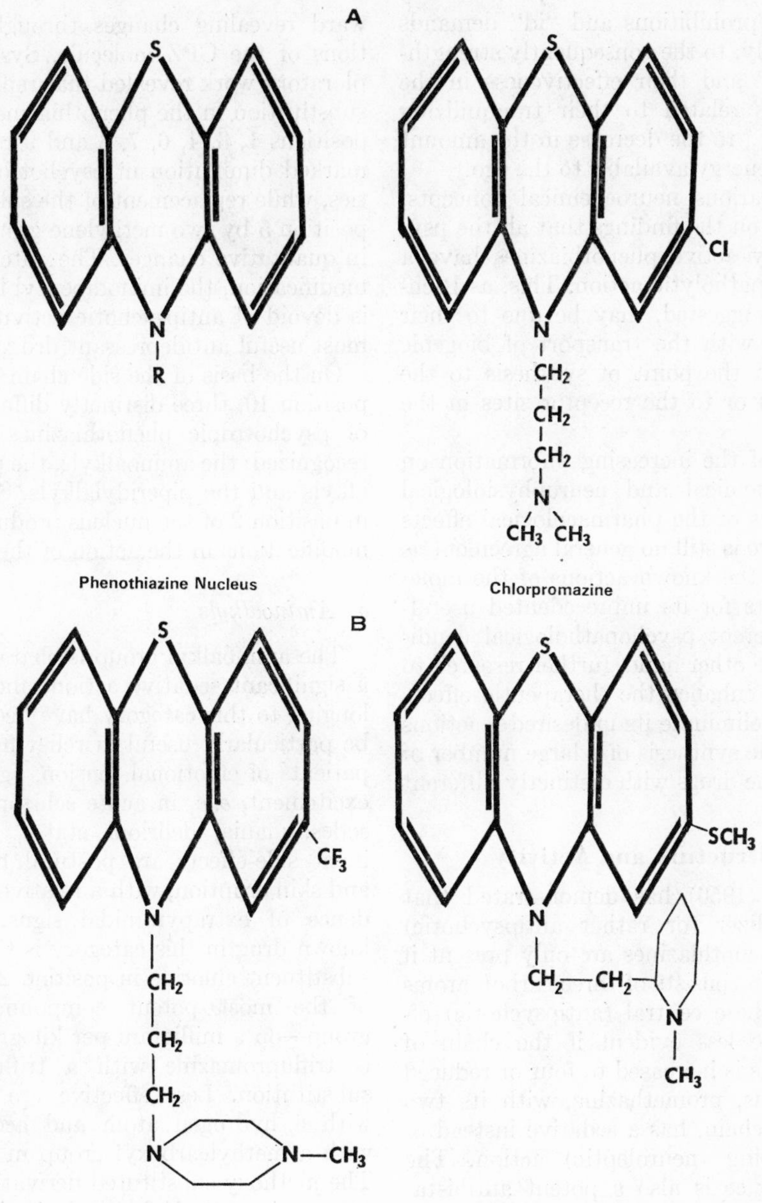

FIG. 10. *a*, The phenothiazine nucleus and chlorpromazine. *b*, Trifluoperazine and thioridazine.

ability to adapt, then CPZ might be able to offer protection from such exhaustion (Paterson, 1963).

2. Action Mechanism

Since these early theories on the action mechanism of CPZ, a number of other hypotheses have been formulated ranging from psychodynamic (Ostow, 1962) to neurochemical (Richter, 1965) concepts.

According to one psychodynamic formulation (Ostow, 1962), the effectiveness of phenothiazines in the psychoneuroses is due to the diminished strength and severity of "superego" prohibitions and "id" demands or, conversely, to the consequently strengthened "ego;" and their effectiveness in the psychoses is related to their tranquilizing property, *i.e.*, to the decrease in the amount of libidinal energy available to the ego.

Of the various neurochemical concepts, one is based on the findings that all the psychotropically active phenothiazines have a central sympatholytic action. This, as Richter (1965) suggested, may be due to their interference with the transport of biogenic amines from the point of synthesis to the storage sites or to the receptor sites in the brain.

In spite of the increasing information on the neurochemical and neurophysiological concomitants of the pharmacological effects of CPZ, there is still no general agreement as to which of the known actions of the molecule accounts for its unprecedented usefulness in different psychopathological conditions. On the other hand, further research to modify and enhance the therapeutic effects of CPZ and eliminate its undesired reactions has led to the synthesis of a large number of phenothiazine drugs with distinctly different properties.

3. Structure and Activity

Himwich (1956) has demonstrated that the tranquilizer (or rather antipsychotic) effects of phenothiazines are only present if the side chain consists of three carbon atoms in a row. These central (antipsychotic) effects become less evident if the chain of carbon atoms is increased to four or reduced to two. Thus, promethazine, with its two carbon side chain, has a sedative instead of a tranquilizing (neuroleptic) action. The same substance is also a potent antihistamine. This, according to Lewis (1962), is related to the amino group attached to the aliphatic chain in β position. Furthermore, of the two carbon side chain containing phenothiazines, diethazine, a diethylamino derivative (in contradistinction to the dimethylamino derivative promethazine), is characterized by antiparkinsonian activity (Sainsbury, 1965).

In the search for a more potent (antipsychotic) and less toxic phenothiazine than CPZ, extensive studies were directed toward revealing changes through modifications of the CPZ molecule. Systematic exploratory work revealed that replacement or substitution in the phenothiazine nucleus in positions 1, 3, 4, 6, 7, 8 and 9 resulted in a marked diminution in psychotropic properties, while replacement of the sulfur atom in position 5 by two methylene groups resulted in qualitative changes. The outcome of this modification, the iminodibenzyl imipramine, is devoid of antipsychotic activity, but is a most useful antidepressant drug.

On the basis of the side chain attached to position 10, three distinctly different groups of psychotropic phenothiazines have been recognized: the aminoalkyls, the piperazinylalkyls and the piperidylalkyls. Substitution in position 2 of the nucleus produced further modifications in the action of these drugs.

a. *Aminoalkyls*

The aminoalkyl group is characterized by a significant sedative action, and drugs belonging to this category have been found to be particularly useful in relieving psychotic patients of emotional tension, agitation and excitement, *e.g.*, in acute schizophrenic episodes, mania, delirious states, etc. Prominent side-effects are postural hypotension and skin eruption, with a relatively low incidence of extrapyramidal signs. The best known drug in this category is CPZ, with a substituent chlorine in position 2, while one of the most potent compounds in this group—on a milligram per kilogram basis—is triflupromazine with a trifluoromethyl substitution. Less effective are promazine with a hydrogen atom and acepromazine with a methylcarboxyl group in position 2. The methoxy-substituted derivative—methopromazine—itself is weak in its psychotropic action, but methotrimeprazine, a methylated levoisomer of this substance, has a characteristically strong sedative effect.

b. *Piperazinylalkyls*

While the aminoalkyl phenothiazines are recommended in excitement and agitation, piperazinylalkyl phenothiazines are used to activate chronic withdrawn schizophrenic patients. Virtually no postural hypotension or skin eruption occurs with drugs in this category, whose prominent side-effects are extrapyramidal manifestations. The least liable to produce extrapyramidal signs and also the least potent in therapeutic action are acetophenazine and carphenazine. Those most likely to produce extrapyramidal signs and also the most potent drugs therapeutically are thioproperazine and fluphenazine, while prochlorperazine, thiopropazate, trifluoperazine, perphenazine and butaperazine are in between the two extremes in extrapyramidal effects.

c. Piperidylalkyls

The piperidyl group consists of only two well known members: thioridazine and propericiazine. Thioridazine is recommended for schizophrenics with depressive mood changes. Closely related to this extensively used substance is propericiazine, a hydroxypiperidyl (in contrast to the methylpiperidyl thioridazine), with a CN group in position 2 on the phenothiazine nucleus. This drug may have a particular effectiveness in personality disorders.

In spite of their distinctive pharmacological and psychological effects, Sainsbury (1965) maintains that the therapeutic efficacy of phenothiazines does not relate consistently to their chemical structure. According to him, the chemical structural features of the phenothiazines thus far have not provided for a sufficiently constant association between pharmacological, psychological and clinical effects to develop a theory of their mode of action.

4. Metabolism

The fate of the different phenothiazine compounds from the time they are first administered until they are excreted from the organism is quite similar. This makes it possible to discuss the metabolism of phenothiazines schematically through the description of the absorption, distribution, inactivation and excretion of any one of the derivatives.

a. Absorption

CPZ, for example, is absorbed in 5 to 10 minutes after parenteral administration and in 30 to 60 minutes after it is taken by mouth. Its immediate sedative action occurs within this period, to a noticeably greater extent with intramuscular than with oral administration. A hypothetical gastrointestinal blood barrier, which may prevent adequate absorption, is held responsible for this discrepancy.

b. Distribution and Storage

Systematic studies have shown that approximately 50 per cent of the daily dose of CPZ is excreted in the urine, with another substantial portion eliminated in the feces. The balance is stored in various body tissues. The largest quantity of stored CPZ is found in keratinous substances (*i.e.*, hair) and in the lungs; less is stored in the pancreas, testes and liver. Some stored CPZ is found in the brain tissue, where drug content varies, being highest in the pituitary gland and lowest in the corpus callosum.

The distribution of CPZ in the organs of the cat after intravenous administration was explored by Gothelf and Karczmar (1963). They demonstrated that the drug shifted rapidly from the blood into the tissues where the highest level was attained, at first in the lungs. After 60 minutes there was equally high concentration in lung, liver and brain and considerably lower concentration in the other organs of the body. At least part of the reason for this, according to Richter (1965), is the lipid solubility of the CPZ molecule, which explains its tendency to adhere to the lipid surfaces of the capillaries (at first in the large vascular bed of the lungs) and its accumulation in organs such as the brain and liver, which are both vascular and have a relatively high lipid content.

Distribution of phenothiazines in the nervous tissues was studied by Murray and Peterson (1964), who were able to demonstrate in tissue cultures of nerve cells under fluorescence microscopy that CPZ was concentrated in the mitochondrial zone of the nerve cell bodies. Roizin *et al.* (1962) have shown by electron micrography that prochlorperazine in low doses induces a reversible alteration of the structure of brain and liver mitochondria, with a partial disintegration of the limiting membranes, which are rich in phospholipids. Richter (1965) suggests that the pharmacological actions of the phenothiazines may be related to their tendency to accumulate at membrane surfaces in the cell.

c. Degradation and Excretion

The main pathways of CPZ metabolism are oxidation, hydroxylation, conjugation, *N*-oxidation and demethylation. The oxidation product of the sulfur atom in position 5 on the phenothiazine ring is sulfoxide, which is a free, *i.e.*, nonconjugated, form together with traces of unoxidized CPZ accounts for approximately 20 per cent of the total daily drug content in the urine. The remaining 80 per cent is accounted for by hydroxylation in positions 3 and 7, most of which appears in the urine in a conjugated form with glucuronic acid.

After discontinuation of drug administration, metabolic products continue to be excreted in the urine for an extended period of time, varying in individual patients from weeks to months. It is known that the ultimate excretion takes place from 6 to 12 months after therapy has been terminated.

5. Chemical and Neurophysiological Correlates of Drug Action

a. Chemical Correlates

The psychotropic property of phenothiazines cannot be reduced to a single chemical concomitant of drug action. There are a number of changes described that are related to the effect of these drugs: phenothiazines inhibit the oxidative phosphorylation of cells, interfere with cortical release of acetylcholine and decrease the utilization of adenosine triphosphate (Beckman, 1958).

Phenothiazines *in vitro* are powerful metabolic blocking agents, and they act in the respiratory chain at the flavoprotein level. However, brain levels *in vivo* of ATP and creatinine phosphate are relatively high after treatment with CPZ, which is the reverse of what would be expected from the findings *in vitro*. Nevertheless, CPZ accelerates the turnover rate of phospholipids *in vivo*. Since this effect is specific for the phospholipids of the brain, it is of particular interest (Richter, 1965).

Another widely recognized activity of these compounds is their ability to counteract the increase in brain monoamines, *i.e.*, serotonin and norepinephrine, after the administration of monoamine oxidase inhibitor (MAOI) substances. Since MAOI's are widely used in the treatment of depression, with particular success in the atypical cases, ignorance of this activity of the phenothiazine compounds may interfere with adequate treatment.

Certain hormonal changes induced by the phenothiazine drugs are chemically measurable. The reduction of pituitary adrenocorticotropic (ACTH) and antidiuretic (ADH) hormone production in turn decreases urinary gonadotropin, estrogen and progestin levels and increases urinary output. By blocking the iodinase system, required for the synthesis of a thyroid hormone (diiodotyrosine), phenothiazines also exert a thiouracil-like action (Grollman, 1965).

In the course of treatment with high dosage CPZ over an extended period, a characteristic purple skin pigmentation was noted in a small number of patients. Studies with these cases suggest that orthostatic hypotension, extrapyramidal signs and skin pigmentation are not entirely unrelated phenomena. They result from the action mechanism of these drugs, which, by interfering with dihydroxyphenylalanine metabolism, decreases dopamine, epinephrine and norepinephrine synthesis. Thus a relatively reduced dopamine level may be correlated with the appearance of extrapyramidal signs and the relatively reduced catecholamine level with orthostatic hypotension. Furthermore, it was assumed that the decreased catecholamime level produces an increased melanocyte-stimulating hormone (MSH) activity of the pituitary (Ban and Lehmann, 1965) and decreased melatonin synthesis in the pineal gland. Probably the same mechanism accounts for the blocking (or reversal) of epinephrine action described in the course of administration of various phenothiazine drugs.

b. Neurophysiological Correlates

Just as the psychotropic property of phenothiazines could not be reduced to a single chemical concomitant, but had to be described in a number of simultaneous chemical changes, so there is no single neurophysiological phenomenon which can fully account for the multifold activities of these drugs. The functional alterations in the nervous system due to phenothiazine compounds are here described from the lowest level of integration to the cerebral cortex.

i. Autonomic Nervous System. The influence of phenothiazine drugs on the autonomic nervous system was described in the early nineteen-fifties and characterized as gangliolytic and strongly adrenolytic but also as mildly anticholinergic with antifibrillatory action. It is usually the antiadrenergic effect of these drugs that is considered to be primarily correlated with their therapeutic effectiveness. Although sympatholytic to the extent that some of these drugs may cause severe orthostatic hypotension at the commencement of treatment, phenothiazine compounds do not interfere with the hyperglycemic response to adrenaline administration. There is a differential balance—dependent on the side chain attached to the phenothiazine nucleus—between the degree of sympatholytic and parasympatholytic activity of different phenothiazine drugs. Compounds with an aminoalkyl group seem to be prominently adrenolytic (*e.g.*, CPZ), while the aminopiperidyl substances (*e.g.*, thioridazine) are equally anticholinergic in their action.

ii. Medulla Oblongata. The effect of phenothiazine drugs on the medulla oblongata is manifest in the antiemetic effect of these compounds (the vomiting center is located in this region). It has been shown that the sensitivity of the trigger zone of the vomiting center is differentially elevated under the influence of the different phenothiazines. High antiemetic potency is ascribed to compounds containing a piperazine side chain, particularly those with a halogen substituted in position 2 in the phenothiazine ring. Interestingly, these drugs are also the most potent (on a milligram per kilogram basis) in antipsychotic action.

iii. Brain Stem Reticular Formation. It has long been considered that the most prominent effect of phenothiazine drugs is their influence on the arousal reaction related to brain stem reticular formation function. This action is correlated with blockage of adrenergic intrareticular mechanisms and with depression in the cortical release of acetylcholine. In later studies, however, arousal to peripheral stimulation has been differentiated from the arousal produced by direct stimulation through implanted electrodes. In the case of barbiturates, it has been shown that the arousal effects to both peripheral and direct stimulation are equally decreased, whereas with CPZ the arousal reaction is diminished to peripheral stimulation only. This implies that, while barbiturates have a direct effect on these brain stem structures, the action of CPZ takes place on the afferent pathways to the reticular formation.

iv. Hypothalamus. The effect of phenothiazines on the hypothalamus is complex. A reaction specific to the hypothalamus is "sham rage." This is characterized by violent outbursts of sympathetic functions in decorticated animals. Sham rage can be controlled by CPZ, which indicates that phenothiazine drugs may have an effect on the hypothalamic centers. This is further supported by the ptosis and miosis (which occur even more after reserpine administration) when CPZ is given. The inhibitory effect of central heat regulation (artificial hibernation) and the endocrine changes produced by phenothiazines give further support to hypothalamic action.

More recently, through implanted microelectrode techniques in self-stimulation experiments, it has been noted that CPZ has very little effect on self-stimulation if the electrodes are in the anterior hypothalamus, but there is complete inhibition of self-stimulation with electrodes in the ventral posterior hypothalamus.

v. Other Structures. Other neurophysiological effects of phenothiazine administration are enhancement or inhibition of the thalamic recruiting responses by small or large doses of CPZ, respectively; shortening of the duration of the characteristic seizure-like discharges from the amygdala and blockage of input from the amygdala to the brain stem; a tendency for rhythmical protracted waves, desynchronization and increased delta activity with induction of spontaneous seizures; or, in general, decreased frequency with relatively increased amplitude (voltage) on the surface electroencephalogram.

Himwich (1965) summarized the action of phenothiazines on the various CNS structures as follows: no effect on the respiratory center and the neocortex; blocking of neurohormones; inhibition of limbic structures; and an acute block and chronic arousal of the mesodiencephalic activating system.

6. Behavioral Pharmacology

Phenothiazines induce behavioral changes over a wide range of functions in animals and man. For example, the prolongation of hexobarbital sleeping time is correlated with the potentiation of the analgesic and sedative action of narcotics, which in turn reduces the necessary opiate dosage in malignancies and brings about a condition in which the patient experiences the pain just as if it were any other objective phenomenon.

a. Animal Studies

The most characteristic effects of phenothiazines on animal behavior were described on a behavioral continuum. There is at first a taming effect. While this lasts, all manifest aggressiveness disappears, and the animals willingly permit any stranger to handle or caress them. In higher doses the animals pass subsequently into a second stage of abnormal behavior, which is characterized by a decrease of spontaneous motor activity. At a certain dose level this passes into immobility, characterized by a particular dissociation, in which the animal becomes fixated in unusual positions with maintenance of its righting reflex. This particular change was called catalepsy since, to the first investigators, it resembled experimentally (bulbocapnine) induced catatonia. Some believe that the cataleptic potency of psychoactive drugs is directly proportionate to their extrapyramidal sign producing effect, which in turn is directly proportionate to the clinically seen neuroleptic syndrome characterized by psychomotor slowing, emotional quieting and affective indifference.

While the correlation between the catalepsy producing effect and therapeutic potency applies to a number of phenothiazine drugs, the beneficial action of some of these compounds in different psychiatric disorders is more closely related to the influence of the substance on conditioned reflexes. Unlike the barbiturates, which, above a certain dosage, suppress the response to both unconditional and conditional stimuli, phenothiazine drugs exert a selective inhibitory effect on the conditioned (*e.g.*, avoidance) response. Furthermore, they also interfere with the acquisition of new conditioned responses and accelerate the extinction of the nonreinforced ones already acquired. Since different psychopathologies have different conditional reflex profiles, these particular properties of phenothiazines can be applied in indicating treatment for psychiatric patients.

In other pharmacological experiments it has been shown that CPZ increases sociability and decreases defensive hostility in cats and hamsters and also decreases excitement in hamsters and aggressive hostility in cats.

b. Human Studies

In humans there is evidence that CPZ reduces vigilance (as measured by the continuous performance and pursuit rotor tests), although it does not affect intellectual activities, such as digit symbol substitution. Trifluoperazine, on the other hand, causes significant decrease in, or impaired performance on, the Critical Flicker Fusion Frequency, After-Image Disappearance Limen and Tapping Speed tests and a significant improvement in Digits Backwards and in Cancellation accuracy. These results imply that this representative of the piperazinylalkyl phenothiazine category selectively decreases perceptual intake and psychomotor speed and at the same time increases attention, including concentration and vigilance (Lehmann and Knight, 1958).

In studies exploring the action of various phenothiazines on selected physiological and performance functions in normal males, DiMascio *et al.* (1963) found that the aminoalkyls at peak time of action produce confusion, impaired speed and performance on the cognitive tests, along with hypotension and miosis. On the other hand, the piperazines had the opposite effects, *i.e.*, improved performance on motor tests and cognitive tasks.

B. CLINICAL DATA

1. Indications and Contraindications

a. Indications

Phenothiazine drugs are successfully administered in numerous pathological conditions. Besides the psychiatric indications, they are frequently prescribed as antihistaminic (promethazine, parathiazine), antipruritic (trimeprazine) and antiparkinsonian drugs (ethopropazine, diethazine). The antiemetic property (especially of the piperazinylalkyl derivatives) is widely utilized in the treatment of nausea and vomiting, particularly in cases of uremia, brain tumor, radiation sickness, carcinomatosis, hyperemesis gravidarum, gastroenteritis and obstructive gastrointestinal lesions. The same antiemetic effect is utilized to combat the nausea of postconcussion syndrome, nitrogen mustard or antibiotic therapy. Their analgesic action is used in the potentiation of the effect of narcotics in malignancies or in combatting the severe pain associated, for example, with terminal carcinoma or herpes zoster. While phenothiazine drugs have some local anesthetic effect, they are more often used in general anesthesia as both pre- and postanesthetic medications. There are also reports on their successful use in hiccoughs and porphyria; phenothiazine drugs combat the pain and nervous manifestations of the latter.

The psychiatric indications of phenothiazines range from functional and organic psychoses through the neuroses to personality disorders and mental deficiency.

i. Functional Psychoses. *α. Schizophrenias.* The particular effectiveness of these drugs was observed in the group of schizophrenias. Although well designed, systematically conducted studies could not reveal significant differences in the therapeutic efficacy of chemically different phenothiazine compounds (*e.g.*, CPZ, prochlorperazine, trifluoperazine and perphenazine), there might be a differential activity in the respect that the aminoalkyl derivatives seem to be especially effective in agitated schizophrenics with florid delusions and hallucinations and still capable of showing plenty of emotional response, while the dull, apathetic, deteriorated cases may respond better to the piperazinylalkyl compounds. It appears that, in general, the best over-all response is achieved in paranoid cases and that in catatonic and hebephrenic patients the prognosis gradually worsens with the duration of the illness. A generally better response to phenothiazines has been described in females with catatonic excitement and in chronic patients who were predominantly aggressive and manneristic than in males with catatonic stupor or with prevailing apathy (Kalinowsky and Hoch, 1961; and Sargant and Slater, 1963).

Denham (1965) asserts that the value of phenothiazines in the treatment of the acute (or acutely relapsing) schizophrenic cannot be disputed. He maintains that with an effective dosage remissions are obtainable within 10 days to 3 weeks. Furthermore, according to Denham (1965), prolonged follow-up seems to contradict those who state that the outcome of schizophrenia after 5 years is the same irrespective of treatment.

Others consider that the time needed for remission is somewhat longer. For example, according to Benson and Schiele (1962), it requires 8 to 12 weeks. During this period phenothiazines at first relieve emotional tension, agitation and excitement. Consequently, fading of the delusions and hallucinations may occur. Finally, they facilitate the development of a better personal integration and social adaptation.

β. Manic-Depressive Psychosis. In manic-depressive psychosis, phenothiazines are successfully used in the alleviation of the manic syndrome, while in depression, with the exception of methotrimeprazine and possibly thioridazine, they are mainly used for controlling agitation.

At a symposium on The Scientific Basis of Drug Therapy in Psychiatry at St. Bartholomew's Hospital in London (Marks and Pare, 1965), Brook (1965) raised the question whether phenothiazines should be avoided in purely depressive illness. The rationale behind his query was Pletscher's (1965) demonstration of a "central amino block" under the influence of these drugs and consequently the production of depressive manifestations. In the discussion, Hinton (1965) gave an account of experiments in which he compared the use of perphenazine with a barbiturate and placebo in a group of outpatients manifesting depression with anxiety. He found that both active substances helped anxiety but only perphenazine had a therapeutic effect on depression. Brodie (1965) has offered an explanation for Hinton's (1959) findings. As a rule, tertiary amines of the CPZ type lose their sedative effect upon removal of an *N*-methyl group from their structure, which may result in a chemical with antidepressant properties. Since this demethylation does take place under normal circumstances in the liver, he offered this as a partial answer to Hinton's (1965) observations. Denham (1965), however, cannot believe that these differences are as simple as dropping the methyl group, although he too had cases in whom phenothiazines exerted an antidepressant action.

ii. Organic Brain Syndromes. Beneficial effects with these drugs have been described in epileptic and clouded states, in psychoses due to trauma, eclampsia, infection, toxic agents (*e.g.*, alcohol), drug withdrawal (*e.g.*, morphine, barbiturate), cardiovascular disease and thyrotoxicosis. There are also favorable reports in cerebral arteriosclerosis, senile dementia and Huntington's chorea. Phenothiazines block lysergic acid diethylamide (LSG_{25}) or mescaline-induced psychoses.

iii. Psychoneuroses. There is no general concensus on the usefulness of phenothiazines in the treatment of the various psychoneuroses. Rees and Lambert (1955), for example, found that CPZ in small doses often exerts a favorable effect in these cases within a short period of time. Merry *et al.* (1957), on the other hand, reported equivocal and Raymond *et al.* (1957) negative findings with the same drug in similar cases. Similarly, while Denham (1965) found perphenazine (as opposed to CPZ) useful in anxiety, Patridge (1965) considered it ineffective in the psychoneuroses.

There is some general agreement on the usefulness of phenothiazines in some cases of tension and anxiety states, although some patients with anxiety, anxiety hysteria and neurotic depression respond poorly. The anxiety symptoms of asthma are often alleviated by phenothiazines. Some obsessive patients benefit from phenothiazine drugs, whereas others become depressed or show an increase in their obsessional symptoms. Chronic hypochondriasis remains unaffected by treatment, and hysterical symptoms may become more pronounced and bizarre.

iv. Personality Disorders. There is even more disagreement on the use of phenothiazines in personality disorders. While it has been stated repeatedly that personality disorders are unresponsive to these drugs, there is evidence of the therapeutic effectiveness of different phenothiazines, especially CPZ, in postencephalitic personality changes and of prochlorperazine in disturbed mental defectives, and quite recently there have been some claims that propericiazine may be particularly useful in character disorders.

At the Leeds Symposium on Behavioral Disorders (Jenner, 1965), this particular application of propericiazine was extensively discussed. In a review of the accumulated data, Ban (1965) reported that in general there was agreement among the investigators on the therapeutic effectiveness of this substance in the behavioral disorders of children (Ernst *et al.*, 1964; Gayral *et al.*, 1963; and Pommé *et al.*, 1963), in the character disorders of adults (Berthier *et al.*, 1963; Doussot *et al.*, 1963; Millon *et al.*, 1963; Verdeau-Paillès, 1963; and Volmat *et al.*, 1963) and in the personality disorders of the aged (Pommé *et al.*, 1963). On the other hand, findings in the character disorders of epileptics (Gayral *et al.*, 1963; Oulès, 1963; Grambert *et al.*, 1963; and Verdeau-Paillès, 1963) and of the mentally retarded (Gayral *et al.*, 1963; and Grambert *et al.*, 1963) remain equivocal.

b. Contraindications

There are relatively few absolute contraindications of phenothiazine treatment. These are comatose states, history of agranulocytosis, infections in general (but not tuberculosis) and acute alcohol intoxication. Some consider extrapyramidal, liver and cardiovascular diseases, including arteriosclerosis and arterial hypertension, as relative contraindications, although most arteriosclerotic psychiatric patients show remarkable improvement on CPZ treatment. Phenothiazine drugs should be administered cautiously to hysterical and depressed patients, to subjects with endocrine and gastrointestinal disturbances and to those with impaired renal functions.

There is no evidence that these drugs should not be administered during pregnancy or in the period of lactation, nor has any carcinogenic effect of phenothiazine drugs been reported.

2. Therapy with Phenothiazine Drugs Alone and in Combination with Other Treatments

a. Phenothiazines Alone

i. Dosage. While the therapeutic dosage range of each phenothiazine drug differs, it generally holds true that, in the treatment of psychotics, the daily dosage is three times as high as that for psychoneurotics. The latter receives a daily dosage which is approximately four times as high as that which successfully controls nausea or vomiting. For example, the actual average dosages for CPZ are 600 mg. (for psychotics), 200 mg. (for psychoneurotics) and 50 mg. (for nausea or vomiting). Taking CPZ as a unit, the approximate activity of the different phenothiazine drugs of the aminoalkyl and piperidylalkyl groups on a milligram per kilogram basis is as follows: promazine and methoxypromazine are somewhat less active, thioridazine is approximately the same, while triflupromazine is twice as active as CPZ. Consequently, promazine, methoxypromazine and thioridazine are administered in the same (or higher) dosages, and triflupromazine, in one-half the daily dosage of CPZ.

The piperazinylalkyls in general have a greater activity than CPZ on a milligram per kilogram basis. This is particularly true for the compounds with a halogen substitution in position 2 on the phenothiazine ring. Thus, while acetophenazine and carphenazine are only twice as active as CPZ, thiopropazate and prochlorperazine are four times, perphenazine six times, trifluoperazine ten times and fluphenazine and thioproperazine twenty times as active on a milligram per kilogram basis.

These dosages apply to oral administration, usually given in equally divided doses three or four times a day in the acute period of the illness and once or twice a day (preferably at night) as maintenance therapy.

ii. Routes of Administration. Besides the safest and most common oral route, phenothiazines are given intramuscularly and infrequently intravenously. For intramuscular administration it has been noted that a dose given parenterally is about three or four times as potent as the same dose given orally. It seems that for an acutely disturbed psychotic female, 50 mg. of CPZ given intramuscularly three or four times daily are sufficient, while for a male about double this amount is required. CPZ injections are rather painful and have to be given deep in the gluteal muscles since subcutaneous administration may cause necrosis. The femoral muscles may be the second choice, while administration into the deltoid should preferably be avoided. It is recommended that the patient, particularly the elderly, stay in a reclining position for at least half an hour after parenteral phenothiazine administration. Most of the phenothiazine drugs are available as tablets, elixir, suppositories, etc., and recently, fluphenazine has been marketed in a sustained release form in which one injection is therapeutically effective for 2 weeks. A sustained release CPZ spansule has been available for some time.

Phenothiazines, especially CPZ and promazine, are occasionally given intravenously. Usually 25 to 50 mg. of the drug are diluted in 500 to 1000 mg. of physiological saline and administered over a 3- to 4-hour period. Besides the common periphlebitis, the possible hazards of this route of administration include critical blood pressure changes and even fatal complications. Since CPZ reverses epinephrine effect, in case of hypotensive reaction, adrenaline administration should be avoided and noradrenaline used instead.

iii. Treatment Procedures. The most

frequently used clinical procedure is continuous treatment. As the initial dose, one-third of the average daily dosage is usually given. From this starting dose, the dosage of the drug is progressively increased until there is a beneficial response in psychopathological symptoms or troublesome side-effects occur. Others recommend raising the dosage until the onset of a fine tremor (easily recognized by a handwriting test). Sometimes, particularly in severely agitated, uncooperative patients, treatment begins with parenteral administration of the drug, which can usually be replaced by oral drug administration within 3 days. If there is any doubt whether the patient is taking his medication, the amount of phenothiazine ingested during the past 48 hours can be indicated by a simple colorimetric urine test (Forrest *et al.*, 1957, 1958, 1959, 1960). In case of hospitalization, besides the psychopathological indices, the return to normal of a patient's body weight serves as a guiding point for the time of discharge. Others put more emphasis on the increased ascorbic acid levels in the blood, and others again on the so-called "insular vagolytic" effects, *i.e.*, slight mydriasis and dry mouth, which are usually correlated with clinical improvement.

Discontinuous treatment with thioproperazine was found most effective in chronic, intractable schizophrenics and in manic patients. This is conducted with doses from three times 5 mg., raised on alternate days to three times 10, 30 and, if necessary, even three times 40 or 50 mg. In other words, dosage is increased on alternate days until a continuous state of hypertonus of the muscles is produced. After 5 days of muscular hypertonia, the drug is withdrawn for 5 days, and then the procedure is repeated. On the average, three courses of treatment are given (Delay, 1957; Denham and Carrick, 1961; and Ban *et al.*, 1962).

iv. Duration of Treatment. The duration of phenothiazine administration depends on the condition for which the drug is administered. For example, in psychoneuroses, with the exception of therapy-resistant, chronic obsessive cases, the drug should not be given after the symptoms which necessitated its administration remit. Schizophrenic patients, on the other hand, should be kept on a maintenance dosage, which, with each of the compounds, is about one-half or less of the daily dosage they received in the acute period of their illness. The rule of thumb is that after the first episode a schizophrenic patient should be maintained on medication for at least a 1-year period, after the second for at least 2 to 3 years and thereafter for an indefinite time. Early cessation of therapy leads to relapse 8 to 12 weeks after discontinuation of the drug in the majority of the cases.

It is fortunate that phenothiazine drugs can be taken over an extended period. Although the initial drowsiness and orthostatic hypotension which are characteristically present with some of these drugs usually disappear within a short period of time, the response of the organism to the drug otherwise remains unaffected. In spite of the withdrawal syndrome—tension, fear, restlessness, vomiting, insomnia, perspiration—which is attributed to excessive adrenaline liberation after abrupt discontinuation of treatment, there is no psychological dependence on phenothiazine drugs.

In the course of treatment, pathological arousal phenomena usually respond within the first 2 weeks of treatment, and affective psychopathology within the first 2 months; mental integration improves only after a longer period.

b. Phenothiazine Drugs in Combination with Other Treatments

i. Physical Treatments. Both electroconvulsive and insulin therapies are occasionally combined with phenothiazine administration. It was once believed that the addition of phenothiazines in general and CPZ in particular resulted in a better and quicker recovery than treatment with insulin or ECT alone; in addition, the opinion was that, by bringing the schizophrenic process to a rapid halt, the change of chronicity or deterioration of personality was lessened. More recently, there has been increasing evidence that phenothiazines alone are able to achieve the same results in most cases. The majority of therapists now agree that only in drug therapy resistant patients is the combination of phenothiazines and insulin or ECT treatment indicated. In these cases it should be borne in mind that the hypotensive action of CPZ is intensified by ECT, and that cerebral seizures and confusional and hypoglycemic reactions are more frequent in combination with insulin than if the latter is given alone. It is therefore common practice to omit one dose of the drug prior to ECT and to maintain the patient in a lying position for at least 30 minutes after consciousness is regained.

ii. Pharmacological. Although it is known that phenothiazines potentiate the effects of other central nervous system depressant drugs and therefore should only be combined with extreme caution, they are frequently given together with sedative, hypnotic and minor tranquilizer compounds. For example, the combination of CPZ and amobarbital is used in sleep treatment (continuous narcosis), while Equazine (meprobamate and promazine) is quite extensively used in the psychoneuroses. In spite of the fact that phenothiazines should be given for only the shortest possible period of time during treatment with antidepressants, there are several combinations of phenothiazines and antidepressants on the market: *e.g.*, Tofranazine (promazine and imipramine); Etrafon and Triavil (perphenazine and amitriptyline); and Parstelin (trifluoperazine and tranylcypromine). Similarly, in spite of the known adverse effects that antiparkinsonian drugs have on psychotic patients, these drugs are quite often given beyond the period necessary to counteract the extrapyramidal manifestations encountered in the course of phenothiazine treatment.

The advantage of adding a phenothiazine to the anticonvulsant medication of epileptics outweighs in certain cases the disadvantage of the relative lowering of the convulsive threshold.

3. Adverse Reactions and Their Treatment

a. Adverse Reactions

In the course of phenothiazine treatment a number of reactions occur, the nature and severity of which depend on the range of activity of the drug. These adverse reactions may affect any organ or organ system, causing either mild discomfort or severe pathological changes that call for termination of treatment. According to the nature of the undesired manifestation, adverse phenothiazine reactions are classed as psychiatric, neurological, autonomic, endocrine, ophthalmological, cardiovascular, bronchopulmonary, gastrointestinal, genitourinary, hepatobiliary, metabolic, hematological and dermatological.

i. Psychiatric. These range from reduction of spontaneous activity to severe toxic confusional states, the incidence of the latter being approximately 1 per cent of treated cases. More frequent are sleep disturbances, transient drowsiness in the initial period of treatment with piperidylalkyl and aminoalkyl derivatives and, paradoxically, insomnia and vivid dreams, particularly in neurotic patients with the piperazinylalkyl compounds. Under the influence of phenothiazine drugs, manic or catatonic excitement may turn into depression or stupor, respectively (or less frequently, catatonic stupor may turn into excitement). Although some of these drugs, *e.g.*, methotrimeprazine or to a lesser extent thioridazine, may be therapeutic for depressed patients, others, especially CPZ, may cause depression in a considerable number of cases. Similarly, while several phenothiazines have a definite beneficial effect on apathetic schizophrenics, others may induce lassitude, lack of initiative and even apathy itself. Motor restlessness, anxiety and jitters are frequent when drugs of the piperazinylalkyl group are administered.

ii. Neurological. Most frequently discussed of all the reactions induced by phenothiazine drugs are the extrapyramidal manifestations. Whether the occurrence of extrapyramidal signs favors therapy has not yet been unanimously accepted. Extrapyramidal signs range in severity from akathisia, usually described as motor restlessness, through dyskinesia to parkinsonism. The dyskinetic syndromes are usually early and transitory manifestations, which readily respond to treatment. They range from speech and swallowing difficulties to torsion spasms, oculogyric crisis, torticollis and choreiform movements. Less responsive to treatment is phenothiazine-induced parkinsonism, which occurs after a more prolonged period of treatment. It develops twice as often in women as in men, it is always preceded by micrographia and manifests itself in diminished drive, lassitude, rigidity, tremor, salivation, greasy skin, etc. A number of irreversible cases have recently been described, all induced by chronic high dosage administration of phenothiazine drugs.

While extrapyramidal signs are very frequent, phenothiazine-induced pyramidal damage is extremely rare. In between these extremes, cerebral seizures may occur in certain predisposed cases after the first administration of the drug but more often after a sudden increase in dosage.

Paresthesia during phenothiazine therapy has also been described.

iii. Autonomic. Characteristic autonomic effects are depression of the sympathetic nervous system activity and the inability to react to stress, *i.e.*, the failure of the autonomic reflexes to raise blood pressure and increase cardiac output. Troublesome reactions are nasal congestion and dry mouth, and a dangerous reaction is the hypotensive—particularly the orthostatic hypotension producing—action of these drugs. Knowledge of this effect has now virtually eliminated fatal complications in hypertensive and arteriosclerotic cases, which sometimes occurred in the early days of phenothiazine therapy.

iv. Endocrine. The most frequently seen endocrinological effects are amenorrhea, swollen breasts, lactation and glycosuria. Reduced sexual urge in the male, increased sexual urge in the female, pseudopregnancy and infertility are also well known phenomena. Phenothiazines decrease adrenocorticotropic and antidiuretic hormone secretions, exert a thiouracil-like action and reduce urinary gonadotropin, estrogen and progestin levels. They block ovulation and suppress the estrus cycle while maintaining the decidual reactions (Jarvik, 1965).

v. Ophthalmological. Blurred vision, lachrymation and keratoconjunctivitis have been known since the beginning of the phenothiazine era. The most severe effect, pigmentary retinopathy, is rare and is seen mainly with thioridazine. More recently, centrally located stellate-form cataracts, corneal opacities and conjunctival pigmentation have been described in a rather large number of cases. The visual acuity of the affected patients, however, is not seriously interfered with.

vi. Cardiovascular. Adverse cardiovascular effects range from redness and flushing due to cutaneous vasodilatation through cardiac failure with edema to syncope and cardiovascular collapse. Mainly after parenteral administration, tachycardia is frequently recorded, while sinus arrhythmia occurs only occasionally. A quinidine-like effect has also been described with varying frequency. Only with thioridazine, however, does it occur to the degree that may warrant particular care in the therapeutic application of this drug in the higher dosage ranges (Ban and St. Jean, 1964).

vii. Bronchopulmonary. Asthmatic attacks were reported to occur in patients previously free of this condition. In others, the frequency and severity of asthmatic attacks were seen to be increased. The incidence of infections—including bronchopulmonary—is higher in patients on phenothiazines, and the danger is magnified because these drugs may mask the symptoms of infection.

viii. Gastrointestinal. Besides nausea and heartburn, depression of gastrointestinal secretion has been described as an adverse effect of phenothiazine treatment. Constipation is a rather common reaction, which has been known since the very first clinical trials with CPZ. Simultaneous administration of CPZ and antiparkinsonian (parasympatholytic) drugs (particularly if added to tricyclic antidepressants) increases constipation and has led in a number of cases to paralytic ileus (Warnes *et al.*, 1967).

ix. Genitourinary. Besides depressing pituitary antidiuretic hormone secretion, phenothiazine drugs inhibit tubular reabsorption, resulting in a diuretic effect. In some cases an increased frequency of micturition has been described. Inability to ejaculate occurs more frequently with thioridazine than with any of the other phenothiazine drugs.

x. Hepatobiliary. Jaundice—the intrahepatic, obstructive type—occurs in 0.1 to 4 per cent of all phenothiazine-treated cases, usually 2 to 4 weeks after commencement of treatment. This is considered to be an allergic reaction, which is supported by the fact that it is preceded by eosinophilia. Dark urine, pale stool and raised alkaline phosphatase levels are characteristic of phenothiazine-induced jaundice. Chronic alcoholism, pregnancy and hypoproteinemic states predispose to phenothiazine-induced jaundice, which also has a higher incidence with some phenothiazines, *e.g.*, CPZ, than with others.

xi. Metabolic. There is usually increased appetite and weight gain during phenothiazine treatment. Occasionally the first symptoms of diabetes mellitus occur, or symptoms of existing diabetes are aggravated. Altered copper metabolism was discovered in 1956, but its practical and theoretical implications have only recently been investigated (Greiner and Nicolson, 1964).

xii. Hematological. Agranulocytosis occurs in 0.001 per cent of phenothiazine-treated cases. Although it is considered to be an allergic reaction, it starts with sore throat, pyrexia and lymphadenitis at any time (or at any dosage) in the course of treatment.

xiii. Dermatological. Among the numerous dermatological effects, pruritis, dermatitis, maculopapular eruptions, erythema multiforme and urticaria may occur approximately 2 weeks after commencing treatment. There are also well known allergic manifestations, *i.e.*, swelling, itching, angioneurotic edema and, not infrequently, contact dermatitis. Photosensitivity to CPZ was one of the first adverse effects recognized after the introduction of this drug, while the purple skin pigmentation which occurs during long term, high dosage phenothiazine—especially CPZ—administration, although known previously, has only recently attracted widespread attention (Ban and Lehmann, 1965).

xiv. Overdosage. Overdosage results in drowsiness, hypotension, tachycardia, tachypnea, hypothermia, extrapyramidal manifestations, absent tendon reflexes, severe stomatitis, convulsions and coma.

b. Treatment of Adverse Reactions

The physician's response to an adverse drug reaction depends on the dynamics of the situation in which the reaction occurs. If the reaction is considered to be dangerous or is seriously interfering with the desired therapeutic action of the drug, a different decision is made than if the therapeutic efficiency of the drug is greater than the problems posed by the adverse drug effect. Adverse effects are evaluated to determine whether they call for discontinuation of treatment; discontinuation of the drug and the substitution of another medication (which belongs to the same chemical group or to another chemical group with similar therapeutic indications); reduction of dosage; maintaining (or reducing) dosage and the addition of adjuvant medication; or acceptance of the unwanted reaction and continuation of treatment.

Discontinuation of treatment is called for in cases of pigmentary retinopathy, agranulocytosis and jaundice, while acceptance of the adverse effect is suggested in mild cases of nasal congestion, dry mouth and hypotension. Replacement therapy is instituted in toxic psychosis, endocrine disturbances and quinidine-like ECG changes.

Persistent drowsiness, extrapyramidal signs, severe hypotension, nonspecific ECG changes and cerebral seizures usually respond to reduction in dosage, while constipation, insomnia, severe extrapyramidal manifestations, recurring cerebral seizures, disturbing dry mouth or nasal congestion, photosensitivity or skin pigmentation, and cataract or corneal opacities which interfere with vision should be treated with adjuvant medication.

In the management of overdosage, gastric lavage, bed rest, analeptics, noradrenaline (but not adrenaline), paraldehyde or barbiturates are used for the symptomatic control of the varied clinical manifestations.

4. The Use of Phenothiazines in Medical Practice

The choice of drug in treatment is determined by the pathological symptom profile of the patient; response to previous drug treatment; physical condition; the experience of the physician with particular compounds; the experience of others as reported in the literature; and the closeness of supervision (Kline and Lehmann, 1962).

Of the aminoalkyls, CPZ is probably still the drug most frequently used. Particular attention should be paid to the hypotensive, photosensitivity and mood-depressant effects of this drug. While the mood-depressant effect of CPZ is eliminated in methotrimeprazine, this drug produces more intensive drowsiness than the parent compound. In the control of alcohol withdrawal and for patients with impaired liver functions, promazine is frequently used. Other drugs of this category, *e.g.*, triflupromazine or methoxypromazine, are less frequently prescribed than CPZ, methotrimeprazine or promazine.

Among the piperazinylalkyls, prochlorperazine, trifluoperazine and perphenazine are the ones most extensively used, both in outpatient neurotics and in chronically hospitalized psychotics. Thiopropazate is given somewhat less often. The beneficial effect of these drugs on apathy makes them particularly desirable in the treatment of institutionalized schizophrenics, while their relatively strong extrapyramidal sign producing action frequently causes alarm in outpatients. While carphenazine and acetophenazine are the least potent and probably the least frequently prescribed in this group of drugs, the marked extrapyramidal manifestations induced by thioproperazine (and, according to some, also by fluphenazine) restrict the administration of this very effective drug to hospital treatment.

Of the two available piperidylalkyls, thioridazine is the more popular compound. There is, however, no conclusive evidence that it produces less extrapyramidal signs, drowsiness or depression than methotrimeprazine (an aminoalkyl), while a higher incidence of pigmentary retinopathy and inability to ejaculate has been reported with thioridazine than with any of the other phenothiazine drugs. Thioridazine is probably the only currently available phenothiazine which in the high therapeutic dosages may produce ECG changes with possibly serious consequences.

Among the other phenothiazines, propericiazine is increasingly used in the management of behavior disorders, promethazine is successfully used as an antihistaminic and is used in the treatment of certain psychoneurotic patients, while trimeprazine is used not only as an antipruritic but also as an antiparkinsonian agent.

There is no doubt that the introduction of the phenothiazine drugs contributed greatly not only to the changes that have taken place in mental hospitals over the past decade but also to the reunion of psychiatry with the other fields of medical science and practice.

SUMMARY

The introduction of the phenothiazines has brought about far-reaching changes in the treatment of psychiatric patients. A large number of formerly untreatable patients have become accessible to hospital treatment, while others, who would once have been hospitalized, can now be treated in their own homes.

The most significant results have occurred in the treatment of schizophrenic patients. Administration of phenothiazines in adequate dosage over a sufficiently long period of time can, on the one hand, bring the schizophrenic process to a halt in a high percentage of cases and, on the other hand, can improve chronically hospitalized inactive and apathetic patients to the point where they can participate in rehabilitation programs. The administration of these drugs may prevent the admission of a great number of patients to psychiatric hospitals and also makes it possible to protect a large number of patients from relapse.

Of the two major phenothiazine groups used in psychiatric treatment, the aminoalkyl group is particularly useful in treating acute schizophrenic episodes and manic and delirious states. The piperazinylalkyl group is most effective in the chronic, withdrawn type of patient.

The mental changes induced by these drugs are but one aspect of the influence which they exert on the entire organism. In addition to their therapeutic or desired effects, phenothiazines also have other effects—sometimes definitely undesired—of varying consequences. Among these, the most common are the extrapyramidal signs (more prominent with the piperazinylalkyl derivatives), which some believe to mark the onset of therapeutic action. This adverse effect can easily be handled by the transient administration of antiparkinsonian drugs. On the other hand, agranulocytosis should be an absolute indication for termination of treatment. In between these extremes is hypotension, in particular, orthostatic hypotension (more frequent with the aminoalkyl derivatives), which in several elderly hypertensive arteriosclerotic cases has led to serious consequences, and which, because of the epinephrine-reversing effect of phenothiazines, is aggravated and not relieved by adrenaline administration.

A succinct clinical appraisal of phenothiazines was given in a brief comment by Rogers (1965): "I come from a hospital which has been substantially transformed by the use of the phenothiazines. I do not believe that social factors are the whole answer. I can think of a number of patients who have lived for some time in a ward in which the environment has been substantially similar apart from varying degrees of therapeutic social pressures. Among these patients in this relatively static environment some may be found in whom there is a critical dose level of phenothiazines. The astute sister will notice deterioration in these patients when the dose is reduced below this level. Such experience suggests that it is not only the social environment but also the chemical environment that has a part to play.

"The other point which I feel merits more attention is the variation between patients in their response to different members of the phenothiazine group. One man's meat is another man's poison among the phenothiazine drugs."

REFERENCES

BAN, T. A.: Comparative clinical study of the antipsychotic properties of haloperidol versus permitil. Symposium internazionale sull'haloperidol e triperidol. (Inst. Luso Farmaco d'Italia, Milano, 1962.)

BAN, T. A.: Annual report of the research department, Douglas Hospital, Verdun, 1965.

BAN, T. A.: Current psychiatric therapies, Vol. IV (book review). Canad. Psychiat. Ass. J., *10:* 514 (1965).

BAN, T. A.: Human pharmacology and systematic clinical studies with a new phenothiazine. In: Proceedings of the Leeds Symposium on behavioral disorders (ed., Jenner, F. A.). (May and Baker, Dagenham, 1965.)

BAN, T. A.: The action of neuroleptic drugs: a psychiatric, neurologic and pharmacological investigation (book review). Canad. Psychiat. Ass. J., *10:* 320 (1965).

BAN, T. A., AND LEHMANN, H. E.: Skin pigmentation, a rare side effect of chlorpromazine, and a hypothesis concerning one of the mechanisms of its development. Canad. Psychiat. Ass. J., *10:* 112 (1965).

BAN, T. A., AND LEVY, L.: Physiological patterns: a diagnostic test procedure based on the conditioned reflex method. J. Neuropsychiat., *2:* 228 (1961).

BAN, T. A., PAPATHOMOPULOS, E., AND SCHWARZ, L.: Clinical studies with thioproperazine (majeptil). Compr. Psychiat., *3:* 284 (1962).

BAN, T. A., AND ST. JEAN, A.: The effect of phenothiazines on the electrocardiogram. Canad. Med. Ass. J., *91:* 537 (1964).

BECKMAN, H.: Drugs, their nature, action and use. (Saunders, Philadelphia, 1958.)

BENSON, W. M., AND SCHIELE, B. C.: Tranquillizing and antidepressive drugs. (Charles C Thomas, Springfield, 1962.)

BERNTHSEN, A. (1883): In: LEAR, E.: Chemistry and applied pharmacology of tranquilizers. (Charles C Thomas, Springfield, 1966.)

BERTHIER, C., *et al.*: Etude clinique d'un nouveau neuroleptique le 8909 R.P. (Paper presented at the Sixty-first Congress of French Speaking Psychiatrists and Neurologists, Nancy, 1963.)

BRODIE, B. B.: Discussion. In: The scientific basis of drug therapy in psychiatry (eds., Marks, J., and Pare, C. M. B.) (Pergamon Press, Oxford, 1965.)

BROOK, M. F.: Discussion. In: The scientific basis of drug therapy in psychiatry (eds., Marks, J., and Pare, C. M. B.) (Pergamon Press, Oxford, 1965.)

DELAY, J.: Les medicaments neuroleptiques, chimiothérapie des psychoses. (O.M.S. groups d'etudes sur les medicaments psychotropes, Geneve, 1957.)

DENHAM, J.: Clinical use of phenothiazines. In: The scientific basis of drug therapy in psychiatry (eds., Marks, J., and Pare, C. M. B.). (Pergamon Press, Oxford, 1965.)

DENHAM, J.: Discussion. In: The scientific basis of drug therapy in psychiatry (eds., Marks, J., and Pare, C. M. B.). (Pergamon Press, Oxford, 1965.)

DENHAM, J., AND CARRICK, D. J.: Therapeutic value of thioproperazine and the importance of the associated neurological disturbances. J. Ment. Sci., *107:* 326 (1961).

DIMASCIO, A., *et al.*: The psychopharmacology of phenothiazine compounds: A comparative study of the effects of chlorpromazine, trifluoperazine and perphenazine in normal males. J. Nerv. Ment. Dis., *136:* 15 (1963).

Doussot, A., *et al.*: Données expérimentales sur l'action clinique d'un dérivé cyane de la phénothiazine, la propericiazine (8909 R.P.). Rev. Neuropsychiat. l'Ouest, *1:* 47 (1963).

Einhorn, A. (1891): In: The pharmacological basis of therapeutics (eds., Goodman, L. S., and Gilman, A.). (MacMillan, New York, 1956.)

Ernst, J., *et al.*: Intérêt du neuleptil (8909 R.P.) en psychiatrie infantile. (Paper presented at the Sixty-second Congress of French-Speaking Psychiatrists and Neurologists, Marseilles, 1964.)

Forrest, F. M., and Forrest, I. S.: A simple test for the detection of chlorpromazine in urine. Amer. J. Psychiat., *113:* 931 (1957).

Forrest, F. M., Forrest, I. S., and Mason, A. S.: A rapid urinary test for chlorpromazine, promazine and pacatal: a supplementary report. Amer. J. Psychiat., *114:* 931 (1958).

Forrest, F. M., Forrest, I. S., and Mason, A. S.: A rapid semi-quantitative urine color test for piperazine-linked phenothiazine drugs (compazine, trilafon and analogous compounds). Amer. J. Psychiat., *116:* 549 (1959).

Forrest, F. M., Forrest, I. S., and Mason, A. S.: A rapid urine color test for triflupromazine (vesprin). Amer. J. Psychiat., *115:* 114 (1959).

Forrest, I. S., and Forrest, F. M.: A rapid urine color test for imipramine (tofranil, Geigy). Amer. J. Psychiat., *116:* 840 (1960).

Forrest, I. S., and Forrest, F. M.: Urine color test for the detection of phenothiazine compounds. Clin. Chem., *6:* 11 (1960).

Gayral, M. L., *et al.*: Note sur l'emploi de la propériciazine, 8909 R.P. (neuleptil) pour le treatment des troubles du caractère chez les enfants et les adolescents. (Paper presented at the Sixty-first Congress of French-Speaking Psychiatrists and Neurologists, Nancy, 1963).

Gayral, M. L., *et al.*: Treatment of depressed mental states with amitriptyline. Ann. Medico-Psychol., *121:* 447 (1963).

Goodman, L. S., and Gilman, A.: The pharmacological basis of therapeutics. (Macmillan, New York, 1956.)

Gordon, M., Craig, P. N., and Zirkle, C. L.: Molecular modification in the development of phenothiazine drugs. In: Molecular modification in drug design (ed., Gould, R. F.). (American Chemical Society, Washington, 1964.)

Gothelf, B., and Karczmar, A. G. (1963): In: Richter, D.: Mode of action of the phenothiazines. In: The scientific basis of drug therapy in psychiatry (eds., Marks, J., and Pare, C. M. B.). (Pergamon Press, Oxford, 1965.)

Gould, R. F. (ed.): Molecular modification in drug design. (American Chemical Society, Washington, 1964.)

Grambert, G, *et al.*: Etude clinique du 8909 R.P. à l'hopital psychiatrique. (Paper presented at the Sixty-first Congress of French-Speaking Psychiatrists and Neurologists, Nancy, 1963.)

Grambert, G., *et al.*: Résultants cliniques obtemus par le 8909 R.P. dans diverses affections mentales en milieu psychiatrique. (Paper presented at the Sixty-first Congress of French-Speaking Psychiatrists and Neurologists, Nancy, 1963.)

Greiner, A. C., and Nicolson, G. A.: Pigment deposition in viscera associated with prolonged chlorpromazine therapy. Canad. Med. Ass. J., *91:* 627 (1964).

Grollman, A.: Pharmacology and therapeutics. (Lea and Febiger, Philadelphia, 1965.)

Himwich, H. E.: Discussion of papers on basic observations of new psychopharmacological agents. Psychiat. Res. Rep. Amer. Psychiat. Ass., *4:* 24 (1956).

Himwich, H. E.: Anatomy and physiology of emotions. In: The scientific basis of drug therapy in psychiatry (eds., Marks, J., and Pare, C. M. B.). (Pergamon Press, Oxford, 1965.)

Himwich, H. E.: The effect of frenquel on EEG changes produced by LSD-25 and mescaline. In: Lysergic acid diethylamide and mescaline in experimental psychiatry (ed., Cholden, L.). (Grune and Stratton, New York, 1956.)

Hinton, J. M.: A comparison of perphenazine (fentazine), sodium amylobarbitone and a placebo in anxious and depressed out-patients. J. Ment. Sci., *105:* 872 (1959).

Hinton, J. M.: Discussion. In: The scientific basis of drug therapy in psychiatry (eds., Marks, J., and Pare, C. M. B.). (Pergamon Press, Oxford, 1965.)

Jarvik, M. E.: Drugs used in the treatment of psychiatric disorders. In: The pharmacological basis of therapeutics (eds., Goodman, L. S., and Gilman, A.). (Macmillan, Toronto, 1965.)

Jenner, F. A. (ed.): Proceedings of the Leeds symposium. (May and Baker, Dagenham, 1965.)

Kalinowsky, L. B., and Hoch, P. H.: Somatic treatments in psychiatry. (Grune and Stratton, New York, 1961.)

Kline, N. S., and Lehmann, H. E.: Handbook of psychiatric treatment in medical practice. (Saunders, Philadelphia, 1962.)

Kuitunen-Ekbaum, E.: Phenothiazine in the treatment of enterobiasis. Canad. J. Public Health, *32:* 308(1941).

Laborit, H.: L'hibernation artificielle. Acta Anaesth. Belg., *2:* 710 (1951.)

Lear, E.: Chemistry and applied pharmacology of tranquillizers. (Charles C Thomas, Springfield, 1966.)

Lehmann, H. E., and Knight, D. A.: Psychophysiologic testing with a new phrenotropic drug. In: Trifluoperazine clinical and pharmacological aspects. (Lea and Febiger, New York, 1958.)

Levy, L., and Ban, T. A.: Phenothiazine drugs and the general practitioner. Canad. Med. Ass. J., *86:* 415 (1962).

Lewis, J. J.: Introduction to pharmacology. (Livingstone, London, 1962.)

Marks, J., and Pare, C. M. B. (eds.): The scientific basis of drug therapy in psychiatry. (Pergamon Press, Oxford, 1965.)

Merry, J., *et al.* (1957): In: Patridge, M.: Discussion. In: The scientific basis of drug treatment in psychiatry (eds., Marks, J., and Pare, C. M. B.). (Pergamon Press, Oxford, 1965.)

Millon, R., *et al.*: Resultats thérapeutiques d'une nouvelle phènothiazine: la propériciazine, en milieu psychiatrique. (Paper presented at the Sixty-first Congress of French-Speaking Psychiatrists and Neurologists, Nancy, 1963.)

Murray, M. R., and Peterson, E. R. (1964): In: Richter, D.: Mode of action of the phenothiazines. In: The scientific basis of drug therapy in psychiatry (eds., Marks, J., and Pare, C. M. B.). (Pergamon Press, Oxford, 1965.)

Ostow, M.: Drugs in psychoanalysis and psychotherapy. (Basic Books, New York, 1962.)

Oules, J.: Action de 8909 R. P. (propericiazine) sur les troubles caracteriels des èpileptiques. (Paper presented at the Sixty-first Congress of French-Speaking Psychiatrists and Neurologists, Nancy, 1963.)

Paterson, A. S.: Electrical and drug treatment in psychiatry. (Elsevier, Amsterdam, 1963.)

Patridge, M.: Discussion. In: The scientific basis of drug therapy in psychiatry (eds., Marks, J., and Pare, C. M. B.). (Pergamon Press, Oxford, 1965.)

Pletscher, A.: Pharmacology of antidepressants. In: Psychopharmacology (eds., Kline, N. S., and Lehmann, H. E.). (Little, Brown, Boston, 1965.)

Pletscher, A.: Pharmacology of monoamine oxidase inhibitors. In: The scientific basis of drug therapy in psychiatry (eds., Marks, J., and Pare, C. M. B.). (Pergamon Press, Oxford, 1965.)

Pommé, B., *et al.*: Aspect de la sénescence pathologique et traitement par un nouveau neuroleptique le 8909 R.P. Ann. Medico-Psychol., *2:* 793 (1963).

Raymond, M. J., *et al.*: Trial of five tranquillizing drugs in psychoneurosis. Brit. Med. J., *2:* 63 (1957).

Rees, W. L., and Lambert, C.: The value and limitations of chlorpromazine in the treatment of anxiety states. J. Ment. Sci., *101:* 834 (1955).

Richter, D.: Mode of action of the phenothiazines. In: The scientific basis of drug therapy in psychiatry (eds., Marks, J., and Pare, C. M. B.). (Pergamon Press, Oxford, 1965.)

Rogers, P. H.: Discussion. In: The scientific basis of drug therapy in psychiatry (eds., Marks, J., and Pare, C. M. B.). (Pergamon Press, Oxford, 1965.)

Roizin, L., *et al.* (1962): In: Richter, D.: Mode of action of the phenothiazines. In: The scientific basis of drug therapy in psychiatry (eds., Marks, J., and Pare, C. M. B.). (Pergamon Press, Oxford, 1965.)

Sainsbury, P.: Structure functional relationship within the phenothiazine class. In: The scientific basis of drug therapy in psychiatry (eds., Marks, J., and Pare, C. M. B.). (Pergamon Press, Oxford, 1965.)

Sargant, W., and Slater, E.: Introduction to physical methods of treatment in psychiatry. (Livingstone, London, 1963.)

Verdeau-Paillés, J.: Experimentation clinique d'un nouveau neuroleptique du groupe des phènothiazines (8909 R.P.) chez 34 malades presentant des troubles caractériels. (Paper presented at the meeting of the Société Moreau de Tours, 1963.)

Volmat, R., *et al.*: Action du 8909 R.P. (propèriciazine) sur les troubles du caractére. (Paper presented at the Sixty-first Congress of French-Speaking Psychiatrists and Neurologists, Nancy, 1963.)

Warnes, H., *et al.*: Discromias cutaneas y alteraciones oculares observadas en el tratamiento prolongado con la cloropromacins. Acta Psiquiat. Psicol. Amer. Latina, *10:* 204 (1964).

Warnes, H., Lehmann, H. E., and Ban, T. A.: Adynamic ileus during psychoactive medication: a report of three fatal and five severe cases. Canad. Med. Ass. J., *96:* 112 (1967).

Eleven

The Rauwolfias

The snakeroot plant—*Rauwolfia serpentina*—had been used for thousands of years to treat snake bite, epilepsy and other ailments (including insanity). Its "tranquilizing" activity was mentioned by Rumpf in 1755, but this property was to be rediscovered only after the recognition of its antihypertensive properties in the nineteen-thirties. Interest in the antihypertensive properties of *Rauwolfia serpentina* has diminished somewhat, while the study of its psychotropic properties has increased, particularly in the nineteen fifties (Miner, 1955; Goodman and Gilman, 1965; Grollman, 1958, and Kalinowsky and Hoch, 1961).

A. BASIC DATA

1. Historical Data

The "Pagla-ka-dacra" or the "insanity herb" as described in ancient Hindu writings was obtained from herb gatherers and extensively used in Ayurvedic medicine. The roots of the plant were sold by "medicine men" and quacks at village fairs and roadside bazaars. Cultivation was limited to the small gardens of medicinal plants which were maintained by Ayurvedic hospitals. For long centuries thereafter it was successfully administered in the Orient and particularly in India for controlling excitement and anxiety.

a. Botany

The "snakeroot" plant belongs to the Rauwolfias, a tropical genus of woody plants of the natural family of Apocynaceae. In general the Apocynaceae are divided into two subfamilies: the Plumeroideae, which have mainly sedative, and antihypertensive properties, and the Echitoideae, which are exclusively cardiac glycosides. Rauwolfia is a genus of Plumeroideae named by Plumier (1703) in honor of the famous sixteenth-century German traveler and botanist. At least 100 species of the Rauwolfia genus have been described to date, and about 55 of them have been chemically and pharmacologically investigated (Woodson *et al.*, 1957).

b. Isolation of Active Ingredients

Systematic exploratory work led to the isolation of the active ingredients of the Rauwolfia plants. At first only their cardiovascular action (Sen and Bose, 1931) and later also their psychotropic effects (Ray, 1931; and Gupta *et al.*, 1943) were demonstrated.

In 1952 Müller *et al.*, working with 18-hydroxyyohimbines, isolated reserpine, a colorless, crystalline ester alkaloid, which accounts for approximately 50 per cent of the activity (both psychotropic and antihypertensive) of the whole *Rauwolfia serpentina* root. Because of its clinical importance, attempts were made to isolate reserpine from species of the Rauwolfia genus other than *Rauwolfia serpentina* and also from the other closely related Apocynaceous plants. Success was reported in all but six of the Rauwolfia species. It was found particularly feasible to extract reserpine from *Rauwolfia vomitoria* of Africa and *Rauwolfia tetraphylla* of America. Finally, Woodward (1956) succeeded in synthesizing this substance.

c. Clinical Discovery

Studies with preparations of the whole root received great impetus by Vakil's (1949) report which gave an account of the successful treatment of high blood pressure in patients previously unresponsive to other therapies. These results were confirmed by Wilkins (1954).

The first paper on the therapeutic effects of *Rauwolfia serpentina* in schizophrenic patients was presented by Hakim (1953). This prompted Kline to undertake clinical investigations with reserpine—the active principle of the *Rauwolfia serpentina* root—in psychiatric patients. Kline's (1954) and Weber's (1954) findings confirmed that reserpine has definite sedative effects as well as ataractic properties. Kline (1954) considered the latter responsible for the particular usefulness of this substance in the treatment of psychotic and especially schizophrenic patients. He also recognized the mood-depressant and extrapyramidal sign producing characteristics of the new drug (Kline and Stanley, 1955; and Kline, 1959).

2. Action Mechanism

Barsa and Kline (1955) and, independently, Landgrabe (1959) clearly delineated three stages of reserpine action. The first is characterized by sedation; the second by "turbulence;" and the third by the dominance of (mental) integrative processes.

A number of hypotheses, ranging from psychodynamic through neurophysiological to chemical concepts, were formulated to account for the clinical changes observed in the course of reserpine treatment.

a. Psychodynamic Hypotheses

Azima *et al.* (1959) considered that the therapeutic action of reserpine in the schizophrenias is associated with a shift toward a more organized state, with a more structured ego system such as seen in the manic-depressive conditions. This formulation is based on the Kleinian (1948) concepts of the schizoid-paranoid-depressive positions.

Ostow and Kline (1959), in another dynamically based hypothesis, maintained that the therapeutic effects of reserpine are associated with a decrease of psychic energy and "motivational impulses." If neuroses and psychoses are the outcome of a break through the repression barrier by instinctual forces, the weakening of these forces may result in attenuation and in some cases elimination of psychopathological symptoms. They considered the depression seen in the course of reserpine administration a consequence of the reduction of psychic energy.

In the course of their dynamic exploration, Ostow and Kline (1959) revealed weird, horrifying dreams in some of their patients. Awakening was slow in these cases and was characterized by a subsequent difficulty in distinguishing "waking reality" from "dream reality." Others gave an account of "flagrantly erotic" or aggressive thoughts and dreams during treatment. Ostow and Kline (1959) concluded that besides its sedative and tranquilizing (decrease of libidinal energy) effects, reserpine also has an ego-intoxicating property.

b. Organically Based Hypotheses

Among these is the neurophysiological concept of Bein (1955), who asserted that reserpine acts on the central regulatory mechanisms which integrate autonomic and somatic functions. Another hypothesis by Brodie (1959) suggests that the psychotropic properties of reserpine result from the depletion of 5-hydroxytryptamine (serotonin) in the brain and other tissues. Supporting this view is the fact that Rauwolfia alkaloids without serotonin-depleting properties have no tranquilizing effects.

In spite of the various hypotheses and of the increasing information on the neurochemical and neurophysiological concomitants of the pharmacological effects of reserpine, there is still no general agreement as to which of the known actions of the molecule accounts for its usefulness in different psychopathological conditions. On the other hand, further research with the aim of modifying and enhancing the therapeutic effects of reserpine and of eliminating its undesirable reactions has led to the isolation, chemical synthesis and pharmacological investigation of a large number of other naturally occurring Rauwolfia alkaloids and synthetically produced related compounds.

3. Structure and Activity

In the search for a more specific, more potent and less toxic substance than reserpine, systematic studies were directed toward isolating numerous alkaloids of the Rauwolfia genus and producing semisynthetic derivatives of the parent compound.

a. Descriptive Aspects

Chemically, extracts of the Rauwolfia root belong to four well defined categories. The yellow-colored anhydronium bases, the tertiary indoline alkaloids and the tertiary indole alkaloids do not have sedative, hypnotic or tranquilizing effects.

To date only tertiary indole alkaloids with carbocyclic ring E have yielded drugs with psychotropic properties (and even in this group, the adrenolytic yohimbine, the sympatholytic corynanthine and the hypotensive rauwolscine are entirely without tranquilizing action). Reserpine is the prototype of the psychoactive substances of this group, although both deserpidine and rescinnamine are also characterized by psychotropic effects.

Reserpine is a 3,4,5-methoxy-benzoylmethyl reserpate. The basic nucleus of reserpine is an indole ethylamine structure resembling serotonin and lysergic acid diethylamide. This led to the assumption that it may exert its action by displacing 5-hydroxytryptamine from the tissues. In addition to the indole nucleus, reserpine also contains six methyl groups and a basic nitrogen which is present as an NH group (Pöldinger and Schmidlin, 1966). Spectral investigation pointed to the presence of two ester linkages in the reserpine molecule: a methoxyindole and a second unsaturated chromophoric system. On alkaline hydrolysis reserpine yielded reserpic acid, 3,4,5-trimethoxybenzoic acid and methanol. It was definitely established that reserpine has mild antihypertensive and predominantly psychotropic properties.

Of the two other naturally occurring psychoactive tertiary indole alkaloids with a carbocyclic ring E, deserpidine (11-desmethoxyreserpine) differs chemically from reserpine only in lacking a methoxy group on ring A in position 11. Clinically this desmethylated analogue is only somewhat less potent in its tranquilizing effect, and it has a somewhat faster onset of action. The other naturally occurring alkaloid, rescinnamine, is a trimethoxycinnemate of reserpic acid methylester. This chemical change resulted in a substance with both cardiovascular and psychotropic effects, similar to those of reserpine but to a considerably decreased extent. Consequently, the incidence and intensity of undesired reactions that may occur in the course of treatment with rescinnamine are also less frequent.

b. Dynamic Aspects

i. General Considerations. Systematic investigations of structure-activity relationships with naturally occurring or semisynthetic analogues of reserpine revealed several patterns. All but one of the stereoisomers of reserpine are of no psychopharmacological interest. The only naturally occurring and pharmacologically active stereoisomer is raujemidine, an unsaturated derivative with approximately half the tranquilizing potential of reserpine.

Changes on ring A showed that the methoxy group in position 11 of reserpine is not essential for its psychotropic effects. Furthermore, it was also seen that while desmethylation reduces the activity of these drugs it probably also shortens the period between the administration of the substance and the onset of therapeutic—or other—effects. It has also been demonstrated that substitution on the same ring may produce profound alterations in the characteristics of the compound. For example, 10-chlorodeserpidine seems to have only tranquilizing (without antihypertensive) action, while 10-methoxydeserpidine seems to have only antihypertensive (without tranquilizing) effect.

Replacement of the hydrogen atom of ring B by a methyl or an alkyl group yield, *N*-methyl and *N*-allyl reserpine. *N*-Allyl

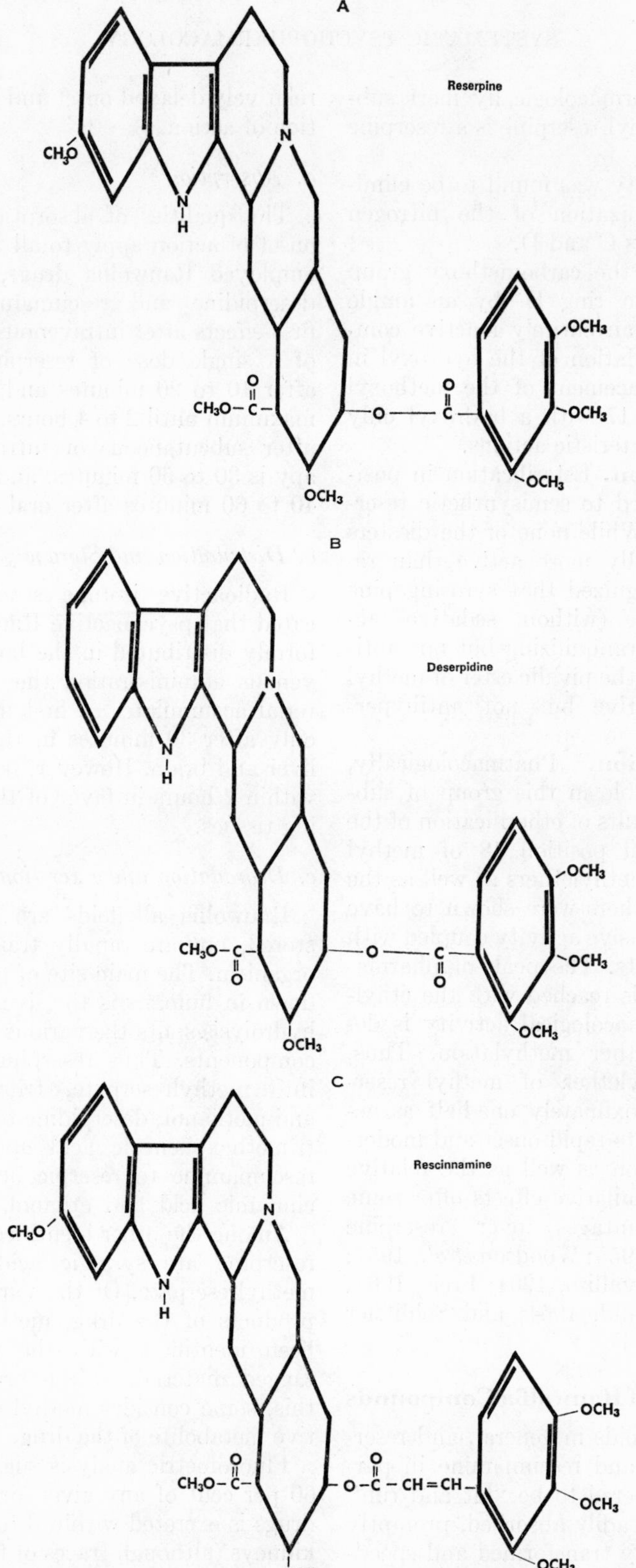

FIG. 11. *a*, Structural formula of reserpine. *b*, Structural formula of deserpidine. *c*, Structural formula of rescinnamine.

reserpine is a pharmacologically inert substance and *N*-methyl reserpine is a reserpine antagonist.

Reserpine activity was found to be eliminated by quaternization of the nitrogen constituent of rings C and D.

Substitution of the carbomethoxy group in position 16—on ring E—by an amide group resulted in an entirely inactive compound, as did acylation of the hydroxyl in position 17. Replacement of the methoxyl group in position 17 with a hydroxyl only reduced the characteristic actions.

ii. Esterification. Esterification in positions 16 and 18 led to semisynthetic reserpine derivatives. While none of the diesters is pharmacologically more active than reserpine, it is recognized that syrosingopine exerts hypotensive (without sedative) action; SU-5171 is tranquilizing but not antihypertensive; and the pivalic ester of methyl reserpate is sedative but not antihypertensive.

iii. Etherification. Pharmacologically, the most remarkable in this group of substances are the results of etherification of the hydroxyl group in position 18 of methyl reserpate. The β-methylethers as well as the epi- or α-methylethers were shown to have slight antihypertensive activity coupled with tranquilizing effects. The peak of pharmacological activity is reached with the ethylethers, and pharmacological activity is decreased with further methylation. Thus, although 18β-ethylether of methyl reserpate is only approximately one-half as active as reserpine, its rapid onset and moderate length of action as well as the relative absence of its cumulative effects offer some therapeutic advantages over reserpine (Schneider *et al.*, 1955; Woodson *et al.*, 1957; Gordon, 1964; Cavallito, 1964; Freis, 1964; Friend, 1964; Gould, 1964; and Schlittler and Plummer, 1964).

4. Metabolism of Rauwolfia Compounds

Rauwolfia alkaloids in general, and reserpine, deserpidine and rescinnamine in particular, are considered to be "hit and run" drugs. They are readily absorbed, promptly distributed, rapidly transformed and speedily excreted. In spite of this, they have a relatively delayed onset and prolonged duration of action.

a. Absorption

The qualities of absorption and delayed onset of action apply to all three frequently employed Rauwolfia drugs, *i.e.*, reserpine, deserpidine and rescinnamine. Thus the first effects after intravenous administration of a single dose of reserpine appear only after 10 to 20 minutes and do not reach a maximum until 2 to 4 hours. Onset of action after subcutaneous or intramuscular therapy is 30 to 50 minutes, and it is as long as 40 to 60 minutes after oral ingestion.

b. Distribution and Storage

Radioactive isotope studies have indicated that psychoactive Rauwolfias are uniformly distributed in the body. After intravenous administration the radioactive material accumulates at first in the lungs and only after 30 minutes in the heart, spleen, liver and brain. However, it is redistributed within 2 hours in favor of the lipid-containing tissues.

c. Degradation and Excretion

Rauwolfia alkaloids are not extensively stored, but are rapidly transformed in the organism. The main site of metabolic breakdown in humans is the liver. Here alkaline hydrolysis splits the various drugs into their components. Thus reserpine is catabolized into methylreserpate, trimethoxybenzoate and methanol; deserpidine to deserpide acid, trimethoxybenzoic acid and ethanol; and rescinnamine to reserpic acid, trimethoxycinnamic acid and ethanol.

Among the other identified metabolites of reserpine are syringic acid and siringoyl methylreserpate. Of the various breakdown products of the drug, methylreserpate has been identified, with the use of tritium-tagged material, in the brain. Because of this, some consider methylreserpate the active metabolite of the drug.

Fluorometric analysis suggests that 50 to 60 per cent of any given oral dose of these drugs is excreted within 3 to 4 hours by the kidneys (although traces of the administered substance may be detected in the urine for several days). In spite of this, however, the action of psychoactive Rauwolfias lasts for up to 5 days after a single effective dose and for several weeks after cessation of continuous drug administration.

Interspecies variation of reserpine metabolism has been noted between rats and dogs. Alkaline hydrolysis takes place readily in rats but only after a considerable delay in dogs. Some believe that the relatively great susceptibility of dogs and the very low susceptibility of rats to reserpine is a consequence of this metabolic variation (Woodson *et al.*, 1957; Jarvik, 1965; and Goodman and Gilman, 1965).

5. Chemical and Neurophysiological Correlates of Drug Action

a. Chemical Correlates

There are a number of chemical changes attributed to the action of psychoactive Rauwolfia alkaloids. One of the most significant is a release of various amines, such as 5-hydroxytryptamine or serotonin (5-HT) and norepinephrine (NE), from their cellular storage sites, which ultimately leads to the depletion of these substances from the various organs, including the brain and the adrenals.

It was early shown that after a single dose of reserpine in the rabbit brain serotonin was decreased to 10 per cent of the pretreatment level within 4 hours and remained so for approximately 36 hours. It took about 168 hours before the normal brain concentration was reestablished.

A similar though slower depletion occurred in the intestines. Here a progressive decline of 5-HT content over a period of 16 hours was observed. Blood serotonin levels began to rise, however, only 48 hours after drug administration and were not normalized for about 7 days.

Another consequence of reserpine's interference with the binding of monoamines is the prevention of the uptake of 5-HT at the cellular sites. This has been confirmed by findings in the peripheral blood, where it was demonstrated that the potential of platelets for binding 5-HT is markedly lowered under the influence of these drugs. Experimental evidence of the same phenomenon was demonstrated in the CNS, where it was shown that, when 5-hydroxytryptophan was administered after pretreatment with reserpine, serotonin was rapidly formed but remained in free form *i.e.*, its binding was prevented.

It is debatable whether it is the change in brain 5-HT levels or in brain NE levels which is responsible for the psychotropic properties of these drugs. Brodie (1959) maintains that the sedative, tranquilizer and particularly the mood-depressant effects produced by reserpine are related to the lowered serotonin (and not of norepinephrine) levels. In favor of this is that the central actions of reserpine are characterized by increased parasympathetic activity, *i.e.*, drowsiness, sleep and diminished responsiveness to external stimuli, which is mediated by a neurohormone with trophotropic activity (*e.g.*, 5-HT). Other supporting facts are that NE (and dopamine) can be selectively depleted without sedative action; behavioral depression accompanies lowered 5-HT and not lowered NE levels; and in animals exposed to cold, brain NE levels are lowered without any of the signs of behavioral depression. Carlsson (1960), however, maintains that changes in brain norepinephrine (and not 5-HT) levels are the ones closely related to the depressant effect of psychoactive Rauwolfia alkaloid preparations. This he supports with the experimental finding that dopa, the precursor of NE, can antagonize reserpine-induced depression, while 5-hydroxytryptophan, the precursor of 5-HT, cannot.

Opposed to both views are Sheppard and Zimmerman's (1960) findings in guinea pigs. After 0.1 mg./kg. of subcutaneously injected reserpine, these investigators found no correlation between the pharmacological response to the drug and the amine content of the brain.

As a result of reserpine administration, urinary excretion of 5-hydroxyindoleacetic acid, the principal 5-HT metabolite, is increased, which is attributed to the liberation and rapid disintegration of the freed serotonin in the brain and other tissues. In the course of chronic administration of the drug there is also a decreased concentration of

NE in the blood simultaneously with the diminished urinary catecholamine levels.

Other peripheral findings, as described by Hippius *et al.* (1959), are the transient elevation of globulin and decrease of albumin in the blood followed by a diminution of globulin and an increase in the albumin. There is also a rise of blood (and also CNS) sugar levels, which in a few cases has led to the activation of latent diabetes.

More recently, lowering of γ-aminobutyric acid concentrations—a possible synaptic inhibitor in the central nervous system—has been shown in the course of reserpine treatment. This might be responsible for the lowered seizure threshold to electrical stimulation under the influence of these drugs (Davies, 1964; Jacobsen, 1964; Remen *et al.*, 1962; and Sourkes, 1962).

b. Neurophysiological Correlates

i. Lower Centers. While psychoactive Rauwolfias exert a strong vagotonic effect, they have relatively little direct influence on the spinal cord or medullary structures. On the other hand, they have a profound inhibiting effect on the vasomotor and heat regulating centers of the midbrain.

ii. Reticular Activating System. The effects of psychoactive Rauwolfias on the reticular activating system are complex. Rinaldi and Himwich (1955) demonstrated a persistent electroencephalographic pattern of alertness originating from the reticular formation of the tegmentum and from the the thalamic projection system. On the basis of these findings, it was assumed that these drugs have a stimulating effect on the mesodiencephalic alerting system and that they induce a facilitating effect on the transmission of impulses in these areas. This was supported and further clarified by subsequent studies, which led to the conclusion that, whereas small doses of reserpine have a stimulating influence on reticular activating system structures, large doses exert the opposite, *i.e.*, inhibitory action.

iii. Hypothalamus. The action of Rauwolfias on the hypothalamic centers has been extensively explored. It was recognized that the sedative and hypnotic effects of reserpine (as well as the hypotension, bradycardia, miosis, hypothermia, and stimulation of peristalsis) are similar to those which Hess (1954) obtained upon electrical stimulation of certain diencephalic structures or that are seen in patients with space-occupying lesions of the posterior hypothalamus. All of this is indirect evidence that the principal site of action of reserpine is in the posterior hypothalamic area. In spite of suppressing sympathetic centers (which are located in the posterior hypothalamus), which leaves the parasympathetic centers unopposed (with a consequent rise of cholinergic activity), reserpine neither antagonizes the effects of sympathomimetic substances, such as epinephrine or norepinephrine, nor potentiates the effects of acetylcholine.

"Sham rage" manifests in violent outbursts of sympathetic (hypothalamic) activity. This reaction, which is characteristic of decorticated animals, was shown to be successfully controlled by reserpine (Weiskrantz and Wilson, 1955). Bower (1955) attributed this to a direct diencephalic action, while Schneider (1955) suggested that it was the result of an increased cortical inhibition of diencephalic areas, which is related to the general facilitation of synaptic transmissions due to the predominance of acetylcholine in the serotonin-acetylcholine balance.

iv. Cortex. Other actions of reserpine are the blocking of impulses arising from certain brain areas and characteristic electroencephalographic effects. Thus, impulses from the prepyriform area, anterior temporal lobe, anterior part of the insula, posterior orbital area and amygdaloid nucleus cannot activate the hypothalamus.

Differential electroencephalographic features of various doses of reserpine were demonstrated by Bente and Itil (1959). While no EEG change could be seen with low dosages of the drug, with prolonged use of 7 to 12 mg. daily, protraction of the basal rhythm with theta and delta activity appeared in the fronto-central and temporal regions. With further increase in dosage (to 40 mg. daily) these changes became more prominent, and there were phases of both decreased tension and high tension wave complexes with fronto-central predominance.

6. Behavioral Pharmacology

Psychoactive Rauwolfia alkaloids induce behavioral changes in animals and man over a wide range of functions.

a. Animal Studies

The prodromal changes (excitement in dogs, playfulness in monkeys) are soon followed by a "taming effect," usually accepted as the first behavioral stage of reserpine action characterized by the absence of manifest agressiveness.

At higher doses the animals pass into a second stage of abnormal behavior, characterized by "quiescence." They pay little attention to their surroundings, have no interest in food and sit motionless. Although they appear to be asleep, or actually are asleep when undisturbed, they are easily aroused.

At a certain dose level this decrease in motor activity passes into immobility, characterized by a particular dissociation—called "catalepsy"—in which the animals, while maintaining their righting reflex, become fixated in unusual positions. Other behavioral effects of reserpine are the gradual reduction in the amount of spontaneous activity of animals over a 4- to 6-hour period (frequently quantified in an activity recorder or jiggle cage) and the degree, time of onset and duration of palpebral ptosis and hypothermia.

In various stimulus-response constellations the threshold of responsivity is raised. Unconditional autonomic reflexes are partially suppressed; emotional responsiveness in stressful situations is markedly reduced; and conditioned motor reflexes are depressed.

The animals do not move to another part of the cage, climb a pole, press a lever or carry out any simple task to avoid a painful stimulus (electroshock) following a warning signal, although when they receive the disagreeable impulse they try to escape it. Similarly or even more affected are food-rewarded conditioned motor responses, which are almost entirely inhibited.

Psychoactive Rauwolfias potentiate the action of sedatives, hypnotics, narcotics and antihypertensives in general and barbiturates, opiates and alcohol in particular. They antagonize the stimulating effect of amphetamine, the emetic response to apomorphine and the anticonvulsant action of diphenylhydantoin.

b. Human Studies

In human pharmacological studies a single dose of reserpine lowers critical flicker fusion frequency threshold; impairs paired associate learning; decreases tapping rate; and increases visual or auditory reaction time.

In clinical pharmacological studies a single dose of reserpine induces a state of quietness, with an inner calmness, a condition in which spontaneous activity or responsivity to external stimuli is reduced.

B. CLINICAL DATA

1. Indications and Contraindications

a. Indications

Rauwolfia alkaloids are successfully administered in numerous pathological conditions. In ancient medicine they were used as sedatives, in the treatment of snake bites and, with questionable success, in epilepsy.

Today they are often given alone or in combination with other drugs in hypertension partly to reduce blood pressure and partly to control the associated anxiety. Less frequently, they are prescribed in vascular and allergic headaches; in the treatment of tachycardia; and for the symptomatic control of choreoathetotic movements (Barrett and Hansel, 1955; and Lambros, 1955).

The psychiatric indications of these drugs range from functional psychoses through organic brain syndromes to the various neuroses (including specific psychiatric indications in the young and in the old) (Hollister *et al.*, 1955; DeMacedo, 1959; Mayer-Gross *et al.*, 1960; Gregory, 1961; Noyes and Kolb, 1961; Ostow, 1962; and Valentine, 1962).

i. Functional Psychoses. *α. Schizophrenias.* Whatever the subtype, symptomatic relief is seen in violent and disturbed patients. There is a decrease in assaultiveness and consequently less need for restraint. Delusions, particularly those associated with hallucinations, respond favorably to reserpine, and thus the drug not only is useful for transient sedation or tranquilization but also facilitates the remission of psychopathological symptoms. Reserpine treatment, however, becomes less and less effective with increasing chronicity of the illness. The best results are obtained in cases in which the psychotic manifestations are associated with anxiety. Of the various schizophrenic subgroups, paranoids and catatonics respond the best and hebephrenics the least.

β. Manic-Depressive Psychosis. In manic-depressive psychoses reserpine is successfully used in the treatment of the manic syndrome, although it should be given with caution because of the easy shift into depression. Because of this, reserpine is used only in exceptionally rare cases and even then only for a short time to control restlessness, excitement and agitation.

ii. Organic Brain Syndromes. Of the acute and chronic organic brain syndromes, beneficial effects with Rauwolfias have been described in patients suffering from both hereditary and acquired conditions such as Huntington's chorea and general paresis of the insane. There are also favorable reports of their efficacy in posttraumatic confusional states and in the control of psychopathological manifestations resulting from alcohol or drug withdrawal (Carey, 1955; and Miner, 1955).

iii. Psychoneuroses. The therapeutic value of psychoactive Rauwolfias in the various psychoneuroses is controversial. Beneficial results have, however, been reported in the symptomatic control of compulsive aggressive manifestations and also for anxiety and tension, especially when they accompany somatic disorders such as chronic asthma, premenstrual tension and menopausal manifestations.

iv. Other Indications. Reserpine has been successfully used in ortho- and geriatric psychiatry. It is therapeutic for irritable and hypertonic infants, in overactive brain-injured children and in erratic mental defectives. It has been tried with questionable success in the control of nocturnal enuresis and in behavioral adjustment problems of children and adolescents (Talbot, 1955).

In geriatrics, reserpine has been used in senile and arteriosclerotic cases. Irritable, irascible, demanding, quarrelsome, hostile patients respond most favorably, while no therapeutic effect is seen in apathetic, negativistic, depressed or withdrawn patients. It has been noted that nocturnal restlessness is usually well controlled (Sainz, 1955).

b. Contraindications

There are relatively few absolute contraindications. They are comatose states, depression (or history of depression), peptic ulcer (or other ulcers of the gastrointestinal tract, excluding ulcerative colitis) and acute alcoholic intoxication. In various cardiovascular conditions (*e.g.*, aortic insufficiency, cardiac failure with edema, and thrombosis) and gastrointestinal diseases (*e.g.*, gastritis and gastrointestinal hyperirritability), these drugs have to be given with extreme caution. Some consider age, debilitating disease and also epilepsy as relative contraindications, although some of the cases suffering from these conditions have shown remarkably good tolerance and a favorable response to reserpine treatment.

There is evidence that it is dangerous to combine reserpine therapy with a number of other psychiatric, medical and surgical treatments. Irreversible cardiovascular collapse due to parasympathetic predominance has been reported after reserpine-treated patients were given electroshock. The increased sensitivity to insulin of reserpinized patients has led to prolonged comas and to a rise in the frequency of cerebral seizures in the course of insulin coma treatment. Premature ventricular contractions or other cardiac complications have occurred when reserpine was given to digitalized patients (or to cases under quinidine treatment); and bradycardia or dangerous hypotension has occurred in patients under general anesthesia.

When psychoactive Rauwolfias are given to pregnant women or in the period of lactation, they may cause nasal congestion or increased tracheobronchial secretion in the new born. No carcinogenic effects of these drugs have been reported.

2. Therapy with Rauwolfias Alone and in Combination with Other Treatments

a. Rauwolfias Alone

i. Dosage. While the therapeutic dosage range of each Rauwolfia drug differs slightly, it generally holds true that, in the treatment of acute psychotics, a daily dosage which is five times as high as that for psychoneurotics has to be prescribed. The latter receive a daily dosage which is approximately twice as high as that which is used—usually as an adjunct—in the control of hypertension. For example, the average daily dosage of reserpine is between 5 and 10 mg. (for acute psychotics), 1 and 2 mg. (for psychoneurotics) and 0.5 and 1 mg. (for hypertensives).

Respective dosages of preparations of the whole *Rauwolfia serpentina* root are 100 to 200 mg. (for hypertensives), 200 to 400 mg. (for psychoneurotics) and 1000 to 2000 mg. (for psychotics), although in some cases doses as high as 10,000 mg. a day have had to be given for the successful control of certain agitated patients. The preparation of the alseroxylon alkaloid fraction is given in dosages of 2 to 4 mg. (for hypertensives) and 4 to 8 mg. (for psychoneurotics). Deserpidine is administered in approximately the same amounts as reserpine itself, while rescinnamine is given in approximately twice as high dosages to obtain similar effects.

With particular indications the dosages of these drugs differ. This applies, for example, to irritable and hypertonic infants, enuretic children and disturbed geriatric, especially arteriosclerotic, patients. In these cases reserpine is prescribed in the daily amount of 0.15 to 0.3 mg. and 5 to 7.5 mg., respectively.

All the dosages discussed are for oral administration, usually given in equally divided doses three or four times a day, *i.e.*, every 8 or 6 hours, in the acute period of the illness and once or twice a day in a reduced dosage (preferably at night) later on as maintenance therapy.

ii. Treatment Procedures. Continuous treatment is the most frequently used clinical procedure with psychoactive Rauwolfias. This commences with the intramuscular administration of a 0.25-mg. testing dose to detect potentially dangerous hypotensive effects.

In acutely disturbed psychotics the starting treatment dose of reserpine is 8 mg. daily given orally in two or three divided doses or as combined intramuscular (5 mg.) and oral (3 mg.) medication. This dosage is maintained for the first 10 days. Thereafter in therapy-responsive cases the intramuscular route of drug administration is replaced by oral treatment for a further 2 to 3 weeks and then slowly reduced to a maintenance dosage that may be as low as one-fifth or even one-tenth of the initial dosage. If after 10 days there is no improvement, the starting dosage is gradually increased until there is a therapeutic response or troublesome side-effects occur. Some recommend raising the dosage in accordance to Haase's (1965) specification, *i.e.*, until the onset of a fine tremor that can easily be recognized by repeated handwriting tests.

Psychoneurotic and also most of the geriatric cases require only small amounts of reserpine (*e.g.*, 1 mg. a day). The daily dosage of the drug is gradually raised until therapeutic effects are noted or troublesome side-effects occur (Sainz, 1955).

iii. Duration of Treatment. The duration of administration depends on the condition which is being treated. In psychoneuroses medication should only be given until symptomatic remission takes place. Schizophrenics should be kept on a "maintenance" dosage after their first episode for at least a 1-year period; after the second for at least 2 to 3 years; and thereafter for an indefinite time. Early cessation of therapy may lead to relapse. It takes a considerable length of time after commencement of treatment for the first therapeutic effects to be observed. Thus the sedative and hypotensive effects may be present within the first week, affective indifference within a fortnight and facilitation of integrative processes and consequently therapeutic action in chronic schizophrenics thereafter (and not rarely only in the third month of treatment). On the other hand, it takes at least 2 weeks after cessation of reserpine treatment for the parasympathetic predominance to wear off and 1 month or even longer for some of the other reserpine-induced effects to disappear.

It is fortunate that Rauwolfia drugs can be taken over an extended period of time (Ayd, 1959). Clinically there is no evidence of the development of drug tolerance or habituation with continued drug administration. If anything, there is an increase in sensitivity observed, which in certain cases may necessitate reduction in dosage. This effect, which is opposite to tolerance, is seen more clearly in animals in the shortening of the onset of reserpine action after repeated doses.

Although there are physical withdrawal symptoms after abrupt discontinuation of prolonged reserpine administration, there is no psychological dependency.

b. Rauwolfias in Combination with Other Treatments

Not infrequently, Rauwolfia drugs are administered in conjunction with other treatments: physical, pharmacological and psychological.

i. Physical. Both electroconvulsive and insulin therapies have been given in combination with reserpine. Only in rare cases are these combinations better than treatment with either reserpine or with electroconvulsions (or insulin) alone. Lowering of convulsive threshold together with lowering of blood pressure (and with increased sensitivity to insulin) may lead to dangerous complications, *e.g.*, severe hypotensive reaction and death after ECT. Physical therapies, especially electroshock, are therefore only rarely combined with reserpine treatment. In these occasional cases the cerebral convulsion is elicited by lower milliamperage and shorter duration of stimulation, and the coma is produced with much less insulin than is usually required.

ii. Pharmacological. Rauwolfias potentiate the effect of other central nervous system depressant drugs, and they should therefore be combined only with extreme caution. An exception to this is glutethimide, a popular hypnotic substance, which reverses (or counteracts) instead of aggravating some of the effects of Rauwolfia drugs (Bussow and Lindner, 1959).

Whereas the combination of reserpine with chlorpromazine offers some advantages in certain psychiatric conditions, the combination of Rauwolfias with antihypertensives results in new and useful medical preparations. At the present the combination of thiazides with Rauwolfia alkaloids is widely used in the management of mild to moderate hypertension.

iii. Behavior Therapy. A combination of reserpine (a single dose of 0.75 mg. at night) and behavior therapy has been used in the treatment of nocturnal enuresis with equivocal success.

3. Adverse Reactions and Their Treatment

a. Adverse Reactions

i. Psychiatric. These range from reduction of spontaneous activity to severe toxic confusional states, although the occurrence of the latter is rare. The main psychiatric complication of reserpine administration is depression. Dysthymic mood changes may take place and are attributed to the effect of prolonged administration of Rauwolfia drugs in certain cases, while in others underlying mild depressions are accentuated to the extent of suicidal ideation, threats or attempts. In the initial period of treatment drowsiness and fatigue or, paradoxically, insomnia and excitement are not infrequent; withdrawal, anhedonia and apathy or inner restlessness, irrational behavior and disturbing nightmares are more common at a later stage of treatment.

ii. Neurological. Headache and dizziness are not infrequently experienced with reserpine, but the most common neurological side-effects are extrapyramidal manifestations. These range in severity from akathisia through dyskinesia to parkinsonism.

While extrapyramidal signs are frequent, a midbrain syndrome—characterized by hyperpyrexia, ocular palsy and decerebrate rigidity—is extremely rare. In between, in occurrence, are cerebral seizures, cerebellar signs and paresthesias.

iii. Autonomic. The most common autonomic side-effects with Rauwolfia drugs are related to the parasympathetic predominance that is produced. Nasal congestion is rather frequent in the course of treatment, as are excessive salivation (although occasionally there is dryness of mouth) and reduction of perspiration.

iv. Endocrinological. Rauwolfias have a blocking effect on pituitary gonadotropins along with a stimulating effect on pituitary antidiuretic hormone secretion. They may precipitate latent or aggravate active diabetes, although not infrequently the high blood sugar levels of excited patients are normalized by these drugs. This is probably related to the effect of reserpine on the endocrines whereby stress reactions (which reflect adrenocortical functions) are reduced. For example, the intramuscular administration of 25 mg. of adrenocorticotropic hormone produces only a 20 to 30 per cent drop in blood eosinophiles instead of a 50 per cent decrease.

v. Ophthalmological. Ptosis of the eyelids and constriction of pupils (miosis) are frequent concomitants of reserpine treatment. Other ophthalmological side-effects are lacrimation and conjunctival vasodilation.

vi. Cardiovascular. In animal experiments on isolated hearts, antiveratrinic and antiarrhythmic actions of Rauwolfias have been described; in humans hypotension and bradycardia are the most common. Occasionally cutaneous vasodilation or epistaxis have occurred in the course of reserpine treatment.

vii. Bronchopulmonary. While small doses of reserpine increase the amplitude of respiration, high doses decrease not only the rate but also the depth and minute volume. Aggravation or precipitation of bronchial asthma may occur. This is not attributed to a direct effect of Rauwolfia drugs but rather to allergic mechanisms.

viii. Gastrointestinal. Besides nausea and heartburn, increased gastric secretion and intestinal motility (diarrhea) are also frequent concomitants of Rauwolfia treatment. Activation of peptic ulcers has been attributed to reserpine administration, and less frequently perforation of gastrointestinal ulcers has been described. All these adverse effects are presumably related to the central enhancement of parasympathetic activity.

ix. Genitourinary. Partly as a consequence of the stimulation of pituitary antidiuretic hormone secretion and partly by a direct effect on the kidneys, water and salt retention are not infrequent in the course of reserpine administration. As a consequence, edema of the face and extremities may develop concomitantly with a weight gain. Other adverse effects are frequency of micturition, nocturnal incontinence and renal colic. Decreased concentration and dilution of the urine have been described based on Volhard's test of renal function.

x. Others. Other infrequently occurring side-effects are biliary colic, thrombocytopenia with purpura, skin rash, seborrheic dermatitis, urticaria, and angioneurotic edema.

xi. Overdosage. Overdosage results in a confusional state which leads to drowsiness and in certain cases to coma. Hypotension, bradycardia, bradypnoea, hypothermia, extrapyramidal signs and convulsions are all indicators of overdosage with these drugs.

b. Treatment of Adverse Reactions

Depending on the nature and severity of the adverse drug reaction and also on the dynamics of the situation in which it occurs, adverse reactions may call for discontinuation of the medication; reduction of the dosage; adjuvant medication; or acceptance of the unwanted reaction and continuation of treatment.

Discontinuation of treatment is indicated in toxic confusional states, depression, midbrain syndrome, activation of gastrointestinal ulcers, biliary colic and thrombocytopenic purpura. Acceptance of the adverse effect and continuation of treatment are suggested in mild cases of nasal congestion, excessive salivation (or dry mouth), lacrimation and conjunctival vasodilation.

Persistent drowsiness, inner restlessness, disturbing nightmares, extrapyramidal signs, cerebral seizures, paresthesia and hypotension usually respond to reduction in dosage. Severe extrapyramidal manifestations, recurring cerebral seizures, disturbing nasal congestion, bradycardia, diarrhea and the dermatological (particularly the allergic) reactions are treated with adjuvant drugs. The marked vagotonic effects frequently seen in the course of treatment with these drugs can be counteracted by orphenadrine.

Rauwolfia-produced bradycardia is abolished by atropine; gastrointestinal symptoms are properly treated by belladonna substances and antacids; and nasal congestion and seborrheic dermatitis, by antihistamines, with or without hydrocortisone. It has been suggested that methylphenidate counteracts reserpine-induced drowsiness and depression (Ferguson, 1955) and that glutethimide may be therapeutic in reserpine-induced extrapyramidal manifestations. The latter reaction responds also to antiparkinsonian medication.

In the management of overdosage, gastric lavage, bedrest, analeptics, paraldehyde or barbiturates are used according to the symptoms manifested. Intravenous administration of 5 per cent glucose in saline with noradrenaline is usually recommended.

4. The Use of Rauwolfias in Medical Practice

At first the powdered preparation of the whole root of *Rauwolfia serpentina* (Raudixin) was used in the therapy of psychiatric patients. Later on, the partially purified mixture of the alseroxylin fraction (Rauwiloid) and isolated single alkaloid preparations were introduced into treatment. Of them, reserpine, deserpidine and rescinnamine are of psychiatric interest. Finally, semisynthetic analogues were prepared and introduced in treatment, *e.g.*, syrosingopine.

Clinical experience with the various Rauwolfia preparations revealed that of the clinically used psychoactive preparations Raudixin and Rauwiloid are the weakest. Therefore their usage had been restricted to psychoneurotic patients. Better results in psychotic patients were obtained with reserpine, deserpidine and rescinnamine, although the last compound is probably more useful in acute anxiety neuroses than in the functional psychoses. Of the two other drugs there are some indications that deserpidine may have a somewhat more rapid onset of action and less adverse effects than reserpine. Clinically, syrosingopine—the semisynthetic analogue—is without psychotropic action, and its usage remains restricted to the treatment of hypertensive patients.

Approximately 15 per cent of the chronic, restless schizophrenics responded to psychoactive Rauwolfias to the extent that they could be discharged from the hospital. Furthermore, the ward adjustment of approximately 70 per cent of chronic schizophrenics improved. The disadvantages of Rauwolfias are their slow onset of action, the production of gastric hypersecretion, which is sometimes accompianed by activation of peptic ulcers, and a relatively high frequency of depression that may occur in the course of treatment. Because of these their use has been restricted primarily to patients who cannot tolerate or are unresponsive to phenothiazine drugs.

However, the introduction of Rauwolfias in psychiatric treatment contributed greatly to the over-all changes which have taken place in psychiatry in the past decade. Besides their therapeutic value they also contributed to psychopathological understanding and opened new avenues for research by recognizing at least one of the neurochemical concomitants of the particular type of depression produced by these drugs.

SUMMARY

While Rauwolfias have been therapeutically used since ancient times, their reassessment in the nineteen fifties and their introduction in the treatment of various psychiatric conditions contributed greatly to the reunion of psychiatry with the other fields of medical science and practice.

At first it was believed that psychoactive Rauwolfias and particularly reserpine merely rendered formerly untreatable patients amenable for psychotherapeutic intervention. This gave place to the contention that the combination of these drugs with other forms of treatment potentiates therapeutic success. Finally it is recognized that not only are these therapeutic combinations often unnecessary but they are also dangerous in a considerable number of cases and that Rauwolfias may be therapeutic in themselves.

Of the three most frequently used Rauwolfias in psychiatric treatment reserpine is the most extensively used and the most reliable, at least in the treatment of psychotic patients. However, deserpidine may have a somewhat prompter onset of action; and rescinnamine is probably superior in the control of anxiety in hypertensive patients. The effectiveness of these drugs is related to their sedative, tranquilizing and antipsychotic properties concomitant with their neurophysiological and neurochemical actions. Of these, particular attention has been focused on their effect on posterior hypothalamic centers and on their interference with the normal binding of monoamines and consequently low serotonin and norepinephrine levels in the various areas of the central nervous system.

Important adverse effects in the course of reserpine treatment are depression, extrapyramidal signs, cardiovascular (including hypotensive) and gastrointestinal manifestations.

REFERENCES

Ayd, F. J.,: Prolonged use of reserpine in schizophrenia. In: Psychopharmacology frontiers (ed., Kline, N. S.). (Little, Brown, Boston, 1959.)

Ayd, F. J., *et al.*: Treatment of depressive states in ambulatory patients. Dis. Nerv. Syst., *20:* 34 (1959).

Azima, H., Cleghorn, R. A., and Azima, F. J.: Psychodynamic action of Rauwolfia derivatives. In: Psychopharmacology frontiers (ed., Kline, N. S.). (Little, Brown, Boston, 1959.)

Barrett, B. M., and Hansel, F. K.: Reserpine, a new adjunct in the managment of resistant headache patterns: a preliminary report. In: Reserpine in the treatment of neuropsychiatric, neurological and related clinical problems (ed., Miner, R. W.). (The Academy, New York, 1955.)

Barsa, J. A., and Kline, N. S.: Combined reserpine-chlorpromazine therapy in disturbed psychotics. Amer. J. Psychiat., *111:* 780 (1955).

Bein, H. J.: Significance of selected central mechanisms for the analysis of the action of reserpine. In: Reserpine in the treatment of neuropsychiatric, neurological and related clinical problems (ed., Miner, R. W.). (The Academy, New York, 1955.)

Bente, D., and Itil, T.: Clinical electroencephalographic investigations. In: Psychopharmacology frontiers (ed., Kline, N. S.). (Churchill, London, 1959.)

Bower, H. M.: Clinical evaluation of reserpine in the treatment of chronic mental patients. Med. J. Austr., *2:* 82 (1955).

Brodie, B. B.: Interaction of psychotropic drugs with physiological and biochemical mechanisms in brain. Mod. Med., *4:* 453 (1959).

Bussow, H., and Lindner, W.: Glutethimide (doriden) in reserpine-induced depression. In: Psychopharmacology frontiers (ed., Kline, N. S.). (Little, Brown, Boston, 1959.)

Carey, E. F.: A new approach to the emergency treatment of cancer by narcotic withdrawal. In: Reserpine in the treatment of neuropsychiatric, neurological and related clinical problems (ed., Miner, R. W.). (The Academy, New York, 1955.)

Carlsson, A.: On the problem of the mode of action of some psychoactive drugs. Psychiat. Neurol. (Basel), *140:* 220 (1960).

Cavallito, C. J.: Molecular modifications among antihypertensive agents. In: Molecular modification in drug design (ed., Gould, R. F.). (American Chemical Society, Washington, 1964.)

Davies, B. E. (ed.): Depression. (University Press, Cambridge, 1964.)

DeMacedo, G.: Reserpine in the schizophrenias. In: Psychopharmacology frontiers (ed., Kline, N. S.). (Little, Brown, Boston, 1959.)

Ferguson, J. T.: Treatment of reserpine-induced depression with a new analeptic: phenidylate. Ann. N.Y. Acad. Sci., *61:* 101 (1955).

Freis, E. D.: Antihypertensive therapy: In: Molecular modification in drug design (ed., Gould, R. F.). (American Chemical Society, Washington, 1964.)

Friend, D. G.: Role of synthetic drugs in therapy of mental illness. In: Molecular modification in drug design (ed., Gould, R. F.). (American Chemical Society, Washington, 1964.)

Goodman, L. S., and Gilman, A. (eds.): The pharmacological basis of therapeutics. (Macmillan, Toronto, 1965.)

Gordon, M. (ed.): Psychopharmacological agents. (Academic Press, New York, 1964.)

Gould, R. F. (ed.): Molecular modification in drug design. (American Chemical Society, Washington, 1964.)

Gregory, I.: Psychiatry. (Saunders, Philadelphia, 1961.)

Grollman, A.: Pharmacology and Therapeutics. (Lea and Febiger, Philadelphia, 1958.)

Gupta, J. C., Deb, A. K., and Kaholi, B. S.: Preliminary observations on use of Rauwolfia serpentina benth in treatment of mental disorders. Indian Med. Gaz., *78:* 547 (1943).

Haase, H. J.: Clinical observations on the action of neuroleptics. In: Haase, H. J., and Janssen, P. A.: The action of neuroleptic drugs. (North-Holland Publishing Company, Amsterdam, 1965.)

Hakim, R. A.: Indigenous drugs in the treatment of mental diseases. (Sixth Gujurat and Saurashtra Provincial Medical Conference, Baroda, 1953.)

Hess, W. R.: Das Zwischenhirn, Syndrome, Lokalisationen, Funkzionen. (Schwabe, Basel, 1954.)

HIPPIUS, H., KANIG, K., AND SELBACH, H.: Dynamic actions of phenothiazines and reserpine. In: Psychopharmacology frontiers (ed., Kline, N. S.). (Little, Brown, Boston, 1959.)

HOLLISTER, L. E., *et al.*: Treatment of chronic schizophrenic reactions with reserpine. In: Reserpine in the treatment of neuropsychiatric, neurological and related clinical problems (ed., Miner, R. W.). (The Academy, New York, 1955.)

JACOBSEN, E.: Investigation into the mode of action of substances acting on the central nervous system. In: Depression (ed., Davies, E. B.). (University Press, Cambridge, 1964.)

JARVIK, M. E.: Drugs used in the treatment of psychiatric disorders. In: The pharmacological basis of therapeutics (eds., Goodman, L. S., and Gilman, A.). (Macmillan, Toronto, 1965.)

KALINOWSKY, L. B., AND HOCH, P. H.: Somatic treatments in psychiatry. (Grune and Stratton, New York, 1961.)

KLEIN, M.: Contributions to psychoanalysis 1921–1945. (Hogarth, London, 1948.)

KLINE, N. S.: Use of Rauwolfia serpentina benth in neuropsychiatric conditions. Ann. N.Y. Acad. Sci., *59:* 67 (1954).

KLINE, N. S. (ed.): Psychopharmacology frontiers. (Little, Brown, Toronto, 1959.)

KLINE, N. S.: Use of reserpine, the newer phenothiazines and iproniazid. Res. Publ. Ass. Res. Nerv. Ment. Dis., *37:* 218 (1959).

KLINE, N. S., AND STANLEY, A. M.: Use of reserpine in a neuropsychiatric, hospital. In: Reserpine in the treatment of neuropsychiatric, neurological and related clinical problems (ed., Miner, R. W.). (The Academy, New York, 1955.)

KLINE, N. S., AND STANLEY, A. M.: Use of reserpine in neuropsychiatric hospitals. Ann. N.Y. Acad. Sci., *61:* 85 (1955).

LAMBROS, V. S.: The use of reserpine in certain neurological disorders: organic convulsive states, enuresis and head injuries. In: Reserpine in the treatment of neuropsychiatric, neurological and related clinical problems (ed., Miner, R. W.). (The Academy, New York, 1955.)

LANDGRABE, B.: Reserpine in clinical psychiatry. In: Psychopharmacology frontiers (ed., Kline, N. S.). (Little, Brown, Boston, 1959.)

MAYER-GROSS, W., SLATER, E., AND ROTH, M.: Clinical psychiatry. (Cassell, London, 1960.)

MINER, R. W. (ed.): Reserpine in the treatment of neuropsychiatric, neurological and related clinical problems. (The Academy, New York, 1955.)

MÜLLER, J. M., SCHLITTLER, E., AND BEIN, H. J.: Reserpin, der sedative wirkstoff aus Rauwolfia serpentina benth. Experientia, *8:* 388 (1952).

NOYES, A. P., AND KOLB, L. C.: Modern clinical psychiatry. (Saunders, Philadelphia, 1961.)

OSTOW, M.: Drugs in psychoanalysis and psychotherapy. (Basic Books, New York, 1962.)

OSTOW, M., AND KLINE, N. S.: The psychic action of reserpine and chlorpromazine. In: Psychopharmacology frontiers (ed., Kline, N. S.). (Little Brown, Boston, 1959.)

PLUMIER, C. (1703): In: WOODSON, R. E.: The botany of Rauwolfia. In: WOODSON, R. E., JR., *et al.*: Rauwolfia: botany, pharmacognosy, chemistry and pharmacology. (Little, Brown, Boston, 1957.)

PÖLDINGER, W., AND SCHMIDLIN, P.: Index psychopharmacorum 1966. (Huber, Bern, 1966.)

RAY, P. C.: The hypnotic action of Rauwolfia serpentina. Patna J. Med., *6:* 193 (1931).

REMMEN, E., *et al.*: Psychochemotherapy. (Western Medical Publications, Los Angeles, 1962.)

RINALDI, F., AND HIMWICH, H. E.: A comparison of effects of reserpine and some barbiturates on the electrical activity of cortical and subcortical structures of the brain of rabbits. Ann. N.Y. Acad. Sci., *61:* 27 (1955).

RUMPF, G. E. (1755): In: SCHLITTLER, E., AND PLUMMER, A. J.: Tranquillizing drugs from Rauwolfia. In: Psychopharmacological agents (ed., Gordon, M.). (Academic Press, New York, 1964.)

SAINZ, A.: The use of reserpine in ambulatory and hospitalized geriatric psychotics. In: Reserpine in the treatment of neuropsychiatric, neurological and related clinical problems (ed., Miner, R. W.). (The Academy, New York, 1955.)

SCHLITTLER, E., AND PLUMMER, A. J.: Tranquillizing drugs from Rauwolfia. In: Psychopharmacological agents (ed., Gordon, M.). (Academic Press, New York, 1964.)

SCHNEIDER, J. A.: Further characterization of central effects of reserpine (serpasil). Amer. J. Physiol., *181:* 64 (1955).

SCHNEIDER, J. A.: The acute effects of reserpine and of amytal on central sympathetic reactivity. Ann. N.Y. Acad. Sci., *61:* 160 (1955).

SCHNEIDER, J. A., *et al.*: Neuropharmacological aspects of reserpine. In: Reserpine in the treatment of neuropsychiatric, neurological and related clinical problems (ed., Miner, R. W.). (The Academy, New York, 1955.)

SEN, G., AND BOSE, K. C.: Rauwolfia serpentina, a new Indian drug for insanity and high blood pressure. Indian Med. World, *2:* 194 (1931).

SHEPPARD, H., AND ZIMMERMAN, J. H.: Reserpine and the levels of serotonin and norepinephrine in the brain. Nature (London), *185:* 40 (1960).

SOURKES, T. L.: Biochemistry of mental disease. (Harper and Row, New York, 1962.)

TALBOT, W.: The use of reserpine in irritable and hypertonic infants. In: Reserpine in the treatment of neuropsychiatric, neurological and related clinical problems (ed., Miner, R. W.). (The Academy, New York, 1955.)

VAKIL, R. B. (1949): In: SCHLITTLER, E., AND PLUMMER, A. J.: Tranquillizing drugs from Rauwolfia. In: Psychopharmacological agents (ed., Gordon, M.). (Academic Press, New York, 1964.)

VALENTINE, M.: An introduction to psychiatry. (Livingstone, Edinburgh, 1962.)

WEBER, E.: Ein Rauwolfia Alkaloid in der Psychiatrie: seine Wirkingsähnlichkeit mit chlorpromazin. Schweiz. Med. Wschr., *84:* 968 (1954).

WEISKRANTZ, L., AND WILSON, W. A.: The effects of reserpine on emotional behavior on normal and brain operated monkeys. Ann. N.Y. Acad. Sci., *61:* 36 (1955).

WILKINS, R. W.: Clinical usage of Rauwolfia. Ann. N.Y. Acad. Sci., *59:* 36 (1954).

WOODSON, R. E., JR.: The botany of Rauwolfia. In: WOODSON, R. E. JR., *et al.*: Rauwolfia: botany, pharmacognosy, chemistry and pharmacology. (Little, Brown, Boston, Toronto, 1957.)

WOODSON, R. E., JR., *et al.*: Rauwolfia: botany, pharmacognosy, chemistry and pharmacology. (Little, Brown, Boston, Toronto, 1957.)

WOODWARD, R. B. (1956): In: SCHLITTLER, E. The chemistry of Rauwolfia alkaloids. In: Rauwolfia: botany, pharmacognosy, chemistry and pharmacology (ed., Woodson, R. E., *et al.*). (Little, Brown, Boston, Toronto, 1957.)

Twelve

The Butyrophenones

A. BASIC DATA

1. Historical Aspects

As occurs so often in pharmacological research, the recognition of a certain specific property, in this case the antipsychotic property of the butyrophenones, was incidental. In their efforts to increase the morphine-like potency of drugs, Janssen *et al.* (1959, 1960, 1961) studied a large series of 4-phenylpiperidines related to pethidine (meperidine). Mannich reaction with normeperidine and acetophenone yielded a propriophenone derivative that was 100 times more potent morphine-like drug than meperidine itself. Lengthening the ethylene chain by one methyl group resulted in the first butyrophenone substance found to possess both morphine-like analgesic and chlorpromazine-like neuroleptic properties.

Subsequent systematic exploratory work revealed that replacing the $COOC_2H_5$ group by an OH radical and substituting the ketonic phenyl ring with fluorine in the para-position increased chlorpromazine-like and decreased morphine-like effects. Thus the 4-fluorobutyrophenone derivative of 4-phenylpiperidine-4-ol was shown to be a typical neuroleptic completely devoid of morphine-like actions. Finally, aromatic substitutions on the phenyl ring attached to the piperidine nucleus yielded haloperidol, trifluperidol (triperidol) and other potent neuroleptic (antipsychotic) drugs (Janssen, 1967).

2. Action Mechanism

A number of hypotheses have been formulated. A neurophysiological hypothesis by Venning (1963) postulated that the behavioral effects of neuroleptic drugs are mediated through the inhibitory pathways of the extrapyramidal system (possibly the caudate loop). There is some experimental evidence for this hypothesis from the studies of Magoun (1944, 1950, 1952), who demonstrated certain inhibitory influences of the basal ganglia (caudate loop) upon the functions of the reticular activating system.

This hypothesis suggests a relationship between neuroleptic potency and the pattern of extrapyramidal side-effects. It does not necessarily mean that extrapyramidal motor phenomena *per se* are necessary or useful therapeutically.

A physiochemical hypothesis of the action mechanism of butyrophenones (and also of other neuroleptic antipsychotic drugs) was put forward by Janssen (1966). While he maintained that the crucial action of these drugs is in specific areas of the extrapyramidal system, he also pointed out that their antipsychotic property is likely to be correlated with their surface tension lowering (or membrane permeability lowering) property. Janssen (1966) suggested that neuroleptic drugs are probably blockers of the "inflow" into cells and consequently that they possibly affect the transport function of specialized astrocytes of the blood-brain barrier around the ventricles and inhibit adrenergic neurons in the same areas.

3. Structure and Activity

The basic structure of this group of compounds is the butyrophenone moiety, which consists of a ketonic phenyl ring with a straight propylene chain with a piperidine nucleus. In the para-position the ketonic phenyl ring has a fluorine substituent, and the piperidine nucleus is substituted in position 4 with a tertiary alcohol group with a phenyl ring. In haloperidol this phenyl ring is para-substituted with a chlorine atom, while in trifluperidol it is meta-substituted with a CF_3 group. This structural difference may account for somewhat greater therapeutic effectiveness of the former substance in acute and of the latter in chronic schizophrenic patients.

The prototype drug in the butyrophenone group is haloperidol, a potent blocker of conditioned responses and a specific antagonist of amphetamine and of apomorphine. It is practically devoid of autonomic effects. Haloperidol exerts antipsychotic and antiemetic effects in man when given in daily doses of 1 to 6 mg., and it is capable of inducing the neuroleptic syndrome.

Further studies by Janssen (1963) revealed that isosteric replacement of the ketonic phenyl ring of butyrophenones is possible without any substantial pharmacological change while para-fluorine substitution increases the neuroleptic potency considerably. On the other hand, ortho- or meta-substitutions (on the same ring) as well as shortening, lengthening or branching of the *trimethylene side chain* decreases the psychoactive potential of these drugs.

Substitutions on the *second phenyl ring* attached to the piperidine nucleus result in the following changes: para-substitution with chlorine (as in haloperidol) yields compounds with considerably longer duration of action than para-substitution with methyl- or meta-substitution with CF_3; and poly-substitution or replacement of the phenyl nucleus by other moieties results in the loss of neuroleptic potency (with the exception of floropipamide, a 4-piperidinopiperidine derivative, which remains psychopharmacologically active).

Replacement of the OH group by other groups, the introduction of a third substituent on the piperidine ring, and reduction of the ketone group to a secondary alcohol function generally decrease neuroleptic and increase morphine-like activity of these drugs.

Replacement of the piperidine ring by a pyrolidine or a hexamethylenimine ring results in loss of activity. However, neuroleptic and adrenolytic activity has been shown among several 4-arylpiperazine analogues of haloperidol (*e.g.*, fluanisone).

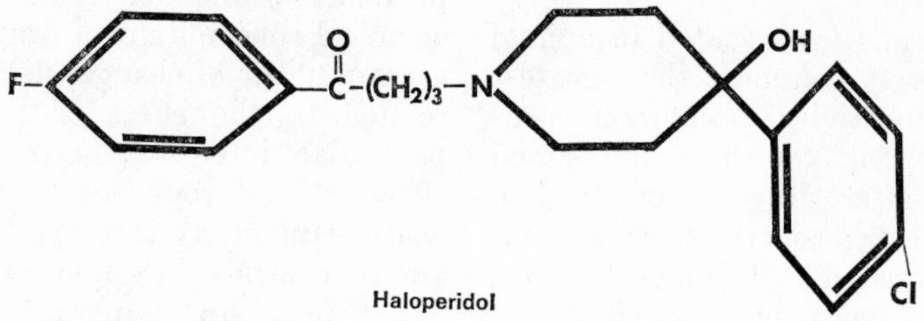

F–C6H4–C(=O)–$(CH_2)_3$–N (piperidine, 4-OH, 4-(4-chlorophenyl))

Haloperidol

F–C6H4–C(=O)–$(CH_2)_3$–N (piperidine, 4-OH, 4-(3-CF_3-phenyl)) .HCl

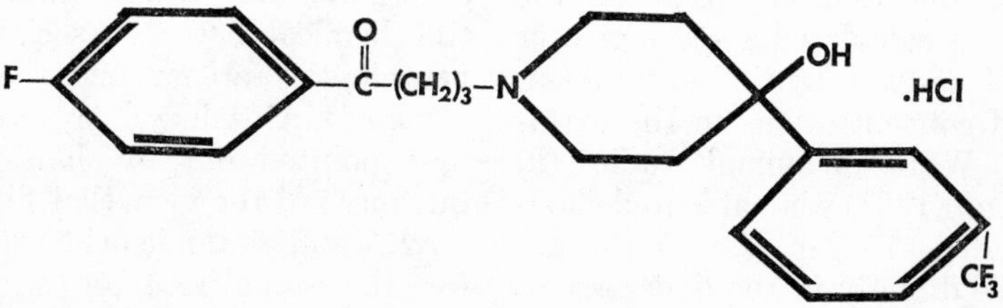

Triperidol

FIG. 12. Haloperidol and triperidol

The neuroleptic (and also antiemetic) potency of the various butyrophenones in decreasing order is as follows: spiroperidol, dihydrobenzperidol, benzperidol, triperidol, haloperidol, ethylperidol, fluanisone and floropipamide (Janssen, 1965).

4. Metabolism

The fate of haloperidol in the organism has been studied both in animal and in man, in normal subjects and in patients with schizophrenic psychopathology (Braun and associates, 1967; and Johnson *et al.*, 1967).

a. Absorption

In animals and humans haloperidol is absorbed promptly. Isotope studies show radioactivity in the blood within the first hour after oral administration. In general, there is a slightly higher plasma concentration in schizophrenics than in normals. There is not only rapid but also nearly complete absorption of the substance. Highest plasma levels are attained 2 to 6 hours after ingestion, which suggests that absorption occurs in the upper gastrointestinal tract. Johnson *et al.* (1967) also demonstrated that plasma levels rapidly reach a plateau and remain nearly the same for about 72 hours and then slowly descend, with significant levels remaining in the circulation for weeks after the ingestion of even small amounts.

b. Distribution

Of all the organs investigated in animal studies, the liver contains the greatest quantity of radioactivity, reaching a maximum of 15 per cent (of the administered dose) 3 hours after drug administration. At the same time a considerably less amount could only be detected in the lungs, kidneys, brain, spleen and heart, in that order.

When total distribution space of the radioactivity was calculated a space greater than the total body weight was obtained. This indicated concentrations in the extravascular sites. While in animal studies (in rats) Braun *et al.* (1967) were able to demonstrate as much as 15 per cent of the administered dose directly in the liver tissues, in humans only the biliary excretion of the radioactivity gave indirect evidence of hepatic drug concentrations.

In rats significant quantities of radioactivity were found in the urine within the first 8 hours after drug administration. However, by 96 hours the amount of radioactivity excreted in the feces approximated that found in the urine. Biliary elimination accounted for approximately 15 per cent of the administered dose.

In humans, urinary excretion of the radioactivity begins rapidly, with a significant amount appearing within 2 hours of ingestion. Although the peak excretion rate is reached within the first 4 hours, only 40 per cent of the radioactivity can be recovered from the urine at the end of the first 5 days. The slow urinary excretion of butyrophenone drugs, combined with the low plasma levels, suggests the binding of these substances in the organism to tissue proteins and especially to cell membranes.

The amount of radioactivity in the feces is less than that in the urine (in humans). Thus even where the urinary and fecal excretions are combined, only 24 to 60 per cent of the ingested dose is recovered. Small amounts of radioactivity are excreted even 28 days after drug administration.

5. Chemical and Neurophysiological Correlates of Drug Action

a. Chemical Correlates

The psychotropic properties of butyrophenones cannot be reduced to a single chemical concomitant of drug action. There are a number of changes described that are related to the effect of these drugs. Of particular interest among these are the effects of butyrophenones on the glutamic acid/γ-aminobutyric acid (GABA) system and on central adrenergic neurons.

i. Effect on Glutamic Acid/GABA System. The striking similarity between the chemical features associated with strong neuroleptic potency and the chemical features of GABA-like depressant activity was first pointed out by Janssen (1966). He put forward the view that "if it is true that GABA and glutamic acid are in competition for the same receptor site on neuronal transmitter receptor membranes; that glutamic acid excites certain neurons by a membrane polarization effect; that GABA depresses these cells and antagonizes glutamic acid without altering membrane potential; that the action of both amino-acids are mediated by cellular and subcellular membrane permeability changes (Curtis and Watkins, 1960; Buniatian, 1963) and unrelated to a transmitter function (Ryall, 1964); and furthermore if it is true that the glutamic acid/GABA system is particularly important in areas of the brain belonging to the extrapyramidal motor system (Mueller and Langemann, 1962), it would appear reasonable to advance the working hypothesis that potent neuroleptics would decrease cellular and subcellular membrane permeability processes, particularly in neurons belonging to the extrapyramidal system, by occupying GABA receptors and making them inaccessible to glutamic acid."

Seeman and Bialy's (1963) findings support this view. They were able to demonstrate that neuroleptic drugs, even in small concentrations, reduce surface tension. These substances reduce membrane permeability by the formation of a "diffusion-limiting" monomolecular subfilm on the outer aspect of the cell membrane (increasing its thickness).

Janssen (1966) surmised that neuroleptics, *e.g.*, butyrophenones, have a greater tendency to form a monomolecular film on GABA-receptor-containing membranes than on others and expected to find that low doses of these substances will interfere specifically with transport mechanisms in the extrapyramidal system, where permeability is regulated largely by the GABA/glutamic acid system.

ii. Effects on Central Adrenergic Neurons. (α). *Dopamine.* Knowing that neuroleptic butyrophenones are amphetamine antagonists, and that the locomotor stimulant action of amphetamine is induced by activation of dopamine receptors in the brain, Rossum (1966) hypothesized that a dopamine receptor blockade is an important factor in the mode of action of these drugs.

Dopamine causes a fall in blood pressure after the blockade of sympathetic alpha receptors in the cat. This effect is counteracted by low doses of butyrophenone drugs, *e.g.*, spiroperidol and haloperidol (Rossum, 1966). This suggested that the butyrophenones are specific dopamine antagonist drugs.

β. *Norepinephrine.* Dresse and De Meyer (1964) demonstrated that antipsychotic butyrophenones prevent the increase of brain norepinephrine (NE) concentration usually seen after tranylcypromine administration. They do not counteract the NE depletory effect of reserpine. This suggests that the inhibition of MAOI activity might be related to the neuroleptic activity of these drugs.

γ. *Others.* There is experimental evidence which suggests that antipsychotic butyrophenones induce a prolonged increase of homovanillic acid concentration in the corpus striatum of the rabbit and a transient increase of 3,4-dihydroxyphenylacetic acid. Carlsson and Lindquist (1962) also demonstrated an enhanced accumulation of methoxytyramine and normetanephrine in the CNS with MAOI's after pretreatment with butyrophenone drugs.

Janssen (1966) asserts that this kind of evidence indicates that neuroleptics may exert their characteristic actions by inhibiting the transport mechanism of dopamine, NE, and similar hypothetical CNS transmitters through the cellular membrane into the cytoplasm of the nerve ending or back into the small transmitter pool through the subcellular membrane, through the membranes surrounding the receptor site into the receptor area, and also through the membranes surrounding the whole synaptic area through which *o*-methylated and other metabolites are probably eliminated.

b. Neurophysiological Correlates

There is no single neurophysiological phenomenon which can fully account for the multifold activities of these drugs. They induce functional alterations in the various areas in the nervous system from the lowest level of integration to the cerebral cortex.

i. Medulla Oblongata. It has been shown (in the dog) that behaviorally inactive doses of haloperidol, trifluperidol and other butyrophenone drugs prevent the emetic effect of large doses of apomorphine (Janssen and Niemegeers, 1959). Since the emetic trigger zone is located in the area cinerea at the floor of the fourth ventricle, it has been suggested that butyrophenones act on the medullary centers.

Dresse (1964) surmised that apomorphine probably penetrates into the emetic chemoreceptor trigger zone through the vascular foot of a particular kind of small astrocyte. It was further assumed that apomorphine possibly depolarizes the astrocytic membrane and electrically stimulates an adrenergic neurone which in turn stimulates the cholinergic neurones of the vomiting center, thereby triggering the emetic process. Since circulating butyrophenones probably penetrate the area cinerea through the same astrocytes, Janssen (1966) hypothesized that they prevent released transmitter substances from reaching the receptors by forming a permeability-decreasing monolayer on the surface of the membranes surrounding the vomiting center.

ii. Brain Stem Reticular Formation. In immobilized cats the arousal threshold has been found to be only slightly affected by haloperidol. In unrestrained cats with implanted electrodes, chronic haloperidol administration has produced a slight elevation of the arousal threshold (Monti *et al.*, 1966).

A decreased responsivity of the reticular formation has been reported by Arrigo *et al.* (1962). This decrease was more marked in the caudal portion of this area than rostrally (since the motor response to posterior hypothalamic stimulation was blocked to a greater degree than the cortical response). This selective action distinctly differentiates psychoactive butyrophenones from other neuroleptic drugs, *e.g.*, phenothiazines or Rauwolfia alkaloids, which interfere with both responses equally (Müller and Warnes, 1964).

iii. Hypothalamus. Histological signs of intense functional stimulation of the supraoptic and paraventricular nucleus of the hypothalamus with a corresponding intense activity of the suprarenal cortex are seen in rabbits under the influence of triperidol (Della Beffa *et al.*, 1962).

iv. Extrapyramidal System. The function of the extrapyramidal system was long considered entirely restricted to the control of motor phenomena. In 1946 Magoun and Rhines demonstrated inhibitory influences of the basal ganglia upon the functions of the reticular system and postulated an inhibitory feedback circuit in the "caudate loop." They also showed that the effects of excitation of this "loop" are antagonistic to those of the brain stem reticular arousal system.

With implanted electrodes Buchwald *et al.* (1961) studied the influence of caudate stimulation on behavior (in cats). They found a lengthening of the reaction time during a conditioned avoidance procedure independent of the impairment in the accuracy of the response.

Since Janssen (1962) has shown that haloperidol and other butyrophenones have an inhibitory influence upon behavior (in rats and dogs) which closely resembled that described by Buchwald *et al.* (1961) (*i.e.*, a significant increase in reaction time in conditioned avoidance responses dissociated from impairment of the accuracy of response), Venning (1963) suggested the possibility that one of the sites of action of these drugs is in the area of the caudate nucleus.

v. Hippocampus. In immobilized cats hippocampal seizure thresholds were found to be raised and the duration of afterdischarges reduced under the influence of a single dose of haloperidol (above 8 mg./kg.). On the other hand, in unrestrained cats chronic (8 to 10 days) administration of the same substance (2 mg./kg. per day) failed to modify hippocampal seizure activity (Monti *et al.*, 1966).

vi. Cerebral Cortex. The effects of butyrophenones on the human electroencephalogram have been systematically explored. Meurice (1960) was first to demonstrate that a single intravenous dose (5 and 10 mg.) of haloperidol induces a "pronounced modulation of alpha-waves or appearance of theta-waves (and in one case stabilisation of an extremely unstable electrodermogram)." The same substance when chronically administered (in daily doses of 3 to 6 mg.) for at least a 10-day period produced a slightly decreased frequency, increased amplitude and a greater spatial repartition of the electroencephalogram.

Similar findings were reported by Milani

(1962), Gattuso and Lanteri (1962), and Müller and Warnes (1964). Furthermore, Bente *et al.* (1962) demonstrated that the EEG effects of floropipamide are intermediate between chlorpromazine and piperazinylalkyl side chain ring containing phenothiazines.

It is interesting to note that the best therapeutic effects in schizophrenics were seen by Bente *et al.* (1962) in cases with a poor alpha rhythm which improved in the course of treatment; while in Müller and Warnes' (1964) series, the shifts in the alpha frequency toward the slow side and the appearance of diffuse disturbances were most prominent in patients with a favorable prognosis. On the other hand, Goldwurm and Torrigiani (1962) suggested that low voltage fast records may indicate a poor therapeutic response.

6. Behavioral Pharmacology

a. Animal Studies

Neuroleptic butyrophenones induce behavioral changes in animals and men over a wide range of functions. This was first discovered by Janssen *et al.* (1956) in mice, using a modification of Eddy's hot plate screening method (Janssen and Eddy, 1960). In this procedure, after subcutaneous drug administration the reaction time of a typical licking reflex (elicited by dropping the mouse onto a 55°C hot plate) is determined. The pupil diameter is measured; and the general behavior of the animal is recorded. It was found that butyrophenones shared with other neuroleptics the properties of producing cataleptic immobility and palpebral ptosis. These properties differentiated them from barbiturate-like hypnotics, which induced ataxia and loss of righting reflex; from morphine-like analgesics, which were characterized by excitement and Straub phenomenon; and from atropine-like anticholinergics, which were without any characteristic behavioral effects (Janssen, 1967).

In one of the early animal pharmacological studies, haloperidol was characterized by a strong analgesic action, potent "cataleptogenic" properties and the lack of autonomic effects (Boissier *et al.*, 1964). Repeated daily administration did not induce habituation in the Traction Test, while it did induce a partial habituation of the analgesic action and a total habituation of potentiation of the hypnotic action of a barbiturate.

Today there are a number of pharmacological tests in which neuroleptic drugs in general or antipsychotic butyrophenones in particular exert characteristic effects. The ten most frequently used procedures (Janssen, 1967) may be subdivided into direct and indirect pharmacological methods. Among the direct pharmacological techniques are the Open Field Test (which consists of measuring exploratory ambulation, rearing, preening and "emotional defecation" in rats) and the Catalepsy-Ptosis Method (in rats). The indirect tests are of three different subgroups. In the first of these the interference with physically induced changes are studied, while in the second interference with chemically induced changes are explored, and in the third the effects of the new substance on conditional reflex behavior are investigated. The DW-Test (*i.e.*, the interference with weight increase in a 22-hour food-deprivation schedule) and the Noble and Collip Drumming Procedure (*i.e.*, the interference with shock) in rats are representatives of the first subgroup of tests. The Antiamphetamine Method (*i.e.*, the blocking of compulsory gnawing movements in rats and emesis in dogs), the Antiepinephrine (or norepinephrine) Test (*i.e.*, the protection against the lethal effects of these catecholamines), and the Antitryptamine Test in rats (*i.e.*, the protection against the clonic seizures of the forepaws induced by this substance) belong to the second subgroup of tests. Finally, the Jumping Box method in rats (an Active Avoidance Procedure) is of the third subgroup.

Characteristic effects of antipsychotic butyrophenones are the following. Inhibition of motor phenomena at low dose levels in the Open Field Test, induction of cataleptic immobility and palpebral ptosis; depression of food consumption and weight increase on the DW test and protection against shock-induced mortality in the Noble and Collip Drumming Procedure;

blocking of the amphetamine- and apomorphine-induced gnawing movements (in rats), inhibiting of the apomorphine-induced emesis (in dog), protection against the lethal effects of E and NE and protection against the tryptamine-induced clonic seizures; and inhibition of conditioned avoidance responses at dose levels that are devoid of obvious behavioral effects.

Recently, Oberst and Crook (1967) have shown an inhibitory effect of haloperidol on a sustained Physical Exercise Test (in which dogs were trained to run on a treadmill for 15-minute intervals, followed by a 2-minute rest period, for a maximum of 1 hour). While normal untreated dogs were able to perform this test without difficulty, haloperidol-treated (12.5 mg./kg. to 25 mg./kg.) dogs could not.

b. Human Studies

When given to normal volunteers, in a placebo-controlled double blind experiment, 4 mg. of haloperidol induced a feeling of tiredness. While haloperidol did not interfere with the efficiency of solution of a mathematical problem, it resulted in an overestimation by the subject of his own ability to carry out the task (Eiff and Jesdinsky, 1960).

In the same human pharmacological study a lowering of blood pressure, pulse rate and temperature was noted. Furthermore, while the maximal "ergometric performance" did not change immediately, haloperidol decreased ergometric performance in longer lasting tests. It was also noted that the participating volunteers felt tired more rapidly when receiving the active substance than the placebo.

i. Psychophysical Effects. A battery of seven psychometric tests was administered to a group of chronic schizophrenic patients (on no medication) to measure the relative influences of the butyrophenones haloperidol and trifluperidol and of chlorprothixene and chlorpromazine (St. Jean *et al.*, 1964). The following tendencies appeared in those tested with butyrophenones. On the visual perceptual tasks the mean scores of haloperidol and trifluperidol were virtually equal; *i.e.*, both butyrophenones tended to lower Critical Flicker Fusion Frequency threshold and both raised the threshold of After-Image Disappearance Limen. On the relatively more structured psychomotor and conceptual tasks such as in Track Tracer Time, Time Reproduction and Word Association Time, the direction and even the magnitude of the effects of the two butyrophenone preparations were found to be nearly equal; *i.e.*, they improved performance on the Track Tracer Time and on the Time Reproduction tests, while they increased Word-Assocation Time. On relatively unstructured motor activity tasks such as Tapping Speed and Reaction Time, triperidol and haloperidol produced widely divergent effects, the former tending to increase performance and the latter tending to decrease it.

In the same experiment chlorpromazine increased the latencies of temporal measures of performance, and the effect of chlorprothixene was generally midway between that of the butyrophenones and chlorpromazine. Where the effects of haloperidol and triperidol diverged, chlorprothixene and haloperidol showed some similarities (and the chlorprothixene effect was midway between that of chlorpromazine and triperidol).

ii. Psychophysiological Effects. In Saarma and Saarma's (1966) experiment a single dose of haloperidol, given to chronic schizophrenics, brought about only slight changes "in both the higher nervous activity and vegetative functions."

In a clinical pharmacological study, Saarma and Saarma (1966), administering 6 mg. of haloperidol daily to a group of chronic schizophrenics, noted the first therapeutic shift as a moderate decrease of sympathetic tone. The autonomic changes were followed by "regression of the passive inhibition, improvement of the excitatory process and the equilibrium of the basic nervous processes." Saarma and Saarma (1966) recognized that, compared with chlorpromazine and trifluoperazine, haloperidol is less potent in "lowering the sympathetic tone and reactivity" and also in producing a "regression of external inhibition and improvement of the excitatory and of the internal inhibitory processes."

B. CLINICAL DATA

1. Indications and Contraindications

a. Indications

Butyrophenone drugs can be successfully administered in a variety of psychopathological conditions. Besides the psychiatric indications, they are frequently used in anesthesiology and as antiemetic drugs. Haloperidol has gained favor in obstetric patients to control nausea, vomiting and apprehension associated with labor and delivery and is also occasionally prescribed for the purpose of augmenting the effects of narcotic analgesics.

Psychiatric indications of butyrophenones are as follows.

i. Functional Psychoses. *α. Schizophrenias.* Divry *et al.* (1960) considered haloperidol "a major weapon in the treatment of schizophrenia" without any further elaboration of the responsive or unresponsive cases. Their enthusiasm was shared by Pacquay, Arnould *et al.* (1960), Kristjansen (1960) and others. More specific findings on the effect of haloperidol were reported by Delay *et al.* (1960), who suggested that the drug is satisfactorily therapeutic in cases of acute schizophrenia and paranoid schizophrenia but disappointing in hebephrenic patients. Bishop and Gallant (1965), in their clinical trial with trifluperidol, failed to corroborate the selective efficacy on paranoid schizophrenic patients. They suggested, however, that this compound is of superior efficacy in both paranoid and nonparanoid schizophrenics.

In the course of a comparative clinical trial of haloperidol, chlorpromazine and chlorprothixene in acute schizophrenics, Lehmann *et al.* (1964) were able to demonstrate that during the first 6 weeks of treatment haloperidol produced significant improvement over a wider range of psychopathological symptoms than either of the two other compounds. In an uncontrolled study Gershon (1967) found trifluperidol therapeutic to the extent that 9 of his 14 patients improved sufficiently to be released from hospital, but with a limited (mainly "hallucinolytic") range of action. Sugerman and Williams (1965), in a comparative study of trifluperidol and trifluoperazine, found the two drugs equally effective in the treatment of acute schizophrenic patients.

The results of systematic studies on the effect of butyrophenones in chronic schizophrenics were presented by Ban and Lehmann (1967). In the first of this series the effect of haloperidol was compared with fluphenazine in a 6-week clinical trial. The findings in this study suggest that, while in general both substances are equally effective therapeutically, haloperidol might be the drug of choice if perceptual disorder prevails and fluphenazine if thought disorder is the predominant symptom (Ban, 1962). The effects of haloperidol were compared with butaperazine in a short term clinical trial, and in the third study with trifluoperazine in a long term, clinical evaluation. In these studies haloperidol proved to be therapeutically equal to the phenothiazine drugs. Even more, it seemed to be somewhat faster in its action than butaperazine (Warnes *et al.*, 1966). Similar findings were reported by Gallant *et al.* (1963), while Schiele (1966) found trifluoperazine therapeutically superior to trifluperidol in a group of chronic anergic schizophrenics. Finally, the therapeutic effects of haloperidol, trifluperidol and floropipamide were studied (in a clinical trial which followed a latin square, double blind, cross-over experimental design). Of the three butyrophenones, triperidol was the most potent compound and floropipamide the least, haloperidol occupying an intermediate position (Warnes *et al.*, 1964). Although floropipamide was the least effective of the three drugs in the last study, Sugerman (1964) still found it an effective drug in the treatment of chronic schizophrenic patients.

β. Manic-Depressive Psychosis. Haloperidol is considered to be one of the best of the available substances in the treatment of manic patients (Divry *et al.*, 1960; Delay *et al.*, 1960; Gerle, 1960; Humbeeck, 1960; Loret, 1960; Oles, 1960; Lindquist, 1961; etc). On the other hand, while it may control anxiety and agitation it remains essentially ineffective (or has an adverse effect) in the treatment of depressions (Waelkens, 1960; Oles, 1960; Loret, 1960; etc.). Fink *et al.* (1966), nevertheless, consider trifluperidol an active antipsychotic drug which alleviates depression and ameliorates affective disturbances.

ii. Organic Syndromes. Beneficial effects with butyrophenones have been reported in both acute and chronic organic cases (Harder, 1961). The usefulness of haloperidol in the treatment of delirium tremens was suggested by Oles (1960) and confirmed by Giacobini and Lassenius (1961); its value in the management of confusional states was recognized by Lereboullet *et al.* (1962), and its therapeutic effect in Huntington's chorea was established by Olsson (1961). A particular indication for haloperidol is in Gilles de la Tourette's Disease.

Successful treatment of Tourette's disease with haloperidol was reported by Seignot (1961) and subsequently confirmed by Challas and Brauer (1963) and Chapel *et al.* (1964). However, Chapel (1966) points out that, while the symptoms of Tourette's disease are well controlled in all cases, there is no reason to assume that the great hostility locked within these patients is directly affected by the drug.

iii. Other Conditions. Butyrophenones have been found therapeutically useful in orthopsychiatric and in geriatric practice (Fish and Campbell, 1966; and Sugerman *et al.*, 1964).

A useful sedative action of trifluperidol was reported in hyperactive children by Fish and Campbell (1966). The same substance produced increased motor vigor and initiative in some hypoactive cases. Sleep patterns were improved in all the children.

In agitated, overactive and hostile elderly patients suffering from a chronic brain syndrome with cerebral arteriosclerosis or senile brain disease, Sugerman *et al.* (1964) found haloperidol therapeutically effective.

b. Contraindications

There are relatively few absolute contraindications of butyrophenone treatment. Among these are comatose states, Parkinson's disease and spastic diseases. Some consider the first trimester of pregnancy, infancy and depressive states as relative contraindications. They should not be used in the treatment of patients who are generally sensitive to drugs or in patients with a predisposition for Parkinsonian manifestations.

According to Humbeeck (1960), haloperidol should be used carefully in patients with encephalitic lesions and in aged patients in general, while Waelkens (1960) considers all forms of central paralysis, all forms of depression and neurosis, and coronary sclerosis as contraindications of butyrophenone treatment.

2. Therapy Alone and in Combination

a. Butyrophenones Alone

i. Dosage. While the therapeutic dosage range of the various butyrophenone drugs differs slightly, it generally holds true that of the three clinically most frequently used preparations haloperidol is usually given in dosages twice as high as trifluperidol and floropipamide is usually given in dosages ten to twenty times the dosage of haloperidol (or twenty to forty times the dosage of trifluperidol). Thus haloperidol, longer acting than trifluperidol, is used in a daily dosage of 0.5 mg. to 30 mg.; trifluperidol, 0.25 to 15 mg.; and floropipamide, 200 to 600 mg.

In the psychiatric disorders of old age, haloperidol is usually given in dosages which rarely exceed 5 mg. a day. The same applies to the treatment of Gilles de la Tourette's disease (Chapel, 1966).

In a recent clinical study it was found that on an average the stabilizing (equivalent) dose of haloperidol was $\frac{1}{70}$ of the previous phenothiazine dose in cases in which the patients had received chlorpromazine and $\frac{1}{40}$ of the previous dose in patients who had received methotrimeprazine (Amin *et al.*, 1967).

ii. Routes of Administration. Butyrophenones are most commonly given orally. For intramuscular administration haloperidol is used in a dosage of 2.5 mg. to 5 mg. every 4 to 6 hours until the desired effect is achieved. Thereafter parenteral therapy is replaced by peroral treatment.

Some consider intravenous haloperidol the most potent therapeutic agent in all forms of psychomotor agitation. In a group of 45 agitated psychiatric patients, resistant to the usual sedative drugs, 5 mg. of intravenous haloperidol within 5 to 10 minutes—with a duration of 4 hours—were shown to be effective in nearly all cases (Divry *et al.*, 1960).

iii. Treatment Procedures. Continuous therapy is the clinical procedure most frequently used. As the initial dose, one-fourth of the average daily dosage is usually given. From this starting point the dosage of the drug is progressively increased until there is a beneficial response in the psychopathological symptoms or troublesome side-effects occur. Others recommend raising the dosage until the onset of a fine tremor, easily recognized by Haase's (1965) handwriting test. When treatment in severely agitated, uncooperative patients begins with parenteral (intramuscular or intravenous) administration, this can usually be replaced within 3 days by orally given doses.

According to the Vademecum International Canada (1967) a dosage of 1 to 2 mg. twice or thrice a day orally should be used initially and adjusted upward until the desired effect is achieved or side-effects intervene. Then it is recommended to adjust dosage downward for optimum maintenance treatment.

Haase (1965) suggested, however, that independent of the actual dosage the occurrence of fine motor extrapyramidal signs (EPS) is a condition *sine qua non* for a drug-induced reduction of the "psychoenergetic level." He maintains that where fine motor EPS are absent, the dosage is too low and the drug is psychotherapeutically ineffective.

iv. Duration of Treatment. The duration of butyrophenone administration is dependent on the condition that is being treated. With the exception of manic and schizophrenic psychopathologies, however, they should only be given until symptomatic remission. Manic patients have to be maintained on butyrophenone treatment for the known duration of their manic episodes (a 6- to 12-month period); and schizophrenics after their first episode for at least 1 year, after the second for at least 2 to 3 years and thereafter for an indefinite time.

It is fortunate that butyrophenone drugs can be taken over an extended period of time and that in spite of occasional mild withdrawal manifestations there is no addiction to butyrophenone drugs. Nor has carcinogenicity or teratogenicity thus far been detected.

b. Butyrophenones in Combination with Other Treatments

Not infrequently butyrophenones are administered in conjunction with other—physical and pharmacological—treatments.

i. Physical. Electroconvulsive therapy is only occasionally combined with butyrophenone administration. In these cases the hypotensive action of these drugs is intensified by the ECT. It is common practice to omit one dose of the drug prior to treatment and to maintain the patient in a lying position for at least 30 minutes after consciousness is regained. An advantageous aspect of combined treatment is that haloperidol is reported to shorten the duration of postconvulsive confusion (Milani, 1962). This, according to Müller and Warnes (1964), is similar to the effects of anticholinergic compounds and also of some phenothiazine drugs, such as promethazine (Bente, 1963).

ii. Pharmacological. In the past decade the effectiveness of the various phenothiazines in the treatment of acute and chronic schizophrenic patients has been definitely established. There are still many patients, however, particularly among the chronic schizophrenics, who have shown inadequate therapeutic response. To find out whether these patients would further improve with the addition of a butyrophenone to their treatment regime, Lehmann *et al.* (1967) conducted a placebo-controlled double-blind comparative clinical trial. A butyrophenone—haloperidol or trifluperidol—was added to the patients' regular phenothiazine medication for a period of 6 weeks. It was found that certain patients in the active medication groups responded remarkably well to the addition of the butyrophenone drug. This suggested that the combination is potentially useful in certain therapy-resistant cases. It was not possible, however, to make any prediction of the type of patient who would benefit from the combination.

Haloperidol prolongs only the hypnotic action of barbiturates, but not their anticonvulsant action. Even more, butyrophenones may precipitate cerebral seizures in previously controlled epileptics. The same substances may intensify the primary effect of anesthetics and narcotics; potentiate the effects of alcohol; and interfere with the anticoagulant properties of phenindione, frequently used in the treatment of cardiac cases.

3. Adverse Reactions and Their Treatment

a. Adverse Reactions

Serious side-effects occur mainly with higher doses and in elderly or debilitated patients. It has been noted that of the three most frequently used butyrophenone derivatives the toxicity of floropipamide is the lowest and of trifluperidol, the highest.

Adverse reactions to these drugs may affect any organ or organ system, causing either mild discomfort or severe pathological changes that may call for termination of treatment. Adverse reactions to butyrophenones are classed as psychiatric, neurological, cardiovascular, metabolic and miscellaneous.

A superb account of the side-effects of haloperidol was given by Gerle (1964). His summary is based on 70 published reports including the treatment of 6500 patients. Secondly it includes 40 written or verbal answers to a questionnaire—specially constructed to collect information about toxic effects—covering additional case material of 6000 patients.

i. Psychiatric. There are basically three types of reactions in this category: insomnia, depression and toxic-delirious or confusional states.

α. Insomnia. Mild insomnia in the course of haloperidol treatment was first reported by De Maio *et al.* (1960) and Della Pietra and Fina (1960); and insomnic reactions by Guilbert *et al.* (1961) and Delay *et al.* (1962). Since these first reports, insomnia has been reported in the course of butyrophenone administration by numerous authors (Kristjansen, 1962; Geyer and Mayr, 1962; Sugerman *et al.*, 1964; etc.).

β. Depression. Depressive reactions in the course of treatment with butyrophenones have been reported by Della Pietra and Fina (1960), Harder (1961), Humbeeck (1960) and Kristjansen (1962). Triperidol treatment had to be discontinued in a patient because of a serious suicidal attempt, and floropipamide treatment was promptly terminated in another patient who became depressed and voiced suicidal ideas (Warnes *et al.*, 1964).

Pacquay *et al.* (1962) suggested that the depression which occurs in the course of treatment with butyrophenone drugs is probably caused by the improvement of autistic isolation. On the other hand, Caron (1962) pointed out that depression and extrapyramidal akinesia have symptoms in common, which provide for a difficult differential diagnosis.

γ. Toxic Psychoses. Delirious or confusional states with agitation, disorientation, confabulation and visual hallucinations were described with various neuroleptics and, among the butyrophenones, with floropipamide and trifluperidol (Bobon, *et al.*, 1961; and Warnes *et al.*, 1964).

ii. Neurological. Butyrophenones may induce a variety of adverse neurological reactions. They are capable of reactivating epileptic crises and of producing parkinsonian-like and encephalitic-like reactions. However, most frequently encountered are extrapyramidal signs (EPS) and cerebral seizures.

α. Extrapyramidal Signs. Haase (1954, 1955, 1956, 1961, 1962) considers hypokinesia or akinesia as obligatory signs of adequate neuroleptic treatment, in contradistinction to tremor, rigidity and akathisia, which he considers as facultative signs. Nevertheless, he maintains that all coarse motor symptoms, *e.g.*, marked akinesia, are therapeutically disturbing and undesirable (Wagensommer, 1965).

Marked hypokinesia or akinesia is not

infrequent in the course of treatment with butyrophenone drugs. It is characterized by lack of spontaneous and accompanying movements, bent stance, restricted shuffling gait and expressionless face. Often it appears in the form of akinesia accompanied by rigidity and tremor. It occurs more often in female than in male patients and particularly in adolescents, in leptosomes and in cases with cerebral damage (especially cerebrovascular disease). Although personal disposition plays an important part in its development, within the limits of individual constitutional variations the occurrence of this syndrome is in direct proportion with the dosage (Wagensommer, 1965).

Besides hypokinesia, dyskinetic-dystonic reactions are also common side-effects of neuroleptic treatment. They are characterized by sudden short-lived tonic contractions and myoclonic twitchings, *e.g.*, torticollis, mandibular tic or grimacing, jerking movements and oculogyric crisis.

Dyskinesias have been reported with butyrophenones by Delay *et al.* (1960), Aldeghi and Maderna, (1961), Bobon *et al.* (1961), Cardani and Goldwurm (1961), Collard (1961), Giacobini and Lassenius (1961), Harder (1961), etc.

Finally, akathisia, a fundamentally harmless but extremely unpleasant and distressing generalized restlessness, and drug-induced parkinsonism (also called psychomotor Parkinson syndrome and parkinsonoid reaction) may also occur.

β. Cerebral Seizures. Wagensommer (1965) considers epileptiform convulsions one of the more severe side-effects of neuroleptic treatment. Janssen (1962) found that haloperidol and triperidol produce convulsions in rats at subtoxic dose levels. The same was found in human studies. However, Della Beffa *et al.* (1962) and Gattuso and Lanteri (1962) reported improvement of epilepsy in haloperidol-treated cases.

iii. Cardiovascular. Isolated cases of heart failure (Evrard, 1960), ventricular extrasystoles (Evrard, 1960), hypotension (Alema *et al.*, 1961) and precipitation of angina pectoris (Waelkens, 1960) have been reported in the course of haloperidol treatment. Monceaux (1961), Geyer and Mayr (1962) and Leone (1962), on the other nd,ha found that patients with heart disease tolerate haloperidol remarkably well. Nevertheless, with parenteral administration or excessive oral doses, hypotension (or, rather, orthostatic hypotension) may occur and therefore butyrophenones should only be given with great caution to patients with severe cardiac involvement.

iv. Metabolic. Simpson and Cooper (1966) indicated a significant hypocholesterolemic effect associated with trifluperidol administration. This was confirmed in several laboratories (McNeil Laboratories, Oklahoma Medical Center Laboratory). However, in a subsequent study Simpson (1967) found that haloperidol, unlike triperidol, does not affect cholesterol levels.

v. Miscellaneous. Nausea, heartburn, vomiting, constipation and loss of appetite with these drugs are rare (Delay *et al.*, 1960). On the other hand, Kristjansen (1960) found blurred vision in almost 20 per cent of his treated patients.

In spite of a case of obstructive jaundice (Kivalo and Arnell, 1961) and the reoccurrence of an earlier jaundice during treatment (Caron *et al.*, 1961), Gerle (1964) asserts that haloperidol does not cause liver impairment; and similarly in spite of the reported cases of lymphomonocytosis, leukopenia, leukocytosis and anemia (Delay *et al.*, 1960; and Collard, 1962), Gerle (1964) maintains that the drug has practically no toxicity on the hematopoietic system.

A particular syndrome, called "Syndrome Malin," was reported in five cases (out of several hundred treated patients) by Delay *et al.* (1963). It was characterized by strong perspiration, dehydration, hyperthermia and a dazed state of mind. This syndrome is not a consequence of overdosage and it may arise in patients on moderate doses early in the course of their treatment. Death due to cachexia during treatment with moderate doses of haloperidol was reported by Loret (1960), although the cause of cachexia was not proven to be related to the drug (Gerle, 1964).

b. Treatment of Adverse Reactions

It is rare that treatment with psychoactive butyrophenones has to be discontinued because of side-effects. Insomnia usually responds to a reduction in dosage or, if this is unadvisable, to adjuvant hypnotic medication. More recently, there are indications that the combination of haloperidol (given in the morning) and chlorpromazine (given at night) successfully overcomes this adverse effect (Jones *et al.*, 1968). The addition of a tricyclic antidepressant drug is sufficient in most cases to control depressive side-effects, while the occurrence of toxic psychosis may necessitate the withdrawal of the butyrophenone medication and subsequent replacement with another antipsychotic drug.

Extrapyramidal signs only exceptionally demand discontinuation of treatment or reduction of dosage. They are counteracted by antiparkinsonian drugs which should be administered only for the shortest possible period of time. Similarly, cerebral seizures are well controlled by anticonvulsant medication but quite frequently require a reduction in the butyrophenone dosage.

Cardiovascular side-effects are treated symptomatically; and orthostatic hypotension by intravenous vasopressor substances (but not with epinephrine).

All other adverse reactions can usually be dealt with symptomatically except for the "Syndrome Malin," in which immediate discontinuation of treatment is imperative.

4. Butyrophenones in Psychiatric Practice

Divry *et al.* (1958) were first to report the successful control of motor agitation with haloperidol, the first therapeutically used substance of the butyrophenone series, a prototype neuroleptic drug. The relatively low incidence of autonomic side-effects with the new substance was noted already in the earliest clinical studies. Later on, the differential effects of haloperidol (when compared with other antipsychotic drugs) were established.

A clear definition of the neuroleptic effect and its relationship with desirable clinical effects was succinctly summarized by Haase (1965). He described the direct and nonspecific neuroleptic effect as a lowering of the psychoenergetic level, without impairment of consciousness and judgment. Since psychic energy appears outwardly as movement, it was suggested that "neuroleptic inhibition" is localized in the midbrain, where conation finds its first translation into mass movements. Thus it was surmised (Haase, 1959) that the site of neuroleptic action is in the region of the reticular activating and extrapyramidal systems. Subsequently, neuroleptic effectiveness was regarded as a reduction of extrapyramidal psychokinetic conation (Haase, 1961).

On the basis of this theoretical formulation, Haase (1965) considered those conditions in which motor activity is closely related to psychokinetic conation as the indications for neuroleptic treatment. These are as follows: psychomotor agitation—irrespective of origin—in which the reduction of psychokinetic conation brings about a return to normality, *i.e.*, in cases where psychokinetic conation is raised; affective tension and excitement which are considered to be due to a "rise" in the psychoenergetic level; mania in which the elation is indirectly alleviated by the lowering of the psychoenergetic level; psychotic experiences that include the various schizophrenias; and extrapyramidal hyperkinesias.

Besides haloperidol and triperidol, there are a number of other butyrophenones used in clinical practice. Among them are floropipamide, a substance with a relatively weak (half of chlorpromazine) neuroleptic potency. (The average daily oral dose necessary to cross neuroleptic threshold of this drug is 250 to 600 mg.) Floropipamide was originally recommended as an adjuvant to stronger neuroleptics (in the treatment of psychoses) or tranquilizers (in the treatment of neuroses). Nevertheless, Warnes *et al.* (1964) and particularly Sugerman (1964) found it therapeutically useful when given as the sole medication to chronic schizophrenics.

Another butyrophenone derivative used clinically is methylperidol, a substance with a medium-strong (15 times that of chlorpromazine) neuroleptic potency. With the use of the fine motor manifestations as a guide to correct dosage, Hackstein (1963) found a dosage of 10 to 25 mg. daily effective for neuroleptic action. Other butyrophenones such as benzperidol and spiroperidol, which have neuroleptic potencies 400 times that of chlorpromazine, are still in the stage of clinical investigation (Delay, 1966; and Deniker and Pichot, 1966). The anticipated clinically effective doses of these drugs are between 0.3 to 0.9 mg. a day (Haase, 1965).

The neuroleptic potencies of the two most frequently used butyrophenones, haloperidol and trifluperidol, are, respectively, 50 and 200 times that of chlorpromazine, and the average daily oral dosage which is necessary to cross the neuroleptic threshold is approximately 3 to 6 mg. (for haloperidol) and 0.7 to 1.8 mg. (for trifluperidol). In the treatment of psychotic patients (especially in mania, schizophrenia and alcoholic delirium) they are used in somewhat higher doses (0.5 to 30 mg. in the case of haloperidol and 0.25 to 15 mg. in the case of trifluperidol). Although usually used for the same therapeutic indications, it has been noted that, of the two, trifluperidol is a somewhat shorter acting preparation. There are some indications that trifluperidol may be superior to haloperidol in the treatment of chronic (schizophrenic) patients.

Two other psychotherapeutically less important butyrophenones are dihydrobenzperidol and fluanisone, both used in general anesthesia. The former shows strong neuroleptic potency with an ultrashort duration of action and the latter a low neuroleptic potency and short duration of action.

SUMMARY

The butyrophenones were the first group of psychoactive substances to be introduced in which most of the clinical results obtained were predictable from animal data. Haloperidol and trifluperidol have been reported to be therapeutic in a number of conditions ranging from functional psychoses through organic conditions to the psychoneuroses. Among the primary indications of butyrophenones are manic conditions with extreme psychomotor agitation, alcoholic delirium with excessive hallucinatory experiences and the schizophrenias. There are indications that certain schizophrenic patients who are unresponsive to other antipsychotic treatment may benefit from a butyrophenone preparation alone or by the addition of a butyrophenone drug to their former treatment.

The butyrophenones are the third group of antipsychotic substances. Like the phenothiazines and the Rauwolfias, they exert a considerable neuroleptic action, but they can clearly be differentiated from the phenothiazines and Rauwolfias by some of their neurochemical, neurophysiological and clinical effects.

REFERENCES

Aldeghi, E., and Maderna, A.: Primi risultati sull'impiego terapeutico dell'haloperidol in neuropsichiatria infantile. Riv. Sper. Freniat., *85:* 1 (1961).

Alema, G., and Gianotti, G.: Manifestazioni neurologiche d ahaloperidolo e triperidolo. Symposium internazionale sull'haloperidol e triperidol. (Inst. Luso Farmaco d'Italia, Milano, 1962.)

Alema, G., Gianotti, G., and Fiorito, L.: Confronto clinico fra haloperidolo, triperidolo e tioproperazina. Symposium internazionale sull'-haloperidol e triperidol. (Inst. Luso Farmaco d'Italia, Milano, 1962.)

Alema, G., *et al.:* Chimioshock da haloperidol. Riv. Sper. Freniat., *85:* 2 (1961).

Alema, G., *et al.:* Dati clinicostatistici su 269 casi trattati con haloperidolo. Symposium internazionale sull'haloperidol e triperidol. (Inst. Luso Farmaco d'Italia, Milano, 1962.)

Amin, M., Lehmann, H. E., and Ban, T. A.: Dose equivalent for haloperidol and phenothiazines. Canad. Med. Ass. J., *97:* 465 (1967.)

Amin, M., Lehmann, H. E., and Ban, T. A.: Non-equivalence of antipsychotic drugs. Canad. Med. Ass. J., *98:* 56 (1968.)

Arrigo, A., Savoldi, F., and Tartara, A.: The effects of haloperidol and triperidol on behavior, electric activity and cerebral flow of blood in non-anesthetized rabbits. Symposium internazionale sull'haloperidol e triperidol. (Inst. Luso Farmaco d'Italia, Milano, 1962.)

Ban, T. A.: Clinical studies on the antipsychotic properties of haloperidol versus permitil. Symposium internazionale sull'haloperidol e triperidol. Instituto Luso Farmaco d'Italia, Milan, 1962.)

Ban, T. A., and Lehmann, H. E.: Efficacy of haloperidol in drug refractory patients. Int. J. Neuropsychiat., *3:* 10 (1967).

Bente, D.: Elektroenzephalographie und Psychiatrische Parmacotherapie. In: Anthropologische und Naturwissenschaftliche Grundlagen der Pharmakopsychiatrie (eds., Achelis, T. D., and Ditfurth, H.). (Thieme, Stuttgart, 1963.)

Bente, D., Pfeiffer, W., and Mueller, M. L.: Data on a new derivative of butyrophenone: clinical and electroencephalographic effects of dipiperon (R 3345). (Congr. Psychiat. Neurol. French Lang. Sixtieth Session, Antwerpen, 1962.)

Bishop, M. P., and Gallant, D. M.: Trifluperidol in "paranoid" and "non-paranoid" schizophrenics. Curr. Ther. Res., *7:* 96 (1965).

Bobon, J., Collard, J., and Demaret, A.: Un neuroleptique original à effet hypnogène différé: le dipipérone (R 3345) butyrophenone carbamidée. Acta Neurol. Belg., *61:* 611 (1961).

Boissier, J. R.: A new class of neuroleptics: disubstituted N-N'piperazines. In: Psychopharmacological methods (eds., Votava, Z., Horvath, M., and Vinar, O.). (Pergamon Press, New York, 1963.)

Boissier, J. R., *et al.:* Quelques actions pharmacologiques du halopéridol (R 1625). Acta Neurol. Belg., *60:* 39 (1960).

Boissier, J. R., *et al.:* The use of a particular reaction of mice for the study of psychotropic drugs. Therapie, *19:* 571 (1964).

Boissier, J. R., and Simon, P.: Etude pharmacologique prévisionnelle de deux neuroleptiques apartenant à une série chimique nouvelle. Therapie, *21:* 1491 (1966).

Braun, G. A., Kade, C. F., and Roscoe, E. L.: Metabolism of haloperidol in the rat. Int. J. Neuropsychiat., *3:* 22 (1967).

Braun, G. A., Poos, G. I., and Soudijn, W.: Distribution, excretion and metabolism of neuroleptics of the butyrophenone type. Europ. J. Pharmacol., *1:* 58 (1967).

Buchwald, N. A., *et al.:* Effects of caudate stimulation on visual discrimination. Exp. Neurol., *4:* 23 (1961).

Buniatian, H. C. (1963): In: Janssen, P. A. J.: The pharmacology of haloperidol. Int. J. Neuropsychiat., *3:* 10 (1967).

Cardani, A., and Goldwurm, G. F.: Esperienze cliniche con un nuovo farmaco psicolettico (R-1625). Riv. Sper. Freniat., *85:* 231 (1961).

Carlsson, A., Hillarp, N. A., and Waldeck, B.: Analysis of the Mg^{++}-ATP dependent storage mechanism in the amine granules of the adrenal medulla. Acta Physiol. Scand., *59:* (Suppl. 215) 1, (1963.)

Carlsson, A., and Lindquist, M.: In vivo decarboxylation of α-methyl DOPA and α-methyl metatyrosine. Acta Physiol. Scand., *54:* 87 (1962).

Caron, M. J., *et al.:* Contribution à l'étude de emploi de l'haloperidol. Ann. Medicopsychol., *119:* 966 (1961).

Caron, M. J. (1962): In: Gerle, B.: Clinical observations of the side effects of haloperidol. Acta Psychiat. Scand., *40:* 65 (1964).

Challas, G., and Brauer, W.: Tourette's disease: relief of symptoms with R 1625. Amer. J. Psychiat., *120:* 283 (1963).

Chapel, J. L.: Gilles de la Tourette's disease. Canad. Psychiat. Ass. J., *2:* 324 (1966).

Chapel, J. L., Brown, N., and Jenkins, R. L.: Tourette's disease—symptomatic relief with haloperidol. Amer. J. Psychiat., *121:* 608 (1964).

Collard, J.: Un nouveau neuroleptique à l'effet hypnogéne différé. Le dipipéron (R 3345) butyrophénone carbamidée. Acta Neurol. Belg., *61:* 611 (1961).

Collard, J. (1962): In: Gerle, B.: Clinical observations of the side effects of haloperidol. Acta Psychiat. Scand., *40:* 65 (1964).

Costa, E., *et al.:* On current status of serotonin as a brain neurohormone and in action of reserpine-like drugs. Ann. N. Y. Acad. Sci., *96:* 118 (1962).

Curtis, D. R., and Watkins, J. C. (1960): In: Janssen, P. A. J.: The pharmacology of haloperidol. Int. J. Neuropsychiat., *3:* 10 (1967).

Delay, J.: Butyrophenone group. (Informal ECDEU report from the clinique des maladies mentales et de l'encephale. Paris, 1966.)

Delay, J. *et al.:* L'emploi des butyrophénones en psychiatrie. Etude statistique et psychometrique. Symposium International sull haloperidol et triperidol. (Instituto Luso Farmaco d'Italia, Milano, 1962.)

Delay, J., *et al.:* L'action du halopéridol dans des psychoses. Acta Neurol. Belg., *60:* 21 (1960).

Delay, J., *et al.:* Un neuroleptique majeur non phénothiazinique et non réserpinique, l'halopéridol, dans le traitement des psychoses. Ann. Medicopsychol., *118:* 145 (1960).

Delay, J., *et al.* (1963): In: Gerle, B.: Clinical observations of the side effects of haloperidol. Acta Psychiat. Scand., *40:* 65 (1964).

Della Beffa, A., Ronchi, E., and Barberini, E.: Considerazioni sulla neurosecrezione ipotalamica e neuroipofisaria in conigli, in corso di trattamento con triperidol, indaguata con il metodo di Gomori. Symposium internazionale sull'haloperidol e triperidol. (Inst. Luso Farmaco d'Italia, Milano, 1962.)

Della Pietra, V., and Fina, G.: L'haloperidol R 1625 in terapia psichiatrica. Osped. Psichiat., *1:* 39 (1960).

DeMaio, D., *et al.:* Sulla terapia con R 1625 di talune psicosi acute e su di una rara complicanza extraneurologica (parotite). Gazz. Med. Ital., *119:* 511, 1960.

Deniker, P., and Pichot, P.: Spiroxamide (spirobutyrophenone). (Informal ECDEU report from the clinique des maladies mentales et de l'encephale. Paris, 1966.)

Divry, P., Bobon, J., and Collard, J.: Le R-1625 nouvelle thérapeutique symptomatique de l'agitation psychomotrice. Acta Neurol. Belg., *58:* 878 (1958).

Divry, P., Bobon, J., and Collard, J.: Rapport sur l'activité neuropsychopharmacologique du halopéridol (R 1625). Acta Neurol. Belg., *60:* 7 (1960).

Divry, P., *et al.:* Etude psychopharmacologique d'une cinqieme butyrophenone: le "methyl peridide" neuroleptique dérive pyrrolidinamidé et méthylé du halopéridol. Acta Neurol. Belg., *60:* 1073 (1960).

Divry, P., Bobon, J., Collard, J., et Demaret, A.,: Psychopharmacologie d'un troisième neuroleptique de la serie des butyrophénones: Le R2498 ou tripéridol. Acta Neurol. Belg., *60:* 465 (1960).

Dresse, A.: Influence de 15 neuroleptiques (butyrophénones et phénothiazines) sur les variations de la teneur du cerveau en noradrenaline et l'activité du rat dans le test d'antistimulation. Arch. Int. Pharmacodyn., *159:* 353 (1966).

Dresse, A., (1964): In: Janssen, P. A.: The pharmacology of haloperidol. Int. J. Neuropsychiat., *3:* 10 (1967).

Dresse, A., and De Meyer, R.: Influence of four butyrophenone neuroleptics on rat brain noradrenaline depletory effect of reserpine. Life Sci., *3:* 759 (1964).

Eiff, A. W., and Jesdinsky, H. J.: Etude clinicopharmacologique du halopéridol chez des personnes normales. Acta Neurol. Belg., *60:* 63 (1960).

Evrard, E.: Discussione controindicazioni. Symposium internationale sur l'haloperidol, Bruxelles 1959. Acta Med. Belg., *60:* 136 (1960).

Fink, M., *et al.:* Trifluperidol in the treatment of psychoses; observations suggestive of anticholinergic activity at higher dosages. J. New Drugs, *6:* 174 (1966).

Fish, B., and Campbell, M.: Triperidol. (Informal ECDEU report, New York University School of Medicine, New York, 1966.)

Gallant, D. M., *et al.:* A controlled evaluation of trifluperidol: a new potent psychopharmacologic agent. Curr. Ther. Res., *5:* 463 (1963).

Gattuso, R., and Lanteri, G.: Sindromi psichiatriche e neurologiche nel trattamento con haloperidol. Symposium internazionale sull'haloperidol e triperidol. (Inst. Luso Farmaco d'Italia, Milano, 1962.)

Gerle, B.: Clinical trials with R 1625. Acta Neurol. Belg., *60:* 70 (1960).

Gerle, B.: Clinical observations of the side-effects of haloperidol. Acta Psychiat. Scand., *40:* 65 (1964).

Gershon, S.: Personal communication, Montreal, 1967.

Geyer, N., and Mayr, F.: Results of psychiatric therapy with the butyrophenone derivative haloperidol. Wien. Med. Wschr., *112:* 603 (1962).

Giacobini, E., and Lassenius, B.: Haloperidol vid behandling av delirium tremens. Svensk. Läkartidn., *58:* 1429 (1961).

Goldwurm, G. F., and Torrigiani, G. I.: Derivativi butirrofenonici e loro associazioni con cloropromazina, in terapia psichiatrica. Symposium internazionale sull'haloperidol e triperidol. (Inst. Luso Farmaco d'Italia, Milano, 1962.)

Goldwurm, G. F., and Vanni, F.: Two new butyrophenone derivative studies with the conditioned reflex technique. Dis. Nerv. Syst., *22:* 1 (1961).

Guilbert, P., Feron, A., and Monceaux, J. P.: Haloperidol in states of manic excitation. Ann. Medicopsychol., *119:* 543 (1961).

Haase, H. J.: Über Vorkommen und Deutung des Psychomotorischen Parkinson-syndroms bei Megaphen bezw Largactil-Dauerbehandlung. Nervenarzt, *25:* 486 (1954).

Haase, H. J.: Psychiatrische Erfahrungen mit Megaphen (Largactil) und dem Rauwolfia Alkaloid Serpasil unter dem Gesichtspunkt de Psycho-motorischen Parkinson Syndroms. Nervenarzt, *26:* 507 (1955).

Haase, H. J.: Über Begriff und Wirkungsweise des Therapeutisch Erstrebten Psycho-Motorischen Serpasil (Rauwolfia Alkaloid) und Largactil (Megaphen) Parkinson Syndroms. Mschr. Psychiat. Neurol., *131:* 201 (1956).

Haase, H. J.: The role of drug-induced extrapyramidal syndromes. In: Psychopharmacology frontiers (ed., Kline, N. S.). (Little, Brown, Boston, 1959.)

Haase, H. J.: Das Therapeutische Achsensyndrome Neuroleptischer Medikamente und Seine Beziehungen zu Extrapyramidaler Symptomatik. Fortschr. Neurol. Psychiat., *29:* 245 (1961).

Haase, H. J.: Extrapyramidal modification of fine movements, a "condition sine qua non" of fundamental therapeutic action of neuroleptic drugs. Rev. Canad. Biol., *20:* 425 (1961).

Haase, H. J.: Intensitat und Aquivalenz Neuroleptischer Wirkung und Ihre Therapeutische Bedautung. Nervenarzt, *33:* 213 (1962).

Haase, H. J.: Clinical observations on the action of neuroleptics. In: Haase, H. J., and Janssen, P. A J.: The action of neuroleptic drugs. (North-Holland Publishing Company, Amsterdam, 1965.)

Hackstein, F. G.: Klinische Erprobung des Butyrophenon Derivates Methylperidol. Therapiewoche, *13:* 485 (1963).

Harder, A.: Klinische Erfahrungen mit Haloperidol, einem Chemisch und Klinisch Eigenartigen Neuroplegikum. Praxis, *868:* 50 (1961).

Humbeeck, L.: Etude clinique du R 1625 (haloperidol). Acta Neurol. Belg., *60:* 75 (1960).

Janssen, P. A. J.: Comparative pharmacologic data regarding six new basic 4-fluorobutyrophenone derivatives, haloperidol, haloanison, triperidol, methylperidid, haloperidid, and dipiperon. Arztneimittelforschung, *11:* 819 (1961).

Janssen, P. A. J.: The measurement of observed differences between treated and untreated animals using an ordinal scale for ranking the degree of confidence in their judgment of two unbiased observers. Psychopharmacologia (Berlin), *2:* 141 (1961).

Janssen, P. A. J.: The relationship between chemical structures and CNS-depressant activity of basic ketones related to haloperidol. Biochem. Pharmacol., *8:* 144 (1961).

Janssen, P. A. J. (1956): In: Janssen, P. A. J.: A review of the pharmacology of haloperidol and of triperidol. In: Symposium internazionale sull'haloperidol e triperidol. (Inst. Luso Farmaco d'Italia, Milano, 1962.)

Janssen, P. A. J.: A review of the pharmacology of haloperidol and of triperidol. (Paper presented at the International Symposium on Haloperidol and Triperidol, Milan, 1962.)

Janssen, P. A. J.: Pharmacologie comparée du halopéridol et du tripéridol. Encéphale, *582:* 51 (1962).

Janssen, P. A. J.: The relationship between chemical structure and CNS—depressant activity of basic ketones related to haloperidol. Mode of action of Drugs, *7:* 371 (1963).

Janssen, P. A. J.: Screening tests and prediction from animals to man. In: Animal behavior and drug action (eds., Steinberg, H., deRenck, A. V. S., and Knight, J.). (Churchill, London, 1964.)

Janssen, P. A. J.: The evolution of the butyrophenones haloperidol and triperidol from meperidine-like 4-phenylpiperidines. Int. Rev. Neurobiol., *86:* 221 (1965).

Janssen, P. A. J.: The pharmacological and clinical mode of action of neuroleptic drugs. Clin. Trials J., *2:* 370 (1966).

Janssen, P. A. J.: The pharmacology of haloperidol. Int. J. Neuropsychiat., *3:* 10 (1967).

Janssen, P. A. J., *et al.*: Chemistry and pharmacology of CNS depressants related to 4-(4-hydroxy-4-phenyl-piperidino)-butyrophenone. I. Synthesis and screening data in mice. J. Med. Pharm. Chem., *1:* 281 (1959).

Janssen, P. A. J., *et al.:* Compounds related to pethidine. III. Basic ketones derived from norpethidine. J. Med. Pharm. Chem., *2:* 271 (1960).

Janssen, P. A. J., *et al.:* A comparative study of the effect of subcutaneous and oral doses of haloperidol on avoidance-escape habits of rats and dogs in a "jumping box" situation. Arzneimittelforschung, *13:* 401 (1963).

Janssen, P. A. J., *et al.:* The pharmacology of dihydrobenzperidol, a new potent and short acting neuroleptic agent chemically related to haloperidol. Arzneimittelforschung, *13:* 205 (1963).

Janssen, P. A. J., *et al.:* Is it possible to predict the clinical effects of neuroleptic drugs (major tranquilizers) from animal data? IV. An improved experimental design for measuring the inhibitory effects of neuroleptic drugs on amphetamine or apomorphine-induced "chewing" and "agitation" in rats. Arzneimittelforschung, *16:* 2 (1966).

Janssen, P. A. J., and Eddy, N. B.: Compounds related to pethidine. IV. New general chemical methods of increasing the analgesic activity of pethidine. J. Med. Pharm. Chem., *2:* 31 (1960).

Janssen, P. A. J., and Niemegeers, C. J. E.: Chemistry and pharmacology of compounds related to 4-(4-hydroxy-4-phenyl-piperidino)-butyrophenone. I. Inhibition of apomorphine vomiting in dogs. Arzneimittelforschung, *9:* 765 (1959).

Janssen, P. A. J., and Niemegeers, C. J. E.: Haloperidide (R 3201), a highly potent and selective anti-emetic agent in dogs. Nature (London), *190:* 911 (1961).

Johnson, P. C., Charalampous, K. D., and Braun, G. A.: Absorption and excretion of tritiated, haloperidol in man (a preliminary report). Int. J. Neuropsychiat., *3:* 24 (1967).

Jones, B., *et al.:* Treatment of chronic schizophrenic patients with haloperidol and chlorpromazine combined. Curr. Ther. Res., *10:* 276 (1968).

Kivalo, E., and Arnell, G.: Treatment of mentally retarded with haloperidol. Ann. Paediat. Fenn., *7:* 320 (1961).

Kristjansen, P.: Experimentation clinique du R 1625 (halopéridol). Symposium international sur le halopéridol. Acta Med. Belg., *60:* 82 (1960).

Kristjansen, P.: Clinical evaluation of haloperidol and related compounds. In: Symposium internazionale sull'haloperidol e triperidol. (Inst. Luso Farmaco d'Italia, Milano, 1962.)

Lehmann, H. E., Ban, T. A., and Lee, H.: The effectiveness of combined phenothiazine and butyrophenone treatment in chronic schizophrenic patients. Curr. Ther. Res., *9:* 36 (1967).

Lehmann, H. E., *et al.:* The effects of haloperidol on acute schizophrenic patients: a comparative study of haloperidol, chlorpromazine and chlorprothixene. In: The butyrophenones in psychiatry. (eds. Lehmann, H. E., and Ban, T. A.). (Q. P. R. A., Montreal, 1964.)

Leone, B.: Prime osservazioni sull' effetto del serenase nella cura delle psicosi da scompenso cardiaco. Symposium internazionale sull' haloperidol e triperidol. (Inst. Luso Farmaco d'Italia, Milano, 1962.)

Lereboullet, J., Benoit, P., and Ledoux, M.: Medications nouvelles en psychiatrie. Rev. Prat., *965:* 12 (1962).

Lindquist, R.: Clinical testing of haldol in schizophrenics and acute manic states. Svensk. Lakartidn., *58:* 1422 (1961).

Loret, L.: Observation sur l'utilisation du R 1625. Acta Neurol. Belg., *60:* 86 (1960).

Magoun, H. W.: Bulbar inhibition and facilitation of motor activity. Science, *100:* 549 (1944).

Magoun, H. W.: Caudal and cephalic influences of the brain stem reticular formation. Physiol. Rev., *30:* 459 (1950).

Magoun, H. W.: An ascending reticular activating system in the brain stem. Arch. Neurol. Psychiat., *67:* 145 (1952).

Magoun, H. W., and Rhines, R. J.: Inhibitory mechanism in bulbar reticular formation. J. Neurophysiol., *9:* 165 (1946).

Meurice, E.: Electroencephalographic studies with R 1625. Acta Neurol. Belg., *60:* 91 (1960).

MILANI, B.: Prime esperienze sull' impiego dell' haloperidol negli stati confusionali secondari a shockterapia. Symposium internazionale sull' haloperidol e triperidol. (Inst. Luso Farmaco d'Italia, Milano, 1962.)

MONCEAUX, J. P.: Psychoses and haloperidol. (Librairie Maloine S. A., Paris, 1961.)

MONTI, J. M., RANCE, A. J., AND KILLAM, K. F.: CNS effects of haloperidol. Fed. Proc., *25:* 229 (1966).

MUELLER, P. B., AND LANGEMANN, H. (1962): In: Janssen, P. A.: The pharmacology of haloperidol. Int. J. Neuropsychiat., *3:* 10 (1967).

MÜLLER, H. F., AND WARNES, H.: Electrophysiological effects of butyrophenone drugs. In: The butyrophenones in psychiatry (eds., Lehmann, H. E., and Ban, T. A.). (Quebec Psychopharmacological Research Ass., Montreal, 1964.)

OBERST, F. W., AND CROOK, J. W.: Behavioral, physical and pharmacodynamic effects of haloperidol in dogs and monkeys. Arch. Int. Pharmacodyn., *167:* 450 (1967).

OLES, M.: Behandlung von Psychoser mit Haloperidol. Med. Mschr., *7:* 452 (1960).

OLES, M.: Klinische Erfahrung mit dem Neuroleptikum Haloperidol (R 1625). Acta Neurol. Belg., *60:* 100 (1960).

OLSSON, M.: Klinisk provning av haldol. Svensk. Lakartidn., *1433:* 58 (1961).

PACQUAY, J., ARNOULD, E., AND BURTON, P.: Experimentation clinique du halopéridol. Acta Neurol. Belg., *60:* 108 (1960).

PACQUAY, J., *et al.*: Quatre années d'application quotidienne du haloperidol en milieu hospitalier psychiatrique. Symposium internazionale sull' haloperidol e triperidol. (Inst. Luso Farmaco d'Italia, Milano, 1962.)

ROSSUM, J. M. (1966): In: Janssen, P. A.: The pharmacology of haloperidol. Int. J. Neuropsychiat., *3:* 10 (1967).

RYALL, R. W. (1964): In: Janssen, P. A.: The pharmacology of haloperidol. Int. J. Neuropsychiat., *3:* 10 (1967).

SAARMA, J., AND SAARMA, M.: Dynamics of higher nervous activity of chronic schizophrenics under treatment with aminazine, stelazine, haloperidol. (Presented at the Fourth World Congress of Psychiatry, Madrid, 1966.)

SCHIELE, B. C.: Trifluperidol versus trifluoperazine. (Informal ECDEU report from the Dept. of Psychiatry, University of Minnesota Hospital, Minneapolis, 1966.)

SEEMAN, P. M., AND BIALY, H. S. (1963): In: Janssen, P. A.: The pharmacology of haloperidol. Int. J. Neuropsychiat., *3:* 10 (1967).

SEIGNOT, J. N.: Un cas de maladie des tics de Gilles de la Tourette gueré par le R 1625. Ann. Medicopsychol., *578:* 119 (1961).

SIMPSON, G. M.: Butyrophenone and cholesterol. (Informal ECDEU report from the research center, Rockland State Hospital, Orangeburg, 1967.)

SIMPSON, G. M., AND COOPER, T. B.: The effect of three butyrophenones on serum cholesterol levels. Curr. Ther. Res., *8:* 249 (1966).

ST. JEAN, A., *et al.*: The psychophysical effects of the butyrophenones in male schizophrenics. In: The butyrophenones in psychiatry (eds., Lehmann, H. E., and Ban, T. A.). (Quebec Psychopharmacological Research Ass., Montreal, 1964.)

SUGERMAN, A. A.: A pilot study of floropipamide (dipiperon). Dis. Nerv. Syst., *25:* 355 (1964).

SUGERMAN, A. A., *et al.*: EEG and behavioral changes in schizophrenia. Arch. Gen. Psychiat. (Chicago), *10:* 340 (1964).

SUGERMAN, A. A., AND WILLIAMS, B. H.: Trifluperidol and trifluoperazine in acute schizophrenic patients. J. New Drugs, *5:* 318 (1965).

SURGERMAN, A. A., WILLIAMS, B. H., AND ADLERSTEIN, A. M.: Haloperidol in the psychiatric disorders of old age. Amer. J. Psychiat., *120:* 1190 (1964).

Vademacum International Canada. (Morgan Jones Publication, Montreal, 1967.)

VENNING, E. H., AND DYRENFURTH, I.: Effect of stress on the excretion of aldosterone. J. Clin. Endocr., *16:* 961 (1956).

VENNING, G. R.: A hypothesis concerning a site of action of tranquilizing drugs and the significance of associated extrapyramidal motor phenomena. J. New Drugs, *3:* 351 (1963).

WAELKENS, J.: Discussione controindicazioni. Symposium internazionale sur l'haloperidol, Bruxelles 1959. Acta Med. Belg., *60:* 136 (1960).

WAELKENS, J.: Le R 1647 dans les états dépressifs. Acta Neurol. Belg., *60:* 576 (1960).

WAGENSOMMER, J.: Therapeutically undesirable effects of neuroleptic drugs. In: Haase, H. J. and Janssen, P. A.: The action of neuroleptic drugs. (North-Holland Publishing Company, Amsterdam, 1965.)

WARNES, H., LEE, H., AND BAN, T. A.: The comparative effectiveness of butyrophenones in chronic psychotic patients. In: The butyrophenones in psychiatry (eds., Lehmann, H. E., and Ban, T. A.). (Q. P. R. A., Montreal, 1964.)

WARNES, H. *et al.*: Butaperazine and haloperidol: a comparative trial of two antipsychotic drugs. Laval Méd., *37:* 143 (1966).

Thirteen

The Thioxanthenes

A. BASIC DATA

1. Historical Aspects

The unprecedented success of the phenothiazines in psychiatry stimulated the search for new synthetic chemicals with psychoactive properties. Numerous attempts were made to develop new drugs with at least equal (or even more specific) psychoactive properties but without the numerous adverse effects of the phenothiazines. In the course of such exploratory work Petersen *et al.* (1958), by replacing the phenothiazine nucleus with a thioxanthene nucleus, succeeded in synthesizing chlorprothixene, the chlorpromazine analogue of the thioxanthene series. This substance has potent psychotropic action, while its toxic and adverse effects (*e.g.*, blood dyscrasias, liver damage, photosensitivity, extrapyramidal signs, depression) appear to be markedly less than those of the phenothiazines.

In the thioxanthenes the nitrogen (N) atom (in position 10 of the phenothiazine nucleus) is replaced by a carbon (C) atom. Since the C in the thioxanthenes has no free electrons, in contradistinction to the N in the phenothiazines, the newly synthesized structure was found to be less aromatic than the parent substance (Scheckel, 1967).

Study of the pharmacodynamics of the thioxanthene analogues of chlorpromazine, promazine and mepazine (Petersen *et al.*, 1958) was followed by exploration of the pharmacological properties of sixty-six other new thioxanthene preparations (Nielsen *et al.*, 1962).

Chlorprothixene, the first thioxanthene derivative, was introduced in 1959; clopenthixol, the second, in 1961 (Petersen and Nielsen, 1964); and thiothixene, the third, 6 years later.

2. Action Mechanism

There is no specific theory on the action mechanism of thioxanthenes. Kato and Gözsy (1961) have nevertheless presented interesting and potentially significant experimental findings. With the dextran-induced edema model in rats (Voorhees *et al.*, 1951) for studying the effects of drugs on capillary functions, they were able to demonstrate that all antipsychotic substances inhibit the edema produced by the "optimal dose" of dextran and provoke edema formation when injected simultaneously with the "critical dose" of the same substance (Kato *et al.*, 1962).

The "dextran edema" model is based on the recognition that a certain so-called "optimal" dose of dextran provokes maximal edema formation in the rat, while a certain higher so-called "critical dose" does not produce edema at all (Voorhees *et al.*, 1951). Antipsychotic action in this system was conceptualized as a reaction (*in vivo*) with both the edema-provoking and the edema-inhibiting reactive sites of the dextran molecule as reflected by the inhibition and by the provocation of the "dextran syndrome." While antihistaminic, antiserotonin, antiapomorphine and sedative properties alone were not necessarily correlated with

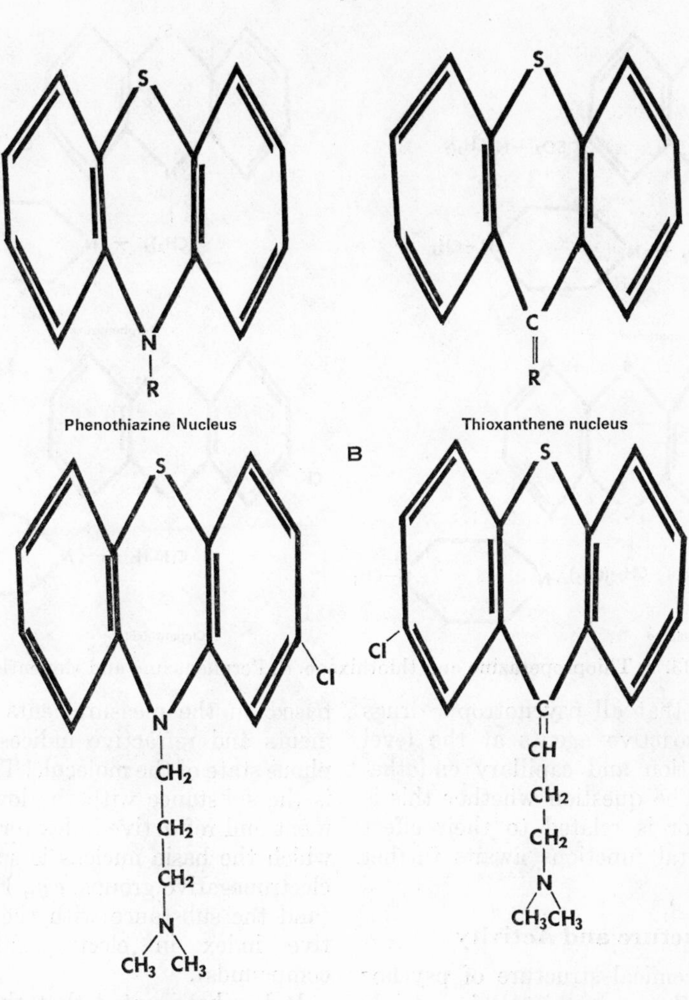

FIG. 13. *a*, The phenothiazine nucleus and the thioxanthene nucleus. *b*, Chlorpromazine and chlorprothixene.

antipsychotic effects, all compounds which inhibited the dextran edema in an arbitrary range of doses lower than 0.5 mg./kg. could be distinguished clinically on the basis of their therapeutic action on such psychotic phenomena as hallucinations, delusions, etc.

Chlorprothixene, the first antipsychotic thioxanthene preparation, was found to fulfill the criteria of an antipsychotic drug in the dextran edema model, occupying an intermediate position between the strongest butyrophenones (*e.g.*, spiroperidol) and the phenothiazines.

More recently, Kato *et al.* (1967), with different techniques, demonstrated that the three clinically used thioxanthene preparations, *i.e.*, chlorprothixene, clopenthixol and thiothixene, had an inhibiting effect on the vascular response to histamine. They were able to show that a subeffective dose of any of the thioxanthene drugs was potentiated by imipramine, but not by tranylcypromine. This suggested that psychoactive thioxanthenes may have an inhibiting effect on catecholamine reuptake. In this respect, the thioxanthenes differ from the antipsychotic phenothiazines (Gözsy *et al.*, 1967).

On the basis of these findings Kato *et al.*

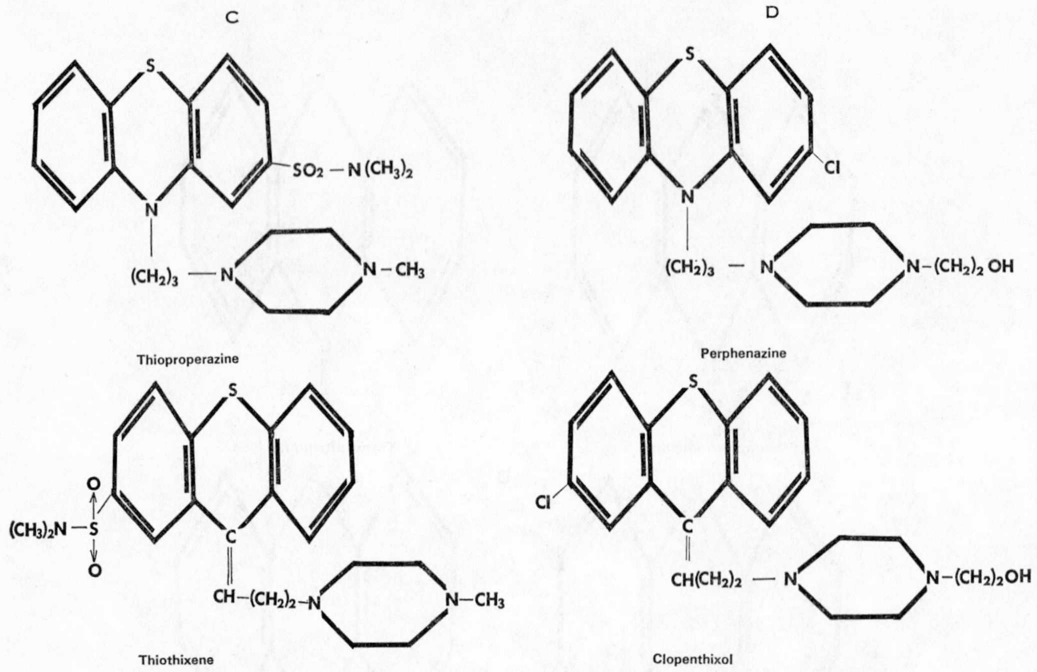

FIG. 13. *c*, Thioproperazine and thiothixene. *d*, Perphenazine and clopenthixol

(1967) suggest that all psychotropic drugs are potent vasoactive agents at the level of microcirculation and capillary endothelial filtration. The question whether this is a coincidence or is related to their effect on higher mental functions awaits further study.

3. Structure and Activity

The basic chemical structure of psychoactive thioxanthenes consists of a triple ring (heterocyclic nucleus) to which a three-carbon side chain (carrying an aliphatic or heterocyclic amine group) is attached. Whereas in phenothiazines the propyl side chain is connected to the nitrogen (of the middle ring in position 10) by a single bond which permits free rotation of every atom in the chain and allows for limitless configurational changes, the side chain in the thioxanthenes is connected to the carbon (of the middle ring in position 9) by a double bond that prohibits any rotation of the first carbon in the side chain and consequently allows for only two (*cis* and *trans*) stereoisomers. Of the two, the *trans* isomer is the biologically more potent.

The assignment of the term *cis* form is based on the measurements of dipole moments and refractive indices in the amorphous state of the molecule. The *trans* isomer is the substance with the lower dipole moment and refractive index for compounds in which the basic nucleus is substituted with electronegative groups, *e.g.*, F, Cl, Br, and I (and the substance with the higher refractive index in electropositive-substituted compounds).

It has been noted that the double bond between the carbon of the thioxanthene ring in position 9 and the side chain is essential for central nervous system action (Petersen and Nielsen, 1964). Thus the saturated analogues have only weak central nervous system activity in contradistinction to the corresponding unsaturated substances.

Systematic changes in the molecule revealed that a halogen and other substitutions in the ring structure in position 2 caused a marked increase in activity. Similarly, when the aliphatic amine group was replaced with a heterocyclic amine group on the side chain, central nervous system action was enhanced. Thus chlorprothixene, the chlorpromazine analogue of the thioxanthene series, was shown to be more active biologically (and also in its psychotropic effects) than N 716, the promazine analogue; and clopenthixol, the perphenazine (piperazinylalkyl) analogue was shown to be more potent than chlorprothixene, which contains a straight side chain.

Of the numerous thioxanthene preparations, only five have been investigated clinically: chlorprothixene (the CPZ analogue), clopenthixol (the perphenazine analogue), SKF10812 (the triflupromazine analogue), thiothixene (the thioproperazine analogue), and flupenthixol (the fluphenazine analogue). Flupenthixol is still at a very early stage of clinical investigation, and the studies with SKF10812 had to be discontinued because of side effects. Thus far, no clear clinical differential indications for chlorprothixene, clopenthixol and thiothixene have been established. On the other hand, their structure-related differential effects in pharmacological tests are well known (Weissman, 1967).

Weissman demonstrated that administration of chlorprothixene to rats induced at first flaccidity and later only catalepsy. On the other hand, both thiothixene (1 mg./kg.) and clopenthixol (2 mg./kg.) induced only catalepsy and no flaccidity. Furthermore, he was also able to show that the selective inhibition of conditioned (discriminated) avoidance responses is more specific with thiothixene than with the other two drugs.

While the onset of action of the CPZ and perphenazine analogues is faster, the duration of action of the thioproperazine analogue is longer.

Both the apomorphine and the amphetamine antagonism effects of thiothixene are stronger than those of either chlorprothixene or clopenthixol. Thiothixene is the least effective in the potentiation of hypnotics, chlorprothixene the most effective, and clopenthixol in between.

4. Metabolism

Among the various thioxanthene derivatives, the metabolic fate of chlorprothixene has been extensively studied in animals and men (Allgén *et al.*, 1960; and Raaflaub, 1967).

a. Absorption and Distribution

Chlorprothixene is promptly absorbed, and its metabolites appear in various organs within 15 to 30 minutes following oral administration. After an intravenous injection, measurable blood levels are present only for a short (few minutes) duration.

Distribution of the substance in the various organs in decreasing order of concentration is as follows: liver, lung, kidney, brain, skeletal muscles, spleen and fat tissues (Petersen and Nielsen, 1964).

b. Degradation and Excretion

Degradation of chlorprothixene occurs via chlorprothixene sulfoxide, which can be either *N*-demethylated or further oxidized (to the *N*-oxide).

Excretion takes place in the urine, the bile and the feces.

5. Chemical and Neurophysiological Correlates of Drug Action

a. Chemical Correlates

There are a number of central and peripheral changes related to the effect of these drugs, *e.g.*, marked inhibitory effect on catecholamines (dopamine, epinephrine, norepinephrine) and serotonin, moderate antihistaminic property, and weak anticholinergic activity.

Most of these effects can only be measured peripherally. In "despinalized" rats, thioxanthenes antagonize the hypertensive reaction to monoamines (*e.g.*, norepinephrine) and interfere with the hypotensive effect of acetylcholine (Nielsen, 1967). Nevertheless, the adrenolytic action of these drugs is considerably less than that of the phenothiazines (*e.g.*, CPZ), and their anticholinergic properties are considerably lower than those of atropine.

It has been noted that the antihistaminic potential of the *cis* analogues is stronger than that of the *trans* analogues (Petersen and Nielsen, 1964).

The end result of these interactions is a shift toward the cholinergic direction (in peripheral autonomic functioning).

Only limited data are available on the biochemical changes induced in the central nervous system by thioxanthene drugs. Roos (1965) demonstrated an increase in homovanillic acid (HVA) concentration in the corpus striatum. This is in variance with Gey and Pletscher's (1961) early findings, according to which there are no significant changes in the cerebral concentrations of dopamine and norepinephrine with thioxanthenes. More recently, it has been recognized that thioxanthenes (like other neuroleptic drugs) significantly enhance the conversion of labeled tyrosine to radioactive catechols, which indicates an increase in the activity of the tyrosine hydroxylase enzyme (Pletscher *et al.*, 1967).

Thus Pletscher *et al.* (1967) suggested that, under the influence of these drugs, the dopamine receptor blockade leads to a compensatory increase in the rate of dopamine synthesis via the "regular" course, *i.e.*, from tyrosine and dopa. The increase in dopamine concentration leads to the excess of homovanillic acid, its breakdown product.

b. *Neurophysiological Correlates*

Parasympathicotonia with a slight depression of the brain stem reticular formation and stimulation of the limbic system structures are the neurophysiological concomitants of thioxanthene drug action.

i. Medulla Oblongata. Inhibition of the chemical trigger zone of vomiting, located in this region, is a common characteristic of thioxanthene drugs. The antiemetic activity of the various thioxanthene preparations was found to be equal to their phenothiazine analogues (Pellmont *et al.*, 1960; and Janssen *et al.*, 1965).

ii. Hypothalamus. Impairment of the temperature-regulating mechanism located in this region is another common characteristic of psychoactive thioxanthene preparations (Pellmont *et al.*, 1960). Thus, in normal room temperature, a hypothermic effect (in mice, rats, dogs and rabbits) has been seen, and a lowering of body temperature could also be shown in hyperthermic conditions induced by LSD and tetrahydronaphthylamine administration or by the intravenous injection of a yeast suspension (Scheckel, 1967).

A correlation between the duration of hypothermia induced in normal temperature and the duration of the effects seen in a conditioned avoidance procedure in rats was indicated by Boff and Scheckel (1964). Furthermore, the hypothermic activity was found to be roughly proportional to the mobility-reducing power (Petersen and Nielsen, 1964).

iii. Cerebral Cortex. The threshold of arousal reactions to electrical stimulation is considerably increased; proprioceptive arousal reaction is inhibited; and the duration of the arousal response produced by physostigmine administration is reduced by thioxanthene drugs (Brucke, 1959).

Synchronous slow waves (3 to 5 c.p.s.) of high voltage and brief periods of low amplitude, high frequency electroencephalographic patterns were seen to be predominantly present (in rabbits and cats) after intravenous administration of psychoactive thioxanthenes.

6. Behavioral Pharmacology

a. *Animal Studies*

i. Direct Tests. Catalepsy and reduction of mobility (in mice and rats) are common characteristics of neuroleptic thioxanthenes.

The effect on spontaneous motor activity (mobility) has been studied in jiggle cages. The exploratory activity normally exhibited by mice in any new environment was found to be interfered with by psychoactive thioxanthenes.

The akinetic (cataleptic) activity was shown in mice with the "vertical rod test," and in rats, with the "rubber stopper method." The akinetic mouse maintained its position instead of climbing up or down; similarly, the akinetic rat maintained its two front paws on the stoppers longer than 30 seconds.

ii. Indirect Tests. Psychoactive thioxanthenes potentiate the sleep-inducing (or hypnotic) effect of alcohol and barbiturates (also reflected in the extended duration of the loss of righting reflex, *i.e.*, the spontaneous adoption of an upright position), and the analgesic effect of morphine-like analgesics. On the other hand, they interfere with the excessive psychomotor stimulation (also reflected in the failure to sniff, lick or gnaw) produced by amphetamines and caffeine (Quinton and Halliwell, 1963; Petersen and Nielsen, 1964; Weissman *et al.*, 1966; and Nielsen, 1967).

iii. Conditioning Tests. The action of these compounds on "discrete trial avoidance," "trace avoidance," "continuous avoidance" and "approach-avoidance conflict" situations has been studied.

In "discrete trial avoidance," animals are presented with a warning (conditional) signal, followed by an electric shock (unconditional stimulus). Lever pressing after the warning signal prevents, and after the electric shock terminates, the electrical current.

In the "trace avoidance" procedure (Heise and McConnell, 1961), a warning (conditional) stimulus (usually a white noise) is followed by a silent period (gap), which ends in a period during which a noise plus shock (unconditional stimulus) is given. As in the discrete trial avoidance procedure, pressing the lever during the noise or silent periods prevented the shock while responses during the last period turned the shock off.

In the "continuous avoidance" procedure as developed by Sidman (1953) and modified for drug research by Heise and Boff (1962), animals are trained to press a lever at a moderate and constant rate to avoid shock. Each lever pressing postponed the shock, and if the animal kept a well defined constant rate (higher than one response per 40 seconds), it was never shocked.

In the "approach-avoidance conflict" procedure (Scheckel and McConnell, 1963), animals are required to press a lever after a conditional stimulus is given to obtain food, but the lever pressing also produces a foot shock (aversive stimulus) in addition to the delivering of the food rewards.

In discrete trial avoidance, thioxanthenes selectively block conditional (avoidance) responses without interfering with the unconditional (escape) reflex. Similarly, in trace avoidance, these drugs suppress responses during the noise or silent periods (while sedatives suppress it in all three and anxiolytics suppress it only in the first period). In the continuous avoidance and in the approach-avoidance conflict situation, a decreased response rate is seen (Scheckel, 1967).

b. Human Studies

The psychophysical effects of chlorprothixene were studied by St. Jean *et al.* (1964). It was found that Critical Flicker Fusion Frequency was reduced (less than with CPZ but more than with haloperidol) and After-Image Disappearance Limen elevated (more than with CPZ and approximately equally with haloperidol) under the influence of the thioxanthene drug. The decrease in Tapping Rate and the increase in Track Tracer Time and Time Reproduction were also midway between CPZ and haloperidol, while the increase in Reaction Time and the decrease in Word-Association Time were less with the thioxanthene preparation than with either phenothiazine or butyrophenones.

B. CLINICAL DATA

1. Indications and Contraindications

a. Therapeutic Indications

Thioxanthenes, particularly chlorprothixene, have been successfully administered in numerous pathological conditions. They have been found useful in the management of nausea and vomiting, especially when associated with radiation therapy, surgery (or emotional disturbance) and also in the alleviation of pain (Cohen *et al.*, 1967, and Petersen and Nielsen, 1964). Nevertheless, the major indications of these substances are in the various psychopathologies.

i. Functional Psychoses. *α. Schizophrenias.* The very first studies with *chlorprothixene* suggested a beneficial action in the schizophrenias (Madsen and Ravn, 1959; Nielsen *et al.*, 1959; Werenberg, 1959; Feldman, 1960; Geller, 1960; and Ravn, 1960, 1961). The early investigators stressed the rapid and pronounced calming effect of this drug and its reliable therapeutic action in paranoid reactions. These findings were supported by Remvis and Sonne (1961), Gayus and Blanchette (1962), Hagopian and Crossfield (1962) and Cahn

(1963). In Cahn's (1963) study of a group of newly admitted paranoid female patients, chlorprothixene was therapeutically equal to chlorpromazine. This is at variance with the findings of Haydu (1961). Lehmann *et al.* (1964) found chlorprothixene inferior to CPZ and to haloperidol in the treatment of acute schizophrenic patients. Kurland and Yazicioglu (1961) found it inferior to trifluoperazine in the therapy of chronic schizophrenic cases.

In the first clinical study, Ravn and Rud (1961) found clopenthixol therapeutically equal to perphenazine, the phenothiazine analogue of the substance, in a group of schizophrenic patients. These findings were confirmed by Ravn (1962), Kaartinen and Sourander (1962), Olsson and Ohnell (1962), Werenberg (1962), Bjørn and Rasmussen (1963), Gartner (1962), Pöldinger (1963) and Sourander and Kaartinen (1963) in subsequent studies. While Gross and Kaltenbäck (1962) suggested that clopenthixol brings about a rapid improvement in acute schizophrenics, particularly in hebephrenic patients, in subsequent studies Lehmann and Ban (1967) emphasized its usefulness in the treatment of chronic schizophrenic cases. In their first study, Ban *et al.* (1963) noted that the drug was therapeutically effective in certain chronic schizophrenic patients in whom previous treatment had failed, while in the second, Bartolucci *et al.* (1966) suggested that clopenthixol is particularly effective in affective psychopathology.

The antipsychotic effects of *thiothixene* were first recognized by Sugerman *et al.* (1965), Simpson and Iqbal (1965) and Gallant *et al.* (1966). Bishop *et al.* (1966) found, however, that treatment with thiothixene in acute schizophrenic cases is less effective than with trifluoperazine, while in chronic schizophrenic cases thiothixene is as effective as thioridazine (Gallant *et al.* 1966). Further studies on the usefulness of thiothixene in schizophrenics have been reported by Wolpert *et al.* (1966), Simeon *et al.* (1967), Hekimian *et al.* (1967) and Oliveros *et al.* (1967).

There was general agreement on the therapeutic value of thiothixene in the treatment of schizophrenic cases at the Groton Symposium (1965) in the United States and at the Paris Symposium (1966) in France. At the Groton meeting (1965), Gallant (1965) stated that no other antipsychotic agent studied in his unit has shown significantly greater therapeutic efficacy than thiothixene in chronic schizophrenics. In the same discussion, Raskin (1965) emphasized that the new substance was as safe as any other neuroleptic drug and more effective than perphenazine. Gilgore (1965), Merlis (1965), Simpson (1965) and Sugerman (1965) independently maintained that it is equal or better therapeutically than trifluoperazine; and Dussik (1965) reported that it is equal or superior to prochlorperazine.

At the Paris Symposium (1966), Gann (1966) described the sequence of therapeutic changes with thiothixene. During the second week, according to him, agitation and agressiveness diminished, and in the fourth week, anxiety and suspiciousness were alleviated. Finally, after 16 weeks in drug-responsive cases, agitation, aggressiveness and excitation disappeared; social adjustment improved; and hallucinations and delusions were virtually eliminated. At the same meeting, Gomez (1966) reported reduction of agitation and excitation with improved environmental adaptation and social contact in his patients. He found a reduction of autistic behavior, aggressiveness, hallucinations and mental confusion. Gomez (1966) described the potent effect of thiothixene, in decreasing order, on the following target symptoms: agitation, excitation, aggressiveness, suspiciousness and depression. Guilmot (1966) emphasized the improvement in social contact. Lambert (1966) characterized thiothixene action as more similar to prochlorperazine than to thioproperazine, and Schmitt (1966) suggested that it is closest to butaperazine and propericiazine. Finally, Deniker (1966) suggested that this drug is particularly effective in hebephrenic cases, while Stockhausen (1966) reported its usefulness in the "apragmatic form of schizophrenia."

β. Mania. Thioxanthenes in the treatment of mania seem to have limited application.

Nevertheless, the therapeutic effectiveness of chlorprothixene in manic patients was suggested by Gross and Kaltenbäck (1961), of clopenthixol by Massaut *et al.* (1962) and of thiothixene by Schiele (1967) and Filotto *et al.* (1967).

γ. *Depression.* Chlorprothixene has been used in the treatment of psychotic depressive cases. The possible antidepressant properties of this substance were first recognized by Madsen and Ravn (1959), and their findings were supported by Feer *et al.* (1960), Hoffet and Cornu (1960), Pöldinger (1960) and, more recently, by Felger (1965). However, Denber *et al.* (1960) were at variance with these reports. At the Thioxanthene Symposium of the Quebec Psychopharmacological Research Association a possible antidepressant effect of thiothixene was suggested (Simpson, 1967).

ii. Others. α. *Psychoneuroses.* Chlorprothixene has been successfully used in the treatment of psychoneurotic patients (Boitelle and Boitelle-Lentulo, 1959; Galeano *et al.*, 1959; Madsen and Ravn, 1959; Werenberg, 1959; Montagut, 1960; Gross and Kaltenbäck, 1961; Korskjaer *et al.*, 1961; Ravn, 1961; Levy *et al.*, 1963; and McCray *et al.* 1963). While clopenthixol in the treatment of psychoneuroses remained ineffective (Holst, 1962), clinical trials with thiothixene are as yet inconclusive.

β. *Organic Brain Syndromes.* There are some indications of the usefulness of chlorprothixene and clopenthixol in the treatment of alcohol-induced psychopathologies as well as in the control of withdrawal manifestations of alcohol, hypnotics or narcotics (Krakowski, 1963; and Fervers, 1964). Others found both these drugs therapeutically effective in disturbed geriatric patients (Nymand and Dahl, 1961; Malmgren and Ohnell, 1963; and Smith and Barron, 1965).

γ. *Childhood Disturbances.* Oettinger (1962) found chlorprothixene therapeutically equal to thioridazine in hyperactive children exhibiting habit and conduct disorders; and Harman *et al.* (1966) suggested that it is therapeutically equal to chlorpromazine.

δ. *Mental Deficiency.* Clopenthixol has been shown to be therapeutically effective in the treatment of mental defectives. In Jensen's (1962) study, however, the treatment of 6 out of 16 patients had to be discontinued because of the severe extrapyramidal manifestations induced by the thioxanthene drug.

b. Contraindications

Contraindications are circulatory collapse and acute intoxication with central depressant substances (*e.g.*, alcohol, hypnotics, opiates). Although no teratogenicity or carcinogenic action has been shown, thioxanthenes should be prescribed with caution in the first trimester of pregnancy.

In animal toxicity studies, a nodular enlargement of the thyroid gland with an increase in the basal metabolic rate was seen in the course of chlorprothixene administration. None of these changes has been reported in patients (Cohen *et al.*, 1967).

2. Therapy Alone and in Combination

a. Thioxanthenes Alone

i. Dosage. The therapeutic dosage range of each thioxanthene preparation differs slightly. It generally holds true, however, that in the treatment of schizophrenics the daily dosage of chlorprothixene is three times that of clopenthixol, and ten times that of thiothixene.

The dosage of *chlorprothixene* varies within a wide range. In depressions, the average daily amount is 45 to 100 mg., while in mania and schizophrenia, oral dosages as high as 1000 mg. daily have been given (Petersen and Nielsen, 1964). The average daily dosage for chlorprothixene in schizophrenics is 400 mg. The dosage of clopenthixol varies within a narrower range. Thus far, the highest daily dosage has been 800 mg., and the average daily dosage in schizophrenics is 150 mg. Least varied is the dosage range of thiothixene. The highest daily dosage has never exceeded 90 mg., and the average daily dosage in schizophrenics is 40 mg.

ii. Routes of Administration. Besides the safest and most common oral route, chlorprothixene and clopenthixol (but not thiothixene) can be given intramuscularly or intravenously. Intramuscular administration of chlorprothixene (100 to 200 mg. per day) or clopenthixol (75 to 150 mg. per day) may be used for controlling agitated patients. In the most severe cases, both drugs can be given intravenously (15 to 30 mg. administered slowly).

iii. Treatment Procedures. Continous therapy is the usual form of treatment with thioxanthene preparations. For *chlorprothixene* and *thiothixene*, the usual initial dose is one-third of the average daily dosage. From this, the daily amount of the drug is progressively increased until therapeutic effects are seen or troublesome side-effects occur.

In severely agitated and/or uncooperative patients, chlorprothixene treatment has to commence with parenteral doses. Once the *calming* effect is achieved, however, this can be replaced by oral medication. The changeover (from parenteral to oral dosing) should be gradual.

Treatment with *clopenthixol*, according to Ravn (1963), should commence with small initial doses. He maintains that by this the occurrence of a considerable number of side-effects can be prevented.

iv. Duration of Treatment. The duration of thioxanthene administration depends on the condition being treated. For example, while psychoneurotics, with the exception of some therapy-resistant chronic obsessive cases, should be treated only until symptomatic remission, schizophrenic patients should be kept on a maintenance dosage over an extended period of time. The rule of thumb is, as with the phenothiazines, that after the first episode, a schizophrenic patient should be maintained on medication for at least a 1-year period, after the second for at least 2 to 3 years, and thereafter for an indefinite period of time.

An account of maintenance therapy with chlorprothixene was reported by Cahn (1963), who treated 47 hospitalized acute paranoid female patients with this drug. Of the 43 cases who were discharged from the hospital, 10 had to be readmitted within 18 months. In these 10 patients, the relapse was intimately related to the withdrawal of their maintenance medication.

It is fortunate that thioxanthenes can be taken over an extended period of time and that, in spite of occasional withdrawal manifestations, there is definitely no addiction to these drugs.

b. Thioxanthenes in Combination with Other Treatments

Not infrequently, thioxanthenes are administered in conjunction with other treatments. When combined with ECT, it should be noted that the hypotensive action of the thioxanthene preparation is intensified; when combined with insulin, the occurrence of cerebral seizures is more frequent. Chlorprothixene has been suggested as an ideal substance for agitated depressive cases in combination with tricyclic antidepressant drugs (Kato *et al.*, 1967; and Ravn, 1961, 1962).

3. Adverse Reactions and Their Treatment

a. Adverse Reactions

In the course of treatment with thioxanthenes, a number of adverse reactions have been described. While side-effects are less often reported with thioxanthene preparations than with any of the other available antipsychotic drugs, this might be due to the fact that they are prescribed less frequently.

According to the nature of the adverse reaction, they are classed as psychiatric, neurological, autonomic, endocrine, cardiovascular, hematological and dermatological.

i. Psychiatric. Besides initial fatigue, somnolence and drowsiness and paradoxical insomnia, no other psychiatric adverse effects have been reported. They are most frequent with chlorprothixene and least common with thiothixene.

ii. Neurological. Most frequently discussed among all the reactions induced by thioxanthene drugs are extrapyramidal (EPS) manifestations. The incidence of these is considerably lower and the severity considerably less than that seen with the corresponding phenothiazine preparations. They are most frequent with thiothixene and the least common with chlorprothixene. Other neurological reactions are cerebral seizures, related to the lowering of the convulsive threshold, and rarely central fever (Ravn *et al.*, 1964).

iii. Autonomic. Among the autonomic reactions, frontal headache, disturbance of accommodation, nasal congestion, dryness of mouth, gastrointestinal disturbances (including constipation) and hyperhydrosis (Deniker, 1966) are the most common.

iv. Endocrine. On the basis of animal experiments, a possible effect of chlorprothixene on the thyroid gland was suggested. More recently, Boris and Stevenson (1967) observed that thioxanthenes may block the secretion of the pituitary antidiuretic hormone in dehydrated rats. Whether these also apply to humans remains to be seen.

v. Cardiovascular. Orthostatic hypotension is not infrequent with thioxanthene preparations. In one of Deniker's (1966) cases, it was severe enough to necessitate drug withdrawal. Occasionally, tachycardia —or paroxysmal tachycardia—occurs but usually only in the higher dosage ranges.

vi. Hematological. Leucopenia and eosinophilia in the course of chlorprothixene administration have been described (Petersen and Nielsen, 1964). Deniker (1966) reported a transient eosinophilia in 5 out of his 20 thiothixene-treated cases; Lambert (1966) noted an inversion of the albumin: globulin ratio; and Gann (1966) detected leucocytosis in the second and third week in some of his patients.

vii. Dermatological. While allergic skin reactions may occur, their incidence is rare.

An attempted suicide with clopenthixol was reported by Nørgaard (1964) in a 30-year-old woman who at the time of her discharge from hospital had been on a 25-mg. daily maintenance dosage. In a suicidal attempt, she took 400 mg. of the drug, which resulted in a cerebral seizure with a short lasting loss of consciousness. Her blood pressure, pulse rate and EEG, however, returned to normal only after a couple of weeks.

b. Treatment of Adverse Reactions

Drowsiness usually subsides spontaneously, but insomnia may necessitate reduction of the dosage. EPS and cerebral seizure respond well to adjuvant (antiparkinsonian or anticonvulsant) medication, but the control of central fever (also of tachycardia) may call for discontinuation of treatment. The therapy of hypotension consists of the administration of vasopressor substances (as with the phenothiazines, excluding epinephrine).

SUMMARY

The introduction of thioxanthenes is another important addition to the clinician's armamentarium in the treatment of psychiatric patients. A number of formerly treatment-resistant cases respond quite favorably to these drugs.

As with the phenothiazines and the butyrophenones, the most significant results have occurred in the treatment of schizophrenic patients. The administration of thioxanthenes in adequate dosage over a sufficiently long period of time can, on the one hand, bring the schizophrenic process to a halt and, on the other hand, improve chronically hospitalized inactive and apathetic patients to the point where they can participate in rehabilitation programs. The administration of these drugs may prevent the admission of patients to psychiatric hospitals and also make it possible to protect patients from relapse.

Of the three major thioxanthene preparations used in psychiatric treatment, chlorprothixene may help when depressive features are present in the schizophrenic illness. Clopenthixol and especially thiothixene may be useful in chronic schizophrenic cases in which other antipsychotics have failed; they are also effective in the treatment of the acutely disturbed patients.

The relatively low incidence of side-effects makes the thioxanthenes an important addition to the presently available antipsychotic preparations.

REFERENCES

ALLGÉN, L. G., *et al.:* On the elimination of chlorprothixene in rat and man. Experientia, *16:* 325 (1960).

BAN, T. A., FERGUSON, K., AND LEHMANN, H. E.: The effect of clopenthixol on chronic psychiatric patients (clinical note). Amer. J. Psychiat., *119:* 984 (1963).

BARTOLUCCI, G., *et al.:* Clinical studies with clopenthixol (sordinol) on chronic psychiatric patients. Curr. Ther. Res., *8:* 581 (1966).

BISHOP, M. P., FULMER, T. E., AND GALLANT, D. M.: Thiothixene versus trifluoperazine in newly admitted schizophrenic patients. Curr. Ther. Res., *8:* 509 (1966).

BJØRN, S., AND RASMUSSEN, C.: Sordinol (clopenthixol) in the treatment of schizophrenics. Acta Psychiat. Scand., *39:* 427 (1963).

BOFF, E., AND HEISE, G. A.: Attenuation of tetrabenazine "reversal" by chlordiazepoxide hydrochloride. Fed. Proc., *22:* 510 (1963).

BOFF, E., AND SCHECKEL, C. L.: Changes in rectal temperature induced by conditional avoidance behavior. Pharmacologist, *6:* 179 (1964).

BOITELLE, M. G., AND BOITELLE-LENTULO, C.: A new neuroplegic agent—taractan. Ann. Medicopsychol., *117:* 515 (1959).

BORIS, A., AND STEVENSON, R. H.: The effects of some psychotropic drugs on dehydration induced antidiuretic hormone activity in the rat. Arch. Int. Pharmacodyn., *166:* 486 (1967).

BRUCKE, F. (1959): In: Petersen, P. V., and Nielsen, M. I. Thioxanthene derivatives. In: Psychopharmacological agents (ed., Gordon, M.). (Academic Press, New York, 1964.)

CAHN, C. H.: Effect of chlorprothixene in patients with paranoid symptoms. Canad. Med. Ass. J., *89:* 719 (1963).

COHEN, S., *et al.:* Psychochemotherapy. (Western Medical Publications, Los Angeles, 1967.)

DENBER, H. C. B., RAJOTTE, P., AND ROSS, E.: Some observations on the chemotherapy of depression: results with "taractan." Compr. Psychiat., *1:* 308 (1960).

DENIKER, P.: Experience with thiothixene. (Presented at the Pfizer Symposium on thiothixene, Paris, 1966.)

DUSSIK, E.: Experience with thiothixene. (Presented at the thioxanthene symposium, Pfizer Medical Research Laboratories, Groton, 1965.)

FEER, H., *et al.:* Klinische Untersuchungen mit Chlorprotixen. Schweiz. Med. Wschr., *90:* 600 (1960).

FELDMAN, P. E.: Clinical evaluation of chlorprothixene. Amer. J. Psychiat., *116:* 929 (1960).

FELGER, H. L.: Depressed hospitalized psychiatric patients treated with chlorprothixene concentrate. J. New Drugs, *5:* 240 (1965).

FERVERS, J.: The treatment of addicts of various kinds with ciatyl. Nervenarzt, *35:* 177 (1964).

FILOTTO, J., *et al.:* Thiothixene in the treatment of affective psychoses: a pilot study. (Presented at the Q.P.R.A. Symposium on Thioxanthenes, Montreal, 1967.)

GALEANO, J., *et al.:* Ensaios clinicos de un derivado de tioxanteno, RO 4-0403. Dia Med. Urug., *26:* 2748 (1959).

GALLANT, D. M.: Experience with thiothixene. (Presented at the thiothixene symposium, Pfizer Medical Research Laboratories, Groton, 1965.)

GALLANT, D. M., BISHOP, M. P., AND SHELTON, W.: A preliminary evaluation of P-4657B: a thioxanthene derivative. Amer. J. Psychiat., *123:* 345 (1966).

GALLANT, D. M., *et al.:* Thiothixene (P-4657B): a controlled evaluation in chronic schizophrenic patients. Curr. Ther. Res., *8:* 153 (1966).

GANN, G.: Experience with thiothixene. (Presented at the Pfizer Symposium on thiothixene, Paris, 1966.)

GARTNER, K.: Experiences with N-746 (sordinol), a psychotropic drug, in a clinical trial. Praxis, *51:* 30 (1962).

GAYUS, I. K., AND BLANCHETTE, J. E.: Effects of chlorprothixene in well established schizophrenic reactions. Amer. J. Psychiat., *119:* 180 (1962).

GELLER, W.: Therapeutic results with the neuroleptic truxal. Med. Klin., *55:* 554 (1960).

GEY, K. F., AND PLETSCHER, A.: Influence of chlorpromazine and chlorprothixene on the cerebral metabolism of 5-hydroxytryptamine, norepinephrine and dopamine. J. Pharmacol. (Kyoto), *133:* 18 (1961).

GILGORE, S. G.: Experience with thiothixene. (Presented at the thiothixene symposium, Pfizer Medical Research Laboratories, Groton, 1965.)

GOMEZ, M. I.: Experiencia clinica con thiothixene un nuevo neuroleptico. (Presented at the Fourth World Congress of Psychiatry, Madrid, 1966.)

GOMEZ, M. I.: Experience with thiothixene. (Presented at the Pfizer Symposium on thiothixene, Paris, 1966.)

GÖZSY, B., KATO, L., AND ST. JEAN, A.: Effect of imipramine on the norepinephrine-induced capillary response in the rat. Experientia, *23:* 210 (1967).

GROSS, H., AND KALTENBÄCK, E.: Erfahrung mit dem Thioxanthenderivat Chlorprothixen in der Klinischen Psychiatrie. Wien. Klin. Wschr., *73:* 64 (1961).

GROSS, H., AND KALTENBÄCK, E.: Sordinol, a new neuroleptic of the thioxanthene series. Wien. Klin. Wschr., *74:* 549 (1962).

GROSS, M., *et al.:* Discontinuation of treatment with ataractic drugs. In: Recent advances in biological psychiatry (ed., Wortis, J.). (Grune and Stratton, New York, 1961.)

GUILMOT, P.: Experience with thiothixene. (Presented at the Pfizer Symposium on thiothixene, Paris, 1966.)

GUILMOT, P.: Experimentation du neuroleptique P-4657 B au thiothixene. (Presented at the Fourth World Congress of Psychiatry, Madrid, 1966.)

HAGOPIAN, P. B., AND CROSSFIELD, R. M.: Experiences with chlorprothixene in a state hospital. Amer. J. Psychiat., *119:* 466 (1962).

HARMAN, C., *et al.:* Clinical experience with chlorprothixene in disturbed children. Int. J. Neuropsychol., *2:* 72 (1966).

HAYDU, G. C.: Effects of metrazol-vitamin administration in chronic psychoses. Curr. Ther. Res., *3:* 255 (1961).

HEISE, G. A., AND BOFF, E.: Behavioral determination of time and dose parameters of monoamine oxidase inhibitors. J. Pharmacol. Exp. Ther., *129:* 155 (1960).

HEISE, G. A., AND BOFF, E.: Continuous avoidance as a base-line for measuring behavioral effects of drugs. Psychopharmacologia (Berlin), *3:* 264 (1962).

HEISE, G. A., AND MCCONNELL, H.: Differences between chlordiazepoxide-type and chlorpromazine-type action in trace avoidance. (Presented at the Third World Congress of Psychiatry, Montreal, 1961.)

HEKIMIAN, L. J., *et al.:* Thioxanthenes: some clinical and physiologic effects of a thioxanthene derivative, thiothixene, in twenty newly hospitalized male schizophrenics. J. Clin. Pharmacol. New Drugs, *7:* 52 (1967).

HOFFET, H., AND CORNU, F.: Klinische Erfahrungen mit dem Thioxanthen derivat, RO 4-0403. Schweiz. Med. Wschr., *90:* 602 (1960).

HOLST, B.: Sordinol in the treatment of neuroses. Ugeskr. Laeg., *125:* 161 (1962).

JANSSEN, P. A. J., NIEMEGEERS, C. J. E., AND SCHELLEKENS, K. H. L.: Is it possible to predict the clinical effects of neuroleptic drugs (major tranquillizers) from animal data? I. "Neuroleptic activity spectra" for rats. Arzneimittelforschung, *15:* 104 (1965).

JENSEN, O.: Sordinol in the treatment of psychic unrest in mental defectives of a low intelligence level. Ugeskr. Laeg., *124:* 1608 (1962).

KAARTINEN, M., AND SOURANDER, C.: Clinical experience with Sordinol (R), a new psychotropic drug. Nord. Psykiat. T., *16:* 130 (1962).

KATO, L., *et al.:* Peripheral vascular effects of thioxanthenes. (Presented at the Q.P.R.A. Symposium on Thioxanthenes, Montreal, 1967.)

KATO, L., AND GÖZSY, B.: Differential and quantitative affinity of psychoactive drugs to mucopolysaccharides. Indian J. Med. Res., *49:* 788 (1961).

KATO, L., *et al.:* Attempt to classify psychotropic drugs based on their affinity to mucopolysaccharides in vivo. J. Clin. Exp. Psychopath., *23:* 75 (1962).

KORSKJAER, G., *et al.:* Truxal as an adjuvant in the treatment of neurosis. Nord. Psykiat. T., *15:* 63 (1961).

KRAKOWSKI, A. J.: Tarasan in a private psychiatric practice. J. New Drugs, *3:* 110 (1963).

KURLAND, A. A., AND YAZICIOGLU, E.: Effect of chlorprothixene on schizophrenic patients. Dis. Nerv. Syst., *22:* 636 (1961).

LAMBERT, P. A.: Experience with thiothixene. (Presented at the Pfizer Symposium on thiothixene, Paris, 1966.)

LEHMANN, H. E., AND BAN, T. A.: Systematic studies with thioxanthenes. (Presented at the Q.P.R.A. Symposium on Thioxanthenes, Montreal, 1967.)

LEHMANN, H. E., AND BAN, T. A.: Studies with new drugs in the treatment of convulsive disorders. Int. J. Clin. Pharmacol., *1:* 231 (1968).

LEHMANN, H. E., *et al.:* The effect of haloperidol in acute schizophrenic patients. A comparative study of haloperidol, chlorpromazine and chlorprothixene. In: The butyrophenones in psychiatry (eds., Lehmann, H. E., and Ban, T. A.). (Québec Psychopharmacological Research Association, Montreal, 1964.)

LEVY, H. A., *et al.:* Chlorprothixene, a new nonphenothiazine ataractic. J. Neuropsychiat., *5:* 138 (1963).

MADSEN, E., AND RAVN, J.: Preliminary therapeutic experiments with a new psychotropic drug, truxal. Nord. Psykiat. Medlemski, *13:* 82 (1959).

MALMGREN, G., AND OHNELL, L. K.: Clinical trial with sordinol on patients with senile dementia. Svensk Lakartidn., *60:* 1630 (1963).

MASSAUT, C., *et al.:* Clinical study of 162 patients treated with a new neuroleptic: clopenthixol (sordinol (R)). Acta Neurol. Belg., *62:* 651 (1962).

MCCRAY, W. E., *et al.:* Long-term drug treatment of psychiatric out-patients. Dis. Nerv. Syst., *24:* 3 (1963).

MERLIS, S.: Experience with thiothixene. (Presented at the thiothixene symposium, Pfizer Medical Research Laboratories, Groton, 1965.)

MONTAGUT, J. B.: Experiencias clinicas con el psicosedativo RO 4-0403. (Presented at the Psychiatric Congress, Barcelona, 1960.)

NIELSEN, M. I.: Pharmacology of clopenthixol. (Presented at the symposium on thioxanthenes, Montreal, 1967.)

NIELSEN, M. I., *et al.:* On truxal, a new psychotropic drug. (Presented at the Danish Psychiatric Association Meeting, Copenhagen, 1959.)

NIELSEN, M. I., *et al.:* Central depressant activity of some thioxanthene derivatives. Acta Pharmacol. (Kobenhavn), *19:* 87 (1962).

NIELSEN, M. I., AND NEUHOLD, K.: The comparative pharmacology and toxicology of tarasan and chlorpromazine. Acta Pharmacol. (Kobenhavn), *15:* 335 (1959).

NØRGAARD, K.: Attempted suicide with clopenthixol (Sordinol). Ugeskr. Laeg., *126:* 597, 1964.

NYMAND, M., AND DAHL, R. (1961): In: Petersen, P. V., and Nielsen, M. I.: Thioxanthene derivatives. In: Psychopharmacological agents (ed., Gordon, M.). (Academic Press, New York, 1964.)

OETTINGER, L.: Chlorprothixene in the management of problem children. Dis. Nerv. Syst., *23:* 568 (1962).

OLIVEROS, R. F., *et al.:* A clinical trial of thiothixene in schizophrenics. Curr. Ther. Res., *9:* 504 (1967).

OLSSON, R., AND OHNELL, L. K.: Sordinol, a new psychotropic drug. Svensk. Lakartidn., *50:* 1778 (1962).

PELLMONT, B., *et al.:* On the pharmacology of taractan, a neuroleptic with special profile of effects. Helv. Physiol. Pharmacol. Acta, *18:* 241 (1960).

PETERSEN, M. C., AND MCBRAYER, J. W. (1959): In: Zirkle, C. L., and Kaiser, C.: Monoamine oxidase inhibitors. In: Psychopharmacological agents (ed., Gordon, M.). (Academic Press, New York, 1964.)

PETERSEN, P. V., *et al.:* Chemical structure and pharmacologic effects of thioxanthene analogues of chlorpromazine, promazine and mephazine. Arzneimittelforschung, *8:* 395 (1958).

PETERSEN, P. V., AND NIELSEN, M. I. (1961): In: Petersen, P. V., and Nielsen, M. I.: Thioxanthene derivatives. In: Psychopharmacological agents (ed., Gordon, M.). (Academic Press, New York, 1964.)

PETERSEN, P. V., AND NIELSEN, M. I.: Thioxanthene derivatives. In: Psychopharmacological agents (ed., Gordon, M.). (Academic Press, New York, 1964.)

PLETSCHER, A., GEY, K. F., AND BURKARD, W. P.: Effects of neuroleptics on the cerebral metabolism of catecholamines. (Presented at the symposium on "Toxicite et effets secondairs des medicaments psychotropes," Paris, 1967.)

PÖLDINGER, W.: Ein Neurolepticum mit Antidepressiver Wirkung, Taractan (RO 4-0403). Praxis, *49:* 468 (1960).

PÖLDINGER, W.: Combined administration of desipramine and reserpine or tetrabenazine in depressive patients. Psychopharmacologia (Berlin), *4:* 308 (1963).

QUINTON, R. M., AND HALLIWELL, G.: Effects of α-methyldopa and dopa on the amphetamine excitatory response in reserpinized rats. Nature (London), *200:* 178 (1963).

RAAFLAUB, J.: Zum Metabolismus des Chlorprothixen. Arzneimittelforschung, *17:* 1393 (1967).

RASKIN, M.: Experience with thiothixene. (Presented at the thiothixene symposium, Pfizer Medical Research Laboratories, Groton, 1965.)

RAVN, J.: Truxal, a new type of psychopharmacological agent. Wien. Klin. Wschr., *72:* 192 (1960).

RAVN, J.: Chlorprothixene: a new psychotropic entity. Amer. J. Psychiat., *118:* 227 (1961).

RAVN, J.: Chlorprothixene for schizophrenia and depression. Chemotherap. Rev., *2:* 187 (1961).

RAVN, J.: A warning against too high an initial dose. Ugeskr. Laeg., *124:* 1707 (1962).

RAVN, J.: Further experience with sordinol. Nord. Psykiat. T., *16:* 136 (1962).

RAVN, J.: On sordinol therapy. Ugeskr. Laeg., *124:* 1707 (1962).

RAVN, J.: Interdependence and development of side effects and dosage of sordinol. Ugeskr. Laeg., *125:* 1200 (1963).

RAVN, J.: Letter to the editor. Acta Psychiat. Scand., *40:* 117 (1964).

RAVN, J., *et al.:* The results of treatment of 252 psychiatric patients with the new psychotropic drug, clopenthixol. (Paper presented at the Third C.I.N.P. Congress, Munich, 1962.)

RAVN, J., AND RUD, C.: Sordinol a new psychotropic drug. Ugeskr. Laeg., *123:* 1663 (1961).

RAVN, J., AND RUD, C.: Clopenthixol (sordinol). Ugeskr. Laeg., *125:* 748 (1963).

RAVN, J., RUD, C., AND WENDELBOE, J.: Psychiatric patients treated with the new psychopharmacological substance clopenthixol (sordinol, ciatyl). Neuropsychopharmacology, *3:* 285 (1964).

REMVIS, J., AND SONNE, L. M.: Chlorprothixene compared to chlorpromazine. Psychopharmacologia (Berlin), *2:* 203 (1961).

ROOS, B. E.: Effects of certain tranquillizers on the level of homovanillic acid in the corpus striatum. J. Pharm. Pharmacol., *17:* 820 (1965).

SCHECKEL, C. L.: Pharmacology and chemistry of the thioxanthenes with special reference to chlorprothixene. (Presented at the Symposium on Thioxanthenes, Montreal, 1967.)

SCHECKEL, C. L., AND BOFF, E.: Behavioral effects of interacting imipramine and other drugs with d-amphetamine, cocaine and tetrabenazine. Psychopharmacologia (Berlin), *5:* 198 (1964).

SCHECKEL, C., AND MCCONNELL, H.: Response latency as a measure of approach and approach-avoidance behavior in the rat. (Presented at the thirty-fourth meeting of the Eastern Psychological Association, New York, 1963.)

SCHIELE, B. C.: Studies with clopenthixol and thiothixene. (Presented at the Symposium on the Thioxanthenes, Montreal, 1967.)

SCHMITT, V.: Experience with thiothixene. (Presented at the Pfizer Symposium on thiothixene, Paris, 1966.)

SIDMAN, M.: Avoidance conditioning with brief shock and no exteroceptive warning signal. Science, *118:* 157 (1953).

SIMEON, J., *et al.:* Clinical trial of navane in schizophrenia. Curr. Ther. Res., *9:* 10 (1967).

SIMPSON, G. M.: Experience with thiothixene. (Presented at the thiothixene symposium, Pfizer Medical Research Laboratories, Groton, 1965.)

SIMPSON, G. M.: Experiences with the thioxanthenes. (Presented at the Q.P.R.A. Symposium on Thioxanthenes, Montreal, 1967.)

SIMPSON, G. M., AND IQBAL, J.: A preliminary study of thiothixene in chronic schizophrenics. Curr. Ther. Res., *7:* 697 (1965).

SMITH, A. J., AND BARRON, A. R.: The use of chlorprothixene in the disturbed geriatric patient. Amer. J. Psychiat., *122:* 213 (1965).

SOURANDER, C., AND KAARTINEN, M.: Further clinical experiences with sordinol, a new psychotropic drug. Nord. Psykiat. T., *17:* 83 (1963).

ST. JEAN, A., *et al.:* The psychophysical effects of the butyrophenones. In: The butyrophenones in psychiatry (eds., Lehmann, H. E., and Ban, T. A.). (Q.P.R.A., Montreal, 1964.)

STOCKHAUSEN, F. G.: Experience with thioxanthenes. (Presented at the Pfizer Symposium on thiothixene, Paris, 1966.)

SUGERMAN, A. A., *et al.*: A pilot study of P-4657B in chronic schizophrenics. Curr. Ther. Res., *7:* 310 (1965).

SUGERMAN, A. A.: Experience with thiothixene. (Presented at the thiothixene symposium. Pfizer Medical Research Laboratories, Groton, 1965.)

VOORHEES, A. B., BAKER, J. H., AND PULANSKY, E. J.: Reaction of albino rats to injections of dextran. Proc. Soc. Exp. Biol. Med., *76:* 254 (1951).

WEISSMAN, A.: A psychopharmacological comparison of thiothixene, chlorprothixene and clopenthixol in rats. (Presented at the Q.P.R.A. Symposium on Thioxanthenes, Montreal, 1967.)

WEISSMAN, A., KOE, B. K., AND TENEN, S. S.: Antiamphetamine effects following inhibition of tyrosine hydroxylase. J. Pharmacol. Exp. Ther., *151:* 339 (1966).

WERENBERG, H.: Truxal. Ugeskr. Laeg., *121:* 1736 (1959).

WERENBERG, H.: The use of sordinol in the treatment of schizophrenia. Nord. Psykiat. T., *16:* 392 (1962).

WOLPERT, A., HAGAMEN, M. B., AND MERLIS, S.: A pilot study of thiothixene in childhood schizophrenia. Curr. Ther. Res., *8:* 617 (1966).

Fourteen

Tricyclic Antidepressants

A. BASIC DATA

1. Historical Aspects

Spontaneous recovery may occur within a month in 20 to 25 per cent of unselected depressed patients. Placebos may increase the chance of significant improvement from 25 to 60 per cent and an *effective antidepressant drug from 50 to 75 per cent* (Lehmann, 1966).

The most extensively used and probably the most reliable of the antidepressant drugs are the tricyclic compounds.

The first tricyclic antidepressant was imipramine. Its basic constituent, the iminodibenzyl nucleus, consists of two benzene rings attached to each other by an ethylene bridge and a nitrogen atom.

This nucleus was synthesized and chemically described by Thiele and Holzinger (1899). It was further explored pharmacologically half a century later, when systematic studies were directed to synthesize iminodibenzyls, particularly aminoalkyls, in the course of searching for new and better antihistaminic compounds (Häfliger and Schindler, 1951).

Pharmacological experiments confirmed the antihistaminic action of the iminodibenzyls and established their sedative effects. Anticholinergic properties, possibly useful in the treatment of parkinsonism, were recognized at the same time. The promising reports of chlorpromazine in the therapy of various psychiatric disorders and especially in the treatment of schizophrenia redirected animal screening toward finding iminodibenzyl derivatives with particularly strong sedative or hypnotic effects which might possibly be useful in the treatment of schizophrenic patients.

A number of drugs were selected for clinical trials. Among them was imipramine, the iminodibenzyl analogue of promazine, which, as Kuhn (1957) discovered, was ineffective in schizophrenics but gave promising results in depression, particularly the endogenous retarded type. The effect of imipramine in these cases was distinctly different from that of stimulant drugs, *e.g.*, amphetamines, which produced only a temporary and superficial euphoria often accompanied by side-effects of overstimulation. Kuhn's (1957) findings were soon confirmed by Lehmann *et al.* (1958).

2. Action Mechanism

A number of hypotheses ranging from the stereochemical to the psychodynamic have been formulated to explain this unexpected antidepressant property.

a. Stereochemical Concept

The stereochemical concept was based on the notion that the molecules of both the antipsychotic phenothiazines and the antidepressant iminodibenzyls have nearly the same spatial volume and shape (Häfliger, 1959). There are only two major differences between the two structures. One of them is the bridge between the two benzene rings, *i.e.*, in phenothiazines, a sulfur (S) atom and in the iminodibenzyls an ethylene (CH_2—CH_2) group. From the chemical point of view, however, this seemingly slight

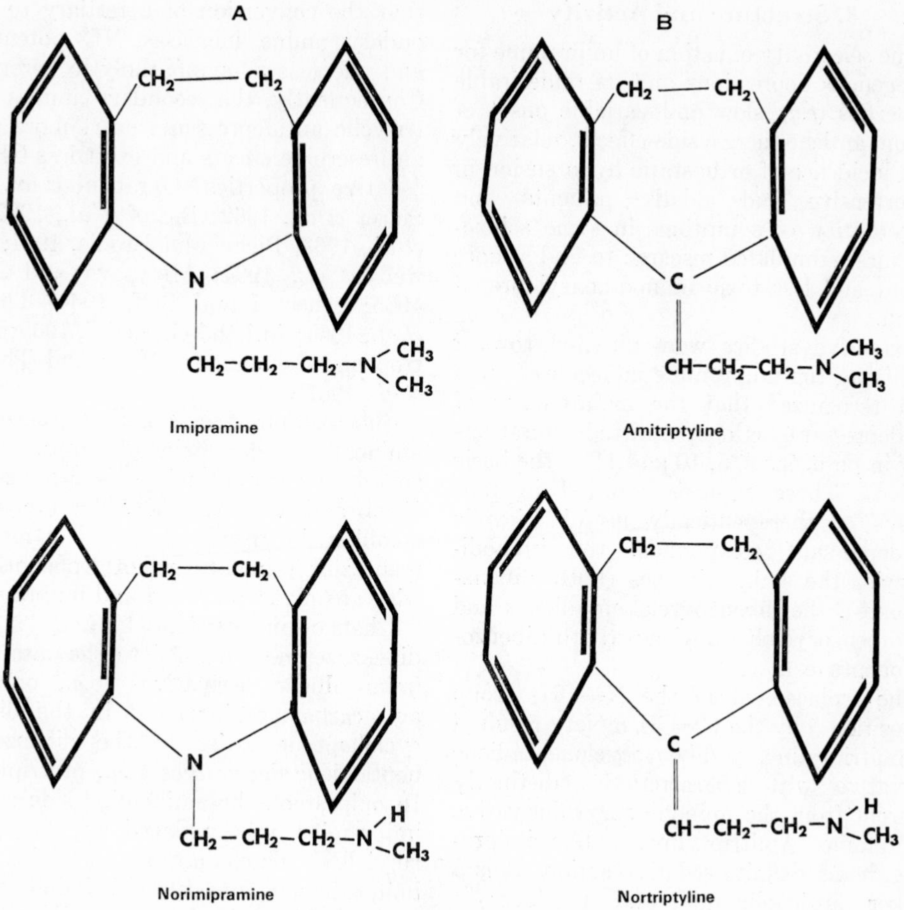

FIG. 14. *a*, Imipramine and norimipramine. *b*, Amitriptyline and nortriptyline

difference implies that, in the phenothiazine ring system, the S atom enables the conjugation of the benzene rings to extend over the bridge, whereas the CH_2—CH_2 group in the iminodibenzyls acts as a barrier to conjugation. The other difference between the two molecules is that imipramine is an asymmetrical molecule in which the two benzene rings are twisted against each other, in contrast to the symmetrical promazine molecule.

b. Psychodynamic Hypothesis

Azima (1961) described a change in the direction of aggressive drives from inward to outward, with a secondary reorganization of libidinal tendencies, a decrease in guilt feelings and a shift from preoccupation with internal object relations to external object relations under the influence of tricyclic antidepressant drugs. He formulated the hypothesis that, under imipramine administration, an economic shift in the aggressive cathectic energies of the superego components of the psyche occurs with a secondary reorganization of libidinal investment resulting in a primary reorganization of aggressive investment from inner to outer objects and relief of the depressive state.

There is still no general agreement on which of the known actions of the molecule accounts for its usefulness in the depressions. Further research to modify and enhance the therapeutic effects of imiprimine and eliminate its undesired reactions has led to the synthesis of a large number of tricyclic antidepressant drugs with distinctly different chemical, pharmacological and clinical properties.

3. Structure and Activity

The selectivity of action of imipramine for endogenous depressions and its undesirable properties (*e.g.*, slow and variable onset of action, anticholinergic side-effects, relatively high incidence of orthostatic hypotension in hypertensive and elderly patients and exacerbation of symptoms in some schizophrenics) stimulated research to find a more potent and less toxic iminodibenzyl preparation.

Extensive studies were directed toward modifying the imipramine molecule. It was soon recognized that the maintenance of antidepressant action permitted alterations only in positions 3, 5, 10 and 11 of the basic nucleus. These changes resulted in four groups of therapeutically useful tricyclic antidepressant compounds, the iminodibenzyls, the iminostilbenes (both dibenzazepines), the dibenzocycloheptadienes and the dibenzocycloheptatrienes (both dibenzocycloheptenes).

The replacement of the N—CH_2 group in position 5 by the C=CH moiety resulted in amitriptyline, a dibenzocycloheptadiene derivative with characteristics distinctly different from the iminodibenzyl derivative imipramine. Amitriptyline, unlike imipramine, has a definite sedative action. It is a weaker anticholinergic and produces a lower incidence of hypotensive and/or adverse psychopathological reactions.

Modifications on the aminoalkyl side chain of both drugs added further quantifiable changes. Desmethylation of imipramine led to desipramine (norimipramine), while desmethylation of amitriptyline resulted in nortriptyline. Both desmethylated drugs showed a more rapid clinical onset of action with probably less severe adverse effects than their parent compounds.

The isolation and identification of desipramine, a "secondary amine" (imipramine metabolite), (Herrmann *et al.*, 1959; Herrmann and Pulver, 1960; and Gillette *et al.*, 1961) and the subsequent demonstration of its potent pharmacological activity stimulated research to explore the potential of other "secondary amines" (Sulser and Dingell, 1966). The results were nortriptyline and protriptyline. It was soon recognized that the conversion of a tertiary to a secondary amine increases NE potentiation and decreases sympatholytic properties. Consequently, the secondary amines of the tricyclic antidepressants exert more potent antireserpine effects and exert less CPZ-like sedative properties (Garattini *et al.* 1962; Sulser *et al.*, 1962; Bickel *et al.*, 1963; Sigg *et al.*, 1963; Bickel and Brodie, 1964; Halliwell *et al.*, 1964; Metysova and Metys, 1965; Scheckel and Boff, 1964; Theobald *et al.*, 1964; Jori and Garattini, 1965; Ribentrop and Schaumann, 1965; and Theobald *et al.*, 1967).

Substitution of an α-methyl group on the aminoalkyl side chain of imipramine resulted in trimipramine (synthesized by Jacob and Messer, 1956). The aim was to combine the beneficial effects of methotrimeprazine (an antipsychotic phenothiazine with anxiolytic activity) and imipramine.

Changes in positions 10 and 11 in the dibenzazepine series led to the unsaturated iminostilbene derivatives (*e.g.*, opipramol and carbamazepine) and in the dibenzocycloheptane series to the dibenzocycloheptatriene derivatives (*e.g.*, protriptyline). In opipramol, the aminoalkyl side chain of imipramine was replaced by the piperazinylalkyl side chain of perphenazine on the iminostilbene (unsaturated iminodibenzyl) nucleus. This added some anxiolytic properties to the molecule while lowering its antidepressant effect. In carbamazepine, the aminoalkyl side chain of the unsaturated nucleus was substituted with a carbomoyl group, resulting in an anticonvulsant with antidepressant properties, useful also in the treatment of trigeminal neuralgia. On the other hand, protriptyline, the unsaturated analogue of nortriptyline, is considered to be a pharmacologically potent and therapeutically promising primarily antidepressant preparation.

More recently, clinical studies with chlorimipramine, the CPZ analogue of the iminodibenzyl series, suggested that the substance may be particularly useful as a "corrector" of the depressant effects of neuroleptics and as an "activator" in chronic apathetic schizophrenic cases. Whether it is this substance which produces the beneficial changes or whether it provides only for the psychic constellation which "shows off the improvement" that occurs in the course of neuroleptic treatment still remains to be seen (Delay, 1967).

4. Metabolism of Tricyclic Antidepressants

The fate of the different tricyclic antidepressant compounds, from the time they are first administered until they are excreted from the organism, at least in part follows similar pathways.

a. Absorption and Distribution

Tricyclic antidepressants are absorbed in 5 to 10 minutes after parenteral administration and in 30 to 60 minutes when taken by mouth. In radioactive isotope studies with imipramine (in rats), it was found that 30 minutes after administration of the drug (via a stomach tube) 65 per cent of the radioactivity had already disappeared from the gastrointestinal tract. A transient sedative action—somewhat more pronounced with amitriptyline than with imipramine—occurs. This is considerably stronger after parenteral administration. The same also hold true for the actual antidepressant action.

Forty to 50 per cent of imipramine—after a single dose administration—is recovered from the urine within 4 days (either unchanged or in the form of metabolites). The balance is transiently stored in the various body tissues, such as the kidney, brain, heart, etc. Relatively high levels have been found in the brain compared with the body fat and in the cardiac muscle compared with skeletal muscles.

b. Degradation and Excretion

The most important metabolic pathways of tricyclic antidepressants are oxidative demethylation, *N*-oxidation, hydroxylation and conjugation. Radioactive isotope studies have shown that oxidative monodemethylation of the side chain is one of the main pathways of metabolism which results in desipramine and nortriptyline (the desmethylated analogues of imipramine and amitriptyline, respectively), which are considered to be the psychopharmacologically active metabolities of these drugs. The *N*-oxidation is also restricted to the side chain.

The major metabolic process of the central ring is hydroxylation, prevailingly in position 2, with subsequent conjugation with glucuronic acid. The resulting glucuronides constitute by far the major part of the urinary excretion products of these drugs.

Tricyclic antidepressants are promptly absorbed and promptly excreted from the organism. It has been noted, however, that relatively low plasma levels and excretion rates are the characteristics of patients with a favorable therapeutic response; and relatively high plasma levels and excretion rates, in therapeutic failures (Berti and Cima, 1962; Bickel *et al.*, 1963; Carr, 1959; Dingell *et al.*, 1961, 1962; Fishman and Goldenberg, 1962; Gillette *et al.*, 1960; Häfliger, 1959; Herrmann *et al.*, 1959; Hermann and Pulver, 1960; Pscheidt, 1962; Pulver *et al.*, 1960; and Ragland, 1962).

c. Differential Features

i. Among Tricyclic Antidepressants. *N*-demethylation and hydroxylation are the two major metabolic pathways for both imipramine and amitriptyline. The hydroxylation of imipramine takes place on one of the aromatic rings (forming phenolic metabolites) and of amitriptyline on the ethylene bridge (leading to alcoholic metabolites) (Herrmann *et al.*, 1959; Hucker and Porter, 1961; and Hucker, 1962).

ii. Interspecies Differences. Dingell *et al.* (1962, 1964) recognized that rat liver preparations metabolize imipramine mainly to desmethylimipramine, whereas rabbit liver microsomes oxidize it to 2-hydroxyimipramine. It was also discovered that rabbits and mice metabolize both imipramine and desmethylimipramine at about the same rate, whereas rats (and humans) metabolize desmethylimipramine slower than imipramine. Consequently, the desmethylated metabolite accumulates in the tissues of rats (and humans) but not in rabbits or mice (Susler and Dingell, 1966; and Leybold and Staudinger, 1962).

On the basis of these striking differences in the metabolism in various animal species, Sulser and Dingell (1966) suggest exploring the possibility of purposefully introducing metabolic alterations, *e.g.*, by slowing metabolism to prolong or enhance therapeutic effects.

5. Chemical and Neurophysiological Correlates of Drug Action

a. Chemical Correlates

The psychoactive effects of tricyclic antidepressants cannot be reduced to a single chemical concomitant of drug action. There are a number of central and peripheral changes related to the action of these drugs. While tricyclic antidepressants as a rule do not have an inhibitory effect on the monoamine oxidase enzyme, they do have an influence on the nervous system transmitter substances, *i.e.*, acetylcholine, norepinephrine and serotonin, that possibly regulate both synaptic transmission and the activity of autonomic nervous system centers.

i. Interaction with Cholinergic Mechanisms. Tricyclic antidepressants exert antiacetylcholine effects and are anticholinergic in their action. Since depression may be related to excessive cholinergic activity in the brain, this anticholinergic action was considered to be intimately related to their therapeutic effects.

The anticholinergic activity of tricyclic antidepressants is considered to be due to the replacement of the sulfur bridge (intimately linked with the sympatholytic action of phenothiazines) by an ethylene bridge. It was recognized that depression frequently accompanies parkinsonism, implicating the importance of a cholinergic dysfunction in both of these conditions. The finding that imipramine improved not only the depression but also the rigidity of patients suffering from parkinsonism is another point in favor of the anticholinergic property of these drugs. The most convincing evidence of the anticholinergic actions of tricyclic antidepressants is, however, the numerous atropine-like side-effects that occur in the course of treatment with these drugs.

ii. Interaction with Adrenergic Mechanisms. Intact CNS catecholamine stores are the prerequisite for the reserpine (or benzoquinolizine) antagonism of tricyclic antidepressants. Thus, depletion of brain catecholamines interferes with this effect, and repletion of brain catecholamines reestablishes it. There is an enhancement of the action of injected norepinephrine (also a potentiation of methylphenidate action) at peripheral sympathetic receptor sites after imipramine, amitriptyline, desipramine or nortriptyline administration. More recently, direct evidence has been obtained that, while both imipramine and amitriptyline antagonize the effect of adrenaline, they enhance the effect of norepinephrine. This enhancement of norepinephrine effect is correlated with a decrease in biogenic amines stored in the brain, which in turn is concomitant with a blockade in the uptake of the administered norepinephrine. This inhibition of re-storage of free biogenic amines—or retardation of inactivation—results in a rise in their available pool manifested in "supersensitization" to catecholamines.

At a Workshop of the NIMH Pharmacology Unit (Sulser and Dingell, 1966; Gyermek, 1966; Vernier, 1966; Lehmann, 1966; and Efron and Kety, 1966), the inhibition of amine uptake mechanisms in the adrenergic neuronal cell membrane was suggested as the central mechanism of tricyclic antidepressant action.

Indirect evidence of this are the findings that tricyclic antidepressants potentiate the central actions of dopa and amphetamine; potentiate the amine releasing action of tetrabenazine and reserpine; and antagonize other reserpine and tetrabenazine effects. The crucial role of NE in these reactions is substantiated by the finding that prior depletion of NE abolishes these effects (Sigg, 1959). Furthermore, it was recognized that, while tricyclic antidepressants inhibit NE uptake both centrally and peripherally, antipsychotic phenothiazines exert this effect only peripherally (Axelrod, 1966).

iii. Other Effects. Tricyclic antidepressants exert antihistaminic and antiserotonin actions. They counteract the spasmogenic effects of these substances on the isolated guinea pig ileus and interfere with the reserpine-produced lowering of brain serotonin levels. Other, peripheral, effects of tricyclic antidepressants are a transient rise in alkaline phosphatase values in the serum, which usually returns to normal with the continuation of treatment. In diabetics, there is a diminution of glycosuria concomitant with imipramine administration. This effect is opposite to that of chlorpromazine on carbohydrate metabolism.

Heuristically more important are the findings of Schildkraut (1965), who demonstrated that clinically effective doses of imipramine decrease vanillylmandelic acid (VMA) excretion, a metabolic product of NE, predominantly. Since the same applies to MAOI antidepressants, Klerman and Cole (1965) suggest the probability of a common action for imipramine and the MAOI's by increasing the amounts of catecholamines available for functional action (at the adrenergic receptor sites). These findings support the crucial role of adrenergic mechanisms in the action of tricyclic antidepressant drugs.

b. Neurophysiological Correlates

There is no single neurophysiological phenomenon which can fully account for the multifold activities of these drugs. It is generally accepted that tricyclic antidepressants selectively affect several subcortical structures, resulting in slow and smooth therapeutic action without appreciable interference with cortical functions.

i. Autonomic Nervous System. The anticholinergic and adrenolytic effects of these drugs were first described in the late nineteen-fifties. In further studies, it was recognized that the anticholinergic action is predominant only with high dosages.

In recent experiments with trimipramine, it has definitely been established that the hypertensive effect of adrenaline is counteracted by pretreatment with this drug, while the norepinephrine-induced hypertension remains unaffected. The same applies for other tricyclic antidepressants. In view of these findings, the ergotropic activity of these drugs is considered to be due to the suppression of the "parasympathetic nervous system" and the sensitization of the "sympathetic nervous system."

Sigg (1959) demonstrated that imipramine interferes with pilocarpine—a parasympathomimetic chemical—induced salivation; with the bradycardia following stimulation of the parasympathetic vagus nerves; and with acetylcholine-induced activity on the isolated intestines. Sulser *et al.* (1960) found that imipramine may also block the centrally mediated increase in parasympathetic output, as seen by the reduction of salivation under the influence of the drug. The first observations of Domenjoz and Theobald (1959) on the cardiovascular system of anesthetized animals, however, indicated a transitory hypotensive action, followed by a more sustained rise of the blood pressure.

ii. Medulla Oblongata. The effect of dibenzazepine and dibenzocycloheptane derivatives on the medulla oblongata is seen as a mild antiemetic effect, which is a common characteristic of all drugs belonging to these categories.

iii. Brain Stem Reticular Formation. Systematic studies revealed the influence of tricyclic antidepressants on the arousal reaction related to brain stem reticular formation function. On the basis of drug-induced changes of the arousal reaction, Himwich (1960) differentiated between two major groups of psychoanaleptics: energizers and antidepressants (suppressant drugs). He calls energizers those drugs which have a stimulating influence on brain stem reticular formation functions, *e.g.*, the amphetamines and methylphenidate, because they increase the electrical activity of the brain and antidepressants those drugs which have an inhibitory (suppressant) effect on the same structures, *e.g.*, imipramine, benactyzine, orphenadrine, etc., because "they act primarily upon depressive affect," diminishing the response to "disturbing beliefs and unpleasant stimuli." All known tricyclic antidepressants belong to this latter category. It has also been noted, however, that the two classical representatives of drugs which are beneficial in depression, the monoamine oxidase inhibitor iproniazid and the dibenzazepine imipramine, are placed in opposite categories, whereas neither benactyzine nor orphenadrine has a comparable antidepressant action with the tricyclic preparations. This implies that the mode of action of these drugs is not exclusively in the depression of the arousal response of the reticular formation in the brain stem. The effect of tricyclic antidepressants was further qualified by psychopharmacological experiments which revealed that chlorpromazine is synergistic with imipramine, evoking a sleep-like brain wave pattern and preventing the alerting response on the electroencephalogram, while reserpine is antagonistic to imipramine in the same areas.

iv. Hypothalamus. The effect of these drugs on the hypothalamus has been extensively investigated with Olds' (1956) method. Under the influence of imipramine, an increase in self-stimulation was seen with electrodes implanted in the lateral hypothalamus, and an augmentation of the methamphetamine-induced increment in the rate of self-stimulation was found with the same method when electrodes were placed in the posterior hypothalamic region. On the basis of the discovery that intravenously given amitriptyline in cats causes a slowing of the spontaneous electrical activity of the brain and attenuation of alerting responses evoked by loud tones and foot pinches, it was postulated that the induced inhibitory effect is due to the blocking of impulses from the anterior hypothalamus to the cortex, thereby increasing the threshold for certain cortical responses, including those involved in depressive states.

v. Others. Other neurophysiological effects concomitant with tricyclic antidepressant administration are inhibition of certain septal areas manifested in decreased duration of after-discharges; slight enhancement of the excitability of the amygdala; rhinencephalic spikes and convulsant brain wave patterns starting from the hippocampus; and desynchronization with a decrease of total electrical activity of the brain, together with an increase in theta rythm and fast beta activity on the surface electroencephalogram (an effect which resembles centrally acting cholinergic blocking agents).

6. Behavioral Pharmacology

Tricyclic antidepressants induce behavioral changes in animals and men over a wide range of functions. Prominent is the reduction of spontaneous motor activity with all tricyclic antidepressants but desipramine. It has been noted that monkeys respond paradoxically to these drugs.

a. Animal Studies

Pharmacological tests on animals with dibenzazepine and dibenzocycloheptane compounds revealed some distinct differences among the drugs of these groups. This was first seen in their effect on body temperature in which only amitriptyline was shown to have a slight hypothermic action. In the operant conditioning model both imipramine and desipramine (both dibenzazepines) increase the speed of pigeons (working to obtain grain by pecking a key) in a Skinner box (1959), while amitriptyline (a dibenzocycloheptene) has the opposite effect. On a Sidman (1959) avoidance schedule, however, both drugs (amitriptyline more and imipramine less) decrease lever pressing (Sigg, 1959; Cook *et al.*, 1962; Cook and Weidley, 1960; Dews, 1962; Hanson, 1961; Kornetsky, 1963; Werner, 1962; and Vernier *et al.*, 1962).

Other pharmacological effects of tricyclic antidepressants are *potentiation* of the behavioral effect of central stimulants and the sleeping time after hexobarbital or ethanol administration (Carlton, 1961; and Hill *et al.*, 1961) and the *antagonism* to cataleptics, morphine, tetrabenazine and reserpine. Reserpine antagonism, however, in the case of imipramine, is clearly evident only when the antidepressant drug is given at least 2 hours prior to reserpine administration, suggesting that this effect is not due to the compound itself but rather to one of its metabolites (desipramine). Protection against the tonic component in convulsions induced by electrostimulation (or pentetrazol administration) is also a common characteristic of these drugs.

A succinct presentation of the pharmacodynamics of tricyclic antidepressants in general and amitriptyline in particular was given by Vernier *et al.* (1962). They differentiated among specifically antidepressant actions, depressant actions and autonomic effects. Among the specific antidepressant actions, they listed the antagonism of tetrabenazine-induced sedation, the antagonism of reserpine-induced hypothermia, the differential sympathomimetic amine blocking response, *i.e.*, potentiation of the NE pressor effect and blockade of the phenethylamine pressor response, and the potentiation of amphetamine effects upon behavior (as noted by Carlton in 1961 and Stein in 1962). On the other hand, the depressant action of tricyclic antidepressants is manifested by a decrease in conditioned avoidance responses (in several species), a protective action against the hind limb tonic extensor component of supramaximal electroshock seizures in mice, and a decrease in the protection against tetrabenazine-induced sedation in mice. Finally, they consider weak anticholinergic properties, some antihistaminic and antiserotonin activity as the characteristic autonomic effects.

b. Human Studies

A self-experimenter has described that, after a latent period of about 30 minutes, 50 or 100 mg. of imipramine caused a sense of tiredness along with the feeling of growing distance between himself and his surroundings. This was followed by an inner restlessness, which he described as "inner quivering." The over-all effect was characterized as a feeling which one experiences when tired and unable to get to sleep. Another introspectionist reported that after a short phase of pleasant relaxation he felt an inner harmony and increased vitality, but without an urge for action "similar to that which one experiences under the influence of amphetamines."

Human pharmacological experiments in healthy volunteers have revealed that imipramine causes a blunting of emotions without loss of initiative. It does not produce euphoria or stimulation but rather engenders a feeling of fatigue accompanied by atropine-like symptoms, *i.e.*, dryness of mouth, palpitation, blurred vision and urinary retention. Continuous administration leads to accentuation of these manifestations and also to difficulty in concentration and thinking. These altered psychological functions resemble those induced by chlorpromazine. Imipramine, however, causes greater impairment of cognitive and affective processes than chlorpromazine, and it does not reduce physical movements to the same degree. It has been noted that desipramine is less potent in this respect than the parent compound (DiMascio *et al.*, 1964; and Idestrom and Cadenius, 1964).

In clinical pharmacological studies, the predominant effect of chronic administration of tricyclic antidepressants in patients with prevailing depressive psychopathology was the "dulling" of the depressive ideation (Pöldinger, 1963). There are occasional reports of manic reactions or hallucinations induced by these drugs, and euphoria or insomnia can occur in the course of treatment. It has been noted that the behavioral alerting and excitement are associated with desynchronization of the electroencephalogram.

B. CLINICAL DATA

1. Therapeutic Indications and Contraindications

a. Therapeutic Indications

Tricyclic antidepressants are successfully administered in numerous pathological conditions. Formerly, it was believed that these drugs are specific for endogenous depressions, but recently several papers have reported equally good therapeutic response in reactive cases. There is increasing evidence that the best therapeutic results are obtained when the depression is "experienced" as a physical ailment and when the mood changes are associated with sleeplessness and loss of appetite. In these patients, tricyclic antidepressants are suggested for the initial pharmacological approach in treatment.

The choice of a particular drug from this group for a particular patient depends upon careful consideration of a number of specific and nonspecific factors. The importance of a hypothetical genetic factor (Angst, 1961) and of personality structure is emphasized by several investigators. The possibility of a genetic factor was raised when a familial responsiveness to imipramine was discovered, and the importance of personality structure was suggested when it was found that passive-dependent individuals fail to respond to these drugs. On the other hand, patients with a good response to a particular drug in a previous depressive episode are likely to respond favorably again in case of relapse.

The actual diagnosis (endogenous-reactive), the quality of depression (typical-atypical) and the prevailing symptomatology (agitated-retarded) in the frame of reference of previous history, including physiological reactivity, however, still remain the most instructive factors in the selection of an antidepressant drug.

The psychiatric indications of tricyclic antidepressants range from functional psychoses through organic conditions and neuroses to personality disorders and mental deficiency.

i. Functional Psychoses. *α. Depressions.* In the functional psychoses, the particular effectiveness of these drugs has been observed in endogenous depressions, including the manic-depressive, recurrent and involutional types. In all these conditions, imipramine, amitriptyline, trimipramine, desipramine, nortriptyline and protriptyline are significantly superior to placebo in their therapeutic effect.

The over-all effectiveness of tricyclic antidepressants in the treatment of depressions was summarized by Lehmann (1966), and the comparative efficacy with other types of therapies in the same conditions was reviewed by Klerman and Cole (1965). According to Lehmann (1966), in 47 uncontrolled studies on the effects of imipramine on a total of 4098 patients, the average percentage improvement was 62.6 (61.1 to 88 per cent), while in 25 uncontrolled studies on the effects of amitriptyline on 2705 patients, the average improvement was 60.6 per cent (23 to 85 per cent). Similarly, in 42 controlled studies with imipramine covering 2705 patients, the average improvement was 66.7 per cent (19 to 100 per cent), while in 16 controlled studies with amitriptyline covering 872 patients, the average improvement was 65 per cent (15 to 81 per cent). Although in 11 studies on the effects of desipramine (covering a total of 355 patients) the average percentage improvement was 72.5 and in the 7 studies on the effects of nortriptyline (covering a total of 250 patients) the average percentage improvement was 78.8, Lehmann (1966) considers the improvement rates on the last two compounds less reliable than the improvements reported in the studies on their parent compounds.

Klerman and Cole (1965) reviewed a number of comparative studies on the treatment of depression with imipramine, electroconvulsive therapy, amitriptyline and desipramine. While in the clinical trials of Greenblatt *et al.* (1964) and also of Robin and Harris (1962) electroconvulsive treatment was found to be significantly superior to imipramine therapy, Delay et al. (1959), Hoff (1959), Hutchinson and Swedberg (1963), Oltman and Friedman (1961) and Wilson *et al.* (1963) found these two forms of treatments equally successful. The therapeutic effects of amitriptyline were found to be significantly superior to imipramine by Burt *et al.* (1962), Hoenig and Visram (1964), Hollister *et al.* (1964), Hordern *et al.* (1963, 1964) and Snow and Rickels (1964), while by others, no significant difference between imipramine and desipramine could be shown (Rose and Westhead, 1964; and Wilson *et al.*, 1963).

β. Schizophrenias. Tricyclic antidepressant drugs are used in schizoaffective and cyclophrenic psychoses and in the depressive hypochondriacal states of some chronic paranoid schizophrenic patients. Amitriptyline and desipramine seem to be equally useful in these conditions. Findings with imipramine and trimipramine are less consistent. It is generally agreed that dibenzazepine derivatives do not help retarded schizophrenics and if they become more active, they also become more hallucinated and deluded. More recently, however, a beneficial effect of chlorimipramine has been suggested in chronic hebephrenic schizophrenic patients.

On the basis of animal data, Stein (1962)

ascribed potential antipsychotic properties to imipramine when administered in high doses. Remmen *et al.* (1962) reported improvement in schizophrenics on the same drug. However, Gallant and Bishop (1967) could not detect antipsychotic activity within the tolerated human dosage range in the course of a clinical trial with imipramine in chronic schizophrenic patients.

ii. Organic Syndromes. In the various chronic organic conditions, tricyclic antidepressants are useful in the treatment of superimposed depressions. Amitriptyline and trimipramine are frequently used in the treatment of depressive manifestations in presenile, senile and arteriosclerotic conditions; and carbamazepine has been found to be particularly useful as an adjuvant for the control of affective psychopathology in epileptics.

iii. Psychoneuroses. For depressed cases with prevailing anxiety, amitriptyline and trimipramine are usually recommended. Patients with psychosomatic reactions respond favorably to nortriptyline, and psychasthenics benefit from desipramine administration. The same drugs have also been reported to be useful in phobic-anxiety states, and they may also be therapeutically successful in helping some therapy-resistant obsessive-compulsive patients.

In the course of a collaborative study, Wittenborn (1967) recognized that those patients who had "schizophrenic qualities, manic depressive history, or an involutional circumstance were found to provide certain relatively unfavourable symptomatic responses, while the remaining patients, including those diagnosed as reactive, responded favourably." These data, according to him, challenge the claims which emphasize a most advantageous response of endogenous patients to imipramine and a less advantageous response of reactive patients. This is in accordance with the results of a former study (Wittenborn, 1962) in which he found the therapeutic effects of imipramine comparable to ECT in a group of premenopausal women with neurotic depression.

iv. Miscellaneous Other Conditions. Favorable therapeutic response in symptomatic reactions of childhood, *e.g.*, nail-biting, hair pulling, tantrums, school phobias, and enuresis, have been described.

Among the different personality disorders, epileptic character changes are beneficially influenced by carbamazepine, while improvement in behavior of psychopaths has been described with desipramine and in passive-aggressive personalities with nortriptyline. Certain alcoholic and mentally deficient cases also benefit from this drug.

The following primary indications of the eight clinically used tricyclic antidepressant compounds were suggested: *imipramine* in endogenous retarded depressions without anxiety, perceptual pathology or thought disorder (particularly in young females); *trimipramine* in depressions in which sedative and anxiolytic effects are desired (particularly in involutional melancholics); *desipramine* in depressions with psychomotor inhibition and lack of drive; *opipramol* in psychoneuroses in which sedative and tranquilizing effects are desired; *carbamazepine* in epilepsy with superimposed affective psychopathology and in trigeminal neuralgia; *amitriptyline* in endogenous depressions (even) with perceptual and cognitive psychopathological changes (particularly in the older age group); *notriptyline* in psychosomatic conditions and reactive depressions; and *protriptyline* in neurotic depression (Ban, 1966).

b. Contraindications

There are relatively few absolute contraindications of tricyclic antidepressants: these are comatose states, history of agranulocytosis and severe liver impairment. Some consider renal and cardiovascular diseases, including arteriosclerosis and arterial hypertension, as relative contraindications, although there is ample evidence that some geriatric psychiatric patients suffering from these conditions do show a remarkably favorable improvement on these drugs. These compounds should definitely not be used in place of hospitalization or electroconvulsive treatment in severely depressed cases in which they may remove psychomotor inhibition prior to lifting the dysthymic mood and thereby increase the risk of suicide.

Particular precautions should be taken in patients with schizophrenia, glaucoma, prostatic hypertrophy, severe constipation or, in general, in all cases where the anticholinergic effect of these drugs is "particularly" undesirable. There are known cases in which schizophrenic episodes, glaucomic attacks and urinary retention have been precipitated, potentiated or aggravated and in which intestinal obstruction with fatal consequences has occurred. The predisposition to these reactions is increased in cases in which the drug is administered together with antiparkinsonian compounds or with phenothiazines, particularly those with piperidylalkyl side chain.

It is the consensus among clinicians that it is better to avoid using tricyclic antidepressant drugs together with monoamine oxidase inhibitors (MAOI's). Furthermore, some recommend that a tricyclic antidepressant should not be used for at least a period of 2 weeks after MAOI treatment is terminated and that MAOI's should not be administered for at least 3 days after the discontinuation of therapy with tricyclic antidepressants. Failure to heed these requirements (except in the case of trimipramine, which may be administered together with MAOI's) has led to serious adverse reactions. These include dizziness, profuse sweating, restlessness, tremor, myoclonic seizure, hyperthermia, vascular collapse, convulsions, delirium, hallucinations and coma.

In addition, these drugs augment the effect of atropine, amphetamines, sympathomimetic amines, thyroid hormone preparations and alcohol, possibly leading to undesired consequences. Particular consideration should be given to the influence of tricyclic antidepressants on cerebral seizure patterns (in epileptics) and on carbohydrate metabolism (in diabetics).

There is no direct evidence that these drugs should not be administered during pregnancy or in the period of lactation, although fetal abnormalities in the course of imipramine administration have been reported in the rabbit (Robson and Sullivan, 1963). No indication of carcinogenic effect has been seen.

2. Therapy Alone and in Combination

a. Tricyclic Antidepressants Alone

i. Dosage. It generally holds true that in the treatment of depressed patients the maximum daily dosage of both of the desmethylated analogues is approximately one-third less than that of their parent compounds. Pediatric and geriatric patients are given a considerably lower dosage, which, in children for example, never exceeds half the maximum adult daily dosage. The recommended therapeutic dosage of these drugs for adults is as follows.

α. Dibenzazepines. Of the three drugs belonging to this category, trimipramine is administered in a slightly higher dosage and desipramine in a dosage which is one-third lower than the parent compound (imipramine). Kuhn (1957) has recommended that treatment with imipramine should commence with a dosage of 25 mg. given at bedtime. If the drug accentuates the tendency to sleep—a vagotonic effect—administration can safely be continued. If its effect is one of insomnia and restlessness—a sympathotonic effect—treatment should progress more cautiously. The dosage usually given for the next 2 days is 75 to 100 mg. in three or four divided doses, which is then gradually increased by 25 mg. daily (or every other day by 50 mg.) until a total daily dose of 250 mg. is reached. This can be continued until pathological symptoms remit, whereupon it is reduced to a maintenance dosage level. The optimal recommended dosage with desipramine and trimipramine is 200 mg. and 300 mg., respectively. The optimal dosage of the two iminostilbenes opipramol and carbamazepine is approximately 200 mg. and 1000 mg., respectively.

β. Dibenzocycloheptenes. Of the two dibenzocycloheptene derivatives, amitriptyline is given in the same dosage as imipramine, but with a somewhat lower optimal dosage—approximately 150 mg. a day—while nortriptyline is given in the same dosage as desipramine but also in a somewhat lower optimal dosage, *i.e.*, 100 mg. a day. In special cases, however, much higher dosages have been successfully administered without any serious adverse effects (*e.g.*, 450 mg. of amitriptyline a day). The optimal dosage of the dibenzocycloheptatriene protriptyline is in the range of 60 mg. daily.

ii. Routes of Administration. Besides the safest and most common oral route, tricyclic antidepressants are given intramuscularly and occasionally intravenously. In severely depressed cases in which a quick therapeutic response is absolutely desired or in uncooperative patients when oral drug administration may be difficult or impossible, it is the accepted practice to commence treatment with intramuscular injections of the drug.

The intramuscular injections are given in the appropriate area of the gluteal muscles (the femoral muscles being the second choice). To prevent hypotensive reactions, it is recommended that patients, especially geriatric cases, stay in a reclining position for at least an hour after parenteral administration. If hypotensive reaction occurs, norepinephrine should be given while epinephrine administration has to be carefully avoided.

Of the different drugs in this group, imipramine and amitriptyline are the ones most frequently administered parenterally (in daily doses of 50 to 100 mg.) for an average of 2 to 3 days, after which the intramuscular doses are replaced with the equivalent oral medication.

Intravenous administration of these drugs is infrequent. When indicated, amitriptyline is usually the drug of choice.

iii. Treatment Procedure. Continuous therapy is the only successful clinical treatment procedure with tricyclic antidepressants. Therapy begins with one-third of the average optimal daily dosage, which then is progressively increased until there is a definite indication of therapeutic action or the optimal dosage is reached. The onset of action varies among the different drugs, and it ranges from 3 days to 6 weeks with an average of 18 days. The most prompt onset of action is observed with opipramol (a tranquilizing action); amitriptyline works somewhat faster than imipramine; and the demethylated analogues usually have a somewhat quicker onset of action than their parent compounds.

The first improvement is almost invariably an objective one (increased activity, greater animation) that is usually noted by the outside observers (unlike ECT, in which a subjective feeling of well-being precedes the signs of objective changes). It is essential that "objective" signs of improvement be present as early as the end of the first week following the commencement of treatment, since patients who do not show any improvement at all during this crucial first week are likely to be therapy resistant (fully or partially). Improvement during the first week of medication, low blood (and also urine) concentrations of the drug, and a decrease in the blood sugar level are good indications for a favorable therapeutic result, but at least 2 or 3 weeks must be allowed before it can definitely be seen that the drug is effective. The time when maximum improvement is reached ranges from 14 to 84 days, and the average patient resumes his normal activities within 3 to 6 weeks.

Imipramine and the other tricyclic antidepressants have a prevailing effect on dysthymic mood and various inhibitory phenomena of depression. In the course of treatment, a general activation takes place first. Movements become faster, and facial expression softens. Slowly, patients acquire a sense of distance from their disturbing—depressing—feelings, become less concerned about themselves and see a brighter future. The effect of these drugs is not cumulative and disappears rather promptly when medication is discontinued.

iv. Duration of Treatment. Since the effect of these drugs wears off quickly, discontinuation of treatment should never be abrupt. The medication should be decreased slowly, thereby permitting observation of changes brought about by the reduction of the dosage. The duration of administration is dependent on both the condition which is being treated and a careful analysis of the previous history of the patient. In schizophrenics, for example, they should be given for only the shortest period of time, while in endogenous depressions antidepressant therapy should be continued beyond the disappearance of symptoms for at least as long as the depressive attack is expected to last.

The adequate maintenance dosage with each of the compounds is approximately two-thirds or less of the optimal daily dosage given in the acute period of the illness. There is no rule of thumb on the length of maintenance therapy, but it is usually accepted that a neurotic depressive should be maintained on his medication for at least 3 to 6 months, a patient suffering from endogenous depression for at least 6 to 12 months and involutional melancholics for at least 12 to 24 months. After several recurring attacks, patients should probably be kept on medication for an indefinite period. Early cessation of therapy may lead to relapse. After the patient is taken off medication, a periodic check-up is recommended. In the course of this regular examination, if reduction of weight or parotid secretion is noted or if the patient is complaining of persistent insomnia, the medication should immediately be resumed.

It is fortunate that tricyclic antidepressants can be taken over an extended period and, in spite of the withdrawal syndrome occasionally seen after abrupt discontinuation of treatment, there is no addiction to these drugs.

b. Tricyclic Antidepressants in Combination with Other Treatments

Not infrequently, tricyclic antidepressants are administered with other treatments: physical or pharmacological.

i. Physical. Both electroconvulsive and fever therapies are occasionally combined with tricyclic antidepressants. It was once believed that the addition of tricyclic antidepressants in general and imipramine in particular results in a better and quicker recovery from depression than treatment with ECT alone. There is now increasing evidence that drugs alone are sufficient in the majority of cases and only in drug-resistant or severely depressed suicidal cases is electroconvulsive (electroshock) therapy recommended.

Instead of ECT, the combination of artificial pyrexia (produced by intravenously given typhoid fever vaccine) and imipramine has been tried successfully in a few drug-resistant cases. The combination has also been useful in acutely suicidal cases. It was assumed that the mechanism which contributed to the favorable response is the lowering of the resistance of the blood brain barrier with the possible result of an increase of drug concentration in the brain. At the same time, the nonspecific anxiety-reducing effect of pyrexia was also noted (Lehmann, 1960).

ii. Pharmacological. Tricyclic antidepressants potentiate the effect of central nervous system stimulant preparations. Combined administration results in a feeling of well-being already in the time lag between the commencement of tricyclic drug administration and the initial signs of antidepressant action. Unnecessarily prolonged administration, however, leads to adverse effects.

There are two symptoms in particular which require additional medication in the course of treatment: insomnia and anxiety. Insomnia is usually controlled by adjuvant hypnotic medication, while anxiety can be successfully counteracted by barbiturates, propanediols or benzodiazepines. The mood-lifting property of some of the drugs in the latter group makes them specially desirable for combined treatment.

There are several combinations of antidepressants and phenothiazines on the market: Tofranazine, which contains 25 mg. of imipramine and 50 mg. of promazine; Triavil, which contains 15 mg. of amitriptyline and 3 mg. of perphenazine; and Etrafon in three different dosage combinations. Etrafon-A consists of 10 mg. of amitriptyline and 4 mg. of perphenazine; Etrafon-D and F contain 25 mg. of amitriptyline and 2 and 4 mg. of perphenazine, respectively.

Combined administration of tricyclic antidepressants and cardiac drugs calls for caution because of the quinidine-like effect of tricyclic antidepressant drugs. The hypoglycemic effect of these drugs may require an adjustment in the insulin dosage of diabetics.

3. Adverse Reactions and Their Treatment

a. Adverse Reactions

In the course of treatment with tricyclic antidepressants, numerous adverse reactions have been reported. Serious side-effects, however, occur mainly with higher doses (300 mg. or higher with imipramine, 200 mg. or higher with amitriptyline). In general, the toxicity of amitriptyline is considered to be lower than that of impramine; adverse effects are less with the desmethylated analogues than with their parent compounds.

Adverse reactions to these drugs may affect any organ or organ system, causing either mild discomfort or severe pathological changes that may call for untimely termination of treatment. According to their nature, adverse reactions to tricyclic antidepressant drugs are classed as psychiatric, neurological, autonomic, ophthalmological, cardiovascular, gastrointestinal, genitourinary, hepatobiliary, metabolic, hematological and dermatological.

i. Psychiatric. These are sympathotonic and vagotonic reactions. The sympathotonic reaction is manifested by insomnia, giddiness, restlessness and agitation; the vagotonic, by weakness, fatigue and somnolence.

Both transient insomnia and somnolence are frequently encountered at an early stage of treatment, the former somewhat more often with desipramine or imipramine and the latter with trimipramine and amitriptyline. Hypomanic and manic reactions as well as toxic confusional states (with or without visual hallucinations) have also been described.

ii. Neurological. While slight dizziness and mild headaches are often encountered, extrapyramidal signs are rather rare. The most common of these is a fine tremor which is seen in approximately 10 per cent of cases. Severe tremors, however, are only seen with high doses. Muscular hypotonia, asthenia, contractions, twitching and dysarthria, all have been reported. Generalized convulsions in epileptics or in patients with pathological EEG's have been seen. There are also occasional reports of peripheral neuropathy, peroneal palsy, dysphagia, central hypothermia and, with toxic doses of imipramine and amitriptyline, respiratory depression.

iii. Autonomic. Most frequently discussed among all the reactions induced by these drugs are the atropine-like parasympatholytic reactions. Among them, dryness of mouth with or without excessive perspiration is the most common. Most serious of the autonomic reactions is orthostatic (postural) hypotension. The incidence of this reaction in different degrees of severity is as high as 24 per cent. There are also occasional reports of nasal stuffiness and flushing.

iv. Ophthalmological. Mydriasis, with consequent disturbance of accommodation is usually seen at the beginning of treatment. Rather disturbing blurred vision has also been reported. The most serious adverse effect in this category is precipitation (of latent) or aggravation of (an existing) glaucoma.

v. Cardiovascular. Adverse cardiovascular effects range from flushing and vasodilation, through congestive cardiac failure with edema, to syncope and cardiovascular collapse. These are somewhat more frequent in elderly patients with damaged circulation. Tachycardia and arhythmia are not infrequently seen. ECG findings resemble a quinidine-like effect with prolongation of the QT interval, flattening of the T waves, a negative inotropic effect and manifestations of vagus blockade. Ventricular tachycardia and fatal fibrillation have been reported. It is fortunate that these adverse cardiovascular effects usually occur at toxic doses and thus drug administration within the therapeutic dosage range remains safe.

vi. Gastrointestinal. Nausea, heartburn, dyspepsia, marked epigastric distress and diarrhea have been described. There are frequent reports of constipation. Concomitant administration of phenothiazines and/or antiparkinsonian drugs aggravate constipation and may lead to paralytic ileus (Warnes *et al.*, 1967).

vii. Genitourinary. Urinary retention is rather common. Difficulty in starting micturition (dysuria) is a bothersome effect that may occur in the therapeutic dosage ranges. Males with a somewhat enlarged prostate are predisposed for this adverse effect. There are reports on cases of nocturia and total bladder paralysis. In the sexual sphere, women may experience a decreased or somewhat heightened libido, while males may complain of impotence or of erections without the ability for orgasm.

viii. Hepatobiliary. Jaundice—the intrahepatic obstructive type—may occur 2 to 3 weeks after commencement of treatment. It is considered to be an allergic reaction.

ix. Metabolic. In therapy-responsive cases, there is usually an increase of appetite and weight gain in the course of treatment. Symptoms of diabetes mellitus are ameliorated.

x. Hematological. Agranulocytosis is rare. It is considered as an idiosyncratic or allergic reaction.

xi. Dermatological. There is a wide range of dermatological reactions, the majority of which are allergic in nature. Generalized rash, itching and urticaria are probably the most frequent. Photosensitization, hyperhydrosis, pruritus and local toxiderma have been described.

There are other reactions more generalized in nature. The first of these is a syndrome which may occur with combined MAOI and tricyclic antidepressant administration. This is manifested by anxiety, headache, nausea, abdominal pain, vomiting, psychomotor agitation, tremor, clonic seizures, dyspnea, cyanosis, labile blood pressure, collapse and, in extreme cases, death.

Another syndrome is related to overdosage. Tricyclic antidepressants are relatively safe, and successful recovery after active therapy has been reported even after ingestion of a dose of 5375 mg. of imipramine. However, there have been fatalities after the ingestion of 350 mg. of imipramine by an infant, over 2500 mg. of the same drug by an adult and a dose of 950 mg. of amitriptyline by a 70-year-old woman. The main clinical findings from the overdosage of imipramine were deep coma, clonic movements, seizures, shock, respiratory depression, hyperpyrexia and disturbance of cardiac rhythm and conduction, while the overdosage of amitriptyline resulted in increased pulse rate and blood pressure, decreased temperature, sluggish pupils, plantar extensor response, deep respiration and coma.

A case of suicide with 5000 mg. of opipramol was reported by Angst *et al.* (1967). It was noted that 12 to 18 hours after the ingestion of the medication patient was fully conscious. However, he died later following a series of epileptic attacks. Biochemical analysis showed the highest opipramol concentrations peripherally in the liver (44 mg. per cent) and in the lungs (40 mg. per cent) and centrally in the pons and thalamus (both 13.1 mg. per cent).

Tolerance develops to the atropine-like effects of these drugs, *i.e.*, to dry mouth, disturbance of accommodation, tachycardia and orthostatic hypotension. Regarding dependence, it is known that while gradual discontinuation results in no noticeable reaction, sudden withdrawal after the drug had been administered over several months above 200 mg. a day may cause malaise, chills, coryza and muscle aches.

b. Treatment of Adverse Reactions

In spite of the accumulated knowledge on adverse effects, there is no way of predicting with certainty whether a new patient will develop an adverse reaction and, if so, when he will do so. The physician's response to this depends on the dynamics of the situation and is based on careful assessment of the relative danger of the adverse effect in comparison to the danger of the untreated psychopathological symptoms. On the basis of this, five different decisions can be made: discontinuation of all psychopharmacological treatment; discontinuation of the drug which is held responsible for the adverse effect and the substitution of another medication with a similar psychotropic action; reduction of dosage; the addition of adjunctive medication; and acceptance of the unwanted reaction.

Discontinuation of all psychopharmacological treatment is suggested in cases of agranulocytosis and jaundice, while acceptance of adverse effects is indicated in libidinal and appetite changes, sweating, dryness of mouth, nasal stuffiness, eosinophilia and mild hypotension. Replacement therapy is instituted in toxic psychoses, in cases in which adjuvant phenothiazine or butyrophenone medication remains ineffective, in glaucomic attacks, progressively increasing cardiac or neurological changes, leukopenia, paralytic ileus or bladder paralysis and impotence.

Persistent giddiness, restlessness, drowsiness, hypotension, mild headache, fatigue, weakness, slight dizziness, extrapyramidal signs, nonspecific ECG changes, mydriasis, blurred vision, difficulty of micturition, nausea and constipation usually respond to reduction in dosage, while persistent constipation, heartburn, dyspepsia, insomnia, severe extrapyramidal manifestations, distressing dry mouth, disturbing perspiration, recurring cerebral seizures or dermatological manifestations call for adjuvant medication. In the treatment of postural hypotension, ACTH or cortisone is recommended.

The management of overdosage is unspecific. Among the different manifestations, cardiac irregularities are most difficult to treat, while convulsions are easily controlled with short acting barbiturate preparations. Hypertension is best treated with short acting adrenergic blocking agents.

4. The Use of Tricyclic Antidepressants in Medical Practice

Of all the dibenzazepine preparations, imipramine is still the drug most frequently prescribed. It is a most reliable drug in endogenous depression, although it may have a somewhat higher incidence of anticholinergic adverse effects and a slower onset of therapeutic action than some of the newer compounds. It remains rather ineffective in agitated cases and in patients with a high anxiety level. If the depressive mood is in the center of the clinical picture, or the depression is experienced as a physical illness (with headache, pressure in the chest, etc.), imipramine is considered to be the drug of choice. If inhibitory phenomena prevail, the somewhat faster acting and more stimulating desipramine is recommended. Finally, when depression is associated with agitation, the more sedative and slightly more anxiety-reducing trimipramine is preferred.

Iminostilbene derivatives are less extensively used than the iminodibenzyl preparations.

The fast acting opipramol is almost exclusively given to patients with various psychosomatic manifestations and carbamazepine to epileptics with dysthymic mood changes (Lehmann and Ban, 1968).

More recently, the dibenzocycloheptene derivative amitriptyline has been used increasingly. It has somewhat less anticholinergic activity than imipramine and is more effective in controlling agitation and relieving anxiety. Both drugs have a better therapeutic effect in women than in men. The desmethylated analogue of amitriptyline, nortriptyline, is somewhat faster acting, less toxic and probably more stimulating than its parent compound. This may also be true for protriptyline.

In a systematic investigation including 137 hospitalized female depressive patients, Hordern *et al.* (1965) found that 81 per cent of the 69 treated with amitriptyline recovered without ECT, as against only 54 per cent of the 68 who received imipramine. On the other hand, they could not show meaningful differences in the adverse effects of the two tricyclic antidepressant compounds. They also recognized that the initial severity of the depressive manifestations in the case of amitriptyline was unrelated to outcome, while with imipramine it was associated with poorer treatment results. The presence of delusions lessened the effectiveness of amitriptyline and nullified the effectiveness of imipramine. Another important finding was that amitriptyline was significantly more effective than imipramine in patients over 50 years of age, in those who were postmenopausal and in those with severe depressions. Although there was a trend that "young severe" patients showed a more favorable immediate (1 week) response to imipramine, after 1 month, even in this group the difference between the two drugs was eliminated.

SUMMARY

The introduction of tricyclic antidepressant compounds brought about significant changes in the treatment of an important group of psychiatric patients. The most important result of therapy with these drugs is that if administered in adequate dosage they are able to shorten the episode of depression in a high percentage of cases. The administration of these drugs may prevent the admission of a great number of patients to psychiatric hospitals and also makes it possible to protect a large number of cases from relapse.

Of the two major antidepressive groups used in psychiatric treatment, the dibenzazepines are particularly useful in treating patients in whom depressive mood manifests itself as a feeling of a physical disease, while the dibenzoheptene group is also effective when anxiety is present. The desmethylated analogues of each group are considered to be more useful in counteracting inhibitory phenomena.

Among the adverse effects, the most common are anticholinergic manifestations (more prominent with dibenzazepines). The majority of these adverse effects are transient, and a great percentage of them are easily handled by reduction in dosage or by adjuvant medication. On the other hand, agranulocytosis is an absolute indication for termination of treatment. In between is hypotension, in particular, orthostatic hypotension, which usually occurs at the commencement of drug administration and has led to serious consequences in several elderly hypertensive arteriosclerotic cases.

REFERENCES

Angst, J.: A clinical analysis of the effects of tofranil in depression. Psychopharmacologia, (Berlin), *2:* 381 (1961).

Angst, J., Brandenberger, H., and Herrmann, B.: Suicid mit opipramol (insidon). Psychopharmacologia (Berlin) *11:* 174 (1967).

Axelrod, J.: Discussion. In: Antidepressant drugs of non-MAO inhibitor type (eds., Efron, D. H., and Kety, S. S.). (U.S. Dept. of Health, Education and Welfare, Bethesda, 1966.)

Azima, H.: Imipramine (tofranil): a new drug for the depressed. Canad. Med. Ass. J., *80:* 535 (1959).

Azima, H.: Psychodynamic and psychotherapeutic problems in connection with imipramine (tofranil) intake. J. Ment. Sci., *107:* 74 (1961).

Ban, T. A.: Clinical pharmacology of tricyclic antidepressants. I. Appl. Ther., *8:* 779 (1966).

Ban, T. A.: Clinical pharmacology of tricyclic antidepressants. II. Appl. Ther., *9:* 66 (1967).

Berti, T., and Cima, L.: Influence of species, sex and environmental temperature on the metabolism of phenothiazine and structurally related psychoactive drugs. (Presented at the Conference on the action, mechanism and metabolism of psychoactive drugs from phenothiazine and structurally related compounds, Paris, 1962.)

Bickel, M. H., and Brodie, B. B.: Structure and antidepressant activity of imipramine analogues. Int. J. Neuropharmacol., *3:* 611 (1964).

Bickel, M. H., Sulser, F., and Brodie, B. B.: Conversion of tranquillizers to antidepressants by removal of one N-methyl group. Life Sci., *4:* 247 (1963).

Burt, C., *et al.:* Amitriptyline in depressive states. J. Ment. Sci., *108:* 711 (1962).

Carlton, P. L.: Potentiation of the behavioral effects of amphetamine by imipramine. Psychopharmacologia (Berlin), *2:* 364 (1961).

Carr, J.: The pharmacology of the psychotomimetic agents. Int. Rec. Med., *172:* 702 (1959).

Cook, L., Kelleher, R. T., and Fellows, E. J.: Pharmacodynamics of chlorpromazine and other phenothiazines. In: Psychosomatic medicine (eds., Nodine, J. H., and Moyer, J. H.). (Lea and Febiger, Philadelphia, 1962.)

Cook, L., and Weidley, E.: Effects of a series of psychopharmacological agents on isolation induced attack behavior in mice. Fed. Proc., *19:* 22 (1960).

Delay, J.: Chlorimipramine. (ECDEU progress report from Cliniques des Maladies Mentales, Paris, 1967.)

Delay, J., Deniker, P., and Lemperiere, T.: Le traitement des états dépressifs et malancoliques en fonctions des nouveaux médicaments antidépresseurs. Presse Med., *67:* 1586 (1959).

Dews, P. B.: A behavioral output enhancing effect of imipramine in pigeons. Int. J. Neuropharmacol., *1:* 265 (1962).

DiMascio, A., Heninger, G., and Klerman, G. L.: Psychopharmacology of imipramine and desipramine: a comparative study of their effects in normal males. Psychopharmacologia (Berlin), *5:* 361 (1964).

Dingell, J. W., Duncan, W. A. M., and Gillette, J. R.: Studies on the binding of imipramine and chlorpromazine in various tissues. Fed. Proc., *20:* 173 (1961).

Dingell, J. V., Sulser, F., and Gillette, J. R.: Metabolism of imipramine in rats and rabbits. Fed. Proc., *21:* 184 (1962).

DINGELL, J. V., SULSER, F., AND GILLETTE, J. R.: Species differences in the metabolism of imipramine and desmethylimipramine. J. Pharmacol., *143:* 14 (1964).

DOMENJOZ, R., AND THEOBALD, W.: Zur Pharmakologie des Tofranil [N-(3-dimethylaminopropyl)-iminodibenzyl-hydrochloride]. Arch. Int. Pharmacodyn., *120:* 450 (1959).

EFRON, D. H., AND KETY, S. S. (eds.): Antidepressant drugs of non-MAO inhibitor type. (U.S. Dept. of Health, Education and Welfare, Bethesda, 1966.)

FISHMAN, V., AND GOLDENBERG, H.: Identification of a new metabolite of imipramine. Proc. Soc. Exp. Biol. Med. (New York), *110:* 187 (1962).

GALLANT, D. M., AND BISHOP, M. P.: The use of imipramine in high dosages: an attempt to elicit antipsychotic activity. Curr. Ther. Res., *9:* 309 (1967).

GARATTINI, S., *et al.:* Effect of imipramine, amitriptyline and their monomethyl derivatives on reserpine activity. J. Pharm. Lond., *14:* 509 (1962).

GILLETTE, J. R., DINGELL, J. V., AND QUINN, G. P.: Physiological distribution and metabolism of imipramine (tofranil). Fed. Proc., *19:* 137 (1960).

GILLETTE, J. R., *et al.:* Isolation from rat brain of a metabolic product, desmethylimipramine, that mediates the antidepressant activity of imipramine (tofranil). Experientia, *17:* 417 (1961).

GREENBLATT, M., GROSSER, G. H., AND WECHSLER, H.: Differential response of hospitalized depressed patients to somatic therapy. Amer. J. Psychiat., *120:* 935 (1964).

GYERMEK, L.: Effects of imipramine-like antidepressant agents on the autonomic nervous system. In: Antidepressant drugs of the non-MAO inhibitor type (eds., Efron, D. H., and Kety, S. S.). (U.S. Dept. of Health, Education and Welfare, Bethesda, 1966.)

HÄFLIGER, F.: Chemistry of tofranil. Canad. Psychiat. Ass. J., *4:* 69 (1959).

HÄFLIGER, F., AND SCHINDLER, W. (1951): In: Häfliger, F., and Burckhardt, V.: Iminodibenzyl and related compounds. In: Psychopharmacological agents (ed., Gordon, M.). (Academic Press, New York, 1964.)

HALLIWELL, G., QUINTON, R. M., AND WILLIAMS, F. E.: A comparison of imipramine, chlorpromazine and related drugs in various tests involving autonomic functions and antagonism of reserpine. Brit. J. Pharmacol., *23:* 330 (1964).

HANSON, H. M.: The effects of amitriptyline, imipramine, chlorpromazine and nialamide on avoidance behavior. Fed. Proc., *20:* 396 (1961).

HERRMANN, B., AND PULVER, R.: Der Stoffwechsel des Psychopharmakon Tofranil. Arch. Int. Pharmacodyn., *126:* 454 (1960).

HERRMANN, B., SCHINDLER, W., AND PULVER, R.: Papier chromatographischer Nachweis von Stoffwechsel Produkten des Tofranil. Med. Exp. (Basel) *1:* 381 (1959).

HILL, R. T., *et al.:* Potentiation of methylphenidate by imipramine, amitriptyline and their desmethyl analogues. Pharmacologist, *3:* 75 (1961).

HIMWICH, H. E.: Biochemical and neurophysiological action of psychoactive drugs. In: Drugs and behavior (eds., Uhr, L., and Miller, J. G.). (Wiley, New York, 1960.)

HOENIG, J., AND VISRAM, S.: Amitriptyline versus imipramine in depressive psychoses. Brit. J. Psychiat., *110:* 840 (1964).

HOFF, H.: Indications for electro-shock, tofranil and psychotherapy in the treatment of depressions. Canad. Psychiat. Ass. J. *4:* 55 (1959).

HOLLISTER, L. E., *et al.:* Controlled comparison of amitriptyline, imipramine and placebo in hospitalized depressed patients. J. Nerv. Ment. Dis., *139:* 370 (1964).

HORDERN, A., AND HAMILTON, M.: Drugs and moral treatment. Brit. J. Psychiat., *109:* 500 (1963).

HORDERN, A., *et al.:* Amitriptyline in depressive states: six month treatment results. Brit. J. Psychiat., *110:* 641 (1964).

HORDERN, A., *et al.:* Depressive states. (Charles C Thomas, Springfield, 1965.)

HUCKER, H. B. (1962): In: Sulser, F., and Dingell, J. V.: The role of adrenergic mechanisms in the mode of action of tricyclic antidepressants. In: Antidepressant drugs of non-MAO inhibitor type (eds., Efron, D. H., and Kety, S. S.). (U.S. Dept. of Health, Education and Welfare, Bethesda, 1966.)

HUCKER, H. B., AND PORTER, C. C. (1961): In: Sulser, F., and Dingell, J. V.: The role of adrenergic mechanisms in the mode of action of tricyclic antidepressants. In: Antidepressant drugs of non-MAO inhibitor type (eds., Efron, D. H., and Kety, S. S.). (U.S. Dept. of Health, Education and Welfare, Bethesda, 1966.)

HUTCHISON, J. T., AND SWEDBERG, D.: Treatment of depression: a comparative study of ECT and six drugs. Brit. J. Psychiat., *109:* 536 (1963).

IDESTROM, C. M., AND CADENIUS, B.: Imipramine—desmethylimipramine. A pharmacological study on human beings. Psychopharmacologia (Berlin), *5:* 431 (1964).

JACOB, R. M., AND MESSER, M. (1956): In: Beaulnes, A.: Psychopharmacologie de la trimipramine. In: Trimipramine a new antidepressant (eds., Lehmann, H. E., Berthiaume, M., and Ban, T. A.). (Quebec Psychopharmacological Research Ass., Montreal, 1964.)

JORI, A., AND GARATTINI, S.: Interaction between imipramine-like agents and catecholamine induced hyperthermia. J. Pharm. Pharmacol., *17:* 480 (1965).

KLERMAN, G. L., AND COLE, J. O.: Clinical pharmacology of imipramine and related antidepressant compounds. Pharmacol. Rev., *17:* 101 (1965).

KORNETSKY, C.: A comparison of the effect of desipramine and imipramine on two schedules of reinforcement. Pharmacologist, *5:* 239 (1963).

KUHN, R.: Über die Behandlung Depressiver Zustande mit Einem Iminodibenzylderivat (G-22355). Schweiz. Med. Wschr., *87:* 1135 (1957).

LEHMANN, H. E.: Combined pharmaco-fever treatment with imipramine (tofranil) and typhoid vaccine in the management of depressive conditions. Amer. J. Psychiat., *117:* 356 (1960).

LEHMANN, H. E.: Depression: categories, mechanisms and phenomena. In: Pharmacotherapy of depression (eds., Cole, J. O., and Wittenborn, J. R.). (Charles C Thomas, Springfield, 1966.)

LEHMANN, H. E.: Non MAO-inhibitor antidepressants in clinical perspective. In: Antidepressant drops of non-MAO inhibitor type (eds., Efron, D. H., and Kety, S. S.). (U.S. Department of Health, Education and Welfare, Bethesda, 1966.)

LEHMANN, H. E., and BAN, T. A.: Studies with new drugs in the treatment of convulsive disorders. J. Clin. Pharmacol., *3:* 231 (1968).

LEHMANN, H. E., CAHN, C. H., AND DEVERTEUIL, R.: Treatment of depressive conditions with imipramine (G-22355). Canad. Psychiat. Ass. J., *3:* 155 (1958).

LEYBOLD, K., AND STAUDINGER, H. J. (1962): In: Sulser, F., and Dingell, J. V.: On the role of adrenergic mechanisms in the mode of action of tricyclic antidepressants. In: Antidepressant drugs of non-MAO inhibitor type (eds., Efron, D. H., and Kety, S. S.). (U.S. Dept. of Health, Education and Welfare, Bethesda, 1966.)

METYSOVA, J., AND METYS, J.: Pharmacological properties of the desmethyl derivatives of some antidepressants of imipramine. J. Neuropharmacol., *4:* 111 (1965).

OLDS, J.: Pleasure centers in the brain. Sci. Amer., *195:* 105 (1956).

OLTMAN, J. E., AND FRIEDMAN, S.: Comparison of EST and antidepressant drugs in affective disorders. Clin. Notes, *1:* 355 (1961).

PÖLDINGER, W.: Combined administration of desipramine and reserpine or tetrabenazine in depressed patients. Psychopharmacologia (Berlin), *4:* 308 (1963).

PÖLDINGER, W., AND SCHMIDLIN, P.: Index psychopharmacorum 1966. (Huber, Bern, 1966.)

PSCHEIDT, G. R.: Demethylation of imipramine in male and female rats. Biochem. Pharmacol., *11:* 501 (1962).

PULVER, R., EXER, B., AND HERRMANN, B.: Einige Wirkungen des N-(γ-dimethylaminopropyl)-iminodibenzyl- HCl and Seiner Metabolite auf den Stoffwechsel von Neurohormonen. Arzneimittelforschung, *10:* 530 (1960).

RAGLAND, J. B.: Distribution of phenothiazines in tissues. Psychopharmacol. Serv. Cent. Bull., *2:* 80 (1962).

REMMEN, E., *et al.*: Psychochemotherapy. (Western Medical Publications, Los Angeles, 1962.)

RIBENTROP, A., AND SCHAUMANN, W. (1965): In: Usdin, E., and Efron, D. H.: Psychotropic drugs and related compounds. (PHSP No. 1589, Washington, 1967.)

ROBIN, A. A., AND HARRIS, J. A.: A controlled comparison of imipramine and electroplexy. J. Ment. Sci., *108:* 217 (1962).

ROBSON, J. M., AND SULLIVAN, F. M.: The production of foetal abnormalities in rabbits by imipramine. Lancet, *1:* 638 (1963).

ROSE, J. T., AND WESTHEAD, T. T.: Comparison of desipramine and imipramine in depression. Amer. J. Psychiat., *121:* 496 (1964).

SCHECKEL, C. L., AND BOFF, E.: Behavioral effects of interacting imipramine and other drugs with d-amphetamine, cocaine and tetrabenazine. Psychopharmacologia (Berlin), *5:* 198 (1964).

SCHILDKRAUT, J. J.: The catecholamine hypothesis of affective disorders: a review of supporting evidence. Amer. J. Psychiat., *122:* 509 (1965).

SIDMAN, M.: Behavioral pharmacology. Psychopharmacologia (Berlin), *1:* 1 (1959).

SIGG, E. B.: Imipramine. Canad. Med. Ass. J., *80:* 663 (1959).

SIGG, E. B.: Neuropharmacologic assessment of tofranil (imipramine) a new antidepressant agent. Fed. Proc., *18:* 144 (1959).

SIGG, E. B.: Pharmacological studies with tofranil. Canad. Psychiat. Ass. J., *4:* 75 (1959).

SIGG, E. B., SOFFER, L., AND GYERMEK, L.: Influence of imipramine and related psychoactive agents on the effect of 5-hydroxytryptamine and catecholamines on the cat nictitating membrane. J. Pharmacol. Exp. Ther., *142:* 13 (1963).

SKINNER, B. F.: Animal research in the pharmacotherapy of mental illness. In: Psychopharmacology: problems in evaluation (eds., Cole, J. O., and Gerard, R. W.). (National Academy of Sciences-National Research Council, Washington, 1959.)

SNOW, L. H., AND RICKELS, K.: Controlled evaluation of imipramine and amitriptyline in hospitalized depressed psychiatric patients. Psychopharmacologia (Berlin), *5:* 409 (1964).

STEIN, L.: Effects and interactions of imipramine, chlorpromazine, reserpine and amphetamine on self-stimulation: possible neurophysiological basis of depression. In: Recent advances in biological psychiatry (ed., Wortis, J.). (Plenum Press, New York, 1962.)

STEIN, L.: New methods for evaluating stimulants and antidepressants. In: Psychosomatic medicine (eds., Nodine, J. H., and Moyer, J. H.). (Lea and Febiger, Philadelphia, 1962.)

SULSER, F., AND BICKEL, M. H.: On the role of brain catecholamines in the antireserpine action of desmethylimipramine. Pharmacologist, *4:* 178 (1962).

SULSER, F., AND DINGELL, J. V.: The role of adrenergic mechanisms in the mode of action of tricyclic antidepressants. In: Antidepressant drugs of non-MAO inhibitor type (eds., Efron, D. H., and Kety, S. S.). (U.S. Dept. of Health, Education and Welfare, Bethesda, 1966.)

SULSER, F., WATTS, J., AND BRODIE, B. B.: Antagonistic actions of imipramine (tofranil) and reserpine on central nervous system. Fed. Proc., *19:* 268 (1960).

SULSER, F., WATTS, J., AND BRODIE, B. B.: Blocking of reserpine action by imipramine, a drug devoid of stimulatory effects in normal animals. Fed. Proc., *20:* 321 (1961).

SULSER, F., WATTS, J. S., AND BRODIE, B. B.: On the mechanism of antidepressant action of imipramine-like drugs. Ann. N.Y. Acad. Sci., *96:* 279 (1962).

THEOBALD, W., *et al.* (1964): In: Gyermek, L.: Effects of imipramine-like antidepressant agents on the autonomic nervous system. In: Antidepressant drugs of non-MAO inhibitor type (eds., Efron, D. H., and Kety, S. S.). (U.S. Dept. of Health, Education and Welfare, Bethesda, 1966.)

THEOBALD, W., *et al.:* Pharmacology of new centrally active tricyclic compounds. In: Antidepressant drugs (eds., Garattini, S., and Dukes, M. N. G.). (Excerpta Medica Foundation, Amsterdam, 1967.)

THIELE, J., AND HOLZINGER, O.: Über o-Diamidodibenzyl. Ann. Chim., *305:* 96 (1899).

VERNIER, V. G.: Pharmacological evidence of mode of action of antidepressant non-MAOI drugs from behavioral and electrophysiological studies. In Antidepressant drugs of non-MAO inhibitor type (eds. Efron, D. H., and Kety, S. S.). (U.S. Dept. of Health, Education and Welfare, Bethesda, 1966.)

VERNIER, V. G., HANSON, H. M., AND STONE, C. A.: The pharmacodynamics of amitriptyline. In: Psychosomatic medicine (eds., Nodine, J. H., and Moyer, J. H.). (Lea and Febiger, Philadelphia, 1962.)

WARNES, H., LEHMANN, H. E., AND BAN, T. A.: Adynamic ileus during psychoactive medication. Can. Med. Assoc. J., *96:* 1430 (1967).

WERNER, G.: Clinical pharmacology of central stimulant and antidepressant drugs. Clin. Pharmacol. Ther., *3:* 59 (1962).

WILLIAMS, R. T.: Detoxication mechanisms in man. Clin. Pharmacol. Ther., *4:* 234 (1963).

WILSON, I. C., *et al.:* A controlled study of treatments of depression. J. Neuropsychiat., *4:* 331 (1963.)

WITTENBORN, J. R.: The dimensions of psychosis. J. Nerv. Ment. Dis., *134:* 117 (1962).

WITTENBORN, J. R.: Diagnostic classification and response to imipramine. (Presented at the ECDEU meeting, Montreal, 1967.)

Fifteen

Monoamine Oxidase Inhibitor Antidepressants

A. BASIC DATA

1. Historical Aspects

The mood-elevating properties of isoniazid in pulmonary tuberculosis were recognized in 1951. Less than 1 year later Delay *et al.* (1952) reported favorably on the antidepressant properties of this substance. These findings were substantiated by the work of Lurie and Maccagnami (1952). Because of the dangerous concomitant effects of isoniazid, however, further psychiatric investigation of the drug was discontinued.

The history of isoniazid in the chemotherapy of tuberculosis goes back to 1945 when Chorine reported on the "tuberculostatic" action of nicotinamide. This finding was confirmed by McKenzie *et al.* (1948). It was subsequently revealed that many pyridine derivatives related to nicotinamide, for example, isonicotinic acid, and the thiosemicarbazones also, possess "tuberculostatic" activity. In view of this, it was expected that synthesizing the thiosemicarbazone of isonicotinaldehyde might result in a therapeutically useful substance. This synthesis started from the methylester of isonicotinic acid, and the first intermediate of the process was isonicotinylhydrazine (isoniazid). While the thiosemicarbazone of isonicotinaldehyde remained generally ineffective, isoniazid was found to be a potent "antituberculosis" agent.

The isopropyl derivative of isoniazid, iproniazid, has also been used in the treatment of patients with tuberculosis and was noted by Selikoff *et al.* (1952) to have "euphorizing" effects like the parent compound. It was tried in the therapy of twelve psychiatric patients and was found beneficial in depressive cases.

The early pioneering work of Zeller and his collaborators (1952) indicated the potent monoamine oxidase (enzyme) inhibiting effect of iproniazid. They called attention to the possible consequences of monoamine oxidase inhibition, *i.e.*, profound alterations in catecholamine metabolism. This was confirmed by Brodie *et al.* (1956), who showed an actual rise in brain monoamine (serotonin, norepinephrine) levels after the administration of iproniazid.

Clinical interest in iproniazid rapidly increased, and by 1957 three independent teams of psychiatrists (Kline *et al.* at Rockland State Hospital, Crane at Montefiore Hospital and Scherbel *et al.* at the Cleveland Clinic) rediscovered its possible antidepressant properties (Remmen *et al.* 1962). It was Kline (1957) who first attributed the clinical antidepressant effect of iproniazid to monoamine oxidase inhibition, *i.e.*, to the increase in cerebral serotonin and norepinephrine levels. He contrasted the antidepressant effect of iproniazid with that of reserpine-induced depression (which is correlated with a decrease in serotonin and norepinephrine levels in the brain).

The enzyme monoamine oxidase (MAO) was discovered in 1928 by Bernheim. Its action results in the oxidative deamination of amines to pharmacologically inactive acidic derivatives. In the course of this, tyramine is oxidized to *p*-hydroxyphenylacetic acid, dopamine to 3,4-dihydroxyphenylacetic acid, epinephrine to 3,4-dihydroxymandelic acid and serotonin to 5-hydroxyindoleacetic acid. All drugs which interfere with the function of the MAO enzyme are usually referred to as monoamine oxidase inhibitors (MAOI's) regardless of their other pharmacological properties. MAOI's comprise a structurally rather heterogeneous group of compounds which range chemically from aliphatic alcohols and xanthines to methylene blue, amphetamines and ephedrine. Pharmacologically they range from antihistamines and local anesthetics to antidepressants.

The first MAOI antidepressant used psychotherapeutically was iproniazid, which was evolved by the substitution of one of the hydrazine ($H_2N \cdot NH_2$) hydrogens of isoniazid by an isopropyl group. In iproniazid the hydrazine moiety is masked with an acyl radical which seems to protect against the undesirable effects of the benzylhydrazine moiety, particularly its hepatotoxic properties. Iproniazid is, nevertheless, a rather toxic substance and was replaced initially by other hydrazine MAOI compounds, *e.g.*, isocarboxazide, nialamide, phenelzine and subsequently with non-hydrazine MAOI drugs. Clinically the most important non-hydrazine MAOI's are the phenylcyclopropylamines, of which tranylcypromine is the most extensively used.

2. Action Mechanism

A number of hypotheses have been formulated on the action mechanism of MAOI's. They range from psychodynamic to physiochemical concepts. Under the influence of MAOI antidepressants, according to the psychodynamic formulation, there is a "plethora" of id energy, which results in a sense of "joyousness and optimism." With a rise of dosage, the increasingly excessive energy (present as id drives) threatens the integrity of the ego, and anxiety appears; and with a further rise the id pressure may cause a "rupture" of ego defenses, leading to neurotic or psychotic manifestations which are not infrequently seen when MAOI's are administered (Ostow, 1962).

In a physiochemical frame of reference, it was suggested that all the MAOI drugs compete with the biologically present monoamine substrates for the active site of the MAO enzyme. Several new hypotheses have since been added. In one of these, the drug-enzyme interaction is conceived as the result of an electrostatic interaction between the positively charged ammonium ion of the amine group of the drug and a negatively charged group of the enzyme. Another possibility considered was that the binding of the free amino groups of the drug to an "electrophilic center" of the enzyme takes place through unshared electrons in the nitrogen atoms of the amino groups (Belleau and Moran, 1961; Moran, 1962; and Zirkle and Kaiser, 1964).

While the mechanism of interaction between MAOI drugs and MAO enzymes is gradually being revealed, the relationship between this action (or the consequences of this action) and antidepressant properties has not yet been fully clarified.

3. Structure and Activity

Although the relationship between monoamine oxidase inhibiting property and antidepressant effect has not been established, a large number of MAOI drugs have been synthesized. Only a small percentage of these have been used in clinical practice.

a. Hydrazines

The origin of the hydrazine MAOI's is in hydrazine hydrate, a powerful reducing agent with highly corrosive properties which has been described as a "violent poison." The derivative phenylhydrazine is a somewhat less poisonous but still very toxic substance, with a particular affinity for the liver and hematopoietic system. Chemical manipulation of these toxic substances has nevertheless, yielded a variety of useful compounds, *e.g.*, the pyrazolone analgesics and antipyretics, the hydrazinophthalazine antihypertensives and the MAOI antidepressant drugs.

The various classes of hydrazine MAOI's

were reviewed superbly by Biel *et al.*, (1964). They subdivided them into four major classes: alkylhydrazines, aminoalkylhydrazines, aralkylhydrazines and hydrazides (or the salts of hydrazines).

i. Alkylhydrazines. These consist of four subgroups: the monoalkylhydrazines, the cycloalkylhydrazines, the bisalkylhydrazines and the hydroxyalkylhydrazines.

In the *monoalkylhydrazine* subgroup structure-activity relationships have been established. It was recognized that, while hydrazine and methylhydrazine were virtually devoid of any MAOI activity, the addition of straight or branched alkyl groups, *e.g.*, ethyl, propyl, pentyl (up to the 5 carbon-atom chains) conferred powerful MAO enzyme inhibiting properties to the substance. Further increases in the length of the alkyl chain resulted in a sharp decrease—and beyond 8 carbon atoms a complete loss—of MAOI activity. It has also been shown that as the compounds become more highly branched they become less effective as MAOI's.

In general the *cycloalkylhydrazines* were found to be less effective enzyme inhibitors than the corresponding open chain substances.

The same holds true for the *bisalkylhydrazines* regardless of whether the dialkylhydrazine substitution takes place symmetrically or asymmetrically. An exception to this is di-isopropylhydrazine, which exerts a greater MAOI activity than its corresponding monoalkyl substance. Because of this it was surmised that the second alkyl group serves as a transporting moiety and prevents the premature clinical interaction of the free hydrazine groups prior to reaching their target sites.

In the last subgroup of this category, *hydroxylalkylhydrazines*, β-hydroxyethylhydrazine was found in certain tests—particularly in reserpine reversal—to be a potent MAOI compound.

ii. Aminoalkylhydrazines. These consist of three subgroups: the alkylaminoalkylhydrazines, the aralkylaminoalkylhydrazines and the heterocyclic-aminoalkylhydrazines. While the *alkylaminoalkylhydrazines* were found to have weak MAOI potency, the *aralkylaminoalkylhydrazines* were seen to have a powerful MAOI enzyme-inhibiting effect. On the other hand, the *heterocyclic-aminoalkylhydrazines* have no effect on the monoamine oxidase enzyme either *in vitro* or *in vivo*.

iii. Aralkylhydrazines. These comprise four subgroups: the phenylalkylhydrazines, the hydrazinium derivatives, the heterocylic alkylhydrazines and the α-hydrazino acids. The *phenylalkylhydrazines* were recognized as one of the most potent MAOI subgroups. The salient features for optimal activity of these substances are an unsubstituted phenyl ring, an ethyl group on the alpha-carbon atom between the phenyl and hydrazine moieties and a mono-substituted hydrazine group.

Of the other subgroups, the *hydrazinium derivatives* have only a very weak enzyme-inhibiting effect, and both the *heterocylic alkylhydrazines* and *α-hydrazino acids* are entirely inactive.

iv. Hydrazides. Hydrazine salts—or hydrazides—are the most important class of hydrazine derivatives. They were developed with the particular purpose of synthesizing an antidepressant drug which does not exert its effect until it reaches the brain, so that more specific and consequently less toxic effects would result. The combination of an active MAOI substance with a carrier moiety which releases the active hydrazine compound only at the target organ led to the synthesis of a large number of acyl derivatives. Iproniazid was the first MAOI antidepressant drug in which the free hydrazine of isopropyl hydrazine was masked with an acyl radical (isonicotinoyl).

Further chemical and pharmacological exploration revealed that the choice of the acyl group is of particular importance with regard to tissue selectivity, passage of the blood brain barrier, and ease of cleavage of the active moiety. It has been shown that, as a consequence of these, 1-pivaloyl-2-benzyl-hydrazine has a greater affinity for inhibiting cardiac than brain MAO's while *l*-glutamyl has a greater affinity for inhibiting brain than cardiac MAO's. It was also recognized that *d*-glutamyl-β-alanyl derivatives exert only a low grade of activity, presumably because d-glutamic acid has little affinity for brain tissue and the unnatural amino acid (β-alanyl) is not subject to the same degree of metabolic cleavage as d-glutamyl (or isonicotinoyl).

Today there are at least eight structurally different hydrazide subgroups: the alkane-carboxylic acids, the cycloalkanecarboxylic acids, the aryl- and aralkylcarboxylic acids, the heterocylic-carboxylic acids, the amino acids, the sulfonic acids, the semicarbazides and the hydrazones. Of particular importance are the heterocyclic-carboxylic acids, of which isocarboxazide and nialamide are clinically used as antidepressants.

Isocarboxazide [1-benzyl-2-(5-methyl-3-isoxazolylcarbonyl) hydrazine] was synthesized in an attempt to increase the antidepressant potency of iproniazid by increasing its MAOI property while simultaneously reducing its hepatotoxicity. The isoxazolycarbonyl group was introduced to improve the stereo specificity of drug action, to facilitate passage across the blood brain barrier and to allow ready cleavage in the body. While the new substance had a stronger MAOI effect and less toxicity than iproniazid, its increased antidepressant properties remain to be seen.

The aim of the synthesis of nialamide [1-isonicotinyl-2-β-(benzylcarbamyl)ethyl hydrazine] was similar. The isopropyl substituent of iproniazid was replaced with a complex moiety. This reduced toxicity and increased MAOI activity, but it also reduced antidepressant potency.

It seems generally true that among the hydrazines the most potent MAOI compounds are characterized by structural simplicity. Increased substitution often

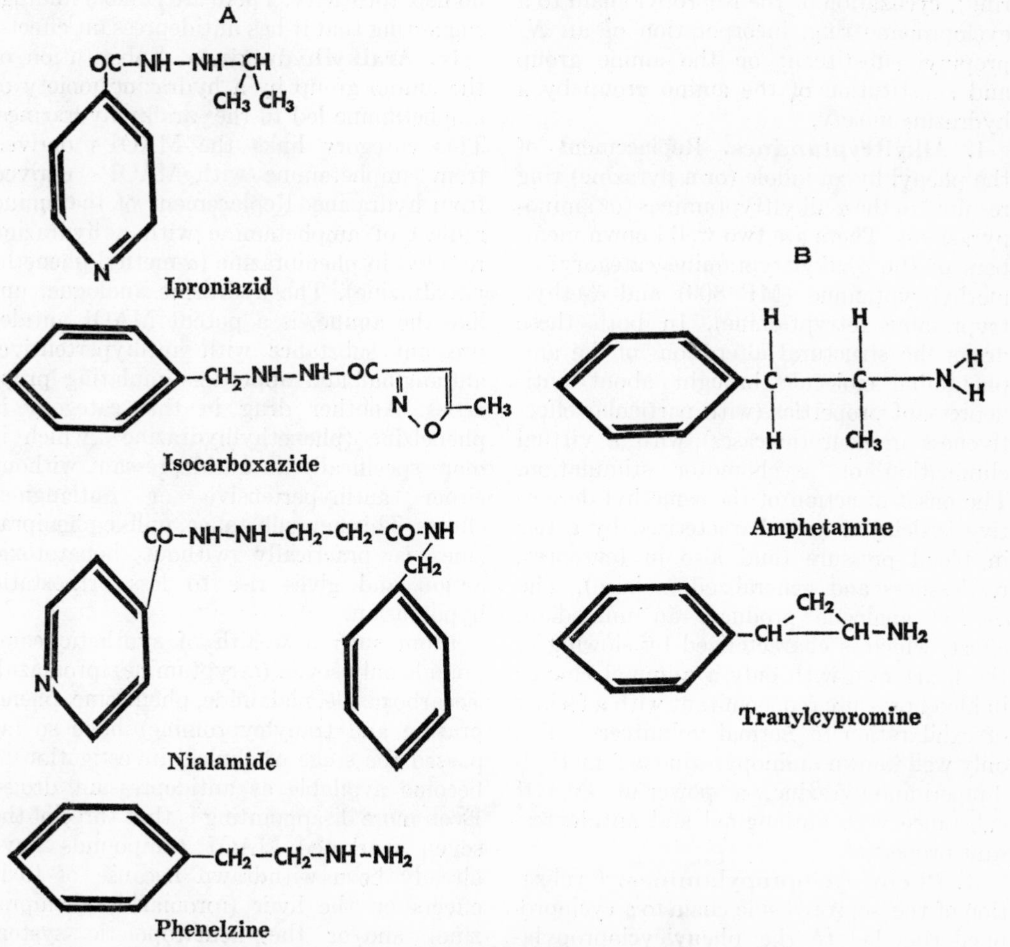

A

OC–NH–NH–CH(CH₃)CH₃

Iproniazid

Isocarboxazide

Nialamide

Phenelzine

B

Amphetamine

Tranylcypromine

FIG. 15. *a*, Hydrazine derivatives. *b*, Amphetamine and tranylcypromine

results in decreased enzyme-inhibiting activity. The aralkyl derivatives display a greater affinity for the brain; the alkyl and aminoalkylhydrazines have a stronger affinity for the liver. Decreased toxicity and greater organ selectivity are achieved by acylating the more active hydrazines. Without the resulting hydrazides the parent hydrazine drugs could not have been introduced into clinical therapeutics, primarily because of toxicity problems (Biel, 1964).

b. Phenylethylamine Derivatives

The origin of the majority of the non-hydrazine MAOI's is in the amphetamines. Structural departures from the original β-phenethylamine skeleton of amphetamine were carried out by replacement of the phenyl by an indole nucleus (or pyrazine ring), cyclization of the isopropyl chain to a cyclopropane ring, incorporation of an *N*-propinyl substituent on the amine group and substitution of the amino group by a hydrazine moiety.

i. Alkyltryptamines. Replacement of the phenyl by an indole (or a pyrazine) ring resulted in the α-alkyltryptamines (or aminopyrazines). There are two well known members of the α-alkyltryptamine category: α-methyltryptamine (MP 809) and α-ethyltryptamine (etryptamine). In both these drugs the structural alteration of the amphetamine molecule brought about antidepressant properties (with particular effectiveness in neurotic cases) with a virtual elimination of psychomotor stimulation. The onset of action of the α-methyl derivative is delayed and characterized by a rise in blood pressure (and also in tenseness, restlessness and generalized malaise). The α-ethyl analogue produces an immediate effect, which is characterized by slowing of the heart rate with only a minimal change in blood pressure (concomitant with a feeling of exhilaration in normal volunteers). The only well known aminopyrazine is 2-methyl-3-piperidino-pyrazine, a powerful MAOI substance with antianginal and antidepressant properties.

ii. Phenylcyclopropylamines. Cyclization of the isopropyl side chain to a cyclopropane ring led to the phenylcyclopropylamines which, in some tests, proved to be 5000 times as potent in MAO enzyme inhibition as the parent amphetamine compounds. The most frequently used member of this group, tranylcypromine, has amphetamine-like pressor and central nervous system stimulating properties, a characteristically rapid onset of therapeutic action (24 to 72 hours) when compared with other MAOI drugs and a particular effectiveness in chronic neurotic depression (and in pseudoneurotic schizophrenia and in schizophrenia with prevailing anhedonia).

iii. Propargylamines. Modifications of the phenylalkylamine side chain to include acetylenic moieties resulted in the propargylamines. Pargyline (*N*-benzyl-*N*-methylpropargylamine), a commonly used antihypertensive of this category, has highly potent MAOI properties with practically no hepatotoxicity. There are clinical findings suggesting that it has antidepressant effects.

iv. Aralkylhydrazines. Substitution of the amino group by a hydrazine moiety of amphetamine led to the aralkylhydrazines. This category links the MAOI's derived from amphetamine with MAOI's derived from hydrazine. Replacement of the amino radical of amphetamine with a hydrazine resulted in pheniprazine (α-methyl-phenethylhydrazine). The hydrazine analogue, unlike the amine, is a potent MAOI antidepressant substance with antihypertensive, antianginal and appetite-stimulating properties. Another drug in this category is phenelzine (phenethylhydrazine), which is more specifically an antidepressant without either antihypertensive or antianginal effects. This new substance, unlike pheniprazine, is practically without hepatotoxic action and gives rise to less orthostatic hypotension.

From such a wealth of synthetic compounds only seven (etryptamine, iproniazid, isocarboxazide, nialamide, phenelzine, pheniprazine and tranylcypromine) have so far passed the stage of clinical investigation to become available as antidepressant drugs. Even more disappointing is that three of the seven marketed MAOI compounds have already been withdrawn because of toxic effects on the liver (iproniazid, pheniprazine) and/or the hematopoietic system (etryptamine) (Bain, 1965; Biel, 1964; Biel *et al.*, 1964; Gordon, 1964; Jarvik, 1965; Pöldinger and Schmidlin, 1966; Remmen *et al.*, 1962; and Zirkle and Kaiser, 1964).

4. Metabolism of Monoamine Oxidase Inhibitor Antidepressants

There is evidence of interspecies differences and of intraspecies variations in the metabolism of MAOI compounds. A good example of *interspecies differences* is the particular sensitivity of the dog to any of the hydrazines. The probable reason for this is that dogs are lacking the ability to produce certain metabolites, *e.g.*, pyruvic acid, glyceraldehyde, hemine and other carbonyl-containing compounds. These metabolites have been found in other species to combine with MAOI agents, resulting in inactive products which no longer have enzyme-inhibiting properties.

In considering *intraspecies variations*, the acetylation mechanism is of utmost importance. Within the human species, for example, there are slow and fast acetylators with distinctly different capacities for metabolizing certain MAOI compounds, such as phenelzine. While this genetically determined mechanism does not seem to have an effect on the therapeutic efficacy of MAOI's, there is ample evidence that toxic and other adverse reactions to these drugs are more common in the slow acetylators.

All the presently available MAOI drugs, regardless of the route given, are readily absorbed. The affinity of the absorbed MAOI substance is toward the MAO enzyme, which is distributed in various organs and tissues, *e.g.*, liver, heart, brain. The particular brain selectivity of some of these compounds is primarily related to their lipid solubility and their ability to penetrate the blood brain barrier, which in the case of hydrazines is strongly influenced by the "protective" acyl radical of the drug.

The organ selectivity of the individual compounds also depends on the route of administration. For example, pheniprazine or phenelzine administered intraperitoneally to rats have an equal affinity toward the brain and liver enzymes, but when administered subcutaneously, they exert a much stronger inhibition on the brain than on the liver enzymes. On the other hand, they have a greater effect on the liver than on the brain when given perorally.

In the course of their activity, the nonhydrazine MAOI's combine directly with the enzyme, while the hydrazide MAOI's have to be cleaved to liberate the active product. The metabolism of these latter drugs consequently follows two main pathways: hydrolysis of the acylhydrazine bound, which yields active biological intermediates, and cleavage of the alkyl or aralkyl substituent whereby hippuric acid and other metabolites of minor importance are formed.

The metabolism of this chemically rather heterogenous group of compounds is best illustrated through the metabolism of representatives of the hydrazine derivatives and of the nonhydrazine drugs.

a. Hydrazine Derivatives

Most extensively investigated in this group is the metabolism of iproniazid by radioactive isotope studies. At first, "radioactive labeling" of the isonicotinic acid group of iproniazid was carried out, which was followed—as a second step in the investigation—by the labeling of the isopropyl portion. As a result, during the "first step," brain and liver radioactivity rose and declined rapidly to the extent that, in a period of 24 hours, no radioactivity could be detected. Within the same time period, 98 per cent of the radioactive substance was "recovered" from the urine; mainly as iproniazid and isonicotinic acid, although MAO inhibition—as revealed through other methods—was still maintained to a considerable extent. In contradistinction to these were findings in the "second step," in which radioactivity in the various organs remained detectable for a longer period than one day and in which the major portion of the administered radioactivity was regained as labeled CO_2 in the expired air. This implies that the CO_2 was formed from radioactive acetone, indicating a preliminary process of dealkylation of the isopropyl group. On the basis of these studies, it was suggested that iproniazid is metabolized by *N*-dealkylation which splits off acetone and isonicotinylhydrazine and by hydrolysis to form isonicotinic acid and isopropylhydrazine.

Radioactive studies with *isocarboxazide* revealed that a large part of this substance is metabolized to hippuric acid, indicating that benzylhydrazine is an intermediate in the *in vivo* degradation of this compound. In experiments with *nialamide* it was found that, while maximum plasma values were reached quickly, they fall to zero within a period of 24 hours. During the same period, up to 44 per cent of the orally administered nialamide was excreted unchanged in the urine and only small amounts of isonicotinic acid were formed. It was suggested that the main metabolic pathway of this drug is cleavage of the amide linkage (since hippuric acid and glucuronic acid monobenzoate are its main metabolites).

b. Phenylethylamine Derivatives

Most investigated and best known in this group is the metabolism of tranylcypromine. It has been shown that a total of 70 to 75 per cent of this phenylcyclopropylamine derivative is excreted within 24 hours in the urine and the feces, of which 4 per cent is tranylcypromine itself (and 13 per cent is hippuric acid). In the subsequent 2 days, only 15 per cent more (totaling approximately 90 per cent in 3 days) is eliminated.

In the metabolism of tranylcypromine, the opening of the cyclopropane ring (or oxidation at the α-carbon atom) takes place prior to the oxidative cleavage at the β-carbon atom. Furthermore, the hydrolytic cleavage of this drug to hydrocinnamaldehyde is followed by the oxidation of this latter substance to hydrocinnamic acid and to benzoic acid. Another alternative pathway of catabolism is a direct oxidative attack on the α-carbon atom, which results in benzoic acid. This primary mechanism is then followed by the opening of the cyclopropane ring or oxidation at the α-carbon atom.

Radioactive studies with *etryptamine* have revealed that maximum plasma concentration after peroral administration is reached in 4 to 5 hours and that 70 to 90 per cent of this α-alkyltryptamine drug is eliminated within 1 day, mainly in the urine. The major metabolic paths are conjugation and deamination, and the major metabolites are the sulfate and glucuronide conjugates, while etryptamine itself is excreted only in small amounts. In radioactive experiments with *pargyline*, it was found that maximum plasma concentration after peroral administration is reached in 1 to 2 hours (*i.e.*, twice as fast as with etryptamine) and that 30 to 90 per cent of this propargylamine drug is eliminated within 1 day. However, metabolites of pargylamine are not detected in the urine before 8 hours, suggesting that the drug is rapidly excreted unchanged and that metabolites are formed only slowly.

It has been noted that for pargyline it takes about 24 hours to produce measurable jejunal inhibition, which then reaches its maximum by the second or third day.

Knowledge of the metabolism of MAOI's led to the classification of these drugs into three pharmacological groups useful from a clinical point of view: the short acting reversible inhibitors (direct stimulants), the long acting irreversible agents (indirect stimulants) and those in between (bimodal stimulants).

Prototypes of the first class are the α-alkyltryptamines (also the harmala alkaloids, the first group of nonhydrazine MAOI's without antidepressant properties) with a characteristically rapid onset (particularly in the case of etryptamine) and brief duration of action.

Prototypes of the second class are the hydrazides and the propargylamines, with characteristically delayed onset and prolonged duration of action.

In between are the phenylcyclopropylamines (*e.g.*, tranylcypromine) and the aralkylhydrazines (*e.g.*, pheniprazine), which have rapid onset (particularly tranylcypromine) but relatively long duration of action (bimodal stimulants). (Benson and Schiele, 1962; Biel *et al.*, 1964; Jarvik, 1965; Kalinowsky and Hoch, 1961; Sourkes, 1962; and Zirkle and Kaiser, 1964).

5. Chemical and Neurophysiological Correlates of Drug Action

a. Chemical Correlates

Since the role of the MAO enzyme is to catalyze oxidative deamination of endogenous (*i.e.*, naturally present) and exogenous (introduced from the outside) monoamines, the primary activity of MAOI drugs is to interfere with this function. There are various means of revealing the chemical changes concomitant with this particular activity. Usually they are subdivided into *in vitro* and *in vivo* procedures, because of the incongruence in the effect of these drugs in the laboratory and in the living animal. This incongruence is commonly attributed to the differential affinity of MAOI substances for the liver or the brain, which in turn is frequently due to the inability (or rather the degree of ability) of these compounds to penetrate the blood brain barrier.

The amount of enzymatic deamination can be measured *in vitro* by at least one of three methods: oxygen uptake and NH_3 release; disappearance of monoamine substrates; and accumulation of deamination products. In these procedures spectrophotometric, spectrophotofluorimetric and fluorimetric techniques are used.

In vivo, MAOI activity is easily determined by a bioassay, e.g., after jejunal biopsy the ability of the jejunal tissue to convert tryptamine to indoleacetic acid is measured. In humans, "less traumatic procedures are employed," such as fluorimetric measurement of the fall in 5-hydroxyindoleacetic acid excretion in subjects treated with an MAOI drug, after administration of a standard dose of 5-hydroxytryptamine (serotonin). The sensitivity of this procedure was markedly increased by the use of tryptamine and measuring the increase in the urinary output of this substance after administering an MAOI drug. By these means a number of MAOI effects on endogenous and exogenous amines were revealed.

i. MAOI Effects on Endogenous Monoamines. Serotonin (5-HT), dopamine and norepinephrine (NE) belong to this group. *5-HT* is primarily found in enterochromaffin cells, platelets and mast cells; it is also naturally present in the neurons of the central nervous system. The site of serotonin is intracellular, where it is partly attached to granular elements and partly found free, *i.e.*, as a mobile pool within the cell. There is a steady balance between the bound and mobile serotonin with a constant leakage from the granular attachment toward the mobile pool, where consequently the excess of 5-HT—catalyzed by an MAO enzyme—is oxidatively deaminated to 5-hydroxyindoleacetaldehyde, which in turn is further transformed into 5-hydroxyindoleacetic acid (5-HIAA). It is the latter substance that diffuses out of the cell and is found excreted in the urine as the end-product of serotonin. Under the influence of an MAOI there is evidence of increased levels of 5-HT in the central nervous system and in the periphery (in the platelets). Simultaneously the amount of 5-HIAA excreted in the urine declines, while the excretion of 5-HT glucuronide is raised due to utilization of alternative pathways of serotonin degradation.

Of the other two endogenous monoamines *dopamine* is found to a large extent in the cytoplasm of cells in the central nervous system, particularly in the putamen and caudate nucleus, and only to a small extent attached to the intracellular storage granules. Dopamine is converted with the help of dopamine oxidase (a MAO enzyme) into norepinephrine, a transformation interfered with by MAOI drugs. As a consequence, there is evidence of an elevated dopamine level in the central nervous system, but with an increase rather than the expected decrease in NE concentration. The reason for this is that MAOI's also block the catabolism of norepinephrine.

Like serotonin, *norepinephrine* also is primarily found intracellularly in granular storages and in mobile pools. There is a constant liberation of bound NE, which freed substance, responding to nervous stimulation, leaks into the synaptic spaces. Within the cell the freed NE is exposed to oxidative deamination—catalyzed by MAO enzymes—into 3-methoxy-4-hydroxymandelic acid (vanillylmandelic acid) (VMA). This inactive metabolite steadily trespasses the cell membrane, where it is further metabolized by catechol-*o*-methyl transferase (COMT) enzymes.

The same enzymes—COMT—play a crucial role in the degradation of extracellular NE (at the synaptic space and also in the circulation) into normetanephrine. Since MAOI's prevent the intracellular deamination of NE but not the extracellular metabolic degradation of the same substance, administration of an MAOI drug simultaneously with increase of brain NE level results in a decrease of 3-methoxy-4-hydroxymandelic acid excretion in the urine, but not of normetanephrine. Because of the balance between the intra and extraneuronal pools of NE, with the intracellular increment of the substance there is also an increase at the extracellular adrenergic receptor sites with a consequent rise of normetanephrine production and its urinary excretion (partly in conjugated form and partly converted to vanillylmandelic acid). It has been noted that the increase of NE—or in general of free monoamines—at the adrenergic receptor sites is nonspecific to MAOI drugs and it is also present with tricyclic antidepressant substances. It has also been noted that the locomotor and sympathetic stimulation parallels the increase in cerebral normetanephrine and not, as formerly believed, the intracellular NE.

ii. MAOI Effects on Exogenous Amines. The effect of MAOI's on parenterally administered exogenous amines has been extensively studied. Particular emphasis was paid to reveal the effects subsequent to pretreatment with the precursors of serotonin and norepinephrine (*i.e.*, tryptophan, 5-hydroxytryptophan, tyrosine and 3,4-dihydroxyphenylalanine) and the effects subsequent to pretreatment with tryptamine and tyramine.

Systematic exploratory work has revealed that the action of MAOI substances is dependent on the presence of oxygen and is augmented by the presence of cyanide. More recently, it has been implied that the presence of copper may also be involved.

It has been recognized that iproniazid and isocarboxazide inhibit MAO activity in two steps: first they exhibit a reversible inhibition; secondly, after hydrolysis, they exhibit an irreversible enzyme-inhibiting effect.

An attempt was subsequently made to find the structural basis of irreversible MAO inhibition. It was Eberson and Persson (1962) who suggested that in the case of hydrazine derivatives this involves the transfer of one electron from the hydrazine to the enzyme and the subsequent oxidation of the hydrazine radical. According to the same authors, the intermediate radicals are the ones which likely react with the active center of the enzyme to produce irreversible changes in its structure.

Whatever the mechanism involved in the action of the reversible or irreversible MAOI substances, the rise in serotonin and dopamine levels in the central nervous system may be explained solely on the basis of their decreased catabolism due to the interference exerted by the drugs on the MAO enzyme. On the other hand, the same explanation seems to be insufficient for the increase of NE or more generally of catecholamine levels which are not particularly good substrates of MAO and which have other pathways of metabolism, probably of greater physiological importance. The question arose whether MAOI's in general and the hydrazine type of MAOI's in particular have other actions besides their inhibitory effect on the MAO enzyme.

Probably the most important finding in this regard was the recognition that, in the course of MAOI (particularly of hydrazine derivative) administration, the diphosphopyridine nucleotide concentration in the brain (and also in the liver) was decreased with a concomitantly increased utilization of pyridoxine. It was soon demonstrated that the hydrazine group of MAOI's readily react with pyridoxal-5-phosphate, which is a coenzyme for several enzyme systems such as amino acid decarboxylase, GABA-transaminase, etc. Finally, it was proved that the hydrazine type of MAOI not only interferes with the breakdown of dopamine, norepinephrine and serotonin but also inhibits the biosynthesis of these amines by interacting with the coenzyme (pyridoxal-5-phosphate) of dopa decarboxylase and of 5-hydroxytryptophan decarboxylase, thus preventing their formation from their precursors. Further support for these was given in the course of studies with γ-aminobutyric acid (GABA), a synaptic inhibitor in the various levels of the central nervous system. The biosynthesis of GABA involves a pyridoxal-dependent enzyme, glutamic acid decarboxylase. The inhibition of glutamic acid decarboxylase results in lowered γ-aminobutyric acid levels in the brain, which in turn leads at first to electrical or even to clinically manifest cerebral seizures. Thus the hydrazine MAOI drug-induced convulsions were thought to be related to the lowered glutamic acid decarboxylase activity in the brain, or in other words, to the lowered GABA concentration. The fact that upon administration of vitamin B_6 (pyridoxin), which is essential to the reactivation of the biosynthesis of GABA, the normal electroshock seizure threshold is reestablished is in favor of this hypothesis.

Other chemical correlates of MAOI drug activity are the inhibition of diamine, methylamine and choline oxidase enzymes by some of the hydrazine derivatives; the inhibition of certain dehydrogenases, *e.g.*, hypothalamic succinic dehydrogenase, particularly by pheniprazine; and the enhancement of glycolysis, which is reflected in the rise in blood pyruvic and lactic acid levels.

The chemically detectable interference of the clinically useful MAOI's with the metabolic degradation of barbiturates, aminopyrine, acetanilid, cocaine and certain narcotics, *e.g.*, meperidine, has important practical implications (Biel, 1964; Jarvik, 1965; Pletscher, 1965; and Sourkes, 1962).

b. Neurophysiological Correlates

Although early electrophysiological studies by Schallek and Kuehn (1960) failed to reveal that iproniazid acted on either the brain stem reticular formation or the cerebral cortex, later investigations were able to detect changes at the various levels of the nervous system.

i. Autonomic Nervous System. The direct effect of MAOI's on autonomic ganglia remained hidden for a while because of the overt sympathotonic action of these drugs. While these are mainly central in origin, the actual effect of all MAOI's on the functioning of autonomic ganglia is depression of nerve impulses, *i.e.*, blockage of ganglionic transmission.

ii. Spinal Cord. There is a differential action among the various groups of MAOI's on spinal cord functions and even a differential action of the same group of drugs in lower or higher dosages. Hydrazines in amounts which produce overt behavioral manifestations depress the transmission of impulses in the spinal cord, whereas α-alkyltryptamines in low or average doses lack the same effect and only when given in higher amounts do they exert inhibitory action on the monosynaptic knee jerk and polysynaptic hind leg reflexes. Etryptamine—a representative of the α-alkyltryptamine category—was found to have a facilitating effect on spinal reflexes in the low or average dosage range. However, all the known therapeutically used MAOI's have a depressant effect on myoneural junctions. Furthermore, some of them (*e.g.*, pheniprazine) are able to induce local anesthesia (as revealed in rabbits) while others, *e.g.*, hydrazines, have a definite analgesic effect.

iii. Brain Stem Reticular Formation. The effect of MAOI's on brain stem reticular formation functions has been extensively explored. While the first experiments of Schallek and Kuehn (1960) did not detect any effect of iproniazid on these structures, later studies by Himwich (1965) showed that "alerting" of the reticular formation was frequently associated with a rise in brain serotonin.

Further investigations, in which parenterally administered α-alkyltryptamines were used, revealed two phases of brain stem reticular formation reaction to MAOI drugs. In the first phase, which occurred immediately after the injection, the type of arousal resembled that produced by amphetamines, *i.e.*, activation of the structures of the midbrain reticular formation. This immediate response was followed by a delayed phase of arousal, which correlates with an increased level of serotonin in the bulbar reticular formation structures.

iv. Septum-Hypothalamus-Amygdala. On the septum-hypothalamus-amygdala triangle, in which the amygdala is the stimulating, certain septal areas the inhibiting and the hypothalamus the conducting part, it was suggested that MAOI's may have a stimulating effect on the amygdala. This was indicated by a lower threshold to electrical stimulation and, in general, an enhanced excitability in this structure. This was complemented by experimental evidence which showed that, under the influence of these drugs, direct stimulation of the amygdala results in prolonged duration of after-discharges (Schallek and Kuehn, 1963; and Kuehn and Schallek, 1965).

While no effects of MAOI's on the septal areas have been shown, indirect evidence (*e.g.*, sympatheticotonia, hyperthermia) of hypothalamic stimulation has been presented. Furthermore, a dissociation in the effects of MAOI's on the amygdala and the hippocampus has been shown. This "inhibitory action" on the hippocampus, manifested in suppressed after-discharges, while the threshold of stimulation remained unchanged.

v. Others. Other neurophysiological effects induced by MAOI's are electroencephalographic changes which are not attributed to the direct effect of these drugs on the cerebral cortex, but are rather the reflection of changes in other structures. Persistent desynchronization of the electroencephalogram has been described with pheniprazine—an aralkylhydrazine—even in low doses, while iproniazid in doses as high as 400 mg./kg. did not produce similar changes. On the other hand, iproniazid and other hydrazines were shown to elicit sleep spindles or seizure-like electrical activities. It has been shown that tranylcypromine, a phenylcyclopropylamine, produces both: first desynchronization lasting a few hours and sleep spindles thereafter. Important for the MAOI-induced electroencephalographic changes are the relative amounts of brain monoamines, particularly 5-HT and NE, and the rate of their synthesis and destruction (Cohen *et al.*, 1967; and Remmen *et al.*, 1962).

6. Behavioral Pharmacology

The behavioral effects of MAOI drugs appear in two or (in the case of irreversible inhibitors) three consecutive phases. The first phase is one of "primary effects," resulting from the direct action of these substances on certain CNS structures. This is followed by a latent period, characterized by a rise in 5-HT and catecholamine levels, leading to pharmacological actions which are dependent upon MAO enzyme inhibition.

In the case of reversible inhibitors, the secondary manifestations wear off shortly after the withdrawal of the MAOI drug, while in the case of irreversible inhibitors, the duration of action is prolonged far beyond the actual presence of the MAOI substance. The sustained activity of these irreversible inhibitors, *e.g.*, hydrazine derivatives, can be antagonized by pretreatment with one of the short acting enzyme inhibitors, such as harmaline, harmine, amphetamine and methylene blue. This phenomenon is probably best explained by the mechanism of competitive antagonism between certain reversible and irreversible MAOI compounds.

a. Animal Studies

The behavioral pharmacology of MAOI's has been extensively investigated in animal experiments and intensively studied in humans through phenomenological explorations. In animal experiments the behavioral effects of MAOI's have been explored after the administration of various MAOI drugs alone and probably even in greater detail after the simultaneous administration of the MAOI with another substance, *e.g.*, with precursors of endogenous monoamines, with exogenous amines, with drugs which have a well established effect on endogenous monoamines, and with convulsants and other pharmaceutical preparations (Jacobsen, 1964; Jarvik, 1965; and Pletscher, 1965).

i. MAOI's Alone. Unrelated to MAO enzyme inhibition is the influence of these drugs on the cardiovascular system. For-example, arylalkylhydrazines (*i.e.*, pheniprazine or phenelzine) possess definite sympathomimetic properties characterized by hypertension and positive inotropic and chronotropic effects on the heart. Other hydrazine derivatives, particularly iproniazid, exert an opposite effect, *i.e.*, a weak adrenergic blockade. This blocking action on sympathetic ganglia leaves the parasympathetic side of the autonomic nervous system unaffected, which is probably responsible for the hypotensive reactions commonly encountered in the course of treatment.

Also independent of the enzyme inhibition are both the convulsant and anticonvulsant effects of some of the hydrazine derivative MAOI's. The *convulsant action* of these compounds has been attributed to the lowering of γ-aminobutyric acid levels, which is a consequence of the reaction between a highly active aldehyde group of pyridoxal (or pyridoxal-5-phosphates) and the carbonyl reagent of hydrazines. As a result of this reaction, pyridoxal, which is a coenzyme of glutamic acid decarboxylase, the enzyme involved in the synthesis of GABA, cannot fulfill its function. The mechanism involved in the *anticonvulsant action* of the same drugs is similar to that responsible for their convulsant action, *i.e.*, the reaction between pyridoxal and hydrazine. Pyridoxal is not only a coenzyme of the enzyme system responsible for the synthesis but also has a coenzyme function to the enzyme system responsible for the degradation of GABA. Thus pretreatment with a hydrazine derivative MAOI prior to reserpine administration, by preventing the fall of GABA concentration seen under natural circumstances with this Rauwolfia alkaloid drug, elevates the threshold for electroshock-induced seizures.

Finally, there are stimulating and excitatory effects observed under the influence of these drugs which are partially attributed to MAO enzyme inhibition. The early stimulation frequently seen with MAOI drugs is usually considered to be a direct amphetamine-like effect. MAO enzyme inhibition is responsible for the excitatory effects superimposed on this early stimulation, as this develops only after a considerable delay, at a time when inhibition of the brain enzyme is almost complete and there is a considerable increase of 5-HT and NE in the central nervous system.

ii. MAOI's in Combination. There is a measurable potentiation of the various behavioral manifestations produced by the precursors of endogenous monoamines in the presence of MAOI drugs. This has been studied in two ways: by measuring the potentiation of the tremor or pyrexia produced by 5-hydroxytryptophan (the precursor of serotonin) and by measuring the potentiation of the central excitement induced by dihydroxyphenylalanine (the precursor of dopamine and norepinephrine). In these tests, isocarboxazide, nialamide and phenelzine were found to be 15 to 20 times more potent than iproniazid. It has been suggested that there is a quantitative relationship between the intensity of the potentiated response and the degree of MAO enzyme inhibition.

A similar, quantitative relationship between the intensity of the potentiated response to exogenous monoamines and MAO enzyme inhibition has been demonstrated. For this purpose, the potentiation of tryptamine-induced tremor (or, less frequently, convulsion) by MAOI drugs was measured (in rats). Maxwell *et al.* (1961), taking the tremor potentiation of iproniazid as the unit, established the following order of potency: iproniazid, 1; nialamide, 1.8; isocarboxazide, 3.1; phenelzine, 18; pheniprazine, 31; and tranylcypromine, 45. It was inferred from these findings that the acylation of a monosubstituted hydrazine will result in a manifold reduction of potency as measured by Maxwell *et al.*'s (1961) test.

Tetrabenazine and reserpine have well established effects on endogenous monoamines. These drugs free the endogenous monoamines from their intracellular granular storages and thus expose them to catabolic processes in which MAO enzymes are involved. Tetrabenazine when given alone produces depression and a characteristic blockade of the conditioned avoidance response. Pretreatment with any of the clinically effective MAOI compounds prevents or even reverses these effects. Only the nonhydrazine MAOI drugs are able to counteract (or reverse) the depression or blockade of the conditioned avoidance response when given *after* tetrabenazine (or reserpine) administration. The various reserpine effects which are prevented or counteracted by various MAOI drugs are the following: depression, sedation, reduced spontaneous motor activity, catalepsy, palpebral ptosis, hypothermia, hypotension, bradycardia, release of catecholamines from the adrenal medulla, prolongation of ethanol sleeping time, facilitation of pentetrazol and electroshock-induced seizure activity. In case of reversal of drug effects by nonhydrazine compounds (in certain animals), manifestations of central and peripheral sympathetic stimulation are observed after reserpine administration, *e.g.*, excitation, mydriasis, exophthalmos, hyperthermia, piloerection, hypertension, tachycardia, etc. It should be noted that MAOI drugs differ in their ability to prevent, counteract or reverse the various reserpine-induced manifestations.

MAOI drugs are able to prevent or alleviate electroshock or pentetrazol-induced cerebral seizures. They are ineffective against strychnine-induced convulsions. There is evidence that they potentiate the effects of various narcotics, analgesics, antipyretics, tricyclic antidepressants, amphetamines and barbiturates. Their interaction with tricyclic antidepressants, particularly with imipramine but not with trimipramine, can be fatal to animals (and may lead to serious consequences in humans). Death is usually preceded by dizziness, sweating, restlessness, excitement and hyperthermia. (The potentiation of barbiturates in some patients led to the aggravation of depressive manifestations.)

b. Human Studies

There are two particular effects of MAOI's which can only be studied in humans: their antianginal and antidepressant effects. The antianginal effect is considered to be the result of coronary dilation. A possible relationship between antianginal action and MAO enzyme inhibition is assumed but has not yet been fully substantiated.

The antidepressant effect of these drugs is of major importance. In those MAOI's which have been synthesized through structural modifications of phenethylamine, the mood-lifting effect is preceded by an amphetamine-like psychomotor stimulating action. With hydrazine derivatives—with the exception of the arylalkylhydrazines—there is a latent period prior to the onset of the antidepressant action. Continuous administration may lead to agitation, talkativeness, hypomania or even manic reactions. Whether this is the drug's effect on the natural history of the illness or a toxic psychokinetic reaction remains undecided. In depressive cases, psychomotor stimulation is followed by an antidepressant action. In normals, however, a euphorizing action precedes a toxic psychokinetic reaction. In some schizophrenic patients, under the influence of MAOI's, hedonia, the ability to experience pleasure, was regained, while in others aggravation of psychopathology, particularly of thought disorder, or the development of a toxic hallucinatory or confusional state, has occurred.

B. CLINICAL DATA

1. Therapeutic Indications and Contraindications

a. Therapeutic Indications

i. Nonpsychiatric. MAOI drugs are successfully administered in numerous pathological conditions. Besides their psychiatric indications, they are prescribed in various cardiovascular, connective tissue and dermatological disorders. The analgesic effect of hydrazines is not infrequently used for pain relief in patients with progressive neoplastic disease; and their antithrombosis effect (prolongation of prothrombin time), particularly in the case of nialamide, may be successfully utilized in depressive cases suffering from coronary thrombosis or peripheral clotting. Among the various cardiovascular indications, MAOI's are probably most useful in angina pectoris, essential hypertension, Reynaud's disease and ischemic ulcers.

The antiphlogistic effect of MAOI's exerted by a direct peripheral action on mesenchymal inflammation and connective tissue growth is utilized in connective tissue disorders such as rheumatoid arthritis, scleroderma, systemic lupus erythematosus, chronic ulcerative colitis and dermatomyositis. Among the dermatological conditions, acne, psoriasis, discoid lupus erythematosis, tuberculoderma and sarcoidosis respond best to MAOI drugs. For a considerable time they were quite frequently prescribed for women suffering from hyperemesis gravidarum in the first trimester of pregnancy. They have also been successfully added to wound-healing preparations.

ii. Psychiatric. There is a great variety of psychiatric indications for MAOI drugs. The most important are the various depressive conditions. Other indications in order of importance are psychoneuroses, functional psychoses, organic brain syndromes and mental retardation.

α. Depressions. There is increasing evidence that the primary therapeutic indications of MAOI's are in reactive, neurotic and stuporous depressions. The best results, however, have been obtained in atypical depressive cases, and the worst in agitated depressive patients.

Of the *hydrazine derivatives*, the therapeutically most potent, iproniazid, had to be withdrawn from clinical application because of its toxicity. Prior to this, however, West and Dally (1959) concluded that patients who responded best to iproniazid were predominantly neurotics with phobic manifestations with a tendency to become depressed. Further characteristics of these patients were absence of guilt feelings and poor responsivity to electroconvulsive treatment. In another analysis, Gallinek (1959) recognized that retarded depressives with somatic complaints and a chronic neurotic background are the best candidates for iproniazid treatment. Favorable responses were subsequently reported in the atypical depressive group, which includes patients with schizophrenic features who are more accurately described as listless rather than depressed. At the same time, Kline and Stanley (1959) reported on favorable therapeutic results with iproniazid in manic-depressive patients. In contradistinction to iproniazid, involutional and also neurotic depressions are considered to be the primary indications for isocarboxazide; and depressions associated with organic disease and also retarded endogenous depressions, for nialamide.

In the four "non-hydrazine" categories, only two preparations are clinically used at present. Of the α-alkyltryptamines, etryptamine, which was particularly indicated in neurotic depressive cases, had to be withdrawn from general use because of toxic effects, and α-methyltryptamine, which was considered to be therapeutically promising for similar patients, had to be abandoned because of its psychogenic action. The phenylcyclopropylamine derivative, tranylcypromine, has a wide range of indications and is probably the most extensively used drug of this entire class. Successful therapeutic results have been reported with this substance in reactive and psychoneurotic depressions, in involutional melancholia and in manic depressive illness.

The application of the propargylamine derivative, pargyline, has been officially limited to antihypertensive therapy. Of the last category in this class (arylalkylhydrazines), phenelzine is the only presently available drug; it is primarily indicated in reactive, atypical or hysterical depressive cases (Sargant and Slater, 1963).

β. Psychoneuroses. Of the various MAOI's, phenelzine is extensively used in psychosomatic and psychophysiological illnesses. Beneficial results with this drug have also been reported in cases with phobic manifestations and hysterical conversion symptoms. There is some evidence that the combination of phenelzine with the benzodiazepine chlordiazepoxide has a superior therapeutic effect in phobic and somatic anxiety, while the combination of phenelzine with the phenothiazine trifluoperazine gives more favorable therapeutic results in free-floating anxiety. Others prefer tranylcypromine alone or in similar combinations for the treatment of the same therapeutic indications.

Beneficial results have been obtained with MAOI's in the "phobic-anxiety syndrome," characterized by recurrent attacks, and also in "inert psychasthenic-anhedonic reactions," which are characterized by chronic depression, anxiety, overactivity and lack of self-confidence. Patients suffering from this condition are usually at their worst at night.

γ. Others. Functional psychoses in general, with the exception of depressed manic-depressive cases, cannot be considered as primary indications for MAOI treatment. Kline and Stanley (1959) had limited success with iproniazid in withdrawn, regressed and burnt-out schizophrenics, while Davies (1964) reported on more favorable findings in a somewhat similar, withdrawn, but probably less regressed group of patients.

Anhedonia, however, a commonly seen symptom in chronic schizophrenia, was seen to be particularly responsive to tranylcypromine administration.

While in chronic brain syndromes MAOI's are used only as symptomatic or adjuvant-medications, more recently, it has been noted that nialamide counteracts certain lysergic acid diethylamide-induced psychopathological manifestations. This important finding, however, needs further clinical confirmation.

There was improvement noted in a group of mongoloids. This was seen in considerable increase in motor and verbal activity (Deniker and Lemperiere, 1964; Greenblatt *et al.*, 1966; Kalinowsky and Hoch, 1961; Kline, 1966; Sargant and Slater, 1963; Smith, 1964; Valentine, 1962; and Votava *et al.*, 1963).

b. Contraindications

While there are relatively few absolute contraindications, there are numerous conditions in which MAOI drugs have to be administered cautiously.

Absolute contraindications are advanced liver damage, pheochromocytoma, impaired renal functions and manifest mania.

Among the relative contraindications are cardiac decompensation, congestive heart failure and cerebral vascular disorders. Here the danger of physical harm usually outweighs the therapeutic expectations. The same applies to most of the schizophrenias and to some of the epilepsies.

Combined administration of an MAOI with a tricyclic antidepressant, narcotic (morphine, pethidine), alcohol, analgesic, antipyretic, adrenaline, amphetamine or barbiturate containing substance may result in severe adverse effects.

Because of their tyramine content, certain foods, *e.g.*, cheese, snails, Chianti, chicken liver, etc., have to be avoided in the course of MAOI antidepressant treatment.

Although there is no evidence that these drugs have a harmful effect on the embryo, some consider it inadvisable to give MAOI's during pregnancy and lactation. No carcinogenic effect of these drugs has been reported.

2. Therapy with MAOI Drugs Alone and in Combination with Other Treatments

a. MAOI Drugs Alone

i. Dosage. While the therapeutic dosage range of each MAOI drug differs slightly, it generally holds true that in the treatment of hypertension a daily dosage which is twice as high as that for depression has to be prescribed.

Of the various presently available MAOI drugs, the hydrazine derivative isocarboxazide and the phenylcyclopropylamine tranylcypromine are clinically the most potent on a milligram per kilogram basis. The antidepressant dosage range for both of these drugs is 10 to 60 mg., with an average daily dosage of 30 mg. in the acute period of treatment and 10 mg. in the maintenance period. (The only MAOI found to be therapeutically effective in a lower dosage was pheniprazine.)

While isocarboxazide and tranylcypromine are the most, nialamide is the least potent on a milligram per kilogram basis. The therapeutic dosage range of this drug is from 75 to 500 mg., with an average daily dosage of 100 to 150 mg. in the acute period of treatment and 50 to 75 mg. in the maintenance period.

In between is the arylalkylhydrazine phenelzine for which therapeutic dosage ranges from 15 to 75 mg. a day, with an average daily dosage of 45 mg. in the acute period of treatment and 15 mg. a day (or every other day) in the maintenance period. These dosages refer to oral administration, usually given in equally divided doses three times a day, *i.e.*, every eight hours in the acute period of the illness and once a day (preferably in the morning) in maintenance therapy.

ii. Routes of Administration. While the safest and most frequently used route of drug administration is the oral, MAOI's can also be given parenterally. The only drugs which are definitely less effective by mouth are the harmala alkaloids (but these substances have more of a psychotogenic than an antidepressant effect). The relatively higher affinity of phenelzine (also pheniprazine) for brain enzymes than for liver enzymes when given subcutaneously to rats apparently does not apply to the clinical situation.

It was noted that intramuscularly administered phenelzine induces a burning sensation at the site of injection which lasts for a few minutes. Neither abscess formation nor induration was subsequently observed. Another interesting finding is the transient decrease in anxiety (and also in insomnia) in depressive cases after intravenous nialamide (and other MAOI) administration. This is in contrast to the worsening of psychopathology which occurs in schizophrenic patients.

iii. Treatment Procedures. The most frequently used clinical procedure with MAOI drugs is continuous therapy. In the course of this, the starting dosage may gradually be raised to four times the initial dosage, and in case of successful treatment, it may be gradually reduced to about one-fourth of this in the maintenance period of treatment.

The course of treatment with the most frequently used hydrazine derivatives (isocarboxazide and nialamide) and the two most frequently used phenylethylamine derivatives (tranylcypromine and phenelzine) is similar. The starting dosage of isocarboxazide is 20 to 30 mg. a day. In the absence of therapeutic response within the first 2 to 3 weeks, the dosage may be gradually raised to a maximum of 60 mg. Isocarboxazide treatment should be terminated if there are no therapeutic effects after 4 weeks. Replacement with a tricyclic antidepressant should not commence before at least 2 weeks.

The initial daily dosage of nialamide is 75 to 100 mg. (or 200 to 300 mg.), which may gradually be increased to 400 or even 500 mg. It has been noted that the first signs of improvement with this drug usually appear a few days later than with isocarboxazide.

Of the phenylethylamine - derivative MAOI's, the course of treatment with tranylcypromine follows exactly the same pattern (and dosage) as with isocarboxazide. The major difference and perhaps advantage of this drug is that the first indications of drug activity may appear within 2 to 4 days. Phenelzine is usually given in twice the dosage of tranylcypromine, and the initial indicators of its action are rarely seen before 10 days.

iv. Duration of Treatment. The duration of MAOI drug therapy depends on the condition being treated. It is generally accepted that treatment should be continued for several months after maximum improvement has been obtained. Premature discontinuation of the medication almost inevitably leads to relapse. It is recommended to continue drug administration, at least on a maintenance level, until the patient has remained well over a 4- to 6-month period, during which time the daily dosage should be decreased slowly. Recurrence of symptoms in the course of reduction of dosage is an absolute indication for resuming the optimal daily amount and also for considerable extension of the contemplated treatment period. In some of the recurrent depressions, maintenance dosage may have to be continued for several years.

It should be noted that the MAO enzyme-inhibiting effect of these drugs may persist for some time after the termination of treatment. This period is thought to be not longer than 48 to 72 hours with tranylcypromine, approximately 10 days with phenelzine and at least 2 weeks with iproniazid.

It is fortunate that, with proper supervision, MAOI drugs can be taken over an extended period. Regular mental and physical examination and simple laboratory tests, which include transaminase estimates (SGOT and SGPT), alkaline phosphatase determinations, urinalysis, blood pressure readings and electrocardiograms are sufficient safeguards. In spite of the physical dependence manifest in blood pressure rise, tachycardia and precordial discomfort upon sudden withdrawal, neither habituation nor addiction has been attributed to these drugs. Because of the risk of cardiac failure or even coronary thrombosis in certain predisposed individuals, termination of MAOI treatment should consist of a slow tapering off rather than abrupt discontinuation of the medication.

b. MAOI Drugs in Combination with Other Treatments

MAOI drugs are often administered in conjunction with other treatments, physical and pharmacological.

i. Physical. *α. ECT.* Both electroconvulsive and insulin therapies are occasionally combined with MAOI drug therapy. It was initially thought that MAOI's should not be given together with electroshock, but it was soon shown that, apart from increasing the seizure threshold to the electrical current, the combination reduces the number of electroshocks required for successful treatment. Thus, after approximately four, instead of eight to ten, electroconvulsions, the patient's condition can often be stabilized or further improved by drug treatment alone.

β. Insulin. Insulin therapy is rarely used in combination with MAOI treatment. Potentiation of insulin effects must be taken into consideration. The enhancement of glycolysis results in an increase in systemic lactic and pyruvic acid levels.

ii. Pharmacological. The potentiating effect of MAOI's on various groups of drugs is well known. Among these are analgesics, anesthetics, antipyretics, narcotics, etc. Particular attention has to be paid to the following interactions: both the sedative and depressant properties of the widely prescribed barbiturates are increased (this also applies to a variety of nonbarbiturate sedatives and hypnotics); blood clotting time with anticoagulants is further delayed; the threshold to the toxic effects of alcohol is decreased; and the anticholinergic effect of antiparkinsonian drugs is increased. There is also some evidence that oral diuretics potentiate the antidepressant and hypotensive effects of MAOI's and that there is an interaction—the nature of which is inconsistent—between MAOI's and steroid preparations.

It was recognized that better results were achieved with a phenelzine and chlordiazepoxide combination in phobic and somatic anxieties and with a phenelzine and trifluoperazine combination in free-floating anxiety than when any of these drugs was given alone. Combinations of MAOI with a benzodiazepine (usually chlordiazepoxide) in the treatment of various neuroses and depressions or with a phenothiazine (usually trifluoperazine, occasionally chlorpromazine) in the treatment of certain schizophrenias (pseudoneurotic, anhedonic) are accepted practice. Parstelin, formerly a commercially available combination containing 10 mg. of tranylcypromine and 1 mg. of trifluoperazine, was for a short period one of the most favored preparations (Benson and Schiele, 1962; and Sargant and Slater, 1963).

In the treatment of severe and unresponsive depressive conditions, orally administered sympathomimetic amines, particularly various amphetamines or methylphenidate increase the therapeutic effect of MAOI's. The prompt action of the sympathomimetic amine helps the patient through the initial period until the MAOI effect sets in and the MAOI prevents the abrupt letdown which is one of the drawbacks of using amphetamines alone. Pretreatment with reserpine may add to the therapeutic efficacy of MAOI treatment; and simultaneous administration of 5-HTP may speed up the therapeutic response. Recently, the originally contraindicated combination of an MAOI with a tricyclic antidepressant has gained increasing acceptance. The way to prevent adverse reactions while potentiating therapeutic effect is to use a very small dosage of one member of the combination with the regular therapeutic dosage of the other (Kline, 1966).

3. Adverse Reactions and Their Treatment

a. Adverse Reactions

Many adverse reactions have been encountered and classified as psychiatric, neurological, autonomic, ophthalmological, cardiovascular, gastrointestinal, genitourinary, hepatobiliary, hematological and dermatological.

i. Psychiatric. These range from inappropriate behavior to rare cases of outright psychosis. The most frequent reactions are diurnal irritability and nocturnal insomnia, which without adjustment of dosage can progress into increased psychomotor activity, motor restlessness and agitation. MAOI's may accentuate or trigger the recurrence of psychotic manifestations in schizophrenics or they may induce a toxic confusional state or a transient hallucinatory reaction.

ii. Neurological. There are both peripheral and central nervous system reactions. Among the former, muscle weakness and tremor are most common with or without hyperreflexia and clonus of the lower extremities. Neuralgias, paresthesias, neuritis and peripheral neuropathies occur only with the hydrazine derivatives.

Of the central neurological effects, headache, dizziness and vertigo are the most common, while convulsions and syncope are rather rare. Special attention is now being paid to the hypertensive crisis first described with tranylcypromine but later also with other MAOI compounds. This usually begins with severe occipital headache, which may radiate frontally. Nausea and vomiting, sweating with fever or cold and clammy skin, dilated pupils and photophobia, neck stiffness, tachycardia with palpitations or bradycardia and constricting chest pain may all be present. The crisis may subside without leaving any major organic damage, or it may lead to intracranial bleeding (subarachnoidal hemorrhage). Consumption of cheese (Cheddar, Camembert or Stilton), Chianti or snails (all with a characteristically high tyramine content) preceded the clinical manifestations in a number of cases. In others the hypertensive crisis could be traced to the ingestion of sympathomimetic amines, methyldopa, dopamine or tryptophan. Whether a special predisposition is also a factor has yet to be decided.

iii. Autonomic. These reactions are rather inconsistent, resulting in a pathological functioning of any of the organ systems. Specific reactions are dryness of the mouth, sweating and headaches (vascular or migraine).

iv. Ophthalmological. With the exception of blurred vision, ophthalmological reactions are rare. There are occasional cases of color blindness. Optic atrophy is exceptionally rare.

v. Cardiovascular. Hypotensive reactions are probably the commonest adverse effects of MAOI drugs. They may be so slight and transient that they do not interfere with treatment or so severe and permanent that they call for emergency measures and withdrawal of medication. They are usually aggravated by simultaneous administration of narcotics, analgesics, diuretics, barbiturates or phenothiazines. A special type of reaction is postural or orthostatic hypotension. The hypotension is preceded by a transient pressor (hypertensive) response with some of the presently available MAOI's, *e.g.*, tranylcypromine.

vi. Gastrointestinal. Adverse gastrointestinal reactions are rare. There are occasional gastrointestinal upsets and infrequent cases of anorexia. Constipation is probably the most common, but it rarely occurs to the extent of causing epigastric or abdominal distress. Diarrhea, a paradoxical reaction, has also been reported.

vii. Genitourinary. These are usually autonomic in nature. Difficulties of micturition and the inability to ejaculate are probably the most frequent. Occasionally edema occurs, while impotence and frigidity are infrequent complaints.

viii. Hepatobiliary. Toxic hepatobiliary reactions were quite common with iproniazid and pheniprazine (both withdrawn from clinical use). While the incidence of hepatocellular damage with iproniazid and pheniprazine was very high, the incidence has markedly decreased with the presently available MAOI drugs. The nature of the hepatocellular damage was described as a balloon puffing of the liver cell with a consequent dissociation of the cytoplasmic content. There were also a mild stasis of bile in the canaliculi and an inflammatory reaction around the injured cells. Laboratory tests showed high transaminase levels; clinically, jaundice appeared on occasions. Any indication of liver involvement has to be handled with extreme caution to prevent the development of irreversible liver necrosis.

ix. Hematological. Etryptamine was withdrawn from therapeutic use because of a few instances of blood dyscrasias which were thought to be related to the administration of this drug. While hematological reactions with the presently available MAOI's are rare, there are cases in which anemia, particularly the hypochromic type, hemolysis, leucopenia or even agranulocytosis have been encountered in the course of treatment.

x. Dermatological. Pathological skin reactions are limited to the occasional case of dermatitis or maculopapular rash.

A special aspect of adverse reactions are those due to overdosage. A case of overdosage with phenelzine (375 mg. in one dose) developed muscular rigidity with hyperreflexia, confusion, pupillary dilation and coma. Another case of overdosage with unknown quantities of isocarboxazide and tranylcypromine developed uncoordinated muscular activity, incoherent speech and hyperthermia, giving place to decerebrate rigidity, carpopedal spasms, myoclonic seizures and coma. The same patient after 4 days manifested overtly psychotic behavior with delusions and auditory hallucinations, which subsided within 3 days. Biochemically there was evidence of elevated blood serotonin levels with increased urinary tryptamine, metanephrine and normetanephrine and decreased urinary 5-hydroxyindoleacetic acid and 3-methoxy-4-hydroxymandelic acid excretion.

In general, overdosage may manifest itself in three distinctly different forms. The least severe is characterized by insomnia, restlessness, anxiety, agitation, confusion and incoherence. In more severe cases, drowsiness, weakness, hypotension, dizziness and possibly shock are in the center of the clinical picture. In the most severe cases, hypertension and headache with or without myoclonic fibrillation of the skeletal muscles are present, as well as hyperpyrexia, progressive generalized rigidity and coma.

b. Treatment of Adverse Reactions

Treatment depends on the nature and severity of the reaction and on the dynamics of the situation, *i.e.*, whether the therapeutic efficiency of the drug is greater than the problems posed by the adverse drug effect. Treatment may consist of discontinuing the medication with or without replacement, reduction of dosage, administration of agents to diminish or eliminate the undesired manifestations and, finally, acceptance of the unwanted reaction and continuation of treatment.

Acceptance of the unwanted reaction (as in the case of dryness of the mouth or excessive perspiration) or discontinuation of all medication without replacement (as in the case of severe hepatic or hematological manifestations) is very rarely indicated. In the majority of cases adverse reactions to MAOI drugs respond well to reduction in dosage. Irritability and insomnia, vascular headaches and migraine and most of the gastrointestinal and genitourinary complaints usually disappear when the dosage is reduced. The neurological, ophthalmological and dermatological reactions generally call for the discontinuation of treatment followed by replacement therapy.

Adverse reactions can be relieved by a number of drugs. In psychoses (toxic or reactivation of process) phenothiazines in general and trifluoperazine in particular are the most useful. Peripheral neuritis may respond to pyridoxine treatment, while chlorpromazine administration with bedrest has been successful in some vascular headaches and migraines. The cardiostimulating action of these drugs (particularly tranylcypromine and phenelzine) is effectively blocked by dichloroisoproterenol, and edema can be controlled by diuretics in general and chlorothiazide in particular.

In the treatment of hypotensive reactions, adrenocorticosteroids are used. Most frequently, intramuscular ACTH (30 to 40 mg.) administration is followed by oral cortisone (12.5 to 37.5 mg.) doses. In certain cases, the addition of dopa to the treatment regime is sufficient to normalize blood pressure.

Hypertensive crises call for the immediate withdrawal of the MAOI medication. As treatment, phentolamine or pentolinium is recommended. Phentolamine is given in a dosage of 5 mg. intravenously, while pentolinium is given in a dosage of 3 mg. subcutaneously. Milder reactions may respond well to intramuscular chlorpromazine administration. It should be noted that, of an estimated three and a half million patients who received tranylcypromine, there were approximately 50 reported cases of cerebrovascular accidents resulting from a hypertensive crisis. Of the 15 reported fatal cases, some might have been saved by adequate counter-measures.

In the management of overdosage, gastric lavage, bedrest and maintenance of proper fluid and electrolyte balance may be of vital importance. Otherwise, the treatment remains mainly symptomatic. Fever is controlled by external cooling. During the fever period, barbiturate or sympathomimetic amine administration should be avoided. Myoclonic seizures may call for barbiturate administration, and levarterenol has been used successfully in the control of hypotension. Since MAOI's may reverse the effect of epinephrine, adrenaline administration in these cases is contraindicated. A case of phenelzine overdosage showed satisfactory response to reserpine administration.

4. The use of MAOI's in Medical Practice

The discovery of MAOI drugs has enabled the clinician to utilize and manipulate the body's monoamine resources in the treatment of various conditions. The application of these substances has gained wide acceptance in psychiatry; they have been less intensively investigated and used elsewhere, *e.g.*, in essential hypertension, angina pectoris, rheumatoid arthritis, local ischemias, skin ulcerations and burns.

There are three different groups of MAOI's used as antidepressants. Drugs of the first group exert their effects by predominantly indirect action, *i.e.*, presumably through enzyme inhibition. Hydrazine derivatives belong to this group. Among them, isocarboxazide is frequently used in both involutional and neurotic depressions, and nialamide is used in organic conditions with depressive manifestations and retarded endogenous depressions.

The second group, known as direct stimulants, consists of the aralkylhydrazines, in which the amino group of the phenethylamine nucleus is substituted by a hydrazine moiety. Drugs of this group have a somewhat faster onset of action than the other hydrazine derivatives, but their clinical effects are more transient. The representative drug of this group is phenelzine, a substance shown to be particularly useful in reactive, atypical or hysterical depressive cases.

The third category is the bimodal stimulant group, which has a phenethylamine nucleus. It is represented by tranylcypromine, a substance which is indicated in a number of depressions but is usually considered to be most valuable in chronic neurotic depressive cases, in depressive manifestations concomitant with somatic illness and (combined with chlordiazepoxide) in numerous neurotic conditions. Parstelin, a combination of tranylcypromine with trifluoperazine, was used successfully in both chronic anhedonic and pseudoneurotic schizophrenias.

Other MAOI drugs are pargyline, phenoxypropazine, iproclozide, mebamazine, 1-pivaloyl-2-benzylhydrazine, 2-methyl-3-piperidinepyrazine, α-methyltryptamine, etc. Pargyline is marketed as an antihypertensive of particular value in hypertensive patients who are also depressed. Mebamazine, α-methyltryptamine and 2-methyl-3-piperidinepyrazine are suggested as useful in the treatment of neurotic depression, although α-methyltryptamine may also exert psychotopathic effects. 1-Pivaloyl-2-benzylhydrazine has definite antianginal but no definite antidepressant properties.

MAOI antidepressants are clinically most effective in the atypical depressive cases. They are ineffective in agitated depressions. In endogenous depressions, tricyclic antidepressant drugs are generally preferred.

Klerman and Cole (1965), in their paper on the clinical pharmacology of imipramine and related antidepressant compounds, reviewed the studies in which imipramine was compared with various MAOI antidepressants. In the six studies in which imipramine was compared with phenelzine, only Martin's (1963) showed statistically significant difference in favor of imipramine. They recognized, however, that in these studies (conducted by Agnew *et al.*, 1961;

Greenblatt *et al.*, 1962; Haydu *et al.*, 1964; Kiloh, 1960; Leitch and Seager, 1963; and Martin, 1963) 138 out of 196 patients improved on imipramine as against 101 out of 164 patients on phenelzine. This difference was shown to be statistically significant. While Rothman's results (1960) slightly favored isocarboxazide over imipramine, Greenblatt *et al.* (1962) and Overall *et al.* (1962) found imipramine superior to isocarboxazide.

The numerous side-effects of MAOI's, their interaction with a great many other frequently used drugs and the dietary precautions necessary are definite drawbacks. On the other hand, by furthering understanding of the neurochemical correlates of depression and actually by being able beneficially to influence reserpine- and tetrabenazine-induced experimental depressions, MAOI's have great heuristic value.

SUMMARY

That MAOI's, by preventing the metabolic breakdown of certain neurotransmitter substances, can induce psychological changes represents a new approach to the treatment of various psychiatric conditions and provides an important tool for further scientific investigations. The best therapeutic results with this new group of drugs have been obtained in the various depressive conditions. When MAOI's were combined with anxiolytic (*e.g.*, chlordiazepoxide) substances, their clinical usefulness was extended to a number of neurotic conditions (*e.g.*, phobias), and when they were combined with neuroleptics (*e.g.*, trifluoperazine), they became beneficial in the treatment of certain schizophrenic symptoms (*e.g.*, anhedonia).

Of the two major MAOI groups used in psychiatry, hydrazine derivatives (*e.g.*, isocarboxazide) are more frequently used in the treatment of psychotic depressions, whereas phenylethylamine derivatives (*e.g.* tranylcypromine) are used primarily in the treatment of neurotic depressive cases. Both groups are considered to be excellent in the treatment of atypical depressions. Hydrazine derivatives have a somewhat delayed onset of therapeutic effects and, after discontinuation of drug administration, a somewhat more prolonged duration of action, which is related to the so-called "irreversible" nature of their MAOI enzyme-inhibiting effect. The onset of primary therapeutic effect is prompt with the phenylethylamine derivatives, due probably to the direct effects of the amphetamine structure of these compounds, and after discontinuation of drug administration, they have a considerably shorter duration of action, which is related to the so-called "reversible" nature of their MAO enzyme-inhibiting effect.

A considerable number of adverse effects have been seen in the course of therapy with these drugs. Hypotensive reactions are the most frequent with both groups, while the most severe reactions are hepatotoxicity with the hydrazines and hypertensive crises with the phenylethylamines. The interaction of MAOI's with other commonly used drugs and with dietary substances calls for careful considerations prior to commencement of treatment with MAOI drugs.

REFERENCES

AGNEW, P. C., *et al.*: A clinical evaluation of four antidepressant drugs (nardil, tofranil, marplan and deprol). Amer. J. Psychiat., *118:* 160 (1961).

BAIN, J.: Mono-amine oxidase inhibitors: a review. Appl. Ther., *7:* 737 (1965).

BELLEAU, B., AND MORAN, J. (1962): In: Zirkle, C. L., and Kaiser, C.: Monoamine oxidase inhibitors. In: Psychopharmacological agents (ed., Gordon, M.). (Academic Press, New York, (1964.)

BENSON, W. M., AND SCHIELE, B. C.: Tranquillizing and antidepressive drugs. (Charles C Thomas, Springfield, 1962.)

BERNHEIM, F. (1928): In: Zirkle, C. L., and Kaiser, C.: Monoamine oxidase inhibitors. In: Psychopharmacological agents (ed., Gordon, M.). (Academic Press, New York, 1964.)

BIEL, J. H.: Some rationales for the development of antidepressant drugs. In: Molecular modification in drug design (ed., Gould, R. F.). (American Chemical Society, Washington, 1964.)

BIEL, J. H., HORITA, A., AND DRUKKER, A. E.: Monoamine oxidase inhibitors (hydrazines). In: Psychopharmacological agents (ed., Gordon, M.). (Academic Press, New York, 1964.)

BRODIE, B. B., PLETSCHER, A., AND SHORE, P. A.: Possible role of serotonin in brain function and in reserpine action. J. Pharmacol., *116:* 9 (1956).

CHORINE, V.: Action de l'amide nicotinique sur les bacilles du gendre mycobacterium. C. R. Acad. Sci. (Paris), *220:* 150 (1945).

COHEN, S., DITMAN, K. S., AND GUSTAFSON, S. R.:

Psychochemotherapy. (Western Medical Publications, Los Angeles, 1967.)

CRANE, G. E.: Psychiatric side effects of iproniazid. Amer. J. Psychiat., *112:* 494 (1956).

CRANE, G. E. (1957): In: Remmen, E., *et al.*: Psychochemotherapy. (Western Medical Publications, Los Angeles, 1962.)

DAVIES, E. B. (ed.): Depression, a Cambridge postgraduate medical course. (University Press, Cambridge, 1964.)

DELAY, J., LAINE, B., AND BUISSON, J. F.: Note concernant l'action de l'isonicotinylhydrazide dans le traitement des etats dépressifs. Ann. Medico Psychol., *110:* 689 (1952).

DENIKER, P., AND LEMPERIERE, T.: Drug treatment of depression. In: Depression, a Cambridge postgraduate medical course (ed., Davies, E. B.). (University Press, Cambridge, 1964.)

EBERSON, L. E., AND PERSSON, K. (1962): In: Biel, J. H., Horita, A., and Drukker, A. F.: Monoamine oxidase inhibitors. In: Psychopharmacological agents (ed., Gordon, M.). (Academic Press, New York, 1964.)

GALLINEK, A.: Marsilid (iproniazid) and electroshock. Amer. J. Psychiat., *115:* 1011 (1959).

GORDON, M. (ed.): Psychopharmacological agents. (Academic Press, New York, 1964.)

GREENBLATT, M., GROSSER, G. H., AND WECHSLER, H.: A comparative study of selected antidepressant medications and EST. Amer. J. Psychiat., *119:* 144 (1962).

GREENBLATT, M., GROSSER, G. H., AND WECHSLER, H.: Drugs in treatment of depression: controlled studies. In: Psychiatric drugs (ed., Solomon, P.). (Grune and Stratton, New York, 1966.)

HAYDU, G. G., *et al.*: Differential therapeutic results of three antidepressant medications according to fixed or flexible schedules. J. Nerv. Ment. Dis., *139:* 475 (1964).

HIMWICH, H. E.: Biochemical and neurophysiological action of psychoactive drugs. In: Drugs and behavior (eds., Uhr, L., and Miller, J. G.). (Wiley, New York, 1960.)

HIMWICH, H. E. (1960): In: Schlittler, E., and Plummer, A. J. Tranquilizing drugs from the Rauwolfia. In: Psychopharmacological agents (ed., Gordon, M.). (Academic Press, New York, 1964.)

HIMWICH, H. E.: Anatomy and physiology of the emotions and their relation to psychoactive drugs. In: The scientific basis of drug therapy in psychiatry (eds., Marks, J., and Pare, C. M. B.). (Pergamon Press, Oxford, 1965.)

HIMWICH, H. E., KETY, S. S., AND SMYTHIES, J. R. (eds.): Amines and schizophrenia. (Pergamon Press, Oxford, 1966.)

HIMWICH, H. E., *et al.*: Correlations between effects of iproniazid on brain activating system with brain neurohormones. Ann. N.Y. Acad. Sci., *80:* 614 (1960).

JACOBSEN, E.: The theoretical basis of depression. In: Depression (ed., Davies, B. E.). (University Press, Cambridge, 1964.)

JARVIK, M. E.: Drugs used in the treatment of psychiatric disorders. In: The pharmacological basis of therapeutics (eds., Goodman, L. S., and Gilman, A.). (MacMillan, Toronto, 1965.)

KALINOWSKY, L. B.: The danger of various types of medication during electric convulsive therapy. Amer. J. Psychiat., *112:* 745 (1956).

KALINOWSKY, L. B.: Appraisal of the "tranquilizers" and their influence on other somatic treatments in psychiatry. Amer. J. Psychiat., *115:* 294 (1958).

KALINOWSKY, L. B.: Prognosis and outcome of somatic treatments in mental disorders. In: Comparative epidemiology of the mental disorders (eds., Hoch, P. H., and Zubin, J.). (Grune and Stratton, New York, 1961.)

KALINOWSKY, L. B.: Electric convulsive therapy after ten years of pharmacotherapy. Amer. J. Psychiat., *120:* 944 (1964).

KALINOWSKY, L. B., AND HOCH, P. H.: Shock treatments and other somatic procedures in psychiatry. (Heinemann, London, 1952.)

KALINOWSKY, L. B., AND HOCH, P. H.: Somatic treatments is psychiatry. (Grune and Stratton, New York, 1961.)

KILOH, L. G.: A controlled trial of iproniazid in the treatment of endogenous depression. J. Ment. Sci., *106:* 1139 (1960).

KLERMAN, G. L., AND COLE, J. O.: Clinical pharmacology of imipramine and related antidepressant compounds. Pharmacol. Rev., *17:* 101 (1965).

KLINE, N. S.: Depression, diagnosis and treatment. Med. Clin. N. Amer., *45:* 1041 (1961).

KLINE, N. S.: The use of psychopharmaceuticals in office practice. Med. Clin. N. Amer., *45:* 1677 (1961).

KLINE, N. S.: Drugs in the treatment of depression: clinical studies. In: Psychiatric drugs (ed., Solomon, P.). (Grune and Stratton, New York, 1966.)

KLINE, N. S., AND LEHMANN, H. E. (eds.): Handbook of psychiatric treatment in medical practice. (Saunders, Philadelphia, 1962.)

KLINE, N. S., AND LEHMANN, H. E. (eds.): Psychopharmacology. International psychiatry clinics. (Little, Brown, Boston, 1965.)

KLINE, N. S., LOOMER, H. P., AND SAUNDERS, J. C. (1957): In: Remmen, E., *et al.*: Psychochemotherapy. (Western Medical Publications, Los Angeles, 1962.)

KLINE, N. S., AND SACKS, W.: Relief of depression within one day using a MAO inhibitor and intravenous 5-HTP. Amer. J. Psychiat., *120:* 274 (1963).

KLINE, N. S., SACKS, W., AND SIMPSON, G.: Further studies on one day treatment of depression with 5-HTP. Amer. J. Psychiat., *121:* 379 (1964).

KLINE, N. S., AND STANLEY, A. M.: Application of psychic energizers such as iproniazid (marsilid). In: Neuropharmacology (eds., Bradley, P., *et al.*). (Elsevier, Amsterdam, 1959.)

KUEHN, A., AND SCHALLEK, W.: Effects of diazepam (valium) on arousal responses from reticular formation and hypothalamus. Fed. Proc., *24:* 516 (1965).

LEITCH, A., AND SEAGER, C. P.: Trial of four antidepressant drugs. Psychopharmacologia (Berlin), *4:* 72 (1963).

LURIE, M. L., AND MACCAGNAMI, G. (1952): In: Deniker, P., and Lemperiere, T. Drug treatment of depression. In: Depression (ed., Davies, E. B.). (University Press, Cambridge, 1964.)

MARTIN, M. E.: A comparative trial of imipramine and phenelzine in the treatment of depression. Brit. J. Psychiat., *109:* 279 (1963).

MAXWELL, D. R., GRAY, W. R., AND TAYLOR, E. M. (1961): In: Biel, J. H. Some rationales for the development of antidepressant drugs. In: Molecular modification in drug design (ed., Gould, R. F.). (American Chemical Society, Washington, 1964.)

MAXWELL, R. A., PLUMMER, A. J., AND ROSS, S.: Response of normotensive and neurogenic hypertensive dogs to ganglionic blocking agents and reserpine. Fed. Proc., *15:* 457 (1956).

MAXWELL, R. A., *et al.*: Pharmacology of [2-(octahydro-1-azocinyl)-ethyl]-guanidine sulfate (SU-5864). J. Pharmacol. Exp. Ther., *128:* 22 (1960).

MCKENZIE, D., *et al.*: The effect of nicotinic acid amide on experimental tuberculosis of white mice. J. Lab. Clin. Med., *33:* 1249 (1948).

MORAN, J. F. (1962): In: Zirkle, C. L., and Kaiser, C.: Monoamine oxidase inhibitors. In: Psychopharmacological agents (ed., Gordon, M.). (Academic Press, New York, 1964.)

OSTOW, M.: Drugs in psychoanalysis and psychotherapy. (Basic Books, New York, 1962.)

OVERALL, J. E., *et al.*: Drug therapy in depression. Clin. Pharmacol. Ther., *3:* 16 (1962).

PEARSON, M. M.: Strecker's fundamentals of psychiatry. (Lippincott, Montreal, 1963.)

PLETSCHER, A.: Alteration of monoamine metabolism caused by drug acting on the CNS. In: Psychopharmacology frontiers (ed., Kline, N. S.). (Little, Brown, Toronto, 1959.)

PLETSCHER, A.: Monoaminoxydasehemmer (monoamine oxidase inhibitors). Deutsch. Med. Wschr., *86:* 647 (1961).

PLETSCHER, A.: Basic aspects of psychotropic drug action. Amer. J. Ment. Defic., *67:* 238 (1962).

PLETSCHER, A.: Pharmacology of antidepressant. In: Psychopharmacology (eds., Kline, N. S., and Lehmann, H. E.). (Little, Brown, Boston, 1965.)

PLETSCHER, A., SHORE, P. A., AND BRODIE, B. B.: Serotonin as a mediator of reserpine action in the brain. J. Pharmacol. Exp. Ther., *116:* 84 (1956).

PLETSCHER, A., *et al.* (1960): In: Biel, J. H., Horita, A., and Drukker, A. E.: Monoamine oxidase inhibitors (hydrazines). In: Psychopharmacological agents (ed., Gordon, M.). (Academic Press, New York, 1964.)

PÖLDINGER, W., AND SCHMIDLIN, P.: Index psychopharmacorum 1966. (Huber, Bern, 1966.)

REMMEN, E., *et al.*: Psychochemotherapy. (Western Medical Publications, Los Angeles, 1962.)

ROTHMAN, T.: Prelimary study of effectiveness of isocarboxazid in depressive syndromes. J. Neuropsychiat., *1:* 148 (1960).

SARGANT, W.: Antidepressant drugs and liver damage. Brit. Med. J., *2:* 806 (1963).

SARGANT, W., AND SLATER, E.: An introduction to physical methods of treatment in psychiatry. (Livingstone, Edinburgh and London, 1963.)

SCHALLEK, W., AND KUEHN, A.: Effects of psychotropic drugs on limbic system of cat. Proc. Soc. Exp. Biol. Med., *105:* 115 (1960).

SCHALLEK, W., AND KUEHN, A.: Effects of trimethadione, diphenylhydantoin, and chlordiazepoxide on after-discharges in the brain of the cat. Proc. Soc. Exp. Biol. Med., *112:* 813 (1963).

SCHALLEK, W., *et al.*: Effects of benzodiazepines on the central nervous system of the cat. Arch. Int. Pharmacodyn., *149:* 467 (1964).

SCHERBEL, A. L.: Clinical experience in treatment of over 2,000 cases with amine oxidase inhibitors. Dis. Nerv. Syst., *21:* 67 (1960).

SCHERBEL, A. L., *et al.* (1957): In: Remmen, E., *et al.*: Psychochemotherapy. (Western Medical Publications, Los Angeles, 1962.)

SELIKOFF, I. J., ROBITZAK, E. H., AND ORNSTEIN, G. G.: Treatment of pulmonary tuberculosis with hydrazine derivatives of isonicotinic acid. J.A.M.A., *150:* 973 (1952).

SMITH, J. A.: The treatment of depression with drugs. In: Depression, a Cambridge post-graduate medical course (ed., Davies, E. B.). (University Press, Cambridge, 1964.)

SOURKES, T. L.: Biochemistry of mental disease. (Harper and Row, New York, 1962.)

SOURKES, T. L., *et al.*: A clinical and metabolic study of dopa (3,4-dihydroxyphenylalanin) and methyldopa in Huntington's chorea. Psychiat. Neurol. (Basel), *149:* 7 (1965).

VALENTINE, M.: An introduction to psychiatry. (Livingstone, Edinburgh, 1962.)

VOTAVA, Z. E., *et al.* (eds.): Psychopharmacological methods. (Pergamon Press, Oxford, 1963.)

WEST, E. D., AND DALLY, P. J.: Effects of iproniazid in depressive syndromes. Brit. Med. J., *2:* 433 (1959).

ZELLER, E. A., *et al.*: Influence of isonicotinic acid hydrazine (INH) and 1-isonicotinyl-2-isopropyl hydrazine (IIH) on bacterial and mammalian enzymes. Experientia, *8:* 349 (1952).

ZIRKLE, C. L., AND KAISER, C.: Monoamine oxidase inhibitors (non-hydrazines). In: Psychopharmacological agents (ed., Gordon, M.). (Academic Press, New York, 1964.)

Sixteen

The Propanediols

A. BASIC DATA

1. Historical Aspects

Prior to the introduction of chlorpromazine and reserpine in the treatment of psychotic patients, mephenesin, a centrally acting muscle relaxant, was used extensively in the therapy of various psychopathological cases.

Mephenesin (3-*o*-toloxy-1,2-propanediol) was the result of the condensation of *o*-cresol with glycerine by Zivkovic in 1908. Almost 40 years passed before its prominent pharmacological properties—muscular relaxation and paralysis—were described by Berger and Bradley (1946). They recognized that, whereas the administration of small amounts of mephenesin resulted in tranquilization, muscular relaxation and a sleep-like condition (from which the animals could easily be aroused), larger doses produced ataxia, which was followed by paralysis.

Mephenesin was first used to produce muscular relaxation during general anesthesia and in the treatment of various neurological disorders. Its use in general anesthesia has been abandoned because of the occurrence of hemolysis and thrombosis (Berger and Ludwig, 1964). It is still used, however, as an adjunct in the treatment of Parkinsonism and for the control of involuntary movements (Berger and Schwartz, 1948; and Schlesinger *et al.*, 1948).

The usefulness of mephenesin in the treatment of psychiatric (reactive depressive and negativistic schizophrenic) patients was first recognized by Gammon and Churchill (1949). These therapeutic indications were extended by Schlan and Unna (1949) and Dixon *et al.* (1950), who were able to demonstrate the beneficial effects of mephenesin in psychoneurotic patients in general and in anxiety states in particular.

Since the rapid oxidation of mephenesin was considered to be a handicap clinically, attempts were made to produce compounds with similar or greater therapeutic effects but with a longer duration of action. This was achieved by structural modifications, firstly by trial and error, and secondly, on the basis of data acquired on mephenesin metabolism (Berger and Ludwig, 1964).

a. First Approach

The compounds which resulted from the first approach were phenaglycodol, mephenoxalone, metaxalone and promoxolane. Phenaglycodol [2-(*p*-chlorophenyl)-3-methyl-2,3-butanediol], a muscle relaxant, differed from mephenesin in its stronger anticonvulsant and weaker anxiolytic effects. It was found to be useful in the treatment of neurotic manifestations in the aged. Mephenoxalone [5-(*o*-methoxy-phenoxymethyl)-2-oxazolidinone], another muscle relaxant, differed from mephenesin in its stronger depressant action on the spontaneous activity of the mice and was also found to have psychotherapeutic effects (Settel, 1957; Carter, 1958; Martinez and Salas, 1960; Friend, 1961; and Furgiuele *et al.*, 1961).

On the other hand, metaxalone [5-(3,5-dimethylphenoxymethyl)-2-oxazolidinone], a centrally acting muscle relaxant, and promoxolane (2,2-diisopropyl-1,3-dioxolane-4-methanol), a muscle relaxant with parasympatholytic action, have no definite psychotropic action (Carroll *et al.*, 1961; Sontag, 1961; Carter, 1962; Kurtzke and Gylfe, 1962; and Lunsford, 1962).

b. Second Approach

Since the short duration of action of mephenesin was thought to be due to the rapid oxidation of its primary hydroxyl group (Riley and Berger, 1949), attempts were made to render the terminal hydroxyl group of the mephenesin molecule less accessible to enzymatic "attack" by esterifying it with a suitable acid. Consequently, substitutions and esterification (Ludwig and Piech, 1951) resulted in meprobamate (2-methyl-2-*n*-propyl-1,3-propanediol dicarbamate), a compound with basically similar but longer duration of action and a wider margin of safety. Although the drug's muscle relaxant and sedative properties were pharmacologically established in 1954, it was not until 1957 that its particular therapeutic action in psychoneurotic patients was shown (Berger, 1954; and Dixon, 1957).

2. Action Mechanism

a. First Hypothesis

The most widely accepted hypothesis on the action mechanism of propanediols in general and meprobamate in particular was formulated by Berger (1954). According to him, by selectively depressing the conductivity of the interneurons, *i.e.*, the neurons which connect the sensory input "lines" and the motor connections leading to the effector organs, meprobamate interferes with the tedious repetitions which are the physiological basis of psychological inflexibility and compulsiveness (characteristics of psychoneuroses).

b. Second Hypothesis

In another hypothesis the effect of propanediols on the thalamus has been implicated for the psychotropic properties of these drugs. This hypothesis is based on the assumption that, "since the ascending reticular activating system impinges on the thalamus and the thalamus also participates in the limbic system through connections with the hypothalamus via the mamillothalamic tract," a noxious stimulus appreciated at the thalamic level can evoke an undesirable emotional response with an accompanying increase in skeletal muscle tone. Thus propanediols were considered to interfere with these responses (Lear, 1966).

3. Structure and Activity

In the search for a more potent and even less toxic propanediol than meprobamate, extensive studies were directed toward discovering the changes through modifications of the meprobamate molecule.

Systematic exploratory work revealed that replacement or substitutions resulted in substances with distinctly different effects. Some of the numerous new compounds were carisoprodol, a muscle relaxant with analgesic properties; mebutamate, a centrally acting blood pressure lowering agent; ethinamate, a hypnotic agent; emylcamate and hydroxyphenamate, both muscle-relaxant and tension-relieving substances; and tybamate, an anxiolytic-sedative drug without dependency-producing effects (Berger, 1959; Melander, 1959; Berger *et al.*, 1960; Hubarta and Hecht, 1961; Young, 1961; Sifferd and Braitberg, 1962; Margolin *et al.*, 1965; and Feldman and Mulinos, 1966).

The structural formula of meprobamate (2-methyl-2-*n*-propyl-1,3-propanediol dicarbamate) is shown in Figure 16*a*.

Carisoprodol (*n*-isopropyl-2-methyl-2-propyl-1,3-propanediol dicarbamate) is obtained from meprobamate by replacing a single hydrogen atom on one of the carbamyl nitrogens with an isopropyl group. Mebutamate (2-methyl-2-*sec*-butyl-1,3-propanediol dicarbamate) is obtained by replacing a single hydrogen atom on the propyl side chain with a methyl group.

Whereas emylcamate (1-ethyl-1-methylpropyl carbamate), hydroxyphenamate (2-hydroxy-2-phenylbutyl carbamate) and ethinamate (1-ethyl-cyclohexane carboxamide) are structurally only distantly related to meprobamate, tybamate (2-methyl-2-propyltrimethylene butylcarbamate carbamate) is structurally close to the parent substance.

Of the various compounds structurally related to meprobamate, the most important psychopharmacologically is tybamate, a substance which shares the sedative, anticonvulsant and muscle relaxant effects of the parent drug but which differs from meprobamate by its ability to suppress the EEG activation induced by LSD_{25} in rabbits; by its antagonism of the rise of blood pressure produced by serotonin in dogs; and by the absence of a stimulatory effect on the microsomal enzymes of the liver (Berger *et al.*, 1964). These differences were attributed to the higher lipid solubility of tybamate. The relatively short half-life of tybamate (approximately 4 hours) in contradistinction to meprobamate (which has a half-life of approximately 11 hours) is considered to be the reason for not attaining truly high plasma levels. This seems to protect against the development of a withdrawal syndrome when drug administration is abruptly discontinued (Shelton and Hollister, 1967).

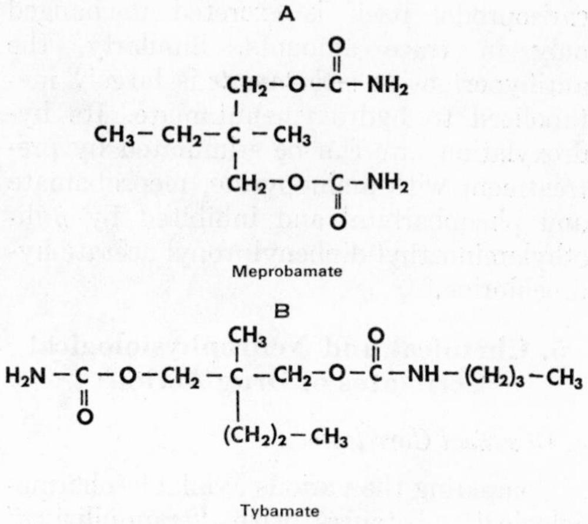

4. Metabolism

a. Meprobamate

Orally administered meprobamate is readily absorbed from the gastrointestinal tract and reaches peak plasma levels 2 hours after ingestion (Hoffman and Ludwig, 1959). Thereafter a steady decline in blood concentrations (half-life, 11 hours) and an increase in body tissue concentrations (with a maximum in the soft organ tissues and a minimum in the brain and fat tissues) occur. About 10 per cent of the total amount of the drug is excreted in the urine unchanged within 24 hours (Berger, 1954; Agranoff *et al.*, 1957; and Walkenstein *et al.*, 1958). Most of the remaining 90 per cent of the drug is also eliminated in the urine over the same time period. The metabolized products are an oxidized derivative, hydroxymeprobamate (a true detoxification product), and a glucuronic acid conjugate (Berger, 1954; Douglas and Ludwig, 1959; and Ludwig *et al.*, 1961).

While there are no interspecies differences in meprobamate metabolism, an increased meprobamate catabolism was shown after the administration of aminopyrine, barbital, chlorpromazine, orphenadrine, phenaglycodol, phenobarbital, phenylbutazone and meprobamate itself (Conney and Burns, 1960; Kato, 1960; Kato and Vassanelli, 1962; and Douglas *et al.*, 1963). That meprobamate increases its own metabolic inactivation is considered to play an important role in the development of tolerance to this drug (Phillips *et al.*, 1962).

A

Meprobamate

B

Tybamate

FIG. 16. *a*, Meprobamate. *b*, Tybamate

b. Tybamate

Tybamate is also readily absorbed from the gastrointestinal tract and reaches peak plasma levels in 6½ hours. Thereafter a sharp decline in blood concentration (half-life, 4 hours) and an increase in body tissue concentrations (with a maximum in the liver and the kidneys and a minimum in the brain) occur. About 7.5 per cent of the total amount of the drug is excreted in the urine unchanged within 24 hours, 60.5 per cent as hydroxytybamate, 30.3 per cent as hydroxymeprobamate and 2.2 per cent as meprobamate (Douglas *et al.*, 1964).

c. Others

Among the various other substances of this group, the analgesic *carisoprodol* is largely metabolized to a compound identified as hydroxycarisoprodol. Hydroxymeprobamate and small quantities of meprobamate also occur in the urine, while carisoprodol itself is excreted unchanged only in trace amounts. Similarly, the antihypertensive *mebutamate* is largely metabolized to hydroxymebutamate. Its hydroxylation rate can be stimulated by pretreatment with aminopyrine, meprobamate and phenobarbital and inhibited by β-diethylaminoethyl-diphenylpropyl acetate-hydrochloride.

5. Chemical and Neurophysiological Correlates of Drug Action

a. Chemical Correlates

Comparing the various available pharmacological substances with "tranquilizing" properties, Berger (1957) distinguished between two distinctly different groups: the "autonomic suppressants" and the "central relaxants." The "autonomic suppressants," which comprise the phenothiazines, reserpine and diphenylmethanes, are characterized by their antagonism to adrenaline, acetylcholine, histamine and serotonin, *i.e.*, substances which regulate certain functions of the autonomic nervous system. On the other hand, the "central relaxants," which comprise mephenesin, meprobamate and related compounds, do not affect autonomic functions and are characteristically free of any adrenolytic, anticholinergic and antihistaminic actions. However, by accelerating the breakdown of acetylcholine at the synaptic junctions, they depress multineuronal reflexes.

There is only limited information available on the chemical correlates of the action of propanediol drugs. Among these, the antiserotonin activity of tybamate is of psychopharmacological importance. This was first shown in anesthetized dogs in which tybamate—like LSD_{25} and also chlorpromazine—counteracted the pressor response (hypertension) induced by serotonin. Another characteristic of tybamate is its high plasma protein binding property. Both of these qualities—antiserotonin effects and plasma protein binding property—are absent in meprobamate (Berger *et al.*, 1964).

b. Neurophysiological Correlates

i. Spinal Cord. Propanediols exert a marked blocking action on the "interneurons." This was first demonstrated at the spinal cord level by Berger (1954). It was shown that under the influence of *meprobamate* the knee jerk, which is a monosynaptic reflex, is virtually unaffected, whereas the flexor and the crossed extensor reflex, which have one or more interneurones interposed between the afferent and efferent limbs of the reflex arc, are decreased or abolished (Abdulian *et al.*, 1957; Berger, 1955, 1957; and Wilson, 1958).

Although meprobamate has little or no effect on the normal patellar reflex, it normalizes a hyperactive and exaggerated knee jerk (Berger and Ludwig, 1964).

An effect similar to that of meprobamate was indicated under the influence of *tybamate*. When given intravenously to chloralosed cats in a dosage of 20 mg./kg. the latter substance blocked or diminished the flexor reflex of the hind limb while it did not affect the patellar reflex (Berger *et al.*, 1964).

A selective inhibition of the spinal-vasoconstrictor tracts was shown under the influence of mebutamate. This could clearly be differentiated from its action on the spinal-motor tracts affecting skeletal muscles (Margolin *et al.*, 1963).

ii. Medulla Oblongata. Mebutamate has been shown to reduce the activity of the stimulated vasomotor areas of the medulla oblongata (Berger and Margolin, 1961; and Margolin *et al.*, 1963).

iii. Brain Stem Reticular Formation. After meprobamate administration, the response of the cerebral cortex to reticular stimulation remains unimpaired. Hence it was assumed that the activity of the brain stem reticular formation is unaffected by this drug (Berger *et al.*, 1957; Hendley *et al.*, 1957, and Kletzkin and Berger, 1959). Gangloff (1959), however, demonstrated that in the effective (and nontoxic) dosage range meprobamate exerts a slight stimulating influence on the brain stem reticular formation structures.

iv. Thalamus. One of the most characteristic effects of meprobamate administration is on the thalamic structures. By implanted electrode techniques it was shown that in low dosages meprobamate decreases the spontaneous electrical activity of the thalamus (and of the caudate nucleus). This was manifested by a slowing of frequency and an increase of voltage (Berger, 1957; Baird *et al.*, 1957; and Hendley *et al.*, 1954, 1955).

It has been noted that although thalamic recruiting responses under the influence of meprobamate are "depressed," they remain unchanged under the influence of tybamate and become enhanced when carisoprodol is given (Berger *et al.*, 1964).

v. Limbic Lobe Structures. The duration of hippocampal seizures induced by electrical stimulation of the fornix was found to be sharply reduced under the influence of tybamate and meprobamate, whereas they remained unaffected after carisoprodol administration. On the other hand, after-discharges are interfered with by carisoprodol and only to a considerably lesser extent by tybamate. Hippocampal after-discharges are unaffected by meprobamate (Berger *et al.*, 1964).

vi. Cerebral Cortex. Psychoactive propanediols in low doses have no direct effect on the cerebral cortex. A decrease of the high frequency components and a slight increase in the amplitude of the slower waves occur only with moderately high doses. Spindles may appear after the administration of high doses (Berger, 1957; and Berger *et al.*, 1964).

6. Behavioral Pharmacology

a. Animal Studies

Psychoactive propanediols induce muscular relaxation in mice and rats which at first leads to the loss of the righting reflex and later on to flaccid paralysis. The same substances induce a slight hind limb ataxia in dogs, which is replaced by flaccid paralysis and prostration. Under these conditions the dog appears to be asleep, but it can be easily aroused in spite of its gross locomotor impairment. It has been noted that all these manifestations are present in a lower milligram per kilogram dosage ratio with tybamate than with meprobamate (Berger *et al.*, 1964).

One of the most characteristic actions of this group of substances is their taming effect, which has been described in vicious monkeys and aggressive cats (Berger, 1954; and Hendley *et al.*, 1954). It has been noted that the taming effect is of a somewhat shorter duration of action with meprobamate than with tybamate.

The dose required for taming varies from animal to animal. This is probably why Gross and Weiskrantz (1961) were unable to obtain taming in rhesus monkeys. On the other hand, Hunt (1957) succeeded in counteracting the irritability and aggressiveness of rats produced by septal lesions. Although psychoactive propanediols in general have no particular effect on conditioned responses, Hess (1957) was able to control fear and avoidance behavior in water fowl with meprobamate.

Other characteristic effects of psychoactive propanediols are the prolongation (synergism) of the duration of hexobarbital-induced anesthesia and the protection (antagonism) from electroshock-, pentetrazol- and strychnine-induced convulsions in mice. As a seizure antagonist, meprobamate proved to be more potent than tybamate.

b. Human Studies

In human pharmacological studies, even in relatively low 400-mg. doses, meprobamate decreased galvanic skin responses to emotionally loaded verbal stimuli but also produced an altered performance on a simulated driving skill test (Loomis and West, 1958). In higher doses (800 mg.) there is a prolongation of visual-motor (also audio-motor) reaction time together with an interference with motor coordination and an impairment of learning tasks (Kornetsky, 1958).

Paterson (1963) reported that, under the influence of these drugs, the frustration threshold is raised, providing a favorable condition for maintaining performance under stressful conditions. This was supported by Lehmann (1968). He demonstrated in an original experiment that the frustration threshold is increased by meprobamate in a conflictual situation.

B. CLINICAL DATA

1. Indications and Contraindications

a. Indications

i. Nonpsychiatric. Propanediols are successfully administered in various pathological conditions. Besides the psychiatric indications, meprobamate is frequently prescribed in the treatment of musculoskeletal disorders in various orthopedic and rheumatic conditions; in the treatment of certain neurological diseases such as cerebral palsy; and in petit mal epilepsy (Tybring, 1957; Perlstein, 1956; Ayd, 1957; Baird and Borofsky, 1957; Eisenberg and Neviaser, 1957; Gillette, 1957; Hermann *et al.*, 1957; Livingstone and Pauli, 1957; Millen, 1957; Schlesinger, 1957; and Sparup, 1957).

Of the other analogues, mebutamate is used for the control of hypertension (Duarte *et al.*, 1960; and Campbell and Kaye, 1962) and carisoprodol for the symptomatic management of pain, muscle spasm and stiffness in a variety of inflammatory, traumatic and degenerative musculoskeletal conditions (Cooper and Epstein, 1959; Friedman, 1957; Gammon and Tucker, 1959; Proctor, 1959; Spears, 1959; Trimpi, 1959, and Wein, 1959).

ii. Psychiatric. *α. Psychoneuroses.* The primary indication for psychoactive propanediol drugs in general and meprobamate in particular is in the various psychoneuroses in which psychic tension and anxiety are associated with irritability and "hyperemotionalism" (Borrus, 1955; Dickel *et al.*, 1957; Gardner, 1957; Hollister *et al.*, 1956; Lemere, 1955; McClendon, 1958; Moyer *et al.*, 1958; Osinski, 1957; Rickels *et al.*, 1959; and Tucker, 1957). Other indications are tension headaches (Blumenthal and Fuchs, 1957; Dixon, 1957; and Friedman, 1957) and insomnia (Dixon, 1957; Lamphier, 1958; Lasagna, 1956; and Prigot *et al.*, 1957).

More recently, the effects of tybamate in various psychoneurotic conditions, including chronic anxiety states, have been systematically explored. Tybamate was found to be significantly superior therapeutically to an inactive placebo (Seeherman, 1964; and Rickels *et al.*, 1967) and more effective in cases of severe anxiety than meprobamate (Chieffi, 1965), particularly in patients with a marked degree of somatization (Raab, *et al.*, 1964). In one comparative study tybamate (750 mg. daily) resulted in a complete disappearance (or marked improvement) of psychoneurotic manifestations in 42 per cent of the patients. Meprobamate (1200 mg. daily) and chlordiazepoxide (30 mg. daily) had the same effect in 40 per cent and 31 per cent, respectively (Vazuka and McLaughlin, 1965).

β. Functional Psychoses. Neither schizophrenia nor manic-depressive psychosis is an indication for propanediol treatment. There is some evidence that the addition of meprobamate and, more recently, of tybamate to antipsychotic or antidepressant treatment may have a beneficial effect on the restlessness and agitation of certain depressive cases (Graffagnino *et al.*, 1957; Hollister *et al.*, 1957; McLaughlin, 1957; Pennington, 1957; and Tucker and Wilensky, 1957).

γ. Chronic Brain Syndromes. Chresrow *et al.* (1965) demonstrated a significant overall improvement and a beneficial action on insomnia, agitation, restlessness and tension as well as on anxiety, depression and behavioral disorders in a placebo-controlled, double-blind study with tybamate conducted on institutionalized male geriatric patients. When compared with meprobamate, Stern (1964) has shown that tybamate produced significantly greater improvement in agitation, anorexia, anxiety, behavioral disorder, depression, insomnia, lack of cooperation, restlessness and tension.

δ. Other Conditions. Meprobamate has been successfully used for the relief of premenstrual tension (as well as pre- and postoperative tension); in the treatment of behavior disorders in children; in the control of chronic alcoholism; and as an adjunct in various cardiac, gastrointestinal, dermatological and allergic conditions (Berger and Ludwig, 1964).

b. Contraindications

The only absolute contraindication to psychoactive propanediol administration is a history of allergic or idiosyncratic reactions to previous administration of these drugs. Caution should be exercised in prescribing these drugs for patients who have previously been addicted to alcohol, narcotics or barbiturates.

To date, no teratogenic or carcinogenic effect attributed to propanediol drug administration has been reported. It has been noted, however, that propanediols trespass the placental barrier (Chambon, 1959).

2. Therapy Alone and in Combination With Other Treatments

a. *Propanediols Alone*

i. Dosage. Although the therapeutic dosage range of each psychoactive propanediol drug differs slightly, it generally holds true that, in the treatment of psychoneurotic patients, 1000 and 2000 mg. daily are the usual therapeutically effective dosages for any of the commercially available compounds. The initial normal adult dosage of meprobamate is 1200 to 1600 mg. (1050 to 1400 mg. of tybamate) for psychoneurotic cases and for the symptomatic relief of anxiety and tension in various psychiatric, general medical or surgical disorders. The maximum recommended dosage of meprobamate is 2400 mg. and of tybamate, 3000 mg. daily, although they have been used in much higher doses without untoward effects. The recommended adult dosage of carisoprodol is 1400 to 1600 mg. and of mebutamate, 900 to 1200 mg.

ii. Treatment Procedure. The most frequently used clinical procedure is continuous treatment. As a starting dose, the average recommended daily amount is prescribed, and this then is adjusted, increased or decreased depending on individual need and tolerance.

The duration of therapy depends upon the condition being treated, but it should continue at least until symptomatic relief is obtained. There are indications, however, that the incidence of dependency on meprobamate increases with the time of drug administration (Billig and Burris, 1957; and Eitinger *et al.*, 1960). Where excessive dosage of meprobamate administration has continued over several months, sudden withdrawal of the drug may precipitate anxiety, insomnia or anorexia (Bulla *et al.*, 1959; and Hollister and Glazener, 1960); or more severe withdrawal reactions such as vomiting ataxia, tremors and muscle twitchings (Ewing and Haizlip, 1958); and occasionally cerebral seizures, particularly in patients with a preexistent CNS abnormality (Barsa and Kline, 1956; Essig and Ainslie, 1957; Ewing and Fullilove, 1957; Greaves and West, 1957; Jonsson, 1959; Lemere, 1956; Mohr and Mead, 1958; Phillips *et al.*, 1957; and Rawitt, 1959).

Animal studies suggested no dependency to carisoprodol or to tybamate (Margolin *et al.*, 1965). This was verified in man for carisoprodol by Fraser *et al.* (1961) and for tybamate by Feldman and Mulinos (1966) and also by Shelton and Hollister (1967).

b. *Propanediols in Combination with Other Treatments*

Psychoactive propanediols can be combined with various other treatments, psychological and pharmacological. Among the propanediol-containing drug combinations frequently used are equagesic (meprobamate, 200 mg.; ethoheptazine citrate, 75 mg.; and acetylsalicylic acid, 250 mg.) for the relief of pain associated with muscle tension and anxiety; equanitrate (meprobamate, 200 mg.; and pentaerythritol tetranitrate, 10 or 20 mg.) for the prevention of angina pectoris in cases of coronary insufficiency; and equazine (meprobamate, 200 mg.; and promazine hydrochloride, 25 mg.) for the symptomatic control of tension, anxiety and agitation.

3. Adverse Reactions and Their Treatment

a. *Adverse Reactions*

Serious adverse reactions are rare in the course of treatment with psychoactive propanediol preparations (Berger and Ludwig, 1964). Two major areas of side-effects are the neuropsychiatric and idiosyncratic (or allergic) reactions (Lear, 1966).

i. Neuropsychiatric. One of the most frequent side-effects is drowsiness, which has been attributed to tybamate administration. In isolated cases the latter drug induced euphoria, while in others it induced a feeling of unreality or panic or a confusional state. Both meprobamate and tybamate may produce ataxia when given in high dosages, and even in medium dosages they may interfere with motor coordination (and consequently with driving skill) when combined with other central nervous system depressant drugs. Grand mal seizures have been described when psychoactive propanediols were administered together with psychoactive phenothiazine preparations (Barsa and Saunders, 1963).

ii. Idiosyncratic or Allergic. These include angioneurotic edema, urticaria, maculopapular rash and bullous dermatitis, (Charkes, 1958; Dixon, 1957; and Selling 1956); nonthrombocytopenic purpura, ecchymoses and peripheral edema (Carmel and Dannenberg, 1956; and Witherspoon, 1957); and fever, fainting spells, bronchial spasm, hypotensive crises, anuria, anaphylaxis, stomatitis and proctitis (Adlin *et al.*, 1958; Bernstein and Klotz, 1957; Blumberg *et al.*, 1959; Brachfeld and Bell, 1959; Charkes, 1958; Holubek *et al.*, 1957; Riising, 1957; and Selling, 1956).

iii. Others. Occasional cases of headache, dizziness, vertigo and paresthesia; nausea, dry mouth, glossitis and gastrointestinal disturbances; and flushing and tachycardia have been reported in the course of tybamate treatment. Agranulocytosis, thrombocytopenic purpura and aplastic anemia have occurred in the course of meprobamate administration, but only when it was given in combination with other drugs (Cummings and Zeluff, 1959; Curran and Barabas, 1961; Meeroff *et al.*, 1959; Meyer *et al.*, 1957; and Zweifler, 1960).

Suicidal attempts with meprobamate have resulted in drowsiness, lethargy, stupor, ataxia, coma, shock and vasomotor and respiratory collapse (Allen and Black, 1956; Fisher, 1957; Hiestand, 1956; Jacobziner and Raybin, 1958, 1959, 1960; Jonsson, 1959; Shane and Hirsch, 1956; Stevens, 1960; Woodward, 1957). No case of tybamate overdosage has yet been reported.

b. Treatment of Adverse Reactions

Treatment of adverse effects is symptomatic. Drowsiness or ataxia respond to reduction in dosage or, if persistent, to the administration of central nervous system stimulants, *e.g.*, amphetamines. Discontinuation of propanediol therapy is the treatment of choice in idiosyncratic or allergic reactions. In these cases, the administration of epinephrine, antihistamines and occasionally hydrocortisone is useful.

SUMMARY

Berger and Bradley (1946), in the course of screening a large number of alpha-substituted glycerol ethers, noted a "significant muscle relaxant and strychnine antagonism without severe embarrassment of respiration" with some of the compounds. Mephenesin was particularly effective in this respect (and also exerted a calming, tranquilizing effect) at dose levels which did not induce narcosis. The brief duration of action, because of its rapid oxidation, limited the clinical value of mephenesin and led to systematic exploratory work which resulted in a number of propanediol substances in which the oxidation of the hydroxyl groups was delayed by converting them into carbamino radicals (Lear, 1966).

Mephenesin was used for a short time in the treatment of numerous psychiatric conditions, including depressions, schizophrenias and psychoneuroses. Although it was one of the first substances used in relieving tension and anxiety without clouding consciousness, its psychiatric applications, as time passed, gradually became more and more restricted. Finally, mephenesin was almost entirely replaced by more potent and less troublesome drugs.

Of the various substances obtained by modifying the basic structure of mephenesin, phenaglycodol and mephenoxalone are used in the treatment of various psychiatric conditions. The consensus is that they are somewhat inferior to meprobamate in their therapeutic effects in the psychoneuroses, although there are indications that phenaglycodol has a definite value in the control of some of the psychopathological manifestations of geriatric cases.

Clinically, the most widely used drug in this category is meprobamate, primarily indicated for various psychoneurotic disorders in which psychic tension prevails. There is an increasing interest in tybamate, which seems to possess a similar range of therapeutic activity but is without dependency-producing properties. Among the other carbamates, emylcamate and hydroxyphenamate are occasionally prescribed in the treatment of various psychosomatic conditions.

Compounds structurally related to meprobamate are ethinamate, which is used as a hypnotic with particular effectiveness as a sleep inducer (Matthews *et al.*, 1964); mebutamate, which is used as an antihypertensive drug; and carisoprodol, which is used as an analgesic.

The propanediol derivatives were among the first of the various groups of psychoactive substances successfully used in the treatment of psychoneurotic patients. Their exact place, however, among the psychotherapeutic substances in general and anxiolytic sedatives in particular has still not been clearly established.

REFERENCES

Abdulian, D. H., Martin, W. R., and Unna, K. R.: Effects of interneuron depressants on inhibition and facilitation of the patellar reflex. Fed. Proc., *16:* 277 (1957).

Adlin, E. V., *et al.*: Fatal reaction following ingestion of meprobamate. Arch. Intern. Med. (Chicago), *102:* 484 (1958).

Agranoff, B. W., Bradley, R. M., and Axelrod, J.: The termination and the physiological disposition of meprobamate. Proc. Soc. Exp. Biol. Med., *96:* 261 (1957).

Allen, A. G., and Black, A. V.: Near fatal case of intoxication with meprobamate, treated with electro-stimulation and levarterenol. Ohio Med. J., *52:* 1303 (1956).

Ayd, F. J.: A clinical report on benactyzine hydrochloride. New Eng. J. Med., *257:* 669 (1957).

Baird, H. W., and Borofsky, L. G.: Infantile myoclonic seizures. J. Pediat., *50:* 332 (1957).

Baird, H. W., *et al.*: The effect of meprobamate on the basal ganglia. Ann. N.Y. Acad. Sci., *67:* 873 (1957).

Barsa, J. A., and Kline, N. S.: Use of meprobamate in the treatment of psychotic patients. Amer. J. Psychiat., *112:* 1023 (1956).

Barsa, J. A., and Saunders, J. C.: Tybamate, a new tranquilizer. Amer. J. Psychiat., *120:* 492 (1963).

Berger, F. M.: The use of cerium oxalate to reduce incidence of emesis in deep insulin therapy. Amer. J. Psychiat., *106:* 865 (1950).

Berger, F. M.: The pharmacological properties of 2-methyl-2-N-propyl-1,3 propanediol dicarbamate (Miltown), a new interneuronal blocking agent. J. Pharmacol. Exp. Ther., *104:* 468 (1952).

Berger, F. M. (1954): In: Berger, F. M., and Ludwig, B. J.: Meprobamate and related compounds. In: Psychopharmacological agents (ed., Gordon, M.). (Academic Press, New York, 1964.)

Berger, F. M.: The pharmacological properties of 2-methyl-2-N-propyl-1,3 propanediol dicarbamate (Miltown), a new interneuronal blocking agent. J. Pharmacol. Exp. Ther., *112:* 412 (1954).

Berger, F. M.: Miltown, a long acting mephenesin-like drug. Fed. Proc., *14:* 318 (1955).

Berger, F. M.: Metabolic reactivity of brain and liver mitochondria towards chlorpromazine. J. Neurochem., *2:* 30 (1957).

Berger, F. M.: The chemistry and mode of action of tranquillizing drugs. Ann. N.Y. Acad. Sci., *67:* 685 (1957).

Berger, F. M.: The muscle-relaxant and analgesic properties of carisoprodol. In: The pharmacology and clinical usefulness of carisoprodol (ed., Miller, J. G.). (Wayne State University Press, Detroit, 1959.)

Berger, F. M.: Classification of psychoactive drugs according to their chemical structures and sites of action. In: Drugs and Behavior (eds., Uhr, L., and Miller, J. G.). (Wiley, New York, 1960.)

Berger, F. M., and Bradley, W.: The pharmacological properties of α:β dihydroxy-γ-(2 methylphenoxy)-propane (myanesin). Brit. J. Pharmacol., *1:* 265 (1946).

Berger, F. M., Kletzkin, M., and Margolin, S.: Pharmacological properties of a new tranquillizing agent, 2-methyl-2 propyltrimethylene butylcarbamate carbamate (tybamate). Med. Exp. (Basel), *10:* 327 (1964).

Berger, F. M., and Ludwig, B. J.: Meprobamate and related compounds. In: Psychopharmacological agents (ed., Gordon, M.). (Academic Press, New York, 1964.)

Berger, F. M., and Margolin, S.: A centrally acting blood pressure lowering agent, (W-583). Fed. Proc., *20:* 113 (1961).

Berger, F. M., and Schwartz, R. P.: Oral myanesin in treatment of spactic and hyperkinetic disorders. J.A.M.A., *137:* 772 (1948).

Berger, F. M., *et al.*: The action of tranquillizers on brain potentials and serotonin. Ann. N.Y. Acad. Sci., *66:* 686 (1957).

Berger, F. M., *et al.*: The pharmacological properties of 2-methyl-2-sec-butyl-1,3-propanediol dicarbamate (mebutamate W-583), a new centrally acting blood pressure lowering agent. J. Pharmacol. Exp. Ther., *134:* 356 (1961).

Berger, F. M., Klotzkin, M., and Margolin, S.: The history, chemistry and pharmacology of carisoprodol. Ann. N.Y. Acad. Sci., *86:* 90 (1960).

BERNSTEIN, C,. AND KLOTZ, S. D.: Allergenicity of tranquillizing drugs. J.A.M.A., *163:* 930 (1957).

BILLIG, O., AND BURRIS, B. L.: Habituation to tranquillizing drugs. J. Tenn. Med. Ass., *50:* 406 (1957).

BLUMBERG, A. G., ROSETT, H. L., AND DOBROW, A.: Severe hypotensive reactions following meprobamate overdosage. Ann. Intern. Med., *51:* 607 (1959).

BLUMENTHAL, L. S., AND FUCHS, M.: Definitive diagnosis and treatment of headache. Southern Med. J., *50:* 1491 (1957).

BORRUS, J. C.: Study of effect of Miltown (2-methyl-2-N-propyl-1,3 propanediol dicarbamate) on psychiatric states. J.A.M.A., *157:* 1596 (1955).

BRACHFELD, J., AND BELL, E. C.: Stomatitis and proctitis as manifestations of meprobamate idiosyncrasy. J.A.M.A., *169:* 1321 (1959).

BULLA, J. D., EWING, J. A., AND BUFFALOE, W. J.: Further controlled studies of meprobamate. Amer. Practit., *10:* 1961 (1959).

CAMPBELL, D. K., AND KAYE, M.: Study of a new antihypertensive agent, (W-583). Appl. Ther., *4:* 143 (1962).

CARMEL, W. J., AND DANNENBERG, T.: Nonthrombocytopenic purpura due to Miltown. New Eng. J. Med., *255:* 770 (1956).

CARROLL, M. N., *et al.*: The pharmacology of a new oxazolidinone with anticonvulsant, analgetic and muscle relaxant properties. Arch. Int. Pharmacodyn., *130:* 280 (1961).

CARTER, C. H.: Phenaglycodol, an anticonvulsant effective in grand mal and petit mal seizures. Antibiot. Med. Clin. Ther., *5:* 675 (1958).

CARTER, C. H.: A new muscle relaxant. Dis. Nerv. Syst., *23:* 98 (1962).

CHAMBON, M.: Determination of procalmadiol in the blood. Therapie, *14:* 771 (1959).

CHARKES, N. D.: Meprobamate idiosyncrasy. Arch. Intern. Med. (Chicago), *102:* 584 (1958).

CHESROW, E. J., *et al.*: Blind study of oxazepam in the management of geriatric patients with behavioral problems. Clin. Med., *72:* 1001 (1965).

CHIEFFI, M. A.: Two-part, double-blind study of the antineurotic action of tybamate. Dis. Nerv. Syst., *26:* 369 (1965).

CONNEY, A. H., AND BURNS, J. J.: Biochemical, pharmacological considerations of zoxazolamine and chlorzoxazone metabolism. Ann. N.Y. Acad. Sci., *86:* 167 (1960).

COOPER, C. D., AND EPSTEIN, J. H.: The clinical evaluation of soma by double-blind technique. In: The pharmacology and clinical usefulness of carisopradol (ed., Miller, J. G.). (Wayne State University Press, Detroit, 1959.)

CUMMINGS, H. W., AND ZELUFF, G. W.: Thrombocytopenic purpura. Med. Rec. Ann. (Houston), *52:* 162 (1959).

CURRAN, T. P., AND BARABAS, E.: Agranulocytosis after imipramine and meprobamate. Brit. Med. J., *5221:* 257 (1961).

DICKEL, H. K., *et al.*: Electromyographic studies of meprobamate and the working anxious patient. Ann. N.Y. Acad. Sci., *67:* 780 (1957).

DIXON, H. H., *et al.*: Clinical observations on tolserol in handling anxiety tension states. Amer. J. Med. Sci., *220:* 23 (1950).

DIXON, N. M.: Meprobamate, a clinical evaluation. Ann. N.Y. Acad. Sci., *67:* 772 (1957).

DIXON, W. E.: On the mode of action of drugs. Med. Mag. Lond., *16:* 454 (1957).

DOUGLAS, J. F., AND LUDWIG, B. J.: Studies on meprobamate metabolism. Fed. Proc., *18:* 385 (1959).

DOUGLAS, J. F., LUDWIG, B. J., AND SMITH, N.: Studies on the metabolism of meprobamate. Proc. Soc. Exp. Biol. Med., *112:* 436 (1963).

DOUGLAS, J. F., *et al.*: Distribution, absorption and metabolic fate of tybamate. Fed. Proc., *23:* 489 (1964).

DURATE, C., *et al.*: Observations on the antihypertensive effectiveness of a new propanediol dicarbamate (W-583). Curr. Ther. Res., *2:* 148 (1960).

EISENBERG, S. H., AND NEVIASER, J. S.: The use of meprobamate in the treatment of skeletal muscle spasm. Ann. N.Y. Acad. Sci., *67:* 853 (1957).

EITINGER, L., RETTERSTOL, N., AND SUND, A.: Habituation and addiction to meprobamate. T. Norsk. Laegeforen., *80:* 914 (1960).

ESSIG, C. F., AND AINSLIE, J. D.: Addiction to meprobamate. J.A.M.A., *164:* 1382 (1957).

EWING, J. A., AND FULLILOVE, R. E.: Addiction to meprobamate. New Eng. J. Med., *257:* 76 (1957).

EWING, J. A., AND HAIZLIP, T. M.: A controlled study of the habit forming propensities of meprobamate. Amer. J. Psychiat., *114:* 835 (1958).

FELDMAN, H. S., AND MULINOS, M.: Lack of addiction from high doses of tybamate. J. New Drugs, *6:* 354 (1966).

FISHER, H. W.: Coma following meprobamate. Hawaii Med. J., *17:* 146 (1957).

FRASER, H. F., ESSIG, C. F., AND WOLBACH, A. B.: Evaluation of carisoprodol and phenyramidol for addictiveness. Bull. Narcotics, *13:* 1 (1961).

FREEDMAN, A. M.: Discussion of L. Eisenberg's paper "Basic issues in drug research with children." In: Child research in psychopharmacology (ed., Fisher, S.). (Charles C Thomas, Springfield, 1959.)

FRIEDMAN, A. P.: Treatment of chronic headaches with meprobamate. Ann. N.Y. Acad. Sci., *67:* 822 (1957).

FRIEND, D. G.: Tranquillizers. III. Meprobamate, phenaglycodal and chlordiazepoxide. New Eng. J. Med., *264:* 870 (1961).

FURGIUELE, A. R., *et al.* Evaluation of certain psychopharmacological compounds. J. Pharm. Sci., *50:* 252 (1961).

GAMMON, G. D., AND CHURCHILL, J. A.: Effects of myanesin upon the central nervous system. Amer. J. Med. Sci., *217:* 143 (1949).

GAMMON, G. D., AND TUCKER, S.: Observations on the use of carisoprodol in various clinical conditions with objective measurement of spasticity. In: The pharmacology and clinical usefulness of carisoprodol (ed., Miller, J. G.). (Wayne State University Press, Detroit, 1959.)

GANGLOFF, H.: Effect of phenaglycodol and meprobamate on spontaneous brain activity, evoked EEG arousal and recruitment in the cat. J. Pharmacol. Exp. Ther., *126:* 30 (1959).

GARDNER, A.: Meprobamate—a clinical study. Amer. J. Psychiat., *114:* 524 (1957).

GILLETTE, H. E.: The effect of meprobamate on cerebral palsy. Ann. N.Y. Acad. Sci., *67:* 859 (1957).

GRAFFAGNINO, P. N., *et al.*: Emotional disorders treated with meprobamate and promazine. Conn. Med., *21:* 1047 (1957).

GREAVES, D. C., AND WEST, L. J.: Convulsions following withdrawal from meprobamate. Report of two cases. Southern Med. J., *50:* 1534 (1957).

GROSS, C. G., AND WEISKRANTZ, L. (1961): In: Berger, F. M., and Ludwig, B. J.: Meprobamate and related compounds. In: Psychopharmacological agents (ed., Gordon, M.). (Academic Press, New York, 1964.)

GUPTA, J. S., *et al.*: A preliminary note on the excretion of Rauwolfia total alkaloids in urine. Indian J. Med. Res., *38:* 67 (1950).

HENDLEY, C. D., *et al.*: Effect of 2-methyl-2-N-propyl-1,3-propanediol dicarbamate (Miltown) on central nervous system. Proc. Soc. Exp. Biol. Med., *87:* 608 (1954).

HENDLEY, C. D., *et al.*: Effect of 2-methyl-2-N-propyl-1,3-propanediol dicarbamate (Miltown) on electrical activity of the brain. Fed. Proc., *14:* 351 (1955).

HENDLEY, C. D., *et al.*: Effect of meprobamate on electrical activity of thalamus and other subcortical areas. In: Tranquillizing drugs (ed., Himwich, H. E.). (A.A.A.S., Washington, 1957.)

HENDLEY, C. D., *et al* (1954): In: Berger, F. M., and Ludwig, B. J. Meprobamate and related compounds. In: Psychopharmacological agents (ed., Gordon, M.). (Academic Press, New York, 1964.)

HERMANN, I. F., *et al.*: Fibrositis: recognition and treatment. (Scientific exhibit at the AMA meeting, Philadelphia, 1957.)

HESS, E. H.: Effects of meprobamate on imprinting in water fowl. Ann. N.Y. Acad. Sci., *67:* 724 (1957).

HIESTAND, E. C.: Overdosage with meprobamate. Presentation of case. Ohio Med. J., *52:* 1306 (1956).

HOFFMAN, A. J., AND LUDWIG, B. J.: An improved colorimetric method for the determination of meprobamate in biological fluids. J. Amer. Pharm. Ass., *48:* 740 (1959).

HOLLISTER, L. E., AND GLAZENER, F. S.: Withdrawal reactions from meprobamate, alone and combined with promazine: a controlled study. Psychopharmacologia (Berlin), *1:* 336 (1960).

HOLLISTER, L. E., *et al.*: Psychiatric use of reserpine and chlorpromazine: results of double-blind studies. In: Psychopharmacology (ed., Kline, N. S.). (A.A.A.S., Washington, 1956.)

HOLLISTER, L. E., *et al.*: Meprobamate in chronic psychiatric patients. Ann. N.Y. Acad. Sci., *67:* 789 (1957).

HOLUBEK, J. E., *et al.*: Toxic reactions to 2-methyl-2-N-propyl-1,3-propanediol dicarbamate. Ann. Intern. Med., *46:* 1002 (1957).

HUBARTA, J. A., AND HECHT, R. A.: Review of clinical use of hydroxyphenamate in 1759 patients. Clin. Med., *69:* 1594 (1961).

HUNT, H. F.: Some effects of meprobamate on conditioned fear and emotional behavior. Ann. N.Y. Acad. Sci., *67:* 712 (1957).

JACOBZINER, H., AND RAYBIN, H. W.: Briefs on accidental chemical poisonings in New York city—adult suicide attempts by poisoning. New York J. Med., *58:* 3326 (1958).

JACOBZINER, H., AND RAYBIN, H. W.: Briefs on accidental poisonings in New York city. Tranquillizer and dye poisonings. New York J. Med., *59:* 4014 (1959).

JACOBZINER, H., AND RAYBIN, H. W.: Briefs on accidental poisoning in New York city. Accidental and intentional poisonings. New York J. Med., *60:* 100 (1960).

JONSSON, B.: Cases of misuse of meprobamate. Svensk Lakaridn., *7:* 445 (1959).

KATO, R.: Induced increase of meprobamate metabolism in rats treated with phenobarbital or phenylglycodol. Med. Exp. (Basel), *3:* 95 (1960).

KATO, R., AND VASSANELLI, P.: Induction of increased meprobamate metabolism in rats pretreated with some neurotropic drugs. Biochem. Pharmacol., *11:* 779 (1962).

KLETZKIN, M., AND BERGER, F. M.: Effect of meprobamate on limbic system of the brain. Proc. Soc. Exp. Biol. Med., *100:* 681 (1959).

KORNETSKY, C.: Effects of anxiety and morphine on the anticipation and perception of painful radiant thermal stimuli. J. Comp. Physiol. Psychol., *47:* 130 (1954).

KORNETSKY, C.: Effects of meprobamate, phenobarbital and dextro-amphetamine on reaction time in learning in man. J. Pharmacol. Exp. Ther., *123:* 216 (1958).

KORNETSKY, C., *et al.*: A comparison of the psychological effects of acute and chronic administration of chlorpromazine and secobarbital (quinalbarbitone) in schizophrenic patients. J. Ment. Sci., *105:* 190 (1959).

KURTZKE, J. F., AND GYLFE, J. C.: A new muscle relaxant in spasticity. Neurology (Minneap.), *12:* 343 (1962).

LAMPHIER, J. A.: Control of tension in general surgery. (Scientific exhibit, Medical Society of the State of New York, New York, 1958.)

LASAGNA, L.: A study of hypnotic drugs in patients with chronic diseases. J. Chronic Dis., *3:* 122 (1956).

LEAR, E.: Chemistry and applied pharmacology of tranquilizers. (Charles C Thomas, Springfield, 1966.)

LEHMANN, H. E.: Experimental psychopathology of depression. (Presented at a Symposium on Depression, Berlin, 1968.)

LEHMANN, H. E.: The influence of neuroleptics

and anxiolytic sedatives on conflict avoidance behavior in human subjects (In press in a special volume dedicated to Professor E. Vencovsky's Anniversary, Prague, 1968.)

Lemere, F.: New tranquillizing drugs. Northwest Med., *54:* 1098 (1955).

Lemere, F.: Drug habituation. J.A.M.A., *160:* 1431 (1956).

Livingstone, S., and Pauli, L.: Meprobamate in the treatment of epilepsy of children. Amer. J. Dis. Child., *94:* 277 (1957).

Loomis, T. A., and West, T. C.: Comparative sedative effect of barbiturate and some tranquillizer drugs in normal subjects. J. Pharmacol. Exp. Ther., *122:* 525 (1958).

Ludwig, B. J., and Piech, E. C.: Some anticonvulsant agents derived from 1,3-propanediols. J. Amer. Chem. Soc., *73:* 5779 (1951).

Ludwig, B. J., *et al.*: Structures of the major metabolites of meprobamate. J. Med. Pharm. Chem., *3:* 53 (1961).

Lunsford, C. D. (1962): In: Berger, F. M., and Ludwig, B. J. Meprobamate and related compounds. In: Psychopharmacological agents (ed., Gordon, M.). (Academic Press, New York, 1964.)

Margolin, F., Plekss, O. J., and Berger, F. M.: Failure of chronic tybamate intoxication to induce withdrawal convulsions in dogs. Pharmacologist, *7:* 143 (1965).

Margolin, S., Plekss, O. J., and Fedor, E. J.: Selective inhibition of dog spinal vasoconstrictor tracts by mebutamate. J. Pharmacol. Exp. Ther., *140:* 170 (1963).

Martinez, M., and Salas, E. A.: Use of a new tranquillizing agent 5-(o-methoxy-phenoxymethol)-2-oxazolidone. Sem. Méd. (B. Air.), *117:* 1142 (1960).

Matthews, V., Lehmann, H. E., and Ban, T. A.: A comparative study of thirteen hypnotic drugs. Appl. Ther., *6:* 806 (1964).

McClendon, S. J.: Management of nocturnal enuresis in childhood. Arch. Pediat., *75:* 101 (1958).

McLaughlin, B. E.: Miltown in the treatment of chronically ill psychiatric patients. Penn. Med. J., *60:* 989 (1957).

Meeroff, M., *et al.*: Thrombocytopenic purpura caused by meprobamate. Dia. Med., *31:* 846 (1959).

Melander, B.: Emylcamate, a potent tranquillizing relaxant. J. Med. Pharm. Chem., *1:* 443 (1959).

Meyer, L. M., *et al.*: Aplastic anemia after meprobamate (2-methyl-2-N-propyl-1,3-propanediol dicarbamate) therapy. New Eng. J. Med., *256:* 1232 (1957).

Millen, F. J.: Miltown—clinical experiences in neuropsychiatric office use. Wisconsin Med. J., *56:* 198 (1957).

Mohr, R. C., and Mead, B. T.: Meprobamate addiction. New Eng. J. Med., *259:* 865 (1958).

Moyer, J. H., *et al.*: A comparative study of four tranquillizing agents, phenobarbital, and inert placebo. Geriatrics, *13:* 153 (1958).

Osinski, W. A.: Treatment of anxiety states with meprobamate. Ann. N.Y. Acad. Sci., *67:* 766 (1957).

Paterson, A. S.: Electrical and drug treatments in psychiatry. (Elsevier, New York, 1963.)

Pennington, V. M.: Use of Miltown (meprobamate) with psychotic patients. Amer. J. Psychiat., *114:* 257 (1957).

Perlstein, M. A.: Use of meprobamate (Miltown) in convulsive and related disorders. J.A.M.A., *161:* 1040 (1956).

Phillips, R. M., *et al.*: Meprobamate addiction. Northwest Med., *56:* 453 (1957).

Phillips, R. M., Miya, T. S., and Yim, G. K. W.: Studies on the mechanism of meprobamate tolerance in the rat. J. Pharmacol. Exp. Ther., *135:* 223 (1962).

Prigot, A., *et al.*: Meprobamate therapy—three years of observation on its use in adaptation and stress induced conditions. Harlem Hosp. Bull., *10:* 63 (1957).

Proctor, R. C.: The headache, backache, and the doctor. In: The pharmacology and clinical usefulness of carisoprodol (ed., Miller, J. G.). (Wayne State University Press, Detroit, 1959.)

Raab, E., Rickels, K., and Moore, E.: A double-blind evaluation of tybamate in anxious neurotic medical clinic patients. Amer. J. Psychiat., *12:* 1005 (1964).

Rawitt, K. C.: The usefulness and effectiveness of equanil in children. Amer. J. Psychiat., *115:* 1120 (1959).

Rickels, K., and Downing, R. W.: Drug and placebo treated neurotic outpatients—pretreatment levels of manifest anxiety, clinical improvement and side reactions. Arch. Gen. Psychiat. (Chicago), *16:* 369 (1967).

Rickels, K., *et al.*: Evaluation of tranquillizing drugs in medical outpatients—meprobamate, prochlorperazine, amobarbital sodium and placebo. J.A.M.A., *171:* 1649 (1959).

Rickels, K., *et al.*: Drug treatment in depression: antidepressant or tranquillizer. J.A.M.A., *201:* 675 (1967).

Riising, P. V.: Shock and anuria after restenil poisoning. Ugeskr. Laeg., *119:* 195 (1957).

Riley, R. F., and Berger, F. M.: Metabolism of myanesin. Arch. Biochem., *20:* 159 (1949).

Schlan, L. S., and Unna, K. R.: Some effects of myanesin in psychiatric patients. J.A.M.A., *140:* 672 (1949).

Schlesinger, E. B.: The value of muscle relaxants in disorders of muscle tone. Ann. N.Y. Acad. Sci., *67:* 833 (1957).

Schlesinger, E. B., *et al.*: Clinical studies in the use of myanesin. Amer. J. Med., *4:* 365 (1948).

Seeherman, R.: Evaluation of tybamate in the clinical management of anxiety. Delaware Med. J., *36:* 213 (1964).

Selling, L. S.: Clinical study of a new tranquillizing drug: use of Miltown. J.A.M.A., *157:* 1594 (1955).

Selling. L. S.: A clinical study of Miltown, a new tranquillizing agent. J. Clin. Exp. Psychopath., *17:* 7 (1956).

SETTEL, E.: Clinical observations on the use of hydroxyzine (atarax) in tension states. Amer. Practit., *8:* 1584 (1957).

SHANE, A. M., AND HIRSCH, S.: Three cases of meprobamate poisoning. Canad. Med. Ass. J., *74:* 908 (1956).

SHELTON, J., AND HOLLISTER, L. E.: Simulated abuse of tybamate in men. J.A.M.A., *100:* 116 (1967).

SIFFERD, R. H., AND BRAITBERG, L. D. (1962): In: Berger, F. M., and Ludwig, B. J.: Meprobamate and related compounds. In: Psychopharmacological agents (ed., Gordon, M.). (Academic Press, New York, 1964.)

SONTAG, K. H.: Pharmacological studies on the mechanism of action of 1,3-dioxolane. Acta Biol. Med. German., *7:* 145 (1961).

SPARUP, K. H.: Meprobamate. Lancet, *2:* 807 (1957).

SPEARS, C. E.: The clinical evaluation of carisoprodol in cerebal palsy. In: The pharmacology and clinical usefulness of carisoprodol (ed., Miller, J. G.). (Wayne State University Press, Detroit, 1959.)

STERN, F. H.: A new drug (tybamate) effective in the management of chronic brain syndrome. J. Amer. Geriat. Soc., *12:* 1066 (1964).

STEVENS, A. E.: Hypotension due to meprobamate overdosage. Brit. Med. J., *2:* 1029 (1960).

TRIMPI, H. D.: Pain control following hemorrhoidectomy. The use of a new analgesic muscle relaxant. In: The pharmacology and clinical usefulness of carisoprodol (ed., Miller, J. G.). (Wayne State University Press, Detroit, 1959.)

TUCKER, K., AND WILENSKY, H.: A clinical evaluation of meprobamate therapy in chronic schizophrenic population. Amer. J. Psychiat., *113:* 698 (1957).

TUCKER, W. J.: The place of Miltown in general practice. Southern Med. J., *50:* 1111 (1957).

TYBRING, G. L.: Experience with the ataractic and alerting drugs at Mendota State Hospital. Wisconsin Med. J., *56:* 430 (1957).

VAZUKA, F. A., AND MCLAUGHLIN, B. E.: Evaluation of new psychopharmacologic agents. A case in point. (A scientific exhibit presented at the Annual Meeting of the American Academy of General Practicioners, San Francisco, 1965.)

WALKENSTEIN, S. S., *et al.*: The excretion and distribution of meprobamate and its metabolites. J. Pharmacol. Exp. Ther., *122:* 80 (1958).

WEIN, A. B.: The use of carisoprodol in orthopedic surgery and rehabilitation. In: The pharmacology and clinical usefulness of carisoprodol (ed., Miller, J. G.). (Wayne State University Press, Detroit, 1959.)

WILSON, V. J.: Action of meprobamate on spinal monosynaptic reflexes and on inhibitory pathways. J. Gen. Physiol., *42:* 29 (1958).

WITHERSPOON, F. G.: Case report: toxic purpura from meprobamate. Amer. Practit., *8:* 270 (1957).

WOODWARD, M. G.: Attempted suicide with meprobamate. Northwest Med., *56:* 321 (1957).

YOUNG, R.: Emylcamate, a new internuncial blocking ataraxic: a study of 203 cases. Intern. Rec. Med., *174:* 345 (1961).

ZIVKOVIC, P.: Formation of ether of glycerol with phenol. Mschr. Chem., *29:* 951 (1908).

ZWEIFLER, A. J.: Agranulocytosis and jaundice during therapy with meprobamate and promazine. New Eng. J. Med., *262:* 1229 (1960).

Seventeen

The Benzodiazepines

In the past 5 years, more patients have received chlordiazepoxide (CDZ) than any other single compound. There is, nevertheless, much controversy as to whether this drug is superior to the best available barbiturate preparations in its "anxiety-relieving" effects. It is usually conceded, however, that the suicidal danger of overdosage with CDZ and its analogues is definitely less than with the barbiturates. At least 5 benzodiazepines are presently available for medical use, the majority of them for the treatment of various neurotic manifestations. One can safely compare their wide application to the use of phenothiazines in the different psychotic conditions, but whether they will have a comparable impact on psychiatry remains to be seen.

A. BASIC DATA

1. Historical Aspects

The basic constituent of CDZ is the benzodiazepine nucleus, which consists of a benzene ring and a seven-membered ring containing two nitrogen atoms in positions 1 and 4 in its structure and, in all of the psychoactive derivatives, a phenyl or pyridyl ring as a substituent.

The benzodiazepines were derived from compounds known in the literature as 3,1,4-benzoxadiazepines, which had no psychiatric use. In the nineteen-fifties, the reaction of one of these substances, chlormethylquinazoline *N*-oxide, with methylamine was studied by Sternbach, who had previously been involved in work with benzoxadiazepines in the nineteen-thirties. The result of this reaction was a well crystallized compound of the expected elemental composition, but without the expected quinazoline *N*-oxide structure. A more detailed analytical investigation revealed that a rearrangement had occurred, resulting in methaminodiazepoxide, a 1,4-benzodiazepine, which later was commonly referred to as chlordiazepoxide (Sternbach *et al.*, 1964).

Even the very first studies revealed the potent taming, anticonvulsant and skeletal muscle relaxing activity of this drug in animals and its definite psychosedative effects in humans. These led to its introduction for the treatment first of anxiety, then of alcoholism, and finally of a variety of psychoneurotic disturbances in general and psychosomatic conditions in particular (Sternbach *et al.*, 1964).

2. Action Mechanism

Since the discovery of CDZ, a large number of 1,4-benzodiazepines have been synthesized, tested in pharmacological experiments and investigated clinically. A number of hypotheses have been formulated on the action mechanism of these drugs. These range from the psychodynamic to the neurophysiological. According to the psychodynamic formulation, CDZ weakens the ego so as to permit psychotic projections. In this respect, the action of CDZ seems to resemble, at least to some extent, the action of hallucinogenic drugs (Ostow, 1962). In the majority of cases, however, the drug has a predominantly anxiolytic effect in the therapeutic dosages without affecting alertness. This can probably be explained by its relatively strong affinity for limbic system structures and its relatively weak affinity for the brain stem reticular activating system (Schallek *et al.*, 1960, 1962, 1963, 1964, 1965).

Since these initial hypotheses, an increasing amount of information on the neurochemical and the neurophysiological concomitants of the pharmacological effects of CDZ has accumulated. In spite of this, there is still no general agreement on which of the known actions of the molecule account for its usefulness in different psychopathological conditions.

3. Structure and Activity

In the search for a more potent and less toxic benzodiazepine than CDZ, extensive studies were directed toward effecting changes through modifications of the CDZ molecule. Chlordiazepoxide, the parent compound, has a methylamino group attached to the carbon atom of the benzodiazepine nucleus in position 2, two hydrogens in position 3, an *N*-oxide group in position 4 and a halogen atom (chlorine) in position 7. It is characterized as a colorless, light-sensitive, crystalline, water-soluble but unstable substance. Pharmacologically, it has pronounced sedative, muscle relaxant and anticonvulsant properties.

Diazepam, the second member of the benzodiazepine family to be extensively studied, differs from CDZ in having a methyl group in position 1 and a carbonyl instead of a methylamino group in position 2 and in not having the *N*-oxide, oxygen characteristic of CDZ. Diazepam is insoluble in water but otherwise has only slightly different physical and chemical properties from its parent compound, although it has a somewhat more potent over-all pharmacological activity. Although diazepam is thought to be more effective in controlling agitation and in lifting depression than CDZ, its drowsiness-producing effect is also more pronounced.

Prazepam, oxazepam and nitrazepam, the three other currently available benzodiazepines, resemble diazepam—and not chlordiazepoxide — structurally. Replacement of the methyl group of diazepam by a cyclopropylmethyl group in position 1 leads to prazepam; and by a hydrogen atom, to oxazepam, a nonhygroscopic crystalline powder. The former is considered to be particularly useful for patients with psychosomatic manifestations, and the latter, in patients in whom the psychopathological changes are associated with an organic damage of the brain.

Replacement of the chlorine atom of CDZ in position 7 by an NO_2 group and attachment of a hydrogen atom to position 1 resulted in nitrazepam, a slightly yellow, crystalline compound, soluble in alcohol,

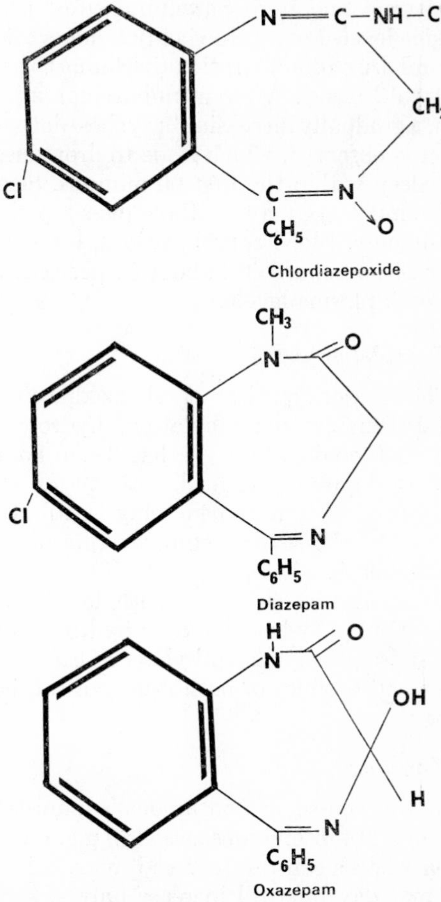

N=C—NH—CH₃ ... CH₂ ... Cl ... C=N→O ... C₆H₅

Chlordiazepoxide

Diazepam

Oxazepam

FIG. 17. Benzodiazepine derivatives

but insoluble in water. Although this substance has a stimulant action on some of the pharmacological tests in animals, it has a striking sleep-inducing property in humans, which makes its indications distinctly different from the other drugs of this family. Whereas the other psychoactive benzodiazepines are primarily prescribed as anxiolytic sedatives, nitrazepam is extensively used as a hypnotic (Lehmann and Ban, 1968; Schallek and Kuehn, 1965; Sternbach, 1959; Sternbach and Reeder, 1961; and Sternbach *et al.*, 1960, 1961, 1962, 1963).

4. Metabolism

a. Absorption

Although psychoactive benzodiazepines are rapidly absorbed from the gastrointestinal tract and from parenteral sites, peak plasma levels are attained only 8 hours after peroral drug administration (declining to half in 1 to 2 days). After intramuscular injection, a gradually increasing "psychosedative" effect is observed, which leads to drowsiness and sleep within the first 60 minutes. Sleep and somnolence may continue over a period of 16 hours. Blood concentrations, however, after 24 hours, are still about 50 per cent of the peak plasma levels.

b. Degradation

The major paths of benzodiazepine metabolism are demethylation, hydroxylation and conjugation. It has been noted that the pharmacological activity of the substance is maintained only until the opening of the seven-membered ring of the basic nucleus.

Diazepam is either demethylated and subsequently hydroxylated or hydroxylated and subsequently demethylated. Oxazepam is the end product of both routes of catabolism.

c. Excretion

In the course of continuous administration of CDZ in high dosages (150 mg. daily) plasma levels can rise to 2 to 6 mcg./ml. on the first day but will increase only slightly following subsequent daily administration of the compound. After discontinuation of medication, as seen by spectrofluorimetric studies with radioactive carbon-tagged material, plasma levels decline rather slowly.

During the first day of drug administration, 1 to 2 per cent of the administered dosage is excreted in the urine unchanged, and 3 to 6 per cent is excreted in a conjugated form. Another considerable portion is eliminated in the feces.

It has been noted that in dogs—also in humans—urinary excretion predominates, while in rats a greater part of the drug is eliminated in the feces.

After discontinuation of benzodiazepine administration, metabolic products may continue to be excreted in the urine and feces for approximately 2 weeks (Baumler and Rippstein, 1961; Koechlin and Schwartz, 1961; Randall, 1961; and Koechlin and D'Arconte, 1963).

5. Chemical and Neurophysiological Correlates of Drug Action

a. Chemical Correlates

Benzodiazepines exert an inhibitory effect on the oxygen uptake of the brain and induce a short lasting increase in the glucose levels of the central nervous system. Furthermore, chlordiazepoxide was shown to block the depression caused by dopa injection and to interfere also with the potentiation of the dopa reaction by iproniazid. On the basis of this it has been suggested that benzodiazepines either prevent the conversion of dopa to dopamine or directly antagonize the effects of the latter substance.

Systematic investigations with nitrazepam have shown that this drug has a slight potentiating influence on the pressor effects of intravenously administered hypertensin and serotonin, without altering the response to epinephrine or histamine. The potentiation of arterial pressure responses to norepinephrine produces an increase in over-all blood flow and cardiac activity.

Other—peripheral—chemical changes are the short lasting increase in glucose, pyruvate and lactate concentrations in the blood stream and the inhibition of oxygen uptake by liver mitochondria.

b. Neurophysiological Correlates

The initial view that the primary site of action of these drugs is upon the visceral brain was supported by Schallek *et al.'s* findings (1960, 1962, 1963, 1964, 1965). They provided experimental evidence that benzodiazepines depress the activity in the limbic system, *i.e.*, septum, amygdala and hippocampus, at a lower dosage than in the reticular activating system. This accounts for the anxiolytic effects of these drugs with the retention of alertness. More recently, functional alterations in the nervous system due to benzodiazepine compounds have been described from the lowest level of integration to the cerebral cortex.

i. Autonomic Nervous System. The slight sympatholytic action, particularly of oxazepam and diazepam, is seen in a minimal ptosis, lacrimation and lowering of blood pressure and pulse rate.

ii. Spinal Cord and Medulla Oblongata. Benzodiazepines have a characteristic inhibitory action on spinal reflexes which can be counteracted by strychnine. Their action, however, on the medullary centers is variable. This was recognized by antiemesis tests in dogs, which revealed that CDZ (in high dosages only) inhibited apomorphine-induced vomiting in approximately 30 to 40 per cent of the animals, while diazepam remained ineffective.

iii. Brain Stem Reticular Formation. The sensitivity of the brain stem reticular formation structures to CDZ and its analogues is relatively low. Whereas in high dosage CDZ blocks the EEG arousal that results from stimulation of the brain stem reticular formation, in low dosage there is sensitization of these structures along with facilitation of transmission of afferent nerve impulses.

iv. Hypothalamus and Thalamus. Benzodiazepines have an inhibitory effect on the sympathetic nuclei of the *hypothalamus* and also on the hypothalamic centers which control pituitary prolactin secretion. This is responsible for the mammotropic effects of these drugs described in rats.

The influence of these drugs on *thalamic* structures is also inhibitory in nature. This is manifested primarily in a raised threshold to stimulation and in a diminished responsivity, *i.e.*, low amplitude and shortened duration of after-discharges, resembling the effects of the anticonvulsants trimethadione and diphenylhydantoin.

v. Septum, Hippocampus and Amygdala. It has been demonstrated that CDZ slows the spontaneous electrical activity of certain *septal areas* of the brain. This is seen only in a somewhat higher dosage than is needed to slow the spontaneous electrical discharges of the hippocampus. This dosage, however, is still somewhat lower than the dosage necessary to slow the spontaneous electrical activity of the cerebral cortex. It has also been noted that the irritability produced by septal lesions is controlled by CDZ in approximately one-half of the dosage necessary for controlling vicious animals after cortical lesion.

The *hippocampus* is more sensitive than the septum to benzodiazepine activity. Even low dosages slow down the spontaneous electrical activity and depress after-discharges to direct stimulation in these structures.

Benzodiazepines slow the spontaneous electrical activity recorded by implanted electrodes in the *amygdaloid areas*. Diazepam and nitrazepam, particularly the latter, increase the threshold of the amygdala to direct stimulation. The same drugs, but particularly diazepam, have a controlling effect on cocaine-induced seizures which spread from the amygdala to other central nervous system structures. Some believe that the anxiolytic effect of benzodiazepines in general and the hypnotic property of nitrazepam in particular are primarily related to their effect on these structures. This theory implies that the amygdala is involved in the production of anxiety, and thus depression of amygdaloid functions reduces anxiety, which in turn provides for an optimal condition for sleep.

vi. Other Structures. Other neurophysiological effects of benzodiazepine administration are the blocking of decerebrate rigidity and the muscle relaxant action. The latter is considered to be due to the effect of these drugs on the extrapyramidal system.

Benzodiazepines induce a shift in the

dominant frequency of the electroencephalogram to fast activity and increase synchronization. This fast activity of 14 to 24 cycles per second spreading posteriorly from the frontal areas to a large extent replaces the normal background activity after a few days. This replacement takes place somewhat sooner with diazepam than with CDZ, and it persists well beyond the disappearance of the drug from the blood plasma after discontinuation of treatment. The fast activity is similar to that seen with barbiturates, meprobamate and other sedatives and is distinctly different from the slow activity usually associated with reserpine, phenothiazine and narcotic administration.

Benzodiazepines tend to normalize some pathological electroencephalograms. The typical three per second spike and wave discharges of petit mal attacks are frequently abolished, together with successful clinical control of the condition, whereas in cases of temporal foci CDZ prevents only the generalization of the abnormality while leaving the foci unaffected (Gordon, 1965; Jarvik, 1965; Müller, 1965; Cohen *et al.*, 1967; and Schallek and Kuehn, 1965).

6. Behavioral Pharmacology

a. Animal Studies

Benzodiazepines induce behavioral changes in animals and man over a wide range of functions. Some of these can be easily seen and assessed, while the measurement of others requires special instruments. On Norton's (1957) behavioral check list, specially designed for monkeys, CDZ proved to be more effective than pentobarbital, meprobamate or even chlorpromazine in reducing aggression. The behavioral effects of CDZ were characterized as "decreased defensive and aggressive hostility and increased sociability." Others indicated that cats were more playful, alert and eager for food after being given a low dosage of CDZ. With increasing dosage, however, this behavior is successively replaced by ataxia.

A taming effect is one of the most characteristic actions of the benzodiazepine drugs. This taming effect was seen in vicious monkeys and in mice stimulated to fight one another by applying electroshocks to their feet.

Benzodiazepines reduced or abolished fighting episodes in amounts far below the ataxic or even the muscle relaxant or sedative dosage. Thus benzodiazepines are different from the barbiturates, *e.g.*, phenobarbital, which, although it blocks fighting below the muscle relaxant dosage, produces a hypnotic effect along with taming. They are also different from meprobamate or chlorpromazine, which produce a reduction in aggression only in ataxic and sedative dosages.

Conditioned lever pressing in monkeys (to avoid a shock, after administering an auditory signal) was found to be inhibited, while conditioned lever pressing (to turn off the shock after receiving it) was maintained. In the same species, the act of pressing of a lever to obtain a pellet to a tone stimulus and accepting with the pellet an electroshock—that is, to perform the conditioned reflex rewarded by food in spite of the electroshock—were facilitated by benzodiazepine drugs. It was also shown that CDZ in general is more effective in decreasing conditioned avoidance behavior than in increasing unconditioned shock tolerance and that it has a positive effect on learning as measured in problem solving experiments.

In rats conditioned to press a lever to avoid electroshock on a warning signal it has been shown that the dosage which first produces a decrement in the conditioned avoidance response is one-third of the dosage which causes the rat to fail to escape the unconditional (shock) stimulus. In trace conditioning when there is a gap between the conditional—noise—stimulus and the unconditional—shock—stimulus there is a strong tendency to respond in the gap (a stronger tendency than with either meprobamate or chlorpromazine) under the influence of chlordiazepoxide (Bernstein and Cancro, 1962; Heise and Boff, 1962, Heise and McConnell, 1961; Randall, 1960, 1961; and Randall *et al.*, 1965).

Another extensively explored property of benzodiazepine drugs is their anticonvulsant action. It is greater than that of meprobamate and, like the taming effect, it is produced below the hypnotic or ataxic dosage, in contrast, for example, to phenobarbital. Although strychnine and pentetrazol convulsions and probably tremorine-induced activity and salivation are antagonized by benzodiazepines, the hypnotic effect of barbiturates, especially phenobarbital, hexobarbital and thiopental, is potentiated, as is that of ether. The central depression produced by excessively high dosages of benzodiazepines in cats was counteracted by bemegride, amphetamine and caffeine administration.

b. Human Studies

In human pharmacological studies diazepam was given in dosages from 15 to 40 mg. a day over a period of a month. With the increase of dosage, drowsiness, slurring of speech and ataxia were seen; and with the increase of time, there was an increasing slowness of mentation with apathy and pronounced impairment of memory functions. On the electroencephalogram a fast—20 to 30 cycles per second—activity was present during the period of drug administration. This reverted to normal only 6 to 8 days after diazepam was withdrawn. Attempts to correlate the behavioral effects with the electroencephalographic changes remained unsuccessful.

In other human experiments chlordiazepoxide produced increased tolerance in a conflict situation, and nitrazepam induced a characteristic reduction of rapid eye movements (DiMascio and Barrett, 1965; Lehmann and Ban, 1968; and Whiteman, 1965).

B. CLINICAL DATA

1. Therapeutic Indications and Contraindications

a. Therapeutic Indications

i. Psychoneuroses. The therapeutic effectiveness of benzodiazepines in the treatment of different psychoneuroses is most convincing.

Benzodiazepines were found to be therapeutically the most useful in anxiety states, phobic conditions and in the mixed forms of psychoneuroses. While results in obsessive-compulsive conditions are less consistent, dissociative and conversion reactions, psychophysiologic disorders (gastrointestinal, cardiovascular, musculoskeletal, dermatological, respiratory, gynecological and neurological) all respond favorably.

The clinical literature on benzodiazepines was excellently reviewed by Sternbach *et al.* (1964) and Cohen *et al.* (1967). The anxiolytic and tension-relieving properties of CDZ were first recognized by Tobin *et al.* (1960) and confirmed by Bowes (1960) and Cohen (1960). Further support was given by Williams (1961), Langston (1962), Dean (1962) and Barsa and Saunders (1962). The therapeutic effectiveness of CDZ in anxiety associated with somatic conditions was reported by numerous authors. Thus Brown (1961), Fishbein and Jones (1961), Scherbel (1960) and Rosenstein and Silverblatt (1961) found it useful in cardiovascular disorders; Hirschleifer *et al.* (1961) and Reinhardt (1962) in gastrointestinal disorders; Thomas (1960), Brown (1961), Rider and Moeller (1961), and Elia (1962) in dermatological disorders; Robinson (1961), Olansky and Olansky (1962), Pernikoff (1960) and Scherbel (1961) in other (respiratory, gynecological and neurological) psychophysiological disorders. Therapeutic actions of diazepam, oxazepam and prazepam in the various psychoneuroses have been indicated by Burdine (1964), Cleckley (1965), Dean (1965), Gilbert (1965), Krakowski (1965), Warner (1965), Kingstone *et al.* (1966), Isham (1966) and Thomas (1966).

ii. Alcoholism. Benzodiazepines are extensively used in alcoholism. CDZ is at least comparable to many other preparations, *e.g.*, paraldehyde and chlorpromazine, in preventing or controlling delirium tremens or acute alcoholic hallucinosis (Ticktin and Schultz, 1960; D'Agostino and Schultz, 1961; Fishbein, 1961; Karolus, 1961; Kissen, 1961; Rosenfeld and Bizzoco, 1961; Chambers *et al.*, 1962; Koutsky and Sletten, 1963; Salzberger, 1964; and Ban *et al.*, 1965) and in the treatment of chronic alcoholism (Mooney *et al.*, 1961; and Smith, 1961). CDZ is also useful as an aid to psychotherapy in the long term rehabilitation of the alcoholic patient, and it has been suggested that drinking episodes are less likely to develop during the course of benzodiazepine treatment.

iii. Epilepsy. Benzodiazepines, particularly diazepam and nitrazepam, are frequently and successfully used—mainly as adjunctive therapy—in the treatment of epileptic patients. Under the influence of these drugs abnormal electroencephalograms are shifted toward normal and seizure frequencies may be reduced. Beneficial effects have been described in patients suffering from grand mal, petit mal, and myoclonic seizures when benzodiazepines were added to their regular medication. In psychomotor epilepsy, benzodiazepines prolong the early sensory phenomena and prevent the development of final automatisms. There are indications that children without actual cerebral seizures but manifesting a characteristic behavior disorder concomitant with electroencephalographic changes have benefited from diazepam treatment.

Benzodiazepines have a striking therapeutic effect on epileptic personality changes. By their inhibitory influence on the amygdala, benzodiazepines ameliorate slowness, perseveration, viscosity, the inadequacy of emotional responses, motor restlessness and decreased attention, while leaving the explosive behavior of the patient unaffected.

The anticonvulsant properties of benzodiazepines were first demonstrated by Randall *et al.* (1961) in animals. Subsequently, the reduction of the frequency or severity of seizures and correction of the pathological behavioral changes under the influence of chlordiazepoxide and diazepam were reported by Bercel (1961), Kaim and Rosenstein (1961), Brodie and Dow (1962), LeVann (1962), and Lehmann and Ban (1968).

iv. Others. Symptomatic relief was reported with CDZ and diazepam in some manic-depressive patients manifesting manic excitement or agitated depression. Diazepam was found to be also useful in involutional melancholia and in the treatment of various psychopathological conditions with prevailing anxiety, depression or paranoid features (Feldman, 1962; Lehmann and Ban, 1964; McCray, 1965; and Stonehill *et al.*, 1966).

b. Contraindications

Shock or coma are the only absolute contraindications of benzodiazepine treatment. It is generally accepted that diazepam should not be given to patients suffering from myasthenia gravis, and it is usually agreed that some of these drugs, especially oxazepam, should be avoided in glaucoma (although evidence of a pronounced anticholinergic action of this substance is lacking).

In certain elderly or debilitated patients, drowsiness, ataxia (or their aggravation) and confusional states have been described even with very low doses. In others, confusional states or precipitation of schizophrenic psychopathology occurred in the course of treatment. In all of these conditions, benzodiazepine administration requires careful supervision.

Combined administration of benzodiazepines with other psychoactive drugs, particularly with barbiturates but also with phenothiazines, tricyclic antidepressants and MAOI's, increases the incidence and the severity of adverse reactions. Although Bowes (1960) and Hoffer (1962) maintain that benzodiazepines do not potentiate alcohol effects, driving skill was shown to be more impaired after a drink or two in benzodiazepine-treated cases.

There is no evidence indicating that benzodiazepines should not be administered during pregnancy (although they definitely cross the placental barrier) or in the period of lactation (Decancq *et al.*, 1965). There has been no carcinogenic effect related to the administration of these drugs.

2. Therapy Alone and in Combination

a. Benzodiazepines Alone

i. Dosage and Routes of Drug Administration. The average daily dosage of the various benzodiazepines for their major indications is as follows: CDZ, 20 to 40 mg.; diazepam, 10 to 30 mg.; oxazepam, 15 to

50 mg.; prazepam, 30 to 60 mg.; and nitrazepam, 5 to 20 mg. Geriatric and pediatric cases and patients suffering from a debilitating disease are given approximately one-quarter the average adult daily dosage.

As a general rule relatively high dosage is administered in alcohol withdrawal and in severe cases of psychoneuroses. Lower dosage is sufficient for controlling psychosomatic manifestations and in conditions where mild to moderate anxiety is present.

Besides the most common oral route, benzodiazepine drugs are quite frequently given intramuscularly and, in certain conditions, intravenously. When the oral route is used, the drug is usually given in three to four divided dosages. For example, CDZ is given in multiples of 5-, 10- or 25-mg. capsules three to four times a day.

It has been noted that a parenterally administered dosage is somewhat faster acting and more potent than the perorally given dosage. Another advantage is that it can be used in cases in which oral administration imposes great difficulties, *e.g.*, delirium tremens. In alcohol withdrawal, massive dosages of CDZ are given parenterally (*e.g.*, 50 to 100 mg. intramuscularly every 4 hours), but more than 300 mg. in any 6-hour period is not recommended.

In other situations, benzodiazepines, especially diazepam, are used intravenously. The substance chosen is dissolved, and the solution is injected slowly. Intravenously administered diazepam may bring about prompt seizure control in status epilepticus with normalization of the electroencephalogram.

ii. Treatment Procedures. The most frequently used clinical procedure is continuous therapy. The average recommended daily dosage is prescribed, and this is then adjusted, increased or decreased, depending on the individual need and tolerance. In most cases it is usually unnecessary to commence treatment with parenteral administration. Even when this is necessary it should be replaced by oral dosage if possible within 3 days.

More recently, successful therapeutic results in chronic drug-resistant psychotic patients have been reported with discontinuous diazepam treatment. In these cases the dosage of the drug was rapidly increased to approximately 100 mg. a day within a week, maintained at this level for a period of 10 days, and then abruptly reduced to a small—5 mg. a day—maintenance dosage (Galambos, 1965; and Lehmann and Ban, 1966).

The duration of therapy is dependent upon the condition which is being treated. The drugs are given until symptomatic relief is obtained and should probably be continued thereafter for a short period of time. It has been observed that patients who respond to these drugs may show at least some improvement within the first 2 or 3 days. Those cases who show no response whatsoever within the first month usually remain therapeutic failures.

As a rule of thumb, these drugs should always be administered in the lowest dosage required for successful therapy and for the shortest period of time necessary. There is evidence that with higher dosage and more prolonged administration the possibility of drug dependence increases. Characteristic of the withdrawal syndrome are agitation, insomnia, loss of appetite, and aggravation or recurrence of the psychopathological state present prior to treatment. Abrupt withdrawal after high dosage administration has led to cerebral seizures. Benzodiazepine dosage should be gradually tapered off whenever treatment is terminated.

b. Benzodiazepines in Combination with Other Treatments

i. Physical. Both electroconvulsive and insulin therapies may be combined with benzodiazepine administration. The combination of diazepam with electroshock has been successfully used in the treatment of agitated depressions; and the combination of CDZ with modified (subcoma) insulin, in various psychoneurotic conditions in which either one of the two therapies alone was ineffective.

ii. Pharmacological. An extensively used commercially available synthetic combination is librax, marketed in capsules containing 5 mg. of CDZ and 2.5 mg. of clinidium bromide. It is used in functional or organic disorders of the digestive tract.

CDZ, diazepam and nitrazepam have been given in association with different anticonvulsant drugs in the treatment of convulsive disorders. The associated administration of CDZ and primidone proved to be particularly effective in the behavior disorders of children with characteristic EEG changes. Other successful drug combinations are CDZ and antihistaminics, which are useful in reducing itching; CDZ and stilbestrol which are successful in controlling the libidinal urges of homosexuals; and CDZ and a monoamine oxidase inhibitor antidepressant recommended for the treatment of various depressive and neurotic conditions.

Of the different monoamine oxidase inhibitors, phenelzine is probably the one most frequently given in association with CDZ. The combination is particularly effective in anxiety and phobic states and in reactive depression accompanied by tension. Combined drug administration has been reported to be useful in recurrent phobic and somatic attacks and in obsessional neuroses with a recurrent course. There are indications that phobic and somatic anxiety, including cardiac neurosis or effort syndrome, respond well to the combination, while free-floating anxiety may respond better to other treatments (Sargant and Slater, 1963).

3. Adverse Reactions and Their Treatment

a. Adverse Reactions

In the course of benzodiazepine treatment a number of reactions occur which are undesired in the particular therapeutic situation. These reactions may cause mild discomfort or pathological changes that call for untimely termination of treatment. According to the nature of the manifestation, adverse reactions are classed as psychiatric, neurological, autonomic and others.

i. Psychiatric. These range from a slight reduction of spontaneous activity to severe toxic confusional states, although the incidence of the latter is well below 1 per cent. The most frequent adverse effect is somnolence and sleep disturbance. In some cases there is transient drowsiness in the initial period of treatment, particularly with nitrazepam and diazepam, which spontaneously wears off with continuation of treatment. In others, drowsiness is dose related and calls for reduction of the dosage.

Infrequently, paradoxical insomnia, hyperexcitability, hyperactivity, agitation, rage or hostility is seen in the course of treatment. Rarely, garrulousness with a heightened sense of well-being resembling inebriation develops, and in others acute "maniacal" behavior, feelings of depersonalization, hallucinations and delusions have been described. Disorientation and toxic delirious or confusional states have also been reported.

Asthenia and apathy are not uncommonly seen, and dysthymic mood frequently becomes overt soon after the commencement of treatment. A significant interference with judgment has been shown on a simulated driving test after 20 mg. of CDZ; and more recently, increased attention has been paid to the nightmares patients have while under treatment, particularly with oxazepam.

ii. Neurological. Ataxia is most frequently discussed among all the reactions induced by benzodiazepines. It is usually dose related, although in some predisposed patients, *i.e.*, geriatric and debilitated cases, it occurs with a rather small daily amount. Headache, dizziness and vertigo are not infrequent, while poor coordination, slurred speech and dysarthria are rather rare. Hyperkinesia, exaggerated reflexes, muscle tenderness, cramps and paresthesia have also been reported.

iii. Autonomic. A relative scarcity of autonomic reactions is characteristic of these drugs. A mild hypotensive reaction and dry mouth, however, are non infrequently seen. Other infrequent autonomic effects, such as constipation, micturition difficulties, pollakisuria, changes in sexual activity and acceleration or deceleration of the heart, are attributed to the administration of benzodiazepine drugs.

iv. Others. Agranulocytosis, menstrual irregularities (missing ovulation) and hepatic dysfunction all have been reported in the course of treatment with benzodiazepines.

It is fortunate that the safety margin of benzodiazepine drugs is wide, and consequently suicidal attempts even with as high a dosage as 2250 mg. of CDZ remained unsuccessful. On the other hand, drowsiness and sedation with slightly depressed blood pressure, pulse rate and respiration were reported with single dosages of 200 to 250 mg.

It has been noted that during the course of combined administration of CDZ with a monoamine oxidase inhibitor, orthostatic hypotensive reactions and edema are frequently seen.

b. Treatment of Adverse Reactions

Discontinuation of all treatment is very rarely indicated (*e.g.*, agranulocytosis). Discontinuation of one specific drug and replacement with another medication are the proper course of treatment for most of the various neurological reactions, which include hyperkinesia, muscle cramps and paresthesia, the most severe autonomic manifestations and disturbances of the menstrual cycle or uncontrollable weight gain.

Drowsiness, dizziness, ataxia, slurred speech and slight hypotension respond to reduction of dosage; and the addition of adjunctive medication is used in the infrequent manifestations of extrapyramidal signs.

In the majority of cases no actual intervention is required in the management of overdosage. In others, bemegrede, caffeine, strychnine or amphetamines are successfully used, for the symptomatic control of specific manifestations.

4. The Use of Benzodiazines in Medical Practice

Common to all the drugs of this category is their usefulness in the various psychoneuroses and ineffectiveness in the functional psychoses. Like most of the drugs that relieve anxiety and tension, they are also liable to cause addiction (dependency).

Among the various benzodiazepines, CDZ is the most extensively used. The average daily dosage of this drug is 30 mg., but there is a wide dosage range (from 10 to 500 mg. a day) in which it can be safely given. CDZ is probably one of the most widely used drugs and also one of the most abused drugs in medical practice. It is primarily indicated in the psychoneuroses in which anxiety prevails. It is also extensively used in the treatment of alcoholism and in the therapy of the psychological concomitants of cardiovascular disease, in functional gastrointestinal illnesses and in the dermatoses of psychogenic origin.

The second benzodiazepine, diazepam, is superior to the parent compound in several clinical conditions. Although the average daily dosage of this drug is approximately 20 mg., it can be given in dosages from 5 to 80 mg. a day. Preference is given to diazepam in different neurological conditions, especially convulsive disorders, in which benzodiazepines are usually prescribed in combination with other treatments. Diazepam is the most useful for pre- and postanesthetic medication. It has also been reported to give excellent therapeutic results in borderline psychiatric conditions and in involutional melancholia. There are more drowsiness and euphoria with it than with CDZ; and the incidence of drug dependence may also be higher.

Oxazepam, the metabolic product of diazepam, is used as an independent compound in treatment. Although the average daily dosage of this drug is 30 mg., it has been administered in dosages from 15 to 60 mg. a day. Stimulation of libido is one of the particular characteristics of this substance, which is also successfully used parenterally in the control of alcohol and drug withdrawal syndromes. Whether the substance has a particular usefulness in chronic organic brain syndromes with superimposed neurotic manifestations will have to be confirmed by further clinical studies.

More recently, nitrazepam has been used with increasing success in the treatment of insomnia in single dosages of 5 to 10 mg. at bedtime. Investigations with another, more recent benzodiazepine, prazepam, have progressed to the point where this drug, in a dosage of 30 to 90 mg. daily, was found to be useful in reducing anxiety in general and somatized anxiety in particular. It has been noted that male patients under the influence of this drug may become more outgoing but some of them may become transiently sexually impotent.

More than half a century intervened between the introduction of the first medically used barbiturate and the introduction of the first psychoactive benzodiazepine compound. The latter made its appearance more than half a decade after chlorpromazine was successfully introduced in the treatment of various psychiatric disorders. Although there is still no general agreement on the superiority of benzodiazepine drugs over the barbiturates, it is generally agreed that the two drug groups exert their action through distinctly different mechanisms.

SUMMARY

The introduction of the first 1,4-benzodiazepine compound, CDZ, led to the extensive use of this drug and its analogues not only in psychiatry but also in general medical practice. The most significant therapeutic effect of these drugs is in the different psychoneuroses.

Of the various benzodiazepine drugs, CDZ is prescribed most frequently. There is increasing evidence, however, that at least in certain conditions, *e.g.*, epilepsy, preanesthetic medication, involutional melancholia, etc., diazepam and, in insomnia, nitrazepam are therapeutically superior to this substance. There are indications of the value of simultaneous administration of benzodiazepines (particularly CDZ) with a monoamine oxidase inhibitor (especially phenelzine) in the treatment of certain depressive and psychoneurotic conditions.

Because of the possibility of addiction, benzodiazepines should be administered in the lowest optimal dosage for the shortest period of time.

Whereas the primary site of action of barbiturates is on the brain stem reticular formation structures and only to a lesser extent on the limbic lobe structures, the primary site of action of the benzodiazepines is on the limbic lobe structures and only to a lesser extent on the brain stem reticular formation structures. Unlike the phenothiazines, both these drug groups remain ineffective in the pathological manifestations of mental integration. On the other hand, both groups have a definite effect on pathological arousal and affective phenomena. In accordance with the brain structures affected, benzodiazepines influence primarily affective and only secondarily arousal manifestations, while barbiturates influence pathological arousal first and pathological affect only thereafter.

REFERENCES

Ban, T. A., *et al.*: Comparative study of chlorpromazine and chlordiazepoxide in the prevention and treatment of alcohol withdrawal symptoms. Clin. Med., *72:* 59 (1965).

Barsa, J. A., and Saunders, J. C.: Chlordiazepoxide in the treatment of psychotics with convulsive disorders. Dis. Nerv. Syst., *23:* 106 (1962).

Baumler, J., and Rippstein, S.: Über dem Nachweis von Metaminodiazepoxide (librium) und seine Metaboliten. Helv. Chim. Acta, *44:* 2208 (1961).

Bercel, N. A.: Clinical experience with a new type of antidepressant drug: ditran. J. Neuropsychiat., *2:* 271 (1961).

Bernstein, B. M., and Cancro, L. P.: Erfahrungen mit Librium in der internische Praxis. Psychopharmacologia (Berlin), *3:* 105 (1962).

Bowes, H. A.: The ataractic drugs: the present position of chlorpromazine, frenquel, pacatal and reserpine in psychiatric practice. Amer. J. Psychiat., *113:* 530 (1956).

Bowes, H. A.: Some observations on milieu-influence in neuroleptic drug therapy. In: The dynamics of psychiatric drug therapy (ed., Sarwer-Foner, G. J.). (Charles C Thomas, Springfield, 1960.)

Bowes, H. A.: The role of librium in an outpatient psychiatric setting. Dis. Nerv. Syst., *21:* 20 (1960).

Brodie, R. E., and Dow, R. S.: Chlordiazepoxide in epilepsy. Northwest Med., *61:* 513 (1962).

Brown, C. H.: Clinical evaluation of librium in gastrointestinal diseases. Amer. J. Gastroen., *35:* 30 (1961).

Burdine, W. E.: Diazepam in general psychiatric practice. Amer. J. Psychiat., *121:* 589 (1964).

Chambers, J. F., *et al.*: Comprehensive care of the acute alcoholic in a municipal hospital. Canad. Med. Ass. J., *86:* 1112 (1962).

Cleckley, H. M.: Use of diazepam as adjunctive therapy in psychiatric disorders. J. So. Carolina Med. Ass., *61:* 1 (1965).

Cohen, I. M.: Discussion of papers of Drs. Randall, Tobin, Bowes, Kinross-Wright, *et al.* Dis. Nerv. Syst., *21:* 35 (1960).

Cohen, S.: Lysergic acid diethylamide: side effects and complications. J. Nerv. Ment. Dis., *130:* 30 (1960).

Cohen, S., and Ditman, K. S.: Complications associated with lysergic acid diethylamide (LSD-25). J.A.M.A., *181:* 161 (1962).

Cohen, S., Ditman, K. S., and Gustafson, S. R.: Psychochemotherapy. (Western Medical Publications, Los Angeles, 1967.)

D'Agostino, A., and Schultz, J. D.: Clinical experience with librium in acute alcoholism. Psychosomatics, *2:* 362 (1961).

Dean, S. R.: Librium as an adjuvant in psychotherapy. Dis. Nerv. Syst., *23:* 27 (1962).

Dean, S. R.: Diazepam as an adjuvant in clinical psychotherapy. Dis. Nerv. Syst., *26:* 181 (1965).

Decancq, H. G., Bosco, G. R., and Townsend, E. H.: Chlordiazepoxide in labor, its effect on the new born infant. J. Pediat., *67:* 836 (1965).

DiMascio, A. and Barrett, J.: Comparative effects of oxazepam in high and low anxious student volunteers. Psychosomatics, *6:* 298 (1965).

Elia, J. C.: Cardiospasm. Clin. Med., *69:* 49 (1962).

Feldman, R. S.: The prevention of fixations with chlordiazepoxide. J. Neuropsychiat., *3:* 254 (1962).

Fishbein, R. E.: Use of intravenous chlordiazepoxide in emergency room treatment. Curr. Ther. Res., *3:* 345 (1961).

Fishbein, R. E., and Jones, F.: Use of librium in general practice. Intern. Rec. Med. Gen. Prac., *174:* 34 (1961).

Galambos, M.: The long term use of valium. Amer. J. Psychiat., *121:* 811 (1965).

Gilbert, M. M.: Clinical trial of a new drug, analog of chlordiazepoxide, for treatment of anxiety and tension. Int. J. Neuropsychiat., *1:* 556 (1965).

Gordon, L.: A review of selected benzodiazepines. (Paper presented at the meeting of the Quebec Psychopharmacological Research Association, Montreal, 1965.)

Hegner, H. L.: Diazepam in the treatment of myalgia, muscle spasm and the anxiety-tension state. Clin. Med., *72:* 1980 (1965).

Heise, G. A., and Boff, E.: Continuous avoidance as a base-line for measuring behavioral effects of drugs. Psychopharmacologia (Berlin), *3:* 264 (1962).

Heise, G. A., and McConnell, H.: Difference between chlordiazepoxide type and chlorpromazine type action in trace avoidance. (Presented at the Third World Congress of Psychiatry, Montreal, 1961.)

Hirschleifer, I., *et al.:* Chlordiazepoxide in cardiovascular disease. Clin. Med., *8:* 926 (1961).

Hoffer, A.: Lack of potentiation by chlordiazepoxide (librium) of depression or excitation due to alcohol. Canad. Med. Ass. J., *87:* 920 (1962).

Isham, A. C.: Office evaluation of diazepam for psychoneurotic anxiety and depressive reactions. Int. J. Neuropsychiat., *2:* 111 (1966).

Jarvik, M. E.: Drugs used in the treatment of psychiatric disorders. In: The pharmacological basis of therapeutics (eds., Goodman, L. S., and Gilman, A.). (MacMillan, Toronto, 1965.)

Kaim, S. C., and Rosenstein, N. N. (1961): In: Sternbach, L. H., *et al.:* 1,4-Benzodiazepines. In: Psychopharmacological agents (ed., Gordon, M). (Academic Press, New York, 1964).

Karolus, H. E.: Librium in the treatment of acute alcoholism. Illinois Med. J., *120:* 96 (1961).

Kingstone, E., Villeneuve, A., and Kossatz, I.: Prazepam in the treatment of anxiety and tension: a clinical study of a new benzodiazepine derivative. Curr. Ther. Res., *8:* 159 (1966).

Kissen, M. D.: The treatment of acute and chronic alcoholism. Quart. J. Stud. Alcohol, *1:* 101 (1961).

Koechlin, B. A., and D'Arconte, L.: Metabolism of chlordiazepoxide. Anal. Biochem., *5:* 195 (1963).

Koechlin, B. A., and Schwartz, M. A.: The metabolic fate of chlordiazepoxide. (Presented at the Federation Meeting, Atlantic City, 1961.)

Koutsky, C. D., and Sletten, I. W.: Chlordiazepoxide in alcohol withdrawal. Minnesota Med., *46:* 354 (1963).

Krakowski, A. J.: Protriptyline in treatment of severe depression. Amer. J. Psychiat., *121:* 807 (1965).

Langston, W. B. (1962): In: Sternbach, L. H., *et al.:* 1,4-Benzodiazepines. In: Psychopharmacological agents (ed., Gordon, M.). (Academic Press, New York, 1964.)

Lehmann, H. E. and Ban, T. A.: Notes from the log-book of a psychopharmacological research unit. I. Canad. Psychiat. Ass. J., *9:* 28 (1964).

Lehmann, H. E. and Ban, T. A.: Notes from the log-book of a psychopharmacological research unit. II. Canad. Psychiat. Ass. J., *9:* 111 (1964).

Lehmann, H. E., and Ban, T. A.: EDCEU progress report, Douglas Hospital, Verdun, 1966.

Lehmann, H., and Ban, T. H.: Effect of hypnotics on rapid eye movement. Int. J. Clin. Pharmacol., *5:* 424 (1968).

Lehmann, H. E., and Ban, T. A.: Studies with new drugs in the treatment of convulsive disorders. Int. J. Clin. Pharmacol., *1:* 231 (1968).

LeVann, L. J.: Chlordiazepoxide, a tranquillizer with anticonvulsant properties. Canad. Med. Ass. J., *86:* 123 (1962).

Markham, C. H.: The treatment of myoclonic seizures of infancy and childhood with LA-1. Pediatrics, *34:* 511 (1964).

McCray, W. E.: Diazepam and combined treatment in outpatients with depressive syndromes. J. Louisiana Med. Soc., *117:* 232 (1965).

Meyler, L. (ed.): Side effects of drugs. (Excerpta Medica Foundation, Amsterdam, 1962.)

Mooney, H. B., *et al.:* Chlordiazepoxide in the treatment of alcoholism. Dis. Nerv. Syst., *22:* 441 (1961).

Müller, H. F.: The benzodiazepines and epilepsy. (Paper presented at the Quebec Psychopharmacological Research Association Meeting, Montreal, 1965.)

Norton, S.: Behavioral patterns as a technique for studying psychotropic drugs. In: Psychotropic drugs (eds., Garattini, S., and Ghetti, V.). (Elsevier, Amsterdam, 1957.)

Olansky, S., and Olansky, M.: Chlordiazepoxide in dermatosis. J. Med. Ass. Georgia, *51:* 349 (1962).

Ostow, M.: Drugs in psychoanalysis and psychotherapy. (Basic Books, New York, 1962.)

Pernikoff, M.: Clinical results with librium in a private non-psychiatric practice. Clin. Med., *7:* 2313 (1960).

Randall, L. O.: Pharmacology of methaminodiazepoxide. Dis. Nerv. Syst., *21:* 7 (1960).

Randall, L. O.: Pharmacology of chlordiazepoxide (librium). Dis. Nerv. Syst., *22:* 7 (1961).

Randall, L. O., Scheckel, C. L., and Banziger, R. F.: Pharmacology of the metabolites of chlordiazepoxide and diazepam. Curr. Ther. Res., *7:* 590 (1965).

Randall, L. O., *et al.:* Pharmacological and clinical studies on valium, a new psychotherapeutic agent of the benzodiazepine class. Curr. Ther. Res., *3:* 405 (1961).

Randall, L. O., *et al.* (1961): In: Remmen, E., *et al.:* Psychochemotherapy. (Western Medical Publications, Los Angeles, 1962.)

Reinhardt, D. J.: Use of chlordiazepoxide as an adjuvant in cardiovascular disorders. Delaware Med. J., *34:* 171 (1962).

Rider, J. A., and Moeller, H. C.: The use of chlordiazepoxide in the treatment of patients with functional gastrointestinal disorders. Amer. J. Gastroent., *36:* 464 (1961).

Robinson, M. M.: The use of chlordiazepoxide to allay preoperative apprehension and anxiety in abrasive surgery. Med. Ann. D.C., *30:* 719 (1961).

Rosenfeld, J. E., and Bizzoco, D. H.: A controlled study of alcohol withdrawal. Quart. J. Stud. Alcohol, *51:* 77 (1961).

Rosenstein, I. N., and Silverblatt, C. W.: Chlordiazepoxide as a broad spectrum psychosedative. J. Amer. Geriat. Soc., *9:* 1003 (1961).

Salzberger, G. J. (1964): In: Cohen, S., *et al.:* Psychochemotherapy. (Western Medical Publications, Los Angeles, 1967.)

Sargant, W., and Slater, E.: An introduction to physical methods of treatment in psychiatry. (Livingstone, London, 1963.)

Schallek, W.: Neurophysiological studies with monoamine oxidase inhibitors. Dis. Nerv. Syst., *21:* 64 (1960).

Schallek, W., and Kuehn, A.: Effects of trimethadione, diphenylhydantoin and chlordiazepoxide on after discharges in brain of cat. Proc. Soc. Exp. Biol. Med., *112:* 813 (1963).

Schallek, W., and Kuehn, A.: An action of mogadon on the amygdala of the cat. Med. Pharmacol. Exp., *12:* 204 (1965).

Schallek, W., and Kuehn, A.: Effects of benzodiazepines on spontaneous EEG and arousal response in cats. Progr. Brain Res., *18:* 231 (1965).

Schallek, W., Kuehn, A., and Jew, N.: Effects of chlordiazepoxide (librium) and other psychotropic agents on the limbic system of the brain. Ann. N.Y. Acad. Sci., *96:* 303 (1962).

Schallek, W., Zabransky, F., and Kuehn, A.: Effects of benzodiazepines on central nervous system of cat. Arch. Int. Pharmacodyn., *149:* 467 (1964).

Scherbel, A. L.: Experimental and clinical effects of amine oxidase inhibitors. Amer. J. Cardiol., *6:* 1125 (1960).

Scherbel, A. L.: Preliminary evaluation of methaminodiazepoxide. Amer. Practitioner Dig. Treat., *12:* 275 (1961).

Smith, R. G.: Evaluation of safety of new drugs by the Food and Drug Administration. J. New Drugs, *1:* 59 (1961).

Snell, W., Corrigan, R. F., and Zimmerman, R. C.: Comparative drug evaluation in treatment of skeletal muscle spasm. Clin. Med., *72:* 957 (1965).

Sternbach, L. H. (1959): In: Sternbach, L. H., *et al.:* 1,4-Benzodiazepines. In: Psychopharmacological agents (ed., Gordon, M.). (Academic Press, New York, 1964.)

Sternbach, L. H., Randall, L. O., and Gustafson, S. R.: 1,4-Benzodiazepines (chlordiazepoxide and related compounds). In: Psychopharmacological agents (ed., Gordon, M.). (Academic Press, New York, 1964.)

Sternbach, L. H., and Reeder, E.: Quinazolines and 1,4-benzodiazepines. II. The rearrangement of 6-chloro-5-phenyl-3H-1,4-benzodiazepine 4-oxide. J. Org. Chem., *26:* 1111 (1961).

Sternbach, L. H., and Reeder, E.: Quinazolines and 1,4-benzodiazepines. IV. Transformations of 7-chloro-2-methylamino-5-phenyl-3H-1,4-oxide. J. Org. Chem., *26:* 4936 (1961).

Sternbach, L. H., *et al.:* Quinazoline 3-oxide structure of compounds previously described in the literature as 3,1,4-benzoxadiazepines. J. Amer. Chem. Soc., *82:* 475 (1960).

Sternbach, L. H., *et al.:* Quinazolines and 1,4-benzodiazepines. VI. Halo-methyl- and methoxy-substituted 1,3-dihydro-5-phenyl-2H-1,4-benzodiazepin-2-ones. J. Org. Chem., *27:* 3788 (1962).

Sternbach, L. H., *et al.:* Quinazolines and 1,4-benzodiazepines. X. Nitro-substituted 5-phenyl-1,4-benzodiazepine derivatives. J. Med. Chem., *6:* 261 (1963).

Stonehill, E., Lee, H., and Ban, T. A.: A comparative study with benzodiazepines in chronic psychotic patients. Dis. Nerv. Syst., *27:* 411 (1966).

Thomas, J. C. (1966): In: Cohen, S., *et al.:* Psychochemotherapy. (Western Medical Publications, Los Angeles, 1967.)

THOMAS, L. J.: Preliminary observation on the use of librium (RO 5-0690) in internal medicine. Dis. Nerv. Syst., *21:* 40 (1960).

TICTIN, H. E., AND SCHULTZ, J. D.: Librium, a new quieting drug for hyperactive alcoholic and psychotic patients. Dis. Nerv. Syst., *21:* 49 (1960).

TOBIN, J. M., BIRD, I. F., AND BOYLE, D. E.: Preliminary evaluation of librium (RO5-0690) in the treatment of anxiety reactions. Dis. Nerv. Syst., *21:* 11 (1960).

WARNER, R. S.: Management of the office patient with anxiety and depression. Psychosomatics, *6:* 347 (1965).

WHITEMAN, E. N.: Approaches to the clinical pharmacology of the benzodiazepines. (Paper presented at the Quebec Psychopharmacological Research Association Meeting, Montreal, 1965.)

WILLIAMS, M. W. (1961): In: Sternbach, L. H., *et al.:* 1,4-Benzodiazepines. In: Psychopharmacological agents (ed., Gordon, M.). (Academic Press, New York, 1964.)

Eighteen

Other Drug Groups

In addition to the ten well established groups of psychoactive substances discussed, there are several other groups of psychotropic drugs, some very new, which have important heuristic or clinical value.

A. SEDATIVES

Most important in this category are the tertiary acetylenic alcohols, the carbamic acid esters of alcohol, the piperidinediones and the quinazolones.

1. Tertiary Acetylenic Alcohols

These are more potent central nervous system depressants than the primary or secondary alcohols. The presence of branched side chains further increases their strength.

Clinically the most frequently used drug of this class is *ethchlorvynol*, the outcome of halogenation of acetylenic carbinols. It is a reliable hypnotic (Ban and McGinnis, 1962; and Matthews *et al.*, 1964) but has dependency-producing properties. Wood and Flippin (1965) reported the occurrence of delirium tremens after ethchlorvynol administration was discontinued. *Methylparafynol*, an unsaturated tertiary carbinol, another member of this class, is a feeble and unreliable soporific drug.

2. Carbamic Acid Esters of Alcohol

Drugs of this group have only limited clinical applications. *Urethan*, the ester of ethyl alcohol, is used in animals only as a general anesthetic because of its toxic—bone marrow depressing—effects.

Ethinamate (Langecker *et al.*, 1953), the carbamic acid ester of an alicyclic alcohol (ethynyl-cyclohexanol), is a reliable hypnotic preparation. Matthews *et al.* (1964) found this substance one of the best sleep-inducing drugs. Occasional cases of thrombocytopenia have been reported in the course of ethinamate administration.

3. Piperidinediones

This class includes *methyprylon* and glutethimide. The latter, an anticholinergic phenylglutarimide, resembles phenobarbital and thalidomide structurally. *Thalidomide* has been shown to produce phocomelia, a malformation of the fetus, when administered during early pregnancy. It is a useful hypnotic in chronic alcoholism and in incurable cancer. *Glutethimide* is one of the most widely used hypnotics today in spite of its dependency-producing properties and the reported case of megaloblastic anemia (Pearson, 1965).

4. Quinazolones

Clinically the only important member of this class is *methaqualone*. The hypnotic property of this substance was an incidental discovery by Gujral *et al.* (1956) while investigating methaqualone as an antimalarial agent. Methaqualone is a potent sleep-inducer, particularly useful in chronic alcoholism and drug addiction (Parsons and Thomson, 1961; Asbell, 1962; Coldrey, 1963; Bordeleau *et al.*, 1965; and Morrison, 1965). Bordeleau *et al.* (1965) found methaqualone a superior hypnotic to *nitromethaqualone;* and it was recognized that *mecloqualone*, another member of this group, is a reliable soporific drug.

5. Miscellaneous

There are indications that γ-aminobutyric acid (GABA) derivatives and *dl*-1-(1-arylalkyl)imidazole-5-carboxylate esters have hypnotic properties.

Among the GABA derivatives, *Na-oxybutyrate* and *β-phenyl-γ-aminobutyric acid* were reported to have soporofic effects (Banschikov and Berezin, 1966).

In the course of animal pharmacological studies with *imidazole carboxylate esters*, Godefroi *et al.* (1965) recognized that some of them exhibit potent but short acting hypnotic properties in rats.

B. STIMULANTS

Most important is the group of piperidyls (or 2-benzylpiperidines) and related compounds.

1. Piperidyls

These are psychomotor stimulants with relatively few autonomic (including cardiovascular) and psychological (including dependency) side-effects. Instrumental in their development was the introduction of chlorpromazine and reserpine in the treatment of psychiatric patients. With the ever increasing use of antipsychotic drugs it became important to find chemicals to antagonize the side-effects (sedation and depression) of neuroleptic treatment. At the same time an effort was made to discover compounds with beneficial effects in chronic, inactive psychiatric patients, therapeutically resistant to the first psychoactive phenothiazine and Rauwolfia alkaloid preparations. This resulted in the piperidyl derivatives in general and methylphenidate and pipradrol in particular.

a. Methylphenidate

2-Benzylpiperidine is the outcome of specific modifications of certain phenylisopropylamines (amphetamines) with CNS stimulating effects; and pyridilacetonitriles are the result of condensation of halopyridines. The transformation of the nitrile function of pyridilacetonitriles and reduction of the pyridine ring yielded a number of new preparations (Krueger and McGrath, 1964), including the methylated derivative methylphenidate (methyl α-phenyl-2-piperidineacetate), synthesized by Hartmann and Panizzon (1950).

The CNS and behavioral stimulating effects of methylphenidate (in animals) were first described by Meier *et al.* (1954). These properties were confirmed by subsequent studies in humans.

In human studies methylphenidate stimulated psychomotor activity; facilitated recall and conditional stimulus discrimination; and increased alertness even in the course of chronic sedative (anxiolytic) or tranquilizer (antipsychotic) drug administration (Ayd, 1957; Ferguson, 1956; Gruber *et al.*, 1956; Plummer *et al.*, 1957; and Ticktin *et al.*, 1958).

The beneficial effect of the drug in chronic, inactive psychiatric patients could not be fully substantiated (Bhaskaran and Nand, 1959; Carey *et al.*, 1956; Lehmann and Ban, 1964; and Pargiter, 1959). Similarly its therapeutic value in mild cases of neurotic depression (Kerenyi *et al.*, 1960) was not confirmed in a controlled trial (Robin and Wiseberg, 1958). Furthermore, Bojanovsky and Chloupkova (1965) reported anhedonia and paranoid traits in a psychotic depressive patient and increase of anxiety in a neurotic depressive patient under the influence of methylphenidate. Since intravenous methylphenidate administration was seen to induce hostile behavior, its therapeutic usefulness became increasingly restricted (Freed, 1958; and Hartert and Browne-Mayers, 1958).

There are definite indications, however, that systemic administration of the drug may have a beneficial effect in certain disturbed—hyperactive—children (Lytton and Knobel, 1959).

b. Pipradrol

Pipradrol (α,α-diphenyl-2-piperidine methanol hydrochloride) increases psychomotor activity and reactivity to environmental stimuli (Brown and Werner, 1954, and Fabing, 1955). Like methylphenidate, the CNS effects of pipradrol are characterized by stimulation of certain hypothalamic, sympathetic centers and brain stem reticular formation structures (Cole and Glees, 1956; and Jouvet and Courjon, 1959). More recently, improvement of memory are shown in animal experiments (Irwin and Benuazizi, 1966) with this drug.

Although the clinical use of pipradrol in the various depressive conditions and schizophrenias remains controversial (Fabing, 1955; Fedotov *et al.*, 1958; and Houston, 1956), the drug was found to be effective in counteracting fatigue regardless of its origin (Antos, 1955; Cohen, 1956; and Levy, 1954) and drowsiness induced by various CNS depressants and anticonvulsants (Antos, 1955; Button, 1956; Fabing, 1957; Kistner and Duncan, 1956; Klingman, 1962; and Ott and McMaster, 1959). Particular usefulness of pipradrol in the treatment of geriatric patients has been suggested by some investigators (LeHew, 1957; Martin *et al.*, 1957; Pomeranze, 1954; and Pomeranze and Gadek, 1957).

2. Miscellaneous

Other CNS stimulants of limited psychopharmacological interest are *strychnine*, which interferes with central inhibitory processes; *picrotoxin*, which blocks postsynaptic inhibition; *bemegride*, a substance chemically related to barbiturates and a potent antidote of barbiturate poisoning; and *nikethamide* (Goodman and Gilman, 1965; and Myschetzky, 1961).

Psychopharmacologically more promising are *1-p-tolyl-1-oxo-2-pyrrolidino-n-pentane hydrochloride*, a substance which in a 60-mg. dose improves motor performance significantly better than 10 mg. of amphetamine; *phacetoperan*, a psychotonic drug which was also found to be useful in depressions without anxiety; and the various auxin derivatives, of which centrophenoxine and mefexamide are of clinical importance. Whereas *centrophenoxine* seems to be of particular value in organic psychopathologies with disturbance of memory and consciousness, *mefexamide* (which in animal studies was shown to have a tranquilizing effect in low, a stimulant effect in medium, and convulsant effects in high doses) seems to possess mood-lifting properties (Bower and McDonald, 1966; Deshaies *et al.*, 1965; Destrem, 1961; Espie, 1966; Giraud, *et al.*, 1961; Heimann and Lukacs, 1965; Launay and Maurey, 1965; Sabbatini, 1964; and Siegfried, 1965).

C. PSYCHOTHERAPEUTIC DRUGS

1. Antipsychotic Drugs

a. Azaphenothiazines

Azaphenothiazines (benzothiazines) are considered by some the fourth phenothiazine group, although the substitution of the pyridine ring for the chlorinated benzene ring differentiates them from the parent phenothiazine compounds.

The benzothiazines were developed in the search for more effective and specific antipsychotic drugs. Pharmacologically they resemble the phenothiazines in general and chlorpromazine in particular. In animal pharmacological experiments it was recognized that members of the new group induce sedation without producing stupor and that they have an inhibitory effect on conditioned avoidance reflexes. Other properties of the new group are antiemetic, antispasmodic, antihistaminic, strong adrenolytic and weak parasympatholytic activity as well as potentiation of the effects of alcohol, barbiturates and analgesics.

Prothipendyl, oxypendyl and isothipendyl have been used clinically with limited success. Although favorable results with *prothipendyl* have been reported in the control of "psychotic overlay" in mental subnormality (McKenzie and Roswell-Harris, 1966), no therapeutic effect could be seen with the same substance in schizophrenic patients (Sugerman and Herrmann, 1966). Sedation with minimal improvement of disturbed behavior was seen with *oxypendyl* in a group of schizophrenics (Simpson and Angus, 1967).

b. Acridanes

This group is closely related chemically to the thioxanthenes. The essential chemical difference is that in the new group the sulfur atom (characteristic of both the phenothiazine and the thioxanthene structures) is replaced by a nitrogen atom and the unsaturated carbon atom of the thioxanthenes is saturated.

Clinically, the most important member of this group is 9-[3-(dimethylamino) propyl]-2-chloracridane. This substance was found to have a therapeutic effect in chronic schizophrenic patients (Freeman and Oktem, 1966). It was shown to be a potent antipsychotic at a dosage considerably lower than that which produces extrapyramidal signs (Simpson *et al.*, 1966).

c. Dibenzoxepines

These are tricyclic compounds chemically similar to both the thioxanthenes and the dibenzocycloheptenes, the main difference being the oxepin ring in place of the cycloheptadien ring.

In animal pharmacological studies dibenzoxepines decrease spontaneous motor activity and the responsiveness to stimulation in mice. They protect against amphetamine-induced death. With increasing dosage, ataxia, ptosis and loss of righting reflex have been described.

Whereas *doxepin*, the promazine analogue of this category, is a thymoleptic, *pinoxepin*, the perphenazine analogue, exerts potent antipsychotic effects. Since pinoxepin beneficially influences irritability, thought disorder, withdrawal and apathy, it is considered to be particularly useful in certain chronic schizophrenics (Gallant *et al.*, 1966; Simpson *et al.*, 1966; and Sugerman *et al.*, 1966).

d. Benzoquinolizines

Drugs of this category resemble the Rauwolfia alkaloid reserpine pharmacologically. Clinically there are two important members of this class: tetrabenazine and benzquinamide.

i. Tetrabenazine. In animal pharmacological studies it was shown that the sedative effect of this substance is accompanied by depletion of brain norepinephrine and serotonin levels. In these experiments tetrabenazine had a faster onset and a shorter duration of action than reserpine.

The antipsychotic properties of tetrabenazine and its therapeutic value in the schizophrenias (and also in hypomanic and manic patients) have been substantiated by Bertolotti and Munarini (1961), Burckard *et al.* (1962) and Kammerer *et al.* (1962).

Tetrabenazine is less and less frequently applied clinically and more and more often used in animal pharmacological studies in the screening for new psychoactive (antidepressant) substances, where its rapid onset and short duration of action are of great advantage.

ii. Benzquinamide. Although this substance does not deplete the monoamine stores in the brain, it was found to be a serotonin antagonist. In animal (also in human) pharmacological studies it reduces anxiety without altering psychomotor performance and depresses conditioned avoidance reflexes (Forney and Hughes, 1963; and Scriabine *et al.*, 1966).

Feldman (1962) indicated that benzquinamide is useful for both functional and organic psychotic patients. This was further supported by Overall *et al.* (1963), Sainz (1963), Scriabine *et al.* (1963) and Settel (1963). However, there is evidence that its toxic behavioral effects outweigh any therapeutic value in schizophrenics (Barsa and Saunders, 1964; Bishop and Gallant, 1963; and Lehmann and Ban, 1963). One of the great drawbacks of this drug is its mood-depressant effect, which may lead to dreams of death and suicidal ideation.

e. Miscellaneous

i. Prediction Based on Animal Pharmacological Studies. There are numerous other substances which have been tried clinically because animal studies and theoretical formulations indicated possible antipsychotic effects. Among them is the antimetabolite *6-aminonicotinamide*, which was found to be effective against audiogenic seizures in mice (Geller *et al.*, 1966); *5-methyl-11-(3-methylamino-propyl)-5,6-dihydromorphanthridine maleate*, which was shown to stimulate chronic schizophrenics (Simpson and Siegler, 1966); *3-ethyl-6,7-dihydro-2-methyl-5-morpholinomethylindole-4-(5H)-one hydrochloride*, a substance which in animal pharmacological experiments curtailed spontaneous activity, disrupted conditioned avoidance responses and antagonized tetrabenazine-induced ptosis and clinically exerted antipsychotic effects (Sugerman and Herrmann, 1967); and *lyopholized yeast*, which at least in one reported study was found to be beneficial for schizophrenic patients (Pedani, 1965).

ii. Prediction Based on Theoretical Grounds. *α. Triiodothyronine.* Triiodothyronine was administered to a group of schizophrenic patients with "diminished" thyroid function. The positive findings of Danziger (1958) and Flack *et al.* (1958), could not be confirmed in more recent studies (Caruso, 1966; and Simpson and Amuso, 1966).

β. Nicotinic Acid. Despite the controversial findings reported with nicotinic acid and nicotinamide adenine dinucleotide in the treatment of schizophrenics—a treatment originally based on the adrenochrome theory of schizophrenia—Ivanova *et al.* (1964) were able to demonstrate that nicotinic acid can successfully control the LSD_{25}-induced "psychotic" state in animals.

γ. Penicillamine. On the basis of the melatonin hypothesis of schizophrenia, elaborated by Greiner *et al.* (1964, 1965) after finding an excess of melanin in certain schizophrenic patients, Nicolson *et al.* (1966) treated schizophrenics successfully with a combination of penicillamine and a copper-free diet. According to them, the negative copper balance is essential to outweigh the imbalance of the melanocyte-stimulating hormone (of the pituitary) and melatonin (of the pineal gland). The negative findings with penicillamine formerly reported by Hollister *et al.* (1959, 1966) were attributed to the lack of a copper-free diet.

2. Antidepressants

Most important in this category are new phenylalkylamines, MAOI's, tricyclic preparations and drugs with an effect on cholinergic mechanisms.

a. Phenylalkylamines

Gamfexine (a phenylpropylamine) and cypenamine (a phenylcyclopentylamine) belong to this group. Of the two, *gamfexine* was found to have a stimulating effect in chronic schizophrenics (Schiele *et al.*, 1966; and Lehmann and Ban, 1966). Its general antidepressant effects, however, are inferior to imipramine (Gershon, 1967). *Cypenamine*, although it does not seem to possess antidepressant properties improves responsiveness, cooperativeness, attention span, verbalization and academic skill in the mentally retarded (Kurland *et al.*, 1967).

b. MAOI's

Of the numerous new MAOI's which have recently been clinically tested, Simpson *et al.* (1966) indicated that *N-[2-(o-chlorphenoxy)ethyl]cyclopropylamine* may have antidepressant effects. Ban *et al.* (1966) were able to demonstrate the thymoleptic properties of *ethyl-N-benzyl-N-cyclopropylcarbamate.*

c. Tricyclic Preparations

Most important are the new dibenzodiazepines, the dibenzothiepines, dibenzoxepines and dihydroanthracenes.

i. Dibenzodiazepines. The only clinically used member of this class is *dibenzepin.* The thymoleptic properties of this substance have been confirmed by Bente *et al.* (1965), Rett *et al* (1965) and Schigutt and Suchanek-Fröchlich (1965).

ii. Dibenzothiepines. A clinically used member of this class is *prothiadene.* The thymoleptic properties of this substance have been confirmed by Pöldinger *et al.* (1966), and Alapin and Zaborowska (1966). Chemically closely related to prothiadene is *4-[3-methylamino-1-propyliden]-9,10-dihydro-4H-benzo[4,5]cyclohepta [1,2-b] thiophene*, another psychoactive propyliden (or thiophene) which was found by Gallant *et al.* (1966) to be therapeutically ineffective in chronic schizophrenic patients.

iii. Dibenzoxepines. The only clinically used antidepressant member of this class is *doxepin.* The thymoleptic properties of this substance have been confirmed by Ribbentrop and Schaumann (1965), Pöldinger *et al.* (1966) and Schaumann and Ribbentrop (1966). Pinoxepin, another member of this class, has been shown to have antipsychotic properties (Gallant *et al.*, 1966).

iv. Dihydroanthracenes. The only clinically used member of this class is *melitra-*

cen. The thymoleptic properties of this substance have been confirmed by Bratlund (1961), Retboll (1963), Bente *et al.* (1966) and Bister *et al.* (1966).

d. Drugs with an Effect on Cholinergic Mechanisms

i. Cholinergic Substances. Deanol and diforene belong to this class. *Deanol* is the para-acetamide benzoic acid salt of 2-dimethylaminoethanol, and consequently it resembles acetycholine structurally. The chemical is the precursor of acetylcholine, and it has a stimulating action on brain stem reticular formation structures. The arousal reaction produced is considered to be responsible for the effectiveness of this substance in fatigue, some of the psychoneuroses (*e.g.*, neurasthenia) and in mild depressions (Pfeiffer *et al.*, 1957; Remmen *et al.*, 1962; Goodhard, 1965; and Malitz *et al.*, 1967).

Less important is *diforene*, another precursor of acetylcholine. Diforene has mild thymoleptic properties, and it improves attention in children (Miletto, 1965).

ii. Anticholinergic Substances. The only clinically important member of this class is Ditran. Ditran is an anticholinergic substance with distinct psychotomimetic effects and antidepressant properties. Its thymoleptic action was first recognized by Abood and Meduna (1958), whose discovery was confirmed by Bercel (1961), Finkelstein (1961) and Davis *et al.* (1964).

e. Miscellaneous

i. Prediction Based on Animal Pharmacological Studies. There are numerous other substances which have been tried clinically because antidepressent effects were predicted on the basis of animal pharmacological studies. Among them are *thozalinone*, an MAOI (*in vitro*) with anticonvulsant, analeptic and anorexogenic action, with still unproven thymoleptic effects (Greenblatt and Osterberg, 1965; and Gallant *et al.*, 1966); *thiazenone*, with a possible beneficial effect in reactive depression (Horovitz, 1965; and Freeman *et al.*, 1965); and *4-phenylcyclo-(2,2,2)-octan-1-amine hydrochloride monohydrate*, a potent antagonist of tetrabenazine with thymoleptic properties (Lehmann *et al.*, 1967). Hematoporphyrin, another substance, was found to be beneficial for depressed patients at least in one reported study (Kröger, 1961).

ii. Prediction Based on Theoretical Grounds. Recognition of lowered corticosteroid levels in a group of depressed patients led McClure (1967) to complement the administration of tricyclic antidepressants with dexamethasone, a substance used in adrenocortical insufficiency. There are indications that the combination has been successful in some therapy-resistant cases.

3. Anxiolytics

a. Diphenylmethanes

Most important in this category are the diphenylmethanes. There are at least seven substances of this class in clinical use: azacyclonol, benactyzine, benztropine, captodiamine, hydroxyzine, orphenadrine and phenyltoloxamine. Only benztropine, captodiamine, orphenadrine and phenyltoloxamine are diphenylmethanes proper; benactyzine is a phenylacetic acid derivative, azacyclonol is a carbinol and hydroxyzine a piperazine.

i. Azacyclonol. This is a substance which is chemically closely related to methylphenidate and pipradrol, but in marked contrast to the latter 2-benzylpiperidine preparations, it has no CNS stimulating properties (Krueger and McGrath, 1964). At one time there was some interest in this drug, which was introduced by Fabing and Hawkins (1955), who found that azacyclonol blocks the psychopathological and electroencephalographic manifestations induced by both LSD_{25} and mescaline sulfate (as well as the peripheral effects of serotonin). For this reason it seemed to be indicated in the treatment of schizophrenic patients, especially for those with real or pseudohallucinations. Although the therapeutic expectations in the schizophrenias were not fulfilled, azacyclonol was found to have a beneficial effect in toxic psychoses and in agitated and agressive patients (Bachann, 1960; Decsi, 1961; Fabing, 1955; Kuziw *et al.*, 1956; Lascelles and Levene, 1959; Rinaldi *et al.*, 1955, 1956; Rosner *et al.*, 1957; and Sarwer-Foner and Koranyi, 1956).

ii. Benactyzine. This is a centrally acting anticholinergic agent which exerts an inhibitory effect on certain higher functions of the central nervous system without having any real sedative action. It was suggested that by acting on the hypothalamic structures and blocking certain nerve impulses by acetylcholine inactivation it raises the threshold of emotional reactions to external stimuli. Since it protects against experimentally induced neuroses in animals, benactyzine was expected to have a therapeutic effect in various psychoneuroses. These expectations were not fulfilled, and although the drug was found useful in the reduction of emotional reactivity to stress, it remained ineffective in the treatment of hysterical patients. In high dosages benactyzine was shown to have psychotomimetic effects (giddiness, difficulty in concentration, a tendency to overestimate the passage of time, and depersonalization) (Ayd, 1957; Feinblatt *et al.*, 1958; Hargreaves *et al.*, 1957; Harrington and Mayer-Gross, 1959; Jacobsen, 1958; Jacobsen *et al.*, 1955; Kinross-Wright and Moyer, 1957; Plichet, 1955; Vojtechovsky, 1958; and Werner, 1958).

iii. Benztropine. This substance is frequently used in the control of drug-induced extrapyramidal manifestations. Like atropine, it may induce a toxic psychosis, which in predisposed individuals may occur even with low dosage at an early stage of treatment.

iv. Captodiamine. On the basis of early clinical trials it was suggested that captodiamine, a diphenhydramine, might have a therapeutic effect in cases of psychoneuroses and in the control of restlessness in children (Sarwer-Foner *et al.*, 1957; and Davidova and Zapletalek, 1965).

v. Hydroxyzine. This is the most widely used member of the diphenylmethane category. It has adrenolytic, anticholinergic, antihistaminic, antiemetic and antispasmodic properties and hypothermic and hypotensive effects; and it also produces a small rise in the arousal threshold by direct stimulation of the brain stem reticular formation structures (Kalinowsky and Hoch, 1961; and Usdin and Efron, 1967).

Clinically hydroxyzine is an anxiolytic which produces psychic relaxation without noticeable decrease in wakefulness and is particularly effective in agitated cases (Darmstadter and Mock, 1965). Although Mock *et al.* (1965) did not find it superior to placebo in a study conducted with outpatient psychoneurotics, Settel (1957) indicated that it normalizes exaggerated responses.

The therapeutic application of hydroxyzine was well reviewed by Morren *et al.* (1964). The primary indications are anxiety, nervous tension, psychoneuroses in general and psychosomatic disorders in particular (Ende, 1956; Funfschilling, 1957; Dolan, 1958; Schram, 1959; Middlefell, 1960; and Gibbon, 1961). The drug has also been successful in alcoholism, behavior disorders of children, geriatrics and dermatological conditions, (Bayart, 1956; Flores, 1957; Freedman, 1958; Rogers, 1959; Cornbleet, 1960; Goldman, 1961; and Shanon, 1962).

vi. Orphenadrine. This is an antihistamine with CNS stimulating properties which has been successfully used in the treatment of psychasthenia and drug-induced extrapyramidal manifestations (Calje, 1961; Blair, 1963; and Zakrzewska *et al.* 1965).

vii. Phenyltoloxamine. This is an infrequently used tranquilizer useful in the control of anxiety-tension, agitation and psychosomatic disorders (Remmen *et al.*, 1962; and Paterson, 1963).

b. Miscellaneous

There are numerous other substances which have been tried clinically because anxiolytic effects were anticipated from animal studies. Among them are dixyrazine, a phenothiazine preparation which was found to be useful in the treatment of some psychoneurotic patients (Dzikowsky, 1961; and Paquay *et al.*, 1961); oxypertine, an indole and fenfluramine, an anorexic agent with an amphetamine-like structure, which were used with equivocal success (Robinson *et al.*, 1965; Skarbek and Jacobsen, 1965; Knowles and Kreitman, 1966; Laubie *et al.*, 1964; and Raich *et al.*, 1966).

D. PSYCHOTOPATHIC DRUGS

Since the turn of the century a great number of psychotopathic substances have been recognized, synthesized and systematically studied. At present there are at least four subclasses of psychotopathic drugs, which are distinctly different chemically and in their psychopathological effects (Downing, 1964).

1. Indole Derivatives

There are five heuristically important major categories in this subclass: the lysergic acid derivatives, the tryptamine derivatives, the reserpine derivatives, the harmine derivatives and the aminochromes.

a. Lysergic Acid Derivatives

i. Lysergic Acid Diethylamide. This is the best known substance in this category and probably the most extensively used and abused of all the psychotopathic substances. Lysergic acid diethylamide, or, as commonly referred to, LSD_{25}, is a synthetic product prepared from lysergic acid, the common nucleus of the ergot alkaloids. It is one of the most active of the psychotopathic substances and one of the most potent drugs ever known (Szara, 1966). In certain predisposed individuals LSD_{25} has induced long term (possibly irreversible) psychopathological changes and may produce chromosomal abnormalities with consequent genetically determined changes.

The history of LSD_{25} dates back to 1938 when Stoll and Hofmann (1943) succeeded in synthesizing ergonovine and also lysergic acid diethylamide. Four years later they discovered the psychotomimetic properties of the latter (Stoll, 1947). One day while exploring the central nervous system stimulating effects of LSD_{25}, in search for nikethamide-like properties, Hofmann (Stoll and Hofmann, 1943) registered a chain of rather unusual experiences. It started with restlessness with increasing difficulty in concentration. It continued with perceptual disturbances. The shape of objects changed; the daylight became unpleasant; disturbing fantastic pictures with extraordinary plasticity and kaleidoscopic colorfulness occurred. This "unusual state" subsided in approximately 2 hours. Since he suspected a relationship between his unusual experiences and the substance he was working with, he intentionally took a small dose of LSD_{25}. A similar reaction verified what he had already suspected.

Lysergic Acid Diethylamide

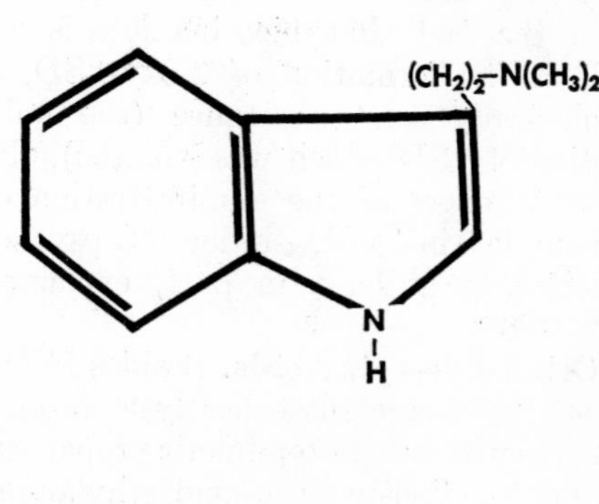

Dimethyltryptamine

FIG. 18. Lysergic acid diethylamide and dimethyltryptamine

The first systematic investigation of LSD_{25} in humans was reported by Stoll (1947). In his analysis of the drug-induced psychopathological changes, he characterized the perceptual pathology as predominantly tactile and visual illusions or hallucinations and the affective psychopathology by the prevalence of one of the following phenomena: euphoria or dysphoria, hyperthymia or dysthymia, laughing or crying and/or emotional lability. He noted passivity, a decrease of adaptive responses with or without thinking difficulties and a dissociation from the environment. Insight was retained in the vast majority of cases, but in some an actual psychotic process was precipitated.

Personality-dependent variability in the responses to LSD_{25} has been noted by DiMascio *et al.* (1961). They found that most of the "athletic" subjects became more anxious and tense under the influence of the drug, while most "aesthetic" individuals rated themselves as less anxious and tense.

These psychotopathic effects have been correlated with elevation of brain serotonin levels (Woolley and Shaw, 1954), with sensitization of the reticular activating system to sensory stimulation (Bradley and Elkes, 1957), with an increase of low voltage fast activity on the electroencephalogram and with centrally mediated sympathetic effects.

The LSD_{25}-induced psychopathological changes can be interfered with by numerous psychoactive drugs. Among them chlorpromazine is probably the most reliable. In view of the fact that nicotinamide is required for the formation of 2-oxy-LSD, a psychologically inert substance (the only derivative of LSD which was isolated), the therapeutic effect of the administration of nicotinamide in LSD_{25}-induced psychopathologies, is at least in part, explained (Hoffer, 1966).

ii. Other Lysergic Acids. Besides LSD_{25} there are at least eight other lysergic acid derivatives with psychotomimetic properties. These are 1-acetyl-lysergic acid ethylamide and diethylamide; 1-methyl-lysergic acid ethylamide and pyrrolidide; lysergic acid ethylamide and morpholide; *d*-lysergic acid dimethylamide; and *N,N*-diethyl-1-methylysergamide dimaleate (Stoll, 1947; Hofmann, 1960; Zsigmond *et al.*, 1961; and Usdin and Efron, 1967).

b. Tryptamine Derivatives

i. N,N-Dialkyl Tryptamines. These substances were first isolated and synthesized by Szara (1956, 1957). The parent compound dimethyltryptamine is present in cohoba, which is prepared by Haitian natives from the *Piptadenia peregrina* seeds. It is a fast acting drug with a short duration of action, which induces introversion, passivity with a feeling of well-being (but lability of mood) and perceptual disturbances accompanied by marked autonomic changes (Szara, 1961; and Arnold *et al.*, 1962). The clinical effects of the diethyl, dipropyl and diallyl analogues are somewhat similar (Böszörmenyi *et al.*, 1959; and Szara and Hearst, 1962).

ii. N,N-Dialkyl-hydroxy-tryptamines. Bufotenine and psilocybin are the two important members of this category. While *bufotenine*, a dimethylserotonin, has been known for some time for its psychotopathic effects (Fabing and Hawkins, 1956), *psilocybin* (also psilocin) was only recently isolated from a mushroom called *Psilocybe mexicana* (Hofmann *et al.*, 1959; Arnold *et al.*, 1962). It induces a dream-like state which has been described as "an unworldly feeling" with clear consciousness. Less important are 4-hydroxy-*N,N*-diethyltryptamine and 4-phosphoryloxy-*N,N*-diethyltryptamine (Leuner and Baer, 1965).

iii. Other Tryptamines. β-Hydroxy-pseudotryptrophan (Sherwood, 1957), nitroserotonin (Woolley, 1960), the 5-methoxy derivatives (gramine, *N*-methyltryptamine, *N,N*-dimethyltryptamine) and α-methyltryptamine belong to this category (Wilkinson, 1958; Hollister *et al.*, 1960; and Gessner *et al.*, 1961). The last is a mild MAOI with some antidepressant properties (Lehmann and Ban, 1963; and Sendbuehler, 1966). It seems that the psychotomimetic potential of this substance outweighs the therapeutic expectations.

c. Reserpine Derivatives

Reserpine and some of its derivatives induce sedation, which gives place to dysthy-

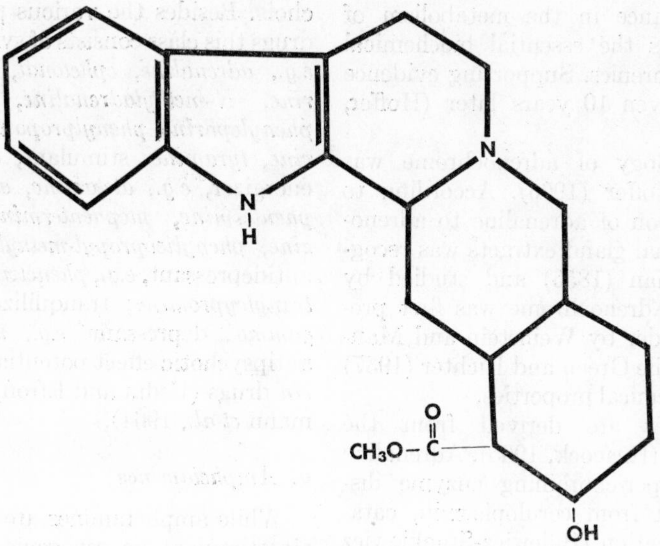

Yohimbine

FIG. 19. Structural formula of yohimbine

mic mood changes. The depression thus produced resembles that seen in stuporous melancholic patients, and there are indications that it is associated with (or dependent upon) the reduction of cerebral monamine (NE, 5-HT) levels. The administration of other reserpine derivatives, *e.g.*, *yohimbine* or *10-acetylyohimbine*, results in psychotomimetic effects (Holmberg and Gershon, 1961; Gershon and Lang, 1962; and Brown *et al.*, 1966).

d. Harmine and Derivatives

This is one of the least explored categories of psychomimetic drugs (Downing, 1964). *Harmine*, an MAOI (Burger and Nara, 1965) was reported to have euphorizing effects in normals (Lewin, 1931) and psychodysleptic effects in psychotic patients (Pennes and Hoch, 1957). The psychotomimetic activity of harmine, however, could not be confirmed (Turner *et al.*, 1955). Nevertheless *harmaline* (another MAOI) and *10-methoxy harmalan* are beyond doubt hallucinogenic agents (Hochstein and Paradies, 1957; and McIsaac *et al.*, 1961); *fenoharman*, a sedative, induces dysthymic mood changes; and *raubasine* and *tetrahydroharmine* have tranquilizing effects (Schmitt and Schmitt, 1958; and Usdin and Efron, 1967).

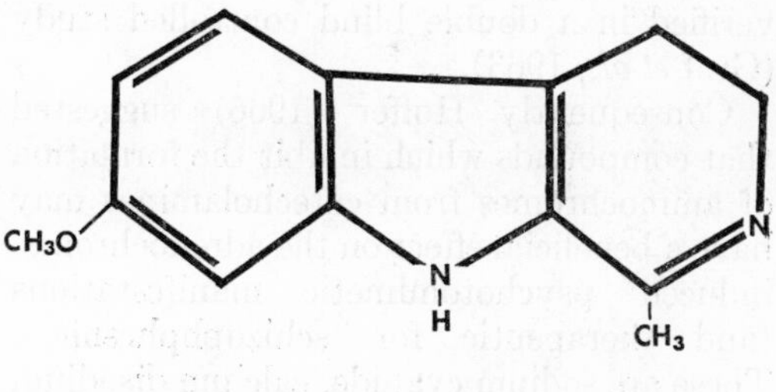

Harmine

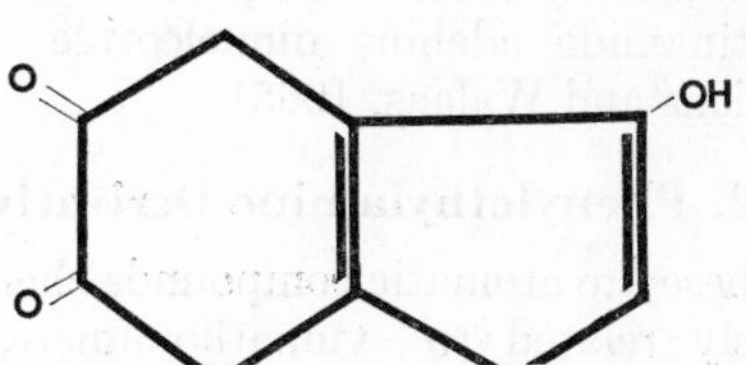

Adrenochrome

FIG. 20. Harmine and adrenochrome

e. Aminochromes

Adrenochrome, *adrenochrome semicarbazone* and *adrenolutin* are of psychopharmacological significance (Hoffer *et al.*, 1954; Hoffer, 1957; Hukki and Seppalainen, 1958; and Buday, 1961). Adrenochrome was reported to be a hallucinogen by Hoffer and his collaborators (1954), who also proposed that a disturbance in the metabolism of adrenochrome is the essential biochemical fault in schizophrenics. Supporting evidence for this was given 10 years later (Hoffer, 1966).

The enzymology of adrenochrome was reviewed by Hoffer (1966). According to him the oxidation of adrenaline to adrenochrome in adrenal gland extracts was recognized by Vulpian (1856) and studied by Kisch (1947). Adrenochrome was first prepared as a powder by Weinstein and Manning (1935), while Green and Richter (1937) described its chemical properties.

Aminochromes are derived from the catecholamines (Heacock, 1965). Adrenaline oxidase, a copper-containing enzyme distinctly different from ceruloplasmin, catalyzes their formation (Billewicz-Stankiewicz *et al.*, 1964). Adrenochrome produces behavioral changes in every mammal. Its hallucinogenic properties in humans have been verified in a double blind controlled study (Grof *et al.*, 1963).

Consequently Hoffer (1966) suggested that compounds which inhibit the formation of aminochromes from catecholamines may have a beneficial effect on the adrenochrome-induced psychotomimetic manifestations (and therapeutic for schizophphrenics). These are sodium cyanide, calcium disodium versenate, ascorbic acid, penicillamine and nicotinamide adenine dinucleotide (NAD) (Walaas and Walaas, 1965).

2. Phenylethylamine Derivatives

These are aromatic compounds chemically closely related to sympathomimetic catechols. Besides the various psychotomimetic drugs this class consists of sympathomimetic, *e.g.*, *adrenaline*, *ephetonal*, *p-hydroxyephedrine*, *N-methyladrenaline*, *norepinephrine*, *phenylephrine*, *phenylpropanolamine*, *synephrine*, *tyramine*; stimulant, *e.g.*, *l-ephedrine*; energizer, *e.g.*, *aletamine*, *aponeuron*, *chlorphentermine*, *mephentermine*, *phendimetrazine*, *phenylisopropyl-methylpropinylalanine*; antidepressant, *e.g.*, *phenelzine*, *pheniprazine*, *tranylcypromine*; tranquilizer, *e.g.*, *phenylgamma*; depressant, *e.g.*, *methyldopa*; and antipsychotic effect potentiating, *e.g.*, *nylidrin* drugs (Usdin and Efron, 1967; and Lehmann *et al.*, 1964).

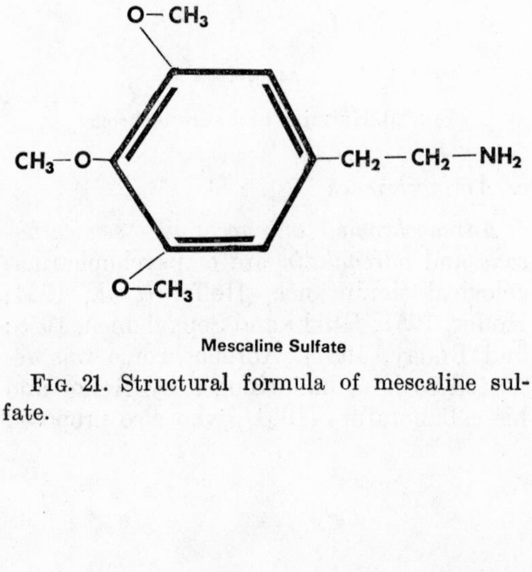

a. Amphetamines

While amphetamines are sympathomimetic, stimulant, anorexogenic and/or analeptic drugs, *e.g.*, *amphetamine phosphate*, *l-amphetamine succinate*, *d-amphetamine sulfate*, *benzphetamine* and *hydroxyamphetamine*, at least four other amphetamine preparations have psychotomimetic effects. These are *amphetamine sulfate*, *methamphetamine*, *3-methoxy-4,5-methylenedioxyamphetamine* and *3,4,5-trimethoxyamphetamine* (Liddel and Weil-Malherbe, 1953; Peretz *et al.*, 1955; Hampton, 1961; and Shulgin *et al.*, 1961). The changes induced by these substances are stimulation, euphoria and hyperthymia, which are soon replaced by fatigue, dysphoria and dysthymia. Finally a reversible condition closely resembling paranoid schizophrenia in its manifestations develops.

b. Mescaline

This is the active ingredient of peyote, the dried tops of the cactus *Lophophora williamsii*. Mescaline was named after the Mescalero Apaches of the Great Plains who used peyote in their religious rituals. The identification of the peyote cactus by Lewin (1888) and the isolation of its active principle led to the elucidation of its structural formula (3,4,5-trimethoxyphenethylamine) by Späth (1919).

Mescaline induces perceptual disturbances in normal subjects, *i.e.*, visual and tactile illusions and hallucinations with or without anxiety, loss of emotional control and inco-

O–CH₃

CH₃–O– –CH₂–CH₂–NH₂

O–CH₃

Mescaline Sulfate

FIG. 21. Structural formula of mescaline sulfate.

ordination of movements. Sense of time and space are characteristically influenced, but the sensorium remains clear (Mayer-Gross, 1951; Reti, 1953; Block, 1958; and Denber, 1958).

A succinct description of mescaline-induced changes is given by Downing (1964). According to him, the unpleasant vegetative symptoms subside within 2 hours. They are followed by a pleasant dream-like condition accompanied by visual (color) hallucinations. Finally depersonalization and time disorientation may occur. The usual duration of mescaline experience is 5 to 12 hours, although Stevenson and Richards (1960) reported reactions which lasted for several months.

Correlated with the mescaline-induced psychological changes is an interference with the epinephrine cycle and an anti-serotonin action. Electroencephalographic changes are present only with relatively high doses. They last for approximately 12 hours after drug ingestion and revert to normal along with the disappearance of the psychopathological symptoms.

c. Other Phenylethylamines

A series of hallucinogenic *N,α-dimethylphenethylamines* were systematically explored by Knoll and his collaborators (1966). Among them are *p*-iodo-; *p*-amino-; *p*-chloro-; *p*-nitro-; and *p*-bromo-*n,α-dimethylphenethylamine*. Other verified hallucinogenics with a phenylethylamine structure are *2,4,5-trimethoxy-α-methyl-4,5-methylenedioxyphenethylamine* (Shulgin, 1964) and *paredrinol* (Knoll *et al.*, 1966).

3. Piperidine Derivatives

The acute organic psychosis-producing effect of *Atropa belladonna* and *Datura stramonium* has been known for a long time and also the euphoric action of *Erythroxylon coca*. The ingredients of these are atropine, scopolamine and cocaine, the parent substances of psychotomimetic piperidine derivatives.

a. Atropine and Related Compounds

Atropine has been reported to induce a toxic psychosis. This effect was utilized in the treatment of various psychoneuroses and psychoses with questionable success (Forrer, 1951; and Forrer *et al.*, 1956). The atropine-induced syndrome starts with a transient acceleration of pulse rate, respiration and a slight rise of blood pressure. These somatic manifestations are soon replaced by psychological changes: restlessness, excitement, giddiness, muscular incoordination, speech disturbance, visual hallucinations, disorientation, confusion and coma (Gordon and Frye, 1955; and Goldenberg, 1957). The coma terminates spontaneously (Kalinowsky and Hoch, 1961).

A large number of substances have been tested whose structure was based on the piperidine ring of the atropine molecule but in which the tropic side chain was replaced by various substituted glycolic acids. Among them Abood *et al.* (1959) recognized psychotomimetic properties in the following: *Ditran* (*N-ethyl-2-pyrrolidylmethylphenylcyclopentyl glycolate*); *N-[2-(N,N-dimethylhydrazino) ethyl]-3-piperidyl benzilate*; *N-cinnamyl-3-piperidyl benzilate*; *4-piperidyl benzilate*; *1-(1-phenyl-2-bromoethyl)-3-piperidyl benzilate*; *1-phenethyl-3-piperidyl benzilate*; and *1-allyl-3-piperidyl benzilate*. Somewhat later Biel *et al.* (1962) suggested that *N-ethyl-3-piperidyl benzilate* and *N-methyl-3-piperidyl benzilate* possess also hallucinogenic properties. More recently, the psychotomimetic properties of (*1-methylpyrrolidin-3-yl*) *α-phenylcyclopentyl glycolate* and of *dexaxadrol*, which is a 2-(2,2-diphenyl-1,3-di-oxolane-4-yl)-piperidine, have also been revealed (Bente *et al.*, 1964; and Lasagna and Pearson, 1965). Other psychodysleptics of this category are Sernyl a (1-(1-phenylcyclohexyl) piperidine (Davies and Beech, 1960) and *N-methyl-2-pyrrolidylmethyl cyclopentylphenyl glycolate*. Of these, Ditran and Sernyl are of heuristic importance.

i. Ditran. This is an anticholinergic substance with distinct hallucinogenic properties. The most prevalent effects are partial (or complete) loss of contact with the environment; altered state of consciousness; and change of behavior under the influence of the hallucinatory experiences. Not infrequently there is a congrade amnesia, which makes at least part of the individual's Ditran experiences inaccessible.

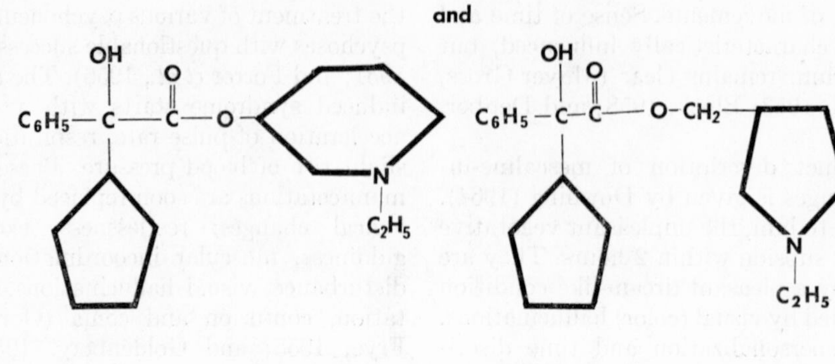

FIG. 22. Structural formula of ditran

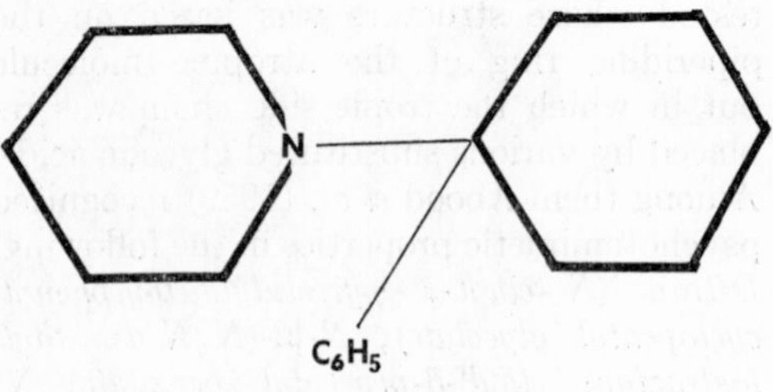

FIG. 23. Structural formula of phencyclidine

ii. Phencyclidine. Like Ditran, Sernyl is also an anticholinergic substance with distinct psychotomimetic properties. Luby *et al.* (1959) described the sensory and cognitive deviations and compared them to schizophrenic symptomatology. They subsequently introduced the term schizophrenomimetic to describe the action of Sernyl. In another study, Ban *et al.* (1961) emphasized the body image disturbance and the associated feelings of unreality (also the estrangement from the environment) under the influence of a certain (0.07 mg./kg.) dosage. Although the Sernyl experience in this dosage was uniformly described as unpleasant and extremely frightening, it was noted that consciousness remained clear throughout the experimental session.

Dose-response relations with Sernyl were described by Ban (1965). According to him, when Sernyl is given below the psychotopathic dose it produces disinhibitory manifestations and when given above the psychotopathic dose it induces narcosis.

4. Tetrahydrocannabinols

These are Cannabis derivatives. Tetrahydrocannibol is the active ingredient of the hemp plant *Cannabis sativa*. All preparations which contain tetrahydrocannibol produce a particular kind of "mental derangement." These preparations have been used for some time under various names, *e.g.*, hashish, bhang, ganjia, charas and churrus. The best known perhaps is marijuana.

The psychopharmacologically most important member of this class is *tetrahydrocannabinol* (Scarlato and Bonaretti, 1959). It induces elation in a dreamy, semiconscious state in which judgment is lost and the imagination is freed of its usual restraints. Other less important Cannabis derivatives with psychotopathic effects are *dimethylheptyl pyran* (Dagirmanjian and Boyd, 1962), *methyloctyl pyran* (Dagirmanjian and Boyd, 1962) and *synhexyl*, which is 1-hydroxy-3-*n*-hexyl-6,6,9-trimethyl-7,8,9,10-tetrahydro-6-dibenzopyran (Loewe, 1946; and Stockings, 1947). The hallucinogenic properties of cannabadiol, cannabiol and dihydrocannabinol have not been substantiated as yet.

5. Other Hallucinogens

There are various other psychotopathic substances of different origin and chemical structure. Among them are diethylaminoethylphenothazine (Courvoisier *et al.*, 1960), a member of the phenothiazine series (most of which are antipsychotic drugs); *anhalamine* and *nalorphine* (Isbell, 1956; and Pennes and Hoch, 1957), both *N*-heterocyclic drugs (the latter frequently used in narcotic withdrawal). Psychotomimetic properties have been attributed to such aromatic compounds as *benactyzine* and *caramiphen* (Kagan, 1956; Vojtechovsky *et al.*, 1958; and Vassiliou *et al.*, 1961) and to aliphatic compounds, for example, *ethyl(1-phenylcyclohexyl)amine*, *dibenamine*, *parathion*, *dimethylacetamide*, *iminodipropionitrile*, *diisopropylfluorophosphate* and *tetraethylpyrophosphate* (Chak and De, 1961; Downing, 1962; Weiss *et al.*, 1962; and Usdin and Efron, 1967).

It is usually agreed that the experience that follows the administration of a hallucinogenic drug depends on external (*e.g.*, therapist, setting, others present) and internal (*e.g.*, disease, motivation, personality, expectations, education, familiarity with the drug) factors. The final reactions are psychotomimetic or psychedelic in nature (Hoffer, 1966). According to Hoffer (1966), plant hallucinogens, *e.g.*, mescaline, LSD_{25} and psiloybin, can produce both, whereas animal hallucinogens, *e.g.*, adrenochrome and adrenolutin, can induce only psychotomimetic responses. On the basis of this, LSD_{25}, psiloybin, mescaline and also Sernyl were tried as pharmacological adjuncts to psychotherapeutic intervention with questionable success. Similarly, attempts to use LSD_{25} in the treatment of alcoholism, character disorders and certain sexual pathologies have remained unrewarding. Toxic psychotic reactions induced by atropine or Ditran for therapeutic purposes in psychotic or psychoneurotic patients have practically been abandoned.

E. PRESENT STATUS

Systematic studies with psychoactive substances of various chemical groups led to the differentiation of the two heuristically and clinically most important basic categories: the category of psychotopathics and the category of psychotherapeutics.

Intensive exploratory work with psychotopathic substances has rendered a variety of artificially induced psychopathological states accessible for direct investigation. Today, a feeling of well-being (or euphoria) can be induced by the administration of monoamine oxidase inhibitors or ketosteroids; dysthymic mood changes and/or depression by reserpine (an indole) or tetrabenazine (a benzoquinolizine), both of which decrease brain NE or 5-HT concentrations; manifestations closely resembling the primary symptoms of schizophrenia by Sernyl, an anticholinergic piperidine; accessory symptoms of schizophrenia by mescaline or LSD_{25}, which interfere with the epinephrine cycle or increase brain serotonin levels, respectively; a paranoid schizophrenia-like state by amphetamine, a sympathomimetic phenethylamine; dream-like semiconscious states by tetrahydrocannabinol; and conditions resembling toxic psychosis (acute brain syndromes) with an altered state of consciousness by atropine or Ditran, both piperidines with anticholinergic properties.

Research with psychotherapeutic drugs has succeeded in differentiating between chemicals with anxiolytic properties particularly useful in the treatment of the psychoneuroses; substances with thymoleptic action, specially indicated in the treatment of depressive illnesses; and compounds with antipsychotic potential, which are used in the treatment of psychotic manifestations in general and schizophrenic psychopathology in particular.

More recently, differential activities among the various groups of substances within these categories have been recognized. The sequence of therapeutic changes differs according to the action of the particular drug. Thus, when given to psychoneurotics, barbiturate action (which has the strongest affinity for brain stem reticular formation structures) is primarily manifested in *sedation* slowly followed by tension relief and anxiety control; propanediol action (which has the strongest affinity for interneuronal connections) produces *tension relief* first and anxiolysis and sedation only thereafter; and benzodiazepine action (which has the strongest affinity for limbic lobe structures) exerts *anxiolytic effects* followed by sedation and relief of tension.

Among the various substances used in the treatment of depressive patients, amphetamines (with predominant affinity for brain stem reticular formation structures) induce primarily *psychomotor stimulation*, which creates a feeling of well-being (euphoria) with or without hyperthymic (elation) mood changes before exhaustion, dysphoria and possibly psychotopathic effects set in; MAOI's (with the simultaneous increase of brain NE and 5-HT concentrations) produce *euphoria* with a subsequent mood lift and not infrequently psychomotor stimulation; and tricyclic antidepressants (which exert a suppressant action on brain stem reticular formation structures together with the interference of monoamine uptake in the brain) induce *elation* which is then followed by a feeling of well-being with or without sedation.

Finally, of the various antipsychotics the phenothiazines (which decrease the utilization of adenosin triphosphate and control the input of the brain stem reticular formation structures) proved to be particularly useful in the treatment of the basic or primary psychopathological symptoms in schizophrenics, the butyrophenones (which, via the caudate loop, have a controlling action on the reticular activating system) are especially effective in the control of the accessory symptoms present in schizophrenics; the thioxanthenes (substances with relatively strong adrenolytic and antiserotonin action but with a relatively weak antiacetylcholine effect) are particularly indicated for pseudoneurotic and schizoaffective cases; and the Rauwolfias (which deplete brain monoamines) seem to be specially useful when recurrent hyperthymic features are associated with the schizophrenic illness, *e.g.*, cyclophrenia.

Although the linkage between psychotopathic and psychotherapeutic substances has not been established, their meeting points become more and more closely defined by systematic psychopharmacological work. This implies that by applying psychopharmacological means a better understanding of the functional alteration "behind" the psychopathological manifestations are obtained. Nevertheless, the primary cause in the etiology of these problems still remains to be elucidated.

REFERENCES

Abood, L. G., and Meduna, L. G. (1958): In: Biel, J. H.: Antidepressant drugs. In: Molecular modification in drug design (ed., Gould, R. F.). (American Chemical Society, Washington, 1964.)

Abood L. G., Ostfeld, A., and Biel, J. H. (1959): In: Downing, D. F.: Psychotomimetic compounds. In: Psychopharmacological agents (ed., Gordon, M.). (Academic Press, New York, 1964.)

Alapin, B., and Zaborowska, E.: Action of prothiadane in depressive states. Neurol. Neurochir. Psychiat. Pol., *16:* 425 (1966).

Antos, R. J. (1955): In: Krueger, G. L., and McGrath, W. R.: 2-Benzylpiperidines and related compounds. In: Psychopharmacological agents (ed., Gordon, M.). (Academic Press, New York, 1964.)

Arnold, O. H., Hift, S. and Hoff, H.: The role of psychotropic drugs in current psychiatric therapy. Compr. Psychiat., *3:* 330 (1962).

Asbell, N.: Clinical evaluation of a new non-barbiturate sedative hypnotic, 2-methyl-3-o-tolyl-4-quinazalone: double blind study. J. Amer. Geriat. Soc., *10:* 1032 (1962).

Ayd, F. J.: Treatment of ambulatory and hospitalized psychiatric patients with perphenazine. Dis. Nerv. Syst., *18:* 394 (1957).

Bachann, K. (1960): In: Usdin, E., and Efron, D. H.: Psychotropic drugs and related compounds. (PHSP No. 1589, Washington, 1967.)

Ban, T. A.: Comments on the use of sernyl. In: Neuropsychopharmacology (eds., Bente, D., and Bradley, P. B.). (Elsevier, Amsterdam, 1965.)

Ban, T. A., Lohrenz, J. R., and Lehmann, H. E.: Observations on the action of sernyl—a new psychotropic drug. Canad. Psychiat. Ass. J., *6:* 150 (1961).

Ban, T. A., and McGinnis, K.: Comparative clinical study of two hypnotic drugs. Canad. Med. Ass. J., *87:* 816 (1962).

Ban, T. A., St. Jean, A., and Lehmann, H. E.: Clinical studies with MO-1255, a new monoamine oxidase inhibitor antidepressant. Curr. Ther. Res., *8:* 614 (1966).

Banschikov, V. M., and Berezin, F. B.: Use of γ-aminobutyric acid derivatives in psychiatric practice. Zh. Nevropat. Psikhiat. Korsakov., *66:* 763 (1966).

Barsa, J. A., and Saunders, J. C.: A double blind study of a new chlorprothixene preparation. Amer. J. Psychiat., *121:* 493 (1964).

Bayart, J. (1956): In: Morren, H. G., *et al.:* Piperazine derivatives. In: Psychopharmacological agents (ed., Gordon, M.). (Academic Press, New York, 1964.)

Bente, D., Hartung, H., and Penning, J. (1964): In: Usdin, E., and Efron, E. H.: Psychotropic drugs and related compounds. (PHSP No. 1589, Washington, 1967.)

Bente, D., *et al.*: Profile of action of an antidepressant of the dibenzodiazepine series—Wander 91/HF 1927 (noveril). In: Neuropsychopharmacology, Vol. IV (eds., Bente, D., and Bradley, P. B.). (Elsevier, Amsterdam, 1965.)

Bente, D., *et al.*: Thymoleptic efficacy represented by melitracene. Arzneimittelforschung, *16:* 319 (1966).

Bercel, N.: Chlordiazepoxide (librium) as an anticonvulsant. Dis. Nerv. Syst., *22:* 17 (1961).

Bertolotti, P., and Munarini, D.: Therapeutic experiences in neuropsychiatry with a derivative of benzoquinolizine (RO 1-9569). Riv. Sper. Freniat., *85:* 185 (1961).

Bhaskaran, K., and Nand, D. S.: Clinical trial with a (2-piperidyl) benzhydrol hydrochloride (meratran) and methylphenidylate (ritalin) in chronic apathetic schizophrenics. Indian J. Med. Sci., *13:* 117 (1959).

Biel, J. H., *et al.*: A cholinergic blockage as an approach to the development of new psychotropic agent. Ann. N. Y. Acad. Sci., *96:* 251 (1962).

Billewicz-Stankiewicz, J., *et al.*: Influencing "adrenaline-oxidases" of blood plasma through biogenic monoamines and neurologically active drugs. Experientia, *20:* 85 (1964).

Bishop, M. P., and Gallant, D. M.: Behavioral toxicity associated with benzquinamide (quantril) therapy in schizophrenic patients. Amer. J. Psychiat., *120:* 180 (1963).

Bister, W., *et al.*: Clinical experience with the new thymoleptic melitracene. Arzneimittelforschung, *16:* 321 (1966).

Blair, D: Drugs for depression. Brit. Med. J., *1* (*5335*): 945 (1963).

Block, W. (1958): In: Downing, D. F.: Psychotomimetic drugs. In: Psychopharmacological agents (ed., Gordon, M.). (Academic Press, New York, 1964.)

Bojanovsky, J., and Chloupkova, K.: Application of ritalin in the differential diagnosis of depression. Activ. Nerv. Sup., *7:* 56 (1965).

Bordeleau, J. M., *et al.*: Study of the hypnotic properties of nitromethaqualone in the psychiatric patient. Canad. Psychiat. Ass. J., *10:* 272 (1965).

Böszörmenyi, Z., Der, P., and Nagy, T. (1959): In: Usdin, E., and Efron, D. H.: Psychotropic drugs and related compounds. (PHSP No. 1589, Washington, 1967.)

Bower, H. B., and McDonald, C.: A controlled trial of A.N.P. 235 (lucidril) in senile dementia. Med. J. Aust., *2:* 270 (1966).

Bradley, P. B., and Elkes, J.: The effects of some drugs on the electrical activity of the brain. Brain, *80:* 77 (1957).

Bratlund, H. (1961): In: Usdin, E., and Efron, D. H.: Psychotropic drugs and related compounds. (PHSP No. 1589, Washington, 1967.)

Brown, B. B., and Werner, H. W.: Pharmacological studies on a new central stimulant: α-(2-piperidyl) benzhydrol HCl (MRD-108). J. Pharmacol., *110:* 180 (1954).

Brown, M. L., *et al.* (1966): In: Usdin, E., and Efron, D. H.: Psychotropic drugs and related compounds. (PHSP No. 1589, Washington, 1967.)

Buday, P. F. (1961): In: Usdin, E., and Efron, D. H.: Psychotropic drugs and related compounds. (PHSP No. 1589, Washington, 1967.)

Burckard, E., *et al.*: Clinical, biological and electroencephalographic study of the action of tetrabenazine (RO 1.9569) in some chronic psychoses. Ann. Medico psychol., *1:* 115 (1962).

Burger, A., and Nara, S. (1965): In: Usdin, E., and Efron, D. H.: Psychotropic drugs and related compounds. (PHSP No. 1589, Washington, 1967.)

Button, J. C. (1956): In: Krueger, G. L., and McGrath, W. R.: 2-Benzylpiperidines and related compounds. In: Psychopharmacological agents (ed., Gordon, M.). (Academic Press, New York, 1964.)

Calje, J. F.: Contribution to the concept of psychasthenia. Ann. Medico Psychol., *119:* 792 (1961).

Carey, B., *et al.*: Methyl-phenidylacetate hydrochloride (ritalin) in the treatment of chronic schizophrenic patients. Amer. J. Psychiat., *113:* 546 (1956).

Caruso, M. J.: Clinical study of the effect of l-Triiodothyronine in chronic, hospitalized schizophrenics. Fôlha Médica, *52:* 129 (1966).

Chak, I. M., and De, N. N. (1961): In: Usdin, E., and Efron, D. H. Psychotropic drugs and related compounds. (PHSP No. 1589, Washington, 1967.)

Cohen, I. M.: Complications of chlorpromazine therapy. Amer. J. Psychiat., *113:* 115 (1956).

Coldrey, P. A.: Hypnotic action of methaqualone. Practitioner, *190:* 368 (1963).

Cole, J., and Glees, P. (1956): In: Krueger, G. L., and McGrath, W. R.: 2-Benzylpiperidines and related compounds. In: Psychopharmacological agents (ed., Gordon, M.). (Academic Press, New York, 1964.)

Cornbleet, T. (1960): In: Morren, H. G., *et al.*: Piperazine derivatives. In: Psychopharmacological agents (ed., Gordon, M.). (Academic Press, New York, 1964.)

Courvoisier, S., *et al.*: Study of the pharmacological properties of 2-diethylaminoethyl phenothiazine-10-dithiocarboxylate (RP 7360). C. R. Soc. Biol. (Paris), *154:* 965 (1960).

Dagirmanjian, R., and Boyd, E. S. (1962): In: Usdin, E., and Efron, D. H.: Psychotropic drugs and related compounds. (PHSP No. 1589, Washington, 1967.)

Danziger, L.: Thyroid therapy of schizophrenia. Dis. Nerv. Syst., *19:* 373 (1958).

Darmstadter, H. J., and Mock, J. E.: Atarax in the treatment of agitation: a pilot study. Dis. Nerv. Syst., *26:* 236 (1965).

Davidova, M., and Zapletalek, M.: Some notes

on the use of captodiamine in pedopsychiatry. Activ. Nerv. Sup., *7:* 298 (1965).

Davies, B. M., and Beech, H. R. (1960): In: Downing, D. F.: Psychotomimetic compounds. In: Psychopharmacological agents (ed., Gordon, M.). (Academic Press, New York, 1964.)

Davis, H. K., *et al.:* Clinical evaluation of JB-329 (ditran). Dis. Nerv. Syst., *25:* 179 (1964).

Decsi, L. (1961): In: Usdin, E., and Efron, D. H.: Psychotropic drugs and related compounds. (PHSP No. 1589, Washington, 1967.)

Denber, H. C. B.: Some preliminary results with a new phenothiazine derivative: prochlorperazine. Psychiat. Res. Rep. Amer. Psychiat. Ass., *9:* 16 (1958).

Deshaies, G., *et al.:* Psychiatric application of a psychotonic drug. Ann. Medico Psychol., *1:* 630 (1965).

Destrem, H.: Clinical trial of centrophenoxine in geriatrics. Presse Med., *69:* 1999 (1961).

DiMascio, A., Rinkel, M., and Lieberman, J.: Personality and psychotomimetic drugs. (Presented at the Third World Congress of Psychiatry, Montreal, 1961.)

Dolan, C. M. (1958): In: Morren, H. G., *et al.:* Piperazine derivatives. In: Psychoparmacological agents (ed., Gordon, M.). (Academic Press, New York, 1964.)

Downing, D. F. (1962): In: Downing, D. F.: Psychotomimetic compounds. In: Psychopharmacological agents (ed., Gordon, M.). (Academic Press, New York, 1964.)

Downing, D. F.: Psychotomimetic compounds. In: Psychopharmacological agents (ed., Gordon, M.). (Academic Press, New York, 1964.)

Dzikowski, H.: New psychiatric remedy, esucos (VCB 3412, dixyrazine). Neurol. Neurochir. Psychiat. Pol., *11:* 543 (1961).

Ende, M. (1956): In: Morren, H. G., *et al.:* Piperazine derivatives. In: Psychopharmacological agents (ed., Gordon, M.). (Academic Press, New York, 1964.)

Espie, M. J.: Pharmacology of centrophenoxine. Application to delirium tremens. Lyon Med., *215:* 935 (1966).

Fabing, H. D.: Clinical experience with Meratran. Dis. Nerv. Syst., *16:* 10 (1955).

Fabing, H. D. (1957): In: Krueger, G. L., and McGrath, W. R.: 2-Benzylpiperidines and related compounds. In: Psychopharmacological agents (ed., Gordon, M.). (Academic Press, New York, 1964.)

Fabing, H. D., and Hawkins, J. R. (1956): In: Usdin, E., and Efron, D. H.: Psychotropic drugs and related compounds. (PHSP No. 1589, Washington, 1967.)

Fabing, H. D., and Hawkins, J. R.: A year's experience with frenquel in clinical and experimental schizophrenic psychoses. Dis. Nerv. Syst., *16:* 329 (1955).

Fabing, H. D., *et al.:* Clinical studies on α-(2-piperidyl) benzylhydrol hydrochloride, a new antidepressant drug. Amer. J. Psychiat., *111:* 832 (1955).

Fedotov, D. D., *et al.:* Preliminary report on the use of meratran in some mental diseases. Zh. Nevropat. Psikhiat. Korsakov., *58:* 592 (1958).

Feinblatt, T. M., *et al.:* A new antipsychotic agent: benactyzine. Dis. Nerv. Syst., *19:* 394 (1958).

Feldman, P. E.: Clinical evaluation of benzquinamide (P-2647) in the control of tension states and "hypersyndromes." Psychosomatics, *3:* 148 (1962).

Ferguson, R. S.: A clinical trail of reserpine in the treatment of anxiety. J. Ment. Sci., *102:* 30 (1956).

Finkelstein, B. A.: Ditran, a psychotherapeutic advance: a review of one hundred and three cases. J. Neuropsychiat., *2:* 144 (1961).

Flack, F. F., *et al.:* Treatment of psychiatric disorders with tri-iodothyronine. Amer. J. Psychiat., *114:* 841 (1958).

Flores, M. (1957): In: Morren, H. G., *et al.:* Piperazine derivatives. In: Psychopharmacological agents (ed., Gordon, M.). (Academic Press, New York, 1964.)

Forney, R. B., and Hughes, F. W.: Behavioral effects on the rat of benzquinamide and benzquinamide-alcohol combinations. Arch. Int. Pharmacodyn., *142:* 237 (1963).

Forrer, G. R.: Atropine toxicity in the treatment of mental disease. Amer. J. Psychiat., *108:* 107 (1951).

Forrer, G. R., *et al.:* Symposium on atropine toxicity therapy. J. Nerv. Ment. Dis., *124:* 256 (1956).

Freed, H.: The use of ritalin intravenously as a diagnostic adjuvant in psychiatry. Amer. J. Psychiat., *114:* 944 (1958).

Freedman, A. M. (1958): In: Morrey, H. G., *et al.:* Piperazine derivatives. In: Psychopharmacological agents (ed., Gordon, M.). (Academic Press, New York, 1964.)

Freeman, H., and Oktem, M. R.: Tranquillizing effects of SKF-14336 in chronic schizophrenic patients. Curr. Ther. Res., *8:* 395 (1966).

Freeman, H., *et al.:* Therapeutic efficacy of a new antidepressant, thiazenone. Curr. Ther. Res., *7:* 655 (1965).

Funfschilling, P. (1957): In: Morren, H. G. *et al.:* Piperazine derivatives. In: Psychopharmacological agents (ed., Gordon, M.). (Academic Press, New York, 1964.)

Gallant, D. M., Bishop, M. P., and Shelton, W.: P-5227: A tricyclic antipsychotic compound. Curr. Ther. Res., *8:* 241 (1966).

Gallant, D. M., *et al.:* DPN (NAD-oxidized forms): a preliminary evaluation in chronic schizophrenic patients. Curr. Ther. Res., *8:* 542 (1966).

Gallant, D. M., *et al.:* Thiothixene: a controlled evaluation in chronic schizophrenic patients. Curr. Ther. Res., *8:* 153 (1966).

Geller, L. M., Cowen, D., and Wolf, A.: Effect of the antimetabolite, 6-aminonicotinamide, on sound-induced seizures in mice. Exp. Neurol., *14:* 86 (1966).

Gershon, S.: Informal EDCEU report from the Department of Psychiatry, New York University School of Medicine, New York, 1967.

Gershon, S., and Lang, W. J.: A psychopharmacological study of some indole alkaloids. Arch. Int. Pharmacodyn., *135:* 31 (1962).

Gessner, P. K., *et al.* (1961): In: Usdin, E., and Efron, D. H.: Psychotropic drugs and related compounds. (PHSP No. 1589, Washington, 1967).

Gibbon, J. (1961): In: Morren, H. G., *et al.*: Piperazine derivatives. In: Psychopharmacological agents (ed., Gordon, M.). (Academic Press, New York, 1964.)

Giraud, J. C., *et al.*: Prolonged post-traumatic coma. Recovery following treatment with ANP 235. Rev. Otoneuroophtal., *33:* 163 (1961).

Godefroi, E. F., *et al.*: dl-1(l-Arylalkyl) imidazole-5-carboxylate esters. A novel type of hypnotic agent. J. Med. Chem., *8:* 220 (1965).

Goldenberg, G.: Atropine psychoses in animals. Novosibersk Govt. Med. Inst., *29:* 7 (1957).

Goldman, H. (1961): In: Morren, H. G., *et al.*: Piperazine derivatives. In: Psychopharmacological agents (ed., Gordon, M.). (Academic Press, New York, 1964.)

Goodhard, R. S. (ed.): Modern drug encyclopedia and therapeutic index. (Reuben H. Donnelly Corporation, New York, 1965.)

Goodman, L. S., and Gilman, A. (eds.): The pharmacological basis of therapeutics. (MacMillan, New York, 1965.)

Gordon, A. S., and Frye, C. W. (1955): In: Downing, D. F.: Psychotomimetic compounds. In: Psychopharmacological agents (ed., Gordon, M.). (Academic Press, New York, 1964.)

Green, D. E., and Richter, D.: Adrenalin and adrenochrome. Biochem. J., *31:* 596 (1937).

Greenblatt, E. N., and Osterberg, A. C.: Some pharmacologic properties of thozalinone, a new excitant. Toxic. Appl. Pharmacol., *7:* 566 (1965).

Greiner, A. C., and Berry, K.: Skin pigmentation and corneal and lens opacities with prolonged chlorpromazine therapy. Canad. Med. Ass. J., *90:* 663 (1964).

Greiner, A. C., and Nicolson, G. A.: New side effects in prolonged chlorpromazine therapy. Canad. Psychiat. Ass. J., *10:* 109 (1965).

Greiner, A. C., and Nicolson, G. A.: Schizophrenia-melanosis. Cause or side effect? Lancet, *2:* 1165 (1965).

Greiner, A. C., *et al.*: Therapy of chlorpromazine melanosis: a preliminary report. Canad. Med. Ass. J., *91:* 636 (1964).

Greiner, J.: Selective patient-participants for drug investigations. J. New Drugs, *2:* 199 (1962).

Grof, S., *et al.*: Clinical and experimental study of central effects of adrenochrome. J. Neuropsychiat., *5:* 33 (1963).

Gruber, K., *et al.* (1956): In: Krueger, G. L., and McGrath, W. R.: 2-Benzylpiperidines and related compounds. In: Psychopharmacological agents (ed., Gordon, M.). (Academic Press, New York, 1964.)

Gujral, M. L., Kohli, R. P., and Saxena, P. N.: Experimental study of hypnotic potency, toxicity and safety margin of 2,3-disubstituted quinazolones. Indian J. Med. Sci., *10:* 871 (1956).

Hampton, W. H.: Observed psychiatric reactions following use of amphetamine-like substances. Bull. N. Y. Acad. Med., *37:* 167 (1961).

Hargreaves, G. R., *et al.* (1957): In: Jacobsen, E.: Benactyzine. In: Psychopharmacological agents (ed., Gordon, M.). (Academic Press, New York, 1964.)

Harrington, J. A., and Mayer-Gross, W. (1959): In: Jacobsen, E.: Benactyzine. In: Psychopharmacological agents (ed., Gordon, M.). (Academic Press, New York, 1964.)

Hartert, D., and Browne-Mayers, A. N.: The use of methylphenidate (ritalin) hydrochloride in alcoholism. J.A.M.A., *166:* 1982 (1958).

Hartmann, M., and Panizzon, L. (1950): In: Krueger, G. L., and McGrath, W. R.: 2-Benzylpiperidines and related compounds. In: Psychopharmacological agents (ed., Gordon, M.). (Academic Press, New York, 1964.)

Heacock, R. A.: The aminochromes (Advances in heterocyclic chem., Vol. 5). (Academic Press, New York, 1965.)

Heimann, H., and Lukacs, G.: Experimental psychological differentiation of the effect of two psychostimulants in man (F-1983 and amphetamine). Psychopharmacologia (Berlin), *8:* 79 (1965).

Hochstein, F. A., and Paradies, A. M. (1957): In: Downing, D. F.: Psychotomimetic drugs. In: Psychopharmacological agents (ed., Gordon, M.). (Academic Press, New York, 1964.)

Hoffer, A.: Epinephrine derivatives as potential schizophrenic factors. J. Clin. Exp. Psychopath., *18:* 27 (1957).

Hoffer, A.: Enzymology of hallucinogens. In: Enzymes in mental health (eds., Martin, G. J., and Kisch, B.). (Lippincott, New York, 1966.)

Hoffer, A.: Laboratory tests for following progress of schizophrenia. Dis. Nerv. Syst., *27:* 466 (1966).

Hoffer, A., Osmond, H., and Smythies, J.: Schizophrenia: a new approach. II. Result of two years' research. J. Ment. Sci., *100:* 29 (1954).

Hofmann, A. (1960): In: Usdin, E., and Efron, D. H.: Psychotropic drugs and related compounds. (PHSP No. 1589, Washington, 1967.)

Hofmann, A., *et al.* (1959): In: Usdin, E., and Efron, D. H.: Psychotropic drugs and related compounds. (PHSP No. 1589, Washington, 1967.)

Hollister, L. E.: Chlorpromazine jaundice. J.A.M.A., *169:* 1235 (1959).

Hollister, L. E., and Hall, R. A.: Phenothiazine derivatives and morphologic changes in the liver. Amer. J. Psychiat., *123:* 2 (1966).

Hollister, L. E., Marazzi, A. S., and Casey, J. F.: Serum oxidase activity in chronic schizophrenics treated with tranquillizing drugs. Amer. J. Psychiat., *116:* 553 (1959).

Hollister, L. E., *et al.* (1960): In: Usdin, E., and

Efron, D. H.: Psychotropic drugs and related compounds. (PHSP No. 1589, Washington, 1967).

Hollister, L. E., *et al.*: Antipyridoxine effect of d-penicillamine in schizophrenic men. Amer. J. Clin. Nutr., *19:* 307 (1966).

Holmberg, G., and Gershon, S.: Autonomic and psychic effects of yohimbine hydrochloride. Psychopharmacologia (Berlin), *2:* 93 (1961).

Horovitz, Z.: Psychoactive drugs and limbic system of the brain. (The Squibb Institute for Medical Research, New Brunswick, 1965.)

Houston, F.: Group behavior in chronic schizophrenics treated with meratran. Brit. Med. J., *1:* 949 (1956).

Hukki, J., and Seppalainen, N. (1958): In: Usdin, E., and Efron, D. H. Psychotropic drugs and related compounds. (PHSP No. 1589, Washington, 1967.)

Irwin, S.: Practical pharmacology of barbiturate sedatives, and related drugs. (Presented at the Sixth Annual Meeting of the ACNP, San Juan, 1967.)

Irwin, S., and Benuazizi, A.: Pentylenetetrazol enhances memory function. Science, *152:* 100 (1966).

Isbell, H. (1956): In: Usdin, E., and Efron, D. H.: Psychotropic drugs and related compounds. (PHSP No. 1589, Washington, 1967.)

Ivanova, R. A., *et al.:* The effect of nicotinic acid on experimental psychosis induced by lysergic acid diethylamide. Zh. Nevropat. Psikhiat. Korsakov. *64:* 1172 (1964).

Jacobsen, E.: The pharmacological classification of central nervous system depressants. J. Pharm. Pharmacol., *10:* 273 (1958).

Jacobsen, E., *et al.:* The autonomic reaction of psychoneurotics to a new sedative: benactyzine, suavitil (benzilic acid diethylaminoethyl-ester hydrochloride). Acta Psychiat. Neurol. Scand., *30:* 627 (1955).

Jouvet, M., and Courjon, J. (1959): In: Krueger, G. L., and McGrath, W. R.: 2-Benzylpiperidines and related compounds. In: Psychopharmacological agents (ed., Gordon, M.). (Academic Press, New York, 1964.)

Kagan, I. S. (1956): In: Downing, D. F.: Psychotomimetic compounds. In: Psychopharmacological agents (ed., Gordon, M.). (Academic Press, New York, 1964.)

Kalinowsky, L. B., and Hoch, P. H.: Somatic treatments in psychiatry. (Grune and Stratton, New York, 1961.)

Kammerer, T. (1962): In: Morren, P., *et al.:* Piperazine derivatives. In: Psychopharmacological agents (ed., Gordon, M.). (Academic Press, New York, 1964.)

Kammerer, T., *et al.*: The use of a new neuroleptic: tetrabenazine. Clinical, biological and electroencephalographic results. Ann. Médico-Psychol., *1:* 106 (1962).

Kerenyi, A. B., *et al.* (1960): In: Krueger, G. L., and McGrath, W. R.: 2-Benzylpiperidines and related compounds. In: Psychopharmacological agents (ed., Gordon, M.). (Academic Press, New York, 1964.)

Kinross-Wright, V., and Moyer, J. H.: Observations upon the therapeutic uses of benactyzine (suavitil). Amer. J. Psychiat., *114:* 74 (1957).

Kisch, B.: Metabolic effects of oxidized suprarenin (omega adrenochrome). Exp. Med. Surg., *5:* 166 (1947).

Kistner, R. W., and Duncan, C. J. (1956): In: Krueger, G. L., and McGrath, W. R.: 2-Benzylpiperidines and related compounds. In: Psychopharmacological agents (ed., Gordon, M.). (Academic Press, New York, 1964.)

Klingman, W. O.: Clinical use of pipradrol. In: Psychosomatic medicine (eds., Nodine, J. H., and Moyer, J. H.). (Lea and Febiger, Philadelphia, 1962.)

Knoll, J., Vizi, E. S., and Ecseri, Z. (1966): In: Usdin, E., and Efron, D. H.: Psychotropic drugs and related compounds. (PHSP No. 1589, Washington, 1967.)

Knowles, J. B., and Kreitman, N.: Trial of oxypertine for anxiety neurosis. Brit. J. Psychiat., *112:* 104 (1966).

Kröger, R.: Treatment of endogenous depression with photodyn. Mat. Med. Nordmark, *8:* 247 (1961).

Krueger, G. L., and McGrath, W. R.: 2-Benzylpiperidines and related compounds. In: Psychopharmacological agents (ed., Gordon, M.). (Academic Press, New York, 1964.)

Kurland, A. A., *et al.:* Cypenamine treatment of mentally retarded children. Curr. Ther. Res., *9:* 293 (1967).

Kurland, A. A., *et al.:* Pilot study of navane in chronic schizophrenics and actue psychotic patients. Curr. Ther. Res., *9:* 298 (1967).

Kuziw, R., *et al.* (1956): In: Usdin, E., and Efron, D. H.: Psychotropic drugs and related compounds. (PHSP No. 1589, Washington, 1967.)

Langecker, H., Schumann, H. J., and Junkmann, K.: Chemische und Pharmacologische Eigenschaften des Aethynyl-Cyclohexylcarbaminsaure-esters. Arch. Exp. Path. Pharmakol., *219:* 130 (1953).

Lasagna, L., and Pearson, J. W. (1965): In: Usdin, E., and Efron, D. H.: Psychotropic drugs and related compounds (PHSP No. 1589, Washington, 1967.)

Lascelles, C. F., and Levene, L. J.: A study of the use of azacyclonal hydrochloride (frenquel) in chronic schizophrenia. J. Ment. Sci., *105:* 247 (1959).

Laubie, M., LeDonarec, J. C., and Schmitt, H.: Experimental studies on a new synthetic coronary dilator: benzydryl-1-piperonyl piperazine. Arch. Int. Pharmacodyn., *151:* 313 (1964).

Launay, J., and Maurey, G.: Psychopharmacological animal study and clinical antidepressant tests of a new auxin derivative: mefexamide (A.N.P. 297). Ann. Medico Psychol., *123:* 141 (1965).

LeHew, L. J. (1957): In: Krueger, G. L., and McGrath, W. R.: 2-Benzylpiperidines and related compounds. In: Psychopharmacological agents (ed., Gordon, M.). (Academic Press, New York, 1964.)

LEHMANN, H. E.: Drug treatment of schizophrenia. In: Psychopharmacology (eds., Kline, N. S., and Lehmann, H E.). (Little, Brown, Boston, 1965.)

LEHMANN, H. E., AND BAN, T. A.: ECDEU progress report, Verdun, 1963.

LEHMANN, H. E., AND BAN, T. A.: Notes from the log-book of a psychopharmacological research unit I. Canad. Psychiat. Ass. J., *9:* 28 (1964).

LEHMANN, H. E., AND BAN, T. A.: ECDEU progress report, Verdun, 1966.

LEHMANN, H. E., BAN, T. A., AND DEBOW, S. L.: A clinical-pharmacological study with EXP 561. Curr. Ther. Res., *9:* 306 (1967).

LEHMANN, H. E., CAHN, C. H., AND DEVERTEUIL, R. L.: The treatment of depressive conditions with imipramine (G 22355). Canad. Psychiat. Ass. J., *3:* 155 (1958).

LEHMANN, H. E., *et al.:* Potentiation of pharmacological and therapeutic action of phenothiazines by nylidrin (Arlidin). Compr. Psychiat., *5:* 36 (1964).

LEUNER, H., AND BAER, G. (1965): In: Usdin, E., and Efron, D. H.: Psychotropic drugs and related compounds. (PHSP No. 1589, Washington, 1967.)

LEVIN, M.: Experimental bromide intoxication: a criticism. Amer. J. Psychiat., *108:* 309 (1951).

LEVY, S. (1954): Krueger, G. L., and McGrath, W. R.: 2-Benzylpiperidines and related compounds. In: Psychopharmacological agents (ed., Gordon, M.). (Academic Press, New York, 1964.)

LEWIN, L. (1888): In: Downing, D. F.: Psychotomimetic compounds. In: Psychopharmacological agents (ed., Gordon, M.). (Academic Press, New York, 1964.)

LEWIN, L.: Phantastica. (Dutton, New York, 1931.)

LIDDEL, D. W., AND WEIL-MALHERBE, H. (1953): In: Downing, D. F.: Psychotomimetic compounds. In: Psychopharmacological agents (ed., Gordon, M.). (Academic Press, New York, 1964.)

LOEWE, S. (1946): In: Usdin, E., and Efron, D. H.: Psychotropic drugs and related compounds. (PHSP No. 1589, Washington, 1967.)

LUBY, E. D. *et al.:* Study of a new schizophrenomimetic drug, sernyl. Amer. Med. Ass. Arch. Neurol. Psychiat., *81:* 363 (1959).

LYTTON, G. J., AND KNOBEL, M.: Diagnosis and treatment of behavior disorders in children. Dis. Nerv. Syst., *20:* 334 (1959).

MALITZ, S., *et al.:* A pilot evaluation of deanol in the treatment of anxiety. Curr. Ther. Res., *9:* 261 (1967).

MARTIN, K. E., *et al.:* Pipradol combined therapy for geriatric and agitated patients. In. Rec. Med. Gen. Pract. Clin., *170:* 33 (1957).

MATTHEWS, V., LEHMANN, H. E., AND BAN, T. A.: A comparative study of thirteen hypnotic drugs. Appl. Ther., *6:* 806 (1964).

MAYER-GROSS, W.: Insulin coma therapy of schizophrenia. J. Ment. Sci., *97:* 132 (1951).

MCCLURE, D. J.: Emotions and endocrines. (Presented at the Services Conference, Allan Memorial Institute, Montreal, 1967.)

MCISAAC, W. M.: Establishment of a new drug addiction program. Psychopharmacology Serv. Cent. Bull., *3:* 40 (1966).

MCISAAC, W. M., *et al.:* 10-Methoxyharmalan, a potent serotonin antagonist which affects conditioned behavior. Science, *134:* 674 (1961).

MCKENZIE, M. E., AND ROSWELL-HARRIS, D.: A controlled trial of prothipendyl (tolnate) in mentally subnormal patients. Brit. J. Psychiat., *112:* 95 (1966).

MEIER, R., *et al.* (1954): In: Krueger, G. L., and McGrath, W. R.: 2-Benzylpiperidines and related compounds. In: Psychopharmacological agents (ed., Gordon, M.). (Academic Press, New York, 1964.)

MIDDLEFELL, R. (1960): In: Morren, H. G., *et al.:* Piperazine derivatives. In: Psychopharmacological agents (ed., Gordon, M.). (Academic Press, New York, 1964.)

MILETTO, G.: Sedative, psychoactive drug, disinhibitor. Remarks on the effects of diforene in neuropsychiatry. Ann. Medico Psychol., *1:* 637 (1965).

MOCK, J. E., RICKELS, K., AND GEE, R.: A clinical evaluation of hydrozyzine and placebo in anxious psychiatric outpatients. Int. J. Neuropsychiat., *1:* 168 (1965).

MORREN, H. G., BIENFET, V., AND REYNTJENS, A. M.: Piperazine derivatives (except phenothiazines). In: Psychopharmacological agents (ed., Gordon, M.). (Academic Press, New York, 1964.)

MORRISON, B. O.: The use of methylquinazolone as a sedative in geriatric patients. Clin. Med., *72:* 347 (1965).

MYSCHETZKY, A.: The significance of megimide in the treatment of barbiturate poisoning. Danish Med. Bull., *8:* 33 (1961).

NICOLSON, G. A., *et al.:* Effect of penicillamine on schizophrenic patients. Lancet, *1:* 344 (1966).

OTT, R. E., AND MCMASTER, R. H. (1959): In: Krueger, G. L., and McGrath, W. R.: 2-Benzylpiperidines and related compounds. In: Psychopharmacological agents (ed., Gordon, M.). (Academic Press, New York, 1964.)

OVERALL, J. E., *et al.:* Benzquinamide in newly admitted schizophrenics: a search for patients best treated with a specific drug. Curr. Ther. Res., *5:* 335 (1963).

PAQUAY, B., *et al.:* Treatment of psychotic and neurotic disorders with dixyrazine. Scalpel (Bruxelles), *114:* 588 (1961).

PACQUAY, P. (1960): In: Morren, H. G., *et al.:* Piperazine derivatives. In: Psychopharmacological agents (ed., Gordon, M.). (Academic Press, New York, 1964.)

PARGITER, R. A.: Parenteral methylphenidate

hydrochloride (ritalin) in chronic underactive schizophrenics. Dis. Nerv. Syst., *20:* 69 (1959).

Parsons, T. W., and Thomson, T. J.: Methaqualone as a hypnotic. Brit. Med. J., *1:* 171 (1961).

Paterson, A. S.: Electrical and drug treatment in psychiatry. (Elsevier, Amsterdam, 1963.)

Pearson, D.: Megaloblastic anaemia due to glutethimide. Lancet, *1:* 110 (1965).

Pedani, M.: First observations on the use of a lyopholized yeast complex intravenously in schizophrenics. Rass. Stud. Psichiat., *54:* 47 (1965).

Pennes, H. H., and Hoch, P. H. (1957): In: Downing, D. F.: Psychotomimetic compounds. In: Psychopharmacological agents (ed, Gordon, M.). (Academic Press, New York, 1964.)

Peretz, D. I., *et al.* (1955): In: Downing, D. F.: Psychotomimetic compounds. In: Psychopharmacological agents (ed., Gordon, M.). (Academic Press, New York, 1964.)

Pfeiffer, C. C., *et al.* (1957): In: Usdin, E., and Efron, D. H.: Psychotropic drugs and related compounds. (PHSP No. 1589, Washington, 1967.)

Plichet, A.: Un nouveau traitement des psychoneuroses: chlorhydrate de l'acide benzilique diéthylaminoethylester. Presse Med., *63:* 1748 (1955).

Plummer, A. J., *et al.:* Some pharmacological interrelationships between methylphenidate (ritalin) and reserpine. Amer. J. Med. Sci., *233:* 719 (1957).

Pöldinger, W., *et al.:* Therapeutical experience with the use of dibenzoxepine derivative in depressive states in five clinics. Arzneimittelforschung, *16:* 650 (1966).

Pomeranze, J. (1954): In: Krueger, G. L., and McGrath, W. R.: 2-Benzylpiperidines and related compounds. In: Psychopharmacological agents (ed., Gordon, M.). (Academic Press, New York, 1964.)

Pomeranze, J., and Gadek, R. J. (1957): In: Krueger, G. L., and McGrath, W. R.: 2-Benzylpiperidines and related compounds. In: Psychopharmacological agents (ed., Gordon, M.). (Academic Press, New York, 1964.)

Raich, W. A., *et al.*: A double blind evaluation of fenfluramine in anxious somatizing neurotic medical clinic patients. Curr. Ther. Res., *8:* 31 (1966).

Remmen, E., *et al.:* Psychochemotherapy. (Western Medical Publications, Los Angeles, 1962.)

Retboll, K. (1963): In: Usdin, E., and Efron, D. H.: Psychotropic drugs and related compounds. (PHSP No. 1589, Washington, 1967.)

Reti, L. (1953): In: Downing, D. F.: Psychotomimetic drugs. In: Psychopharmacological agents (ed., Gordon, M.). (Academic Press, New York, 1964.)

Rett, A., *et al.:* Clinical and psychopharmacological investigations of the actions of 5-methyl-10-β-dimethylaminoethyl-10, 11-dihydro-11-oxo-dibenzo [b,e] [1,4]-diazepine hydrochloride in children. Arzneimittelforschung, *15:* 770 (1965).

Ribbentrop, A., and Schaumann, W. (1965): In: Sulser, F., and Dingell, J. V.: On the role of adrenergic mechanisms in the mode of action of tricyclic antidepressants. In: Antidepressant drugs of non-MAO inhibitor type (eds., Efron, D. H., and Kety, S. S.). (U.S. Dept. of Health, Education and Welfare, Bethesda, 1966.)

Rinaldi, F., Rudy, L. H., and Himwich, H. E.: The use of frenquel in the treatment of distrubed patients with psychoses of long duration. Amer. J. Psychiat., *112:* 343 (1955).

Rinaldi, F., Rudy, L. H., and Himwich, H. E.: Clinical evaluation of azacyclonal, chropromazine and reserpine on a group of chronic psychotic patients. Amer. J. Psychiat., *112:* 678 (1956).

Robin, A. A., and Wiseberg, S. A.: Controlled trial of methylphenidate (ritalin) in the treatment of depressive states. J. Neurol. Neurosurg. Psychiat., *21:* 55 (1958).

Robinson, J. T., *et al.:* A double blind trial of oxypertine for anxiety neurosis. Brit. J. Psychiat., *111:* 527 (1965).

Rogers, E. J. (1959): In: Morren, H. G., *et al.:* Piperazine derivatives. In: Psychopharmacological agents (ed., Gordon, M.). (Academic Press, New York, 1964.)

Rosner, B. S., *et al.:* Clinical evaluation of meratran and frenquel on a chronic psychotic population. Amer. J. Psychiat., *113:* 993 (1957).

Sabbatini, F.: International meeting on the pharmacy of selective psychostimulants. Minerva Med., *55:* 3215 (1964).

Sainz, A.: Benzquinamide: a preliminary report. Amer. J. Psychiat., *119:* 777 (1963).

Sarwer-Foner, G. J., and Koranyi, E. K.: Clinical investigation of azacylonal hydrochloride. Canad. Psychiat. Ass. J., *1:* 92 (1956).

Sarwer-Foner, G. J., Koranyi, E. K., and Dancey, T. E.: Clinical investigation of suvren, a new sedative preparation. Canada. Med. Ass. J., *76:* 933 (1957).

Scarlato, G., and Bonaretti, T. (1959): In: Usdin, E., and Efron, D. H.: Psychotropic drugs and related compounds. (PHSP No. 1589, Washington, 1967.)

Schaumann, W., and Ribbentrop, A.: Interference of central anticholinergic action during testing of potential antidepressants in animal experiments. Arzneimittelforschung, *16:* 646 (1966).

Schiele, B. C., Tredici, L. M., and Zimmerman, R. L.: Clinical trials of a new antidepressant, gamfexine. Curr. Ther. Res., *8:* 565 (1966).

Schigutt, R., and Suchanek-Fröchlich, H.: Treatment of depression with a new benzodiazepine derivative. Wien. Klin. Wschr., *77:* 584 (1965).

Schmitt, H., and Schmitt, H. (1958): In: Usdin, E., and Efron, D. H.: Psychotropic drugs and related compounds. (PHSP No. 1589, Washington, 1967.)

SCHRAM, W. S. (1959): In: Morren, H. G., *et al.:* Piperazine derivatives. In: Psychopharmacological agents (ed., Gordon, M.). (Academic Press, New York, 1964.)

SCHWARZ, L., BAN, T. A., AND SMITH, R.: Clinical trial with cyclopentimine. Amer. J. Psychiat., *118:* 254 (1961).

SCRIABINE, A., *et al.:* Benzquinamide: a new anxiety drug. J.A.M.A., *184:* 276 (1963).

SCRIABINE, A., *et al.:* Antagonism of 5-hydroxytryptamine by benzquinamide. J. Neuropharmacol., *5:* 367 (1966).

SENDBUEHLER, M.: Personal communication, Montreal, 1966.

SETTEL, E.: Clinical observations on the use of hydroxyzine in tension states. Amer. Practit., *8:* 1584 (1957).

SETTEL, E.: A clinical evaluation of benzquinamide with observations on the total activity potential. Clin. Med., *70:* 957 (1963).

SHANON, J. (1962): In: Morren, H. G., *et al.:* Piperazine derivatives. In: Psychopharmacological agents (ed., Gordon, M.). (Academic Press, New York, 1964.)

SHERWOOD, W. K. (1957): In: Usdin, E., and Efron, D. H.: Psychotropic drugs and related compounds. (PHSP No. 1589, Washington, 1967.)

SHULGIN, A. T. (1964): In: Usdin, E., and Efron, D. H.: Psychotropic drugs and related compounds. (PHSP No. 1589, Washington, 1967.)

SHULGIN, A. T., BUNNELL, S., AND SARGANT, T.: The psychotominetic properties of 3,4,5-trimethoxy-amphetamine. Nature, *189:* 1011 (1961).

SIEGFRIED, J.: Therapeutic use of centrophenoxine following surgery for parkinsonism. Ther. Umsch., *23:* 122 (1965).

SIMPSON, G. M.: Experiences with thioxanthenes. (Presented at the Symposium on the Thioxanthenes, Montreal, 1967.)

SIMPSON, G. M., AND ANGUS, J. W.: A preliminary study of oxypendyl in chronic schizophrenia Curr. Ther. Res., *9:* 225 (1967).

SIMPSON, G. M., AND AMUSO, D.: Treatment of chronic schizophrenia with triiodothyronine. Canad. Psychiat. Assn. J., *11:* 303 (1966).

SIMPSON, G. M., AND SIEGLER, A.: A preliminary study of a new dihydromorphanthridine derivative in chronic schizophrenia. Curr. Ther. Res., *8:* 406 (1966).

SIMPSON, G. M., *et al.:* A preliminary study of Lilly-51641. Curr. Ther. Res., *8:* 400 (1966).

SIMPSON, G. M., *et al.:* A preliminary study of SKF 14,336 in chronic schizophrenia. Curr. Ther. Res., *8:* 447 (1966).

SKARBEK, A., AND JACOBSEN, M.: Oxypertine: a review of clinical experience. Brit. J. Psychiat., *111:* 1173 (1965).

SMITH, M. E.: Perphenazine and amitriptyline as adjuncts to psychotherapy. Amer. J. Psychiat., *120:* 76 (1963).

SPÄTH, E. (1919): In: Downing, D. F.: Psychotomimetic compounds. In: Psychopharmacological agents (ed., Gordon, M.). (Academic Press, New York, 1964.)

STEVENSON, I., AND RICHARDS, T. W. (1960): In: Downing, D. F.: Psychotomimetic drugs. In: Psychopharmacological agents (ed., Gordon, M.). (Academic Press, New York, 1964.)

STOCKINGS, G. T. (1947): In: Usdin, E., and Efron, D. H.: Psychotropic drugs and related compounds. (PHSP No. 1589, Washington, 1967).

STOLL, W. A.: Lysergic acid diethylamide, a phantasticum derived from the ergot group of drugs. Schweiz. Arch. Neurol. Psychiat., *60:* 279 (1947).

STOLL, W. A., AND HOFMANN, A.: Partial synthesis of alkaloids of the ergobasin type. Helv. Chim. Acta, *26:* 944 (1943).

SUGERMAN, A. A., AND HERRMANN, J.: A pilot study of dominal in chronic schizophrenics. Curr. Ther. Res., *8:* 487 (1966).

SUGERMAN, A. A., AND HERRMANN, J.: Molindone: an indole derivative with antipsychotic activity. Clin. Pharmacol. Ther., *8:* 261 (1967).

SUGERMAN, A. A., LICHTIGFELD, F. J., AND HERRMANN, J.: A pilot study of clopenthixol in chronic schizophrenics. Curr. Ther. Res., *8:* 220 (1966).

SZARA, S.: The comparison of the psychotic effect of tryptamine derivatives with the effects of mescaline and LSD-25 in self-experiments. In: Psychotropic drugs (eds., Garattini, S., and Ghetti, V.). (Elsevier, Amsterdam, 1957.)

SZARA, S. (1956): In: Böszörmenyi, Z.: Some problems of experimental psychoses. In: Pszichologiai tanulmanyok (eds. Gegesi, K. P., *et al.*). (Akademia; Kiado, Budapest, 1958).

SZARA, S.: Hallucinogenic effects and metabolism of tryptamine derivatives in man. Fed. Proc., *20:* 885 (1961).

SZARA, S.: The hallucinogenic drugs—curse or blessing. (Presented at the 122nd Annual Meeting of the APA, Atlantic City, 1966.)

SZARA, S., AND HEARST, E.: The 6-hydroxylation of tryptamine derivates: a way of producing psychoactive metabolites. Ann. N. Y. Acad. Sci., *96:* 134 (1962).

TICKTIN, H., *et al.:* Effect of methylphenidate hydrochloride in antagonizing barbiturate-induced depressions. Neurology (Minneap.), *8:* 267 (1958).

TURNER, W. J., MERLIS, S., AND CARL, A. (1955): In: Downing, D. F.: Psychotomimetic compounds. In: Psychopharmacological agents (eds. Gordon, M.). (Academic Press, New York, 1964.)

USDIN, E., AND EFRON, D. H.: Psychotropic drugs and related compounds. (National Institute of Mental Health, Public Health Service, U.S. Department of Health, Education and Welfare, Bethesda, 1967.)

USDIN, E., AND USDIN, V. R. (1961): In: Usdin, E., and Efron, D. H.: Psychotropic durgs and related compounds. (PHSP No. 1589, Washington, 1967.)

VASSILIOU, G., *et al.* (1961): In: Usdin, E., and

Efron, D. H.: Psychotropic drugs and related compounds. (PHSP No. 1589, Washington, 1967.)

Vojtechovsky, M. (1958): In: Jacobsen, E., Benactyzine. In: Psychopharmacological agents (ed., Gordon, M.). (Academic Press, New York, 1964.)

Vojtechovsky, M., *et al.* (1958): In: Downing, D. F.: Psychotomimetic compounds. In: Psychopharmacological agents (ed., Gordon, M.). (Academic Press, New York, 1964.)

Vulpian, E. F. A. (1856): In: Hoffer, A.: Enzymology of hallucinogens. In: Enzymes in mental health (eds., Martin, G. J., and Kisch, B.). (Lippincott, New York, 1966.)

Walaas, D., and Walaas, E.: Biochemical aspects of schizophrenia, introduction to session. (NATO Advanced Study Institute, Oslo, 1965.)

Weinstein, S., and Manning, R. J.: Intermediate oxidation product of epinephrine. Proc. Soc. Exp. Biol. Med., *32:* 1096 (1935).

Weiss, A. J., *et al.* (1962): In: Usdin, E., and Efron, D. H.: Psychotropic drugs and related compounds. (PHSP No. 1589, Washington, 1967.)

Werner, H. (1958): In: Jacobsen, E.: Benactyzine. In: Psychopharmacological agents (ed., Gordon, M.). (Academic Press, New York, 1966.)

Wilkinson, S. J. (1958): In Usdin, E., and Efron, D. H.: Psychotropic drugs and related compounds. (PHSP No. 1589, Washington, 1967.)

Wood, H. P., and Flippin, H. F.: "Delirium tremens" following withdrawal of ethchlorvynol. Amer. J. Psychiat., *121:* 1127 (1965).

Woolley, D. W. (1960): In: Usdin, E., and Efron, D. H.: Psychotropic drugs and related compounds. (PHSP No. 1589, Washington, 1967.)

Woolley, D. W., and Shaw, E. (1954): In: Smythies, J. R.: Introduction. In: Amines and schizophrenia (eds., Himwich, H. E., Kety, S. S., and Smythies, J. R.). (Pergamon Press, London, 1967.)

Zakrzewska, F., *et al.:* Electromyographic study of the effect of a single dose of orphenadrine HCl (disipal) or meprobamate on neuroleptic-induced extrapyramidal syndrome. Neurol. Neurochir. Psychiat. Pol., *15:* 107 (1965).

Zsigmond, E. K., Földes, F. F., and Földes, V. M.: The inhibitory effect of psilocybin and related compounds on human cholinesterases. Fed. Proc., *20:* 393 (1961).

Part Three

APPLIED PSYCHOPHARMACOLOGY

Nineteen

Concepts and Definitions

A. NOMENCLATURE

The introduction of chlorpromazine heralded the beginning of a new era in psychiatry. The discoveries and progress which followed in the search for new pharmacological substances that influence human behavior have given an unprecedented impetus to the evolution of new concepts and theories in psychiatry. The need for extension and clearer definition of older terminologies was soon apparent, and it was inevitable that a new nomenclature would arise.

According to this new nomenclature, *psychopharmacological substances* are drugs—in the broadest sense—which have a predominant effect on psychological processes, such as perception, mood, thinking and overt behavior. Since these substances act on human psychological events, they are also referred to as *psychoactive chemicals*.

The now commonly used term *psychotropic drugs* was introduced by Gerard (1957). This term covers the whole spectrum of synthetic and natural compounds which possess "psychic" tropism, *i.e.*, substances capable of modifying mental activity and human behavior. Psychotropic drugs are also defined as substances which act on the central nervous system, directly or indirectly, and thereby affect mental and emotional processes. The latter definition is intended to point out their dominant or exclusive effects on the higher functions of the central nervous system.

Phrenotropic drugs is another term which implies pharmacological activity characterized mainly by the effects on mental or emotional processes.

In practice, the terms psychopharmacological, psychoactive, psychotropic, and phrenotropic are often used interchangeably.

1. Psychotherapeutic Drugs

a. Tranquilizers

The rather new concept of tranquilizing action or *tranquilizers* was introduced into psychiatry with the advent of chlorpromazine and other drugs for treating psychiatric patients. The latter term refers to drugs with the potential of calming disturbed behavior without producing hypnosis. These substances are further characterized by producing selective inhibition of the central nervous system in ascending order; *i.e.*, they inhibit subcortical structures prior to and to a greater extent than the cerebral cortex. Tranquilizers, therefore, imply substances which reduce anxiety and agitation without any clouding of consciousness.

While the concept of tranquilizers gained wide acceptance, the term *ataractic*, which was introduced almost simultaneously for the same group of substances, achieved limited usage. The latter term is derived from the Greek adjective *ataraktos* ("without confusion, cool and collected") and from the noun *ataraxia* ("peace of mind" or "freedom from confusion"). Fabing (1955) proposed that chlorpromazine and other similar drugs which produce *ataraxia*, *i.e.*, the absence of emotional upset and a condition of imperturbability, be called *ataraxics*. Again, in practice, ataractic, ataraxic, and tranquilizer are used almost synonymously, but the last term has remained by far the most popular.

With the introduction of a great number of substances with tranquilizing properties, tranquilizers became a heterogenous group. Consequently they were subdivided into two main categories, *i.e.*, major and minor tranquilizers.

i. Major Tranquilizers. Major tranquilizers are drugs which produce calmness with relatively little hypnotic effect. They are useful for controlling the symptoms of acutely and chronically disturbed psychotic patients. These drugs were found to produce many side reactions but no psychological dependency or habituation.

Other investigators have characterized major tranquilizers as substances which relieve psychotic symptoms and are particularly effective for controlling psychomotor agitation.

More recently, those substances which were categorized as major tranquilizers have often been referred to by two newer terms, *i.e.*, neuroleptics or antipsychotics.

Delay (1961) calls *neuroleptics* those major tranquilizers which can be used effectively to treat psychotic symptoms and are distinguished by their effects on the subcortical ganglia often leading to parkinsonism, akathisia, dystonia or other extrapyramidal signs. On the other hand, Lehmann (1961) calls *antipsychotic* (*or psychotostatic*) those neuroleptics or major tranquilizers which have a therapeutic effect on specifically psychotic symptoms, such as hallucinations, paranoid delusions or autistic behavior, regardless of whether they produce a neurological syndrome or sedation.

ii. Minor Tranquilizers. Minor tranquilizers are substances which produce relaxation, together with mild sedative effects. They are useful in the treatment of psychoneurotic patients and common "nervous tension." They produce relatively few adverse reactions and no extrapyramidal manifestations, but their administration may, however, lead to habituation and dependency.

Minor tranquilizers are further subdivided into *muscle relaxants* and *anxiolytics* depending upon whether the drug primarily relieves psychological (and physical) tension or anxiety *per se*. Some consider minor tranquilizers as "the tranquilizers."

The term *psycholeptics* (Delay, 1961) applies to all drugs which possess sedative or tranquilizing properties. Psycholeptic, therefore, is an all encompassing term, and Delay meant it to include hypnotics (sedatives), neuroleptics (major tranquilizers, antipsychotics or psychotostatics) and the tranquilizers (minor tranquilizers). He defines a psycholeptic as a substance "which depresses mental tonus, slows down mental activity, diminishes alertness, and occasionally produces somnolence. The corresponding decrease in emotional tonus may lead to affective indifference."

b. Thymoleptics

Opposed to the psycholeptics are the psychoanaleptics, which are substances which stimulate mental activity regardless of whether this is caused by "an increase of vigilance, by an increase of intellectual energy, or by an elevation of emotional tonus."

Among the psychoanaleptics are included the direct stimulants, bimodal stimulants and indirect stimulants.

The *direct stimulants* are characterized by a rapid onset and a brief duration of action. They have an over-all excitatory effect on the higher and lower cerebral centers, inducing arousal in general and increased psychomotor activity in particular. Direct stimulants produce relatively few side-effects, but they do produce habituation and dependency.

In contrast, the pharmacological action of the *indirect stimulants* is mediated by their monoamine oxidase enzyme inhibiting properties. These substances are characterized by a slow onset and a prolonged duration of action. Unlike the direct stimulants, they produce a relatively high incidence of side-effects but rarely lead to habituation or dependency.

In between the direct and indirect stimulants are the *bimodal stimulants*. These substances act rapidly at first through direct stimulation of the nervous tissue, but their stimulating effects are sustained mainly through the slower and cumulative indirect action of monoamine oxidase enzyme inhibition.

Bimodal stimulants and indirect stimulants are called also *psychic energizers*. This implies that these drugs increase the electrical activity of the brain by stimulating the reticular formation (Himwich, 1959). It also implies that clinically they have not only stimulating effects but also euphorizing and mood-lifting properties (Kline, 1959). The general term psychic energizer is, however, being increasingly replaced by the specific term *antidepressant,* denoting characteristic mood-lifting properties.

It should be noted that when Himwich (1959) originally referred to antidepressants he meant that group of psychoanaleptic substances which by inhibiting the reticular formation act upon the depressive affect by diminishing the readiness to respond to disturbing beliefs and unpleasant stimuli. These same substances were also referred to as central nervous system *suppressants* by Benson and Schiele (1962), *i.e.*, drugs with sedative properties beneficial in the treatment of certain depressions.

At present, however, in spite of any earlier specific connotations, the term antidepressant refers to all drugs which are useful in the treatment of depression. To emphasize their mood-lifting properties and their therapeutic effectiveness on dysthymic mood, antidepressants are also called *thymoleptics* (*or thymerethics*).

2. Psychotopathic drugs

These are chemicals which may have therapeutic uses but are more important because of their ability artificially to induce psychopathological changes. Usually they are referred to as *psychotogenic drugs*, which by definition can induce psychotic-like behavior by producing perceptual distortion and interfering with normal thought processes; or *psychodysleptics*, which by definition disturb mental activity, create a delusional disturbance of judgment, and distort appreciation of reality values. Psychotogenic drugs are capable of producing a condition which is usually referred to as "*model psychosis*" in normal individuals by causing a severe disturbance in mental integration. Because the "model psychosis" can mimic naturally occurring psychoses, these substances are not infrequently called *psychotomimetic* (or *psychosomimetic*) drugs.

An important group of psychotomimetics are the *hallucinogens*, which were defined by Hoffer (1966) as drugs which induce psychological disturbances similar to those found in schizophrenia without causing clouding of consciousness, confusion or gross physiological disturbances. The experiences induced by a hallucinogen were divided into psychotomimetic and psychedelic reactions (Hoffer, 1965). The psychotomimetic (Gerard, 1956) reactions were characterized as "changes" in thought, perception and mood and sometimes in posture without causing either major disturbances of the autonomic nervous system or addictive "craving," and the *psychedelic* reactions were characterized "by freedom from anxiety and tension, and by unforgettable and even mystical happenings during which insights may be gained" (Osmond, 1957).

In various attempts to describe the nature of the experience induced by these drugs, some investigators have coined such terms as *phantastica* and *mysticomimetics*. Others have tried to introduce terms which imply a more precise description of the experience induced, *e.g.*, *psycholytics*, *i.e.*, drugs which dissolve the homogeneity of psychic experience; *cataleptogenics*, *i.e.*, primarily catalepsy producing; and *schizophrenogenic*, *i.e.*, primarily schizophrenia-like condition producing.

B. CLASSIFICATIONS

Early classifications of psychotropic drugs are from the nineteen-thirties. In this they were divided into two major categories: depressants and stimulants.

This classification was further qualified by the Council of Drugs of the American Medical Association (Kautz, 1958). They proposed that central nervous system depressants should be divided into two categories: (1) nonselective depressants and (2) selective depressants. Nonselective depressants included sedatives, hypnotics, and analgesics; the selective depressants were further subdivided in accordance with their specific action.

In the same year Lehmann (1958) formulated his first clinical classification. He classified psychotropic substances into three major categories, *i.e.*, inhibitory, excitatory and psychotomimetic drugs. He also proposed further subdivisions. For example, the inhibitory class he divided into the older sedatives (*e.g.*, chloralhydrate, paraldehyde and barbiturates) and the newer tranquilizers (*e.g.*, phenothiazines, Rauwolfias and propanediols); and the excitatory drugs, into true stimulants (*e.g.*, caffeine, amphetamines and piperidyls) and pseudostimulants (*e.g.*, alcohol and barbiturates).

Today, the three most widely accepted clinical classifications of psychoactive drugs are Kline's "*pragmatic*" (1959), Delay's "*phenomenological*" (1961) and Lehmann's "*psychophysiological*" (1961).

1. Pragmatic Approach

Kline's (1959) pragmatic classification distinguished psychoactive drugs under three main headings: psychic inhibitors, psychic activators and psychotomimetics.

Psychic inhibitors are the hypnotics (*e.g.*, barbiturates), ataraxics or drugs which produce emotional equilibrium (*e.g.*, phenothiazines) and sedatives (*e.g.*, propanediols). *Psychic activators* include psychomotor stimulants (*e.g.*, amphetamines), psychic stimulants (*e.g.*, tricyclic antidepressants) and psychic energizers or drugs with a dominant antidepressant effect (*e.g.*, MAOI's). He defined *psychotomimetics* (*e.g.*, LSD_{25}) as drugs which produce the so-called "model psychosis," *i.e.*, as drugs which have hallucinogenic and mildly stimulating properties.

2. Phenomenological Approach

Delay (1961) based his classifications on phenomenology and divided all psychoactive drugs into three main classes: psycholeptics, psychoanaleptics and psychodysleptics.

In the psycholeptic class he included all those substances which produce relaxation and depress mental activity. He further distinguished between depressors of vigilance and depressors of affect. *Depressors of vigilance* are the hypnotics (*e.g.*, barbiturates) which depress the level of consciousness, lower intellectual or noetic activity, produce a hypnoid state with slight electroencephalographic changes and induce clinical and electroencephalographic sleep. The *depressors of affect* regulate the oscillation of emotional tonus between the "pathetic" (overresponsive) and the "apathetic" poles. These include all "the tranquilizers" (minor tranquilizers or anxiolytic drugs, *e.g.*, propanediols, benzodiazepines) which by their action substitute an apathetic tone for a pathetic one and the neuroleptics (major tranquilizers, *e.g.*, Rauwolfias, phenothiazines and butyrophenones) which induce a neurological syndrome and improve psychotic behavior.

In contradistinction to psycholeptics are the *psychoanaleptics*. The latter group includes all the substances which stimulate mental activity. These again are distinguished between stimulants of vigilance and stimulants of affect. *Stimulants of vigilance* include all of the sympathomimetic amines, *e.g.*, methylphenidate, while the *stimulants of affect* include all other effective antidepressants.

In the *psychodysleptic* class (mescaline, LSD_{25}) belong all those chemicals which disturb mental activity and are characteristically antagonized by the various psycholeptics.

3. Psychophysiological Approach

Lehmann's (1961) psychophysiological classification developed in two stages. At first he divided psychoactive drugs into five major categories: stimulants (*e.g.*, amphetamines); sedatives (*e.g.*, barbiturates); antipsychotics (*e.g.*, phenothiazines, Rauwolfias); psychotogenics (*e.g.*, LSD_{25}); and antidepressants (*e.g.*, tricyclic antidepressants).

This classification was based on the principal effects of psychoactive drugs on three psychophysiological parameters, *i.e.*, on arousal, mental integration and mood.

On the two extremes of the arousal parameter continuum, he distinguished between stimulants and sedatives, and similarly he distinguished between antipsychotics and psychotomimetics on the mental integration parameter. Regarding the mood parameter continuum, he maintained that only one end can successfully be attacked by antidepressant drugs, whereas no specific drug for the control of elation is available.

This classification was further refined by Lehmann (1963), and thereafter the first category included those drugs which influence the level of arousal as reflected in mental and behavioral activity, *i.e.*, the psychostimulants (*e.g.*, caffeine) and psychoinhibitors. The latter were subdivided into sleep-inducing hypnotics (chloralhydrate) and tension-reducing tranquilizers or sedatives (*e.g.*, barbiturates). The mood parameter became the parameter of affect and included those drugs which affect the quality or intensity of emotional or affective states. These drugs were subdivided into anxiolytic drugs (*e.g.*, benzodiazepines). Finally those drugs which affected the integration of perceptual and cognitive processes were subdivided into psychotomimetics (*e.g.*, LSD_{25}) and antipsychotics (*e.g.*, phenothiazines and butyrophenones).

Recently the following five classes of psychoactive drugs have been adopted by the World Health Organization: neuroleptics, anxiolytic sedatives, antidepressants, psychostimulants and psychodysleptics.

The WHO (1967) adopted the following definitions. *Neuroleptics* (also known as antipsychotics, formerly called major tranquilizers or ataractics) are drugs with therapeutic effects on psychoses and other types of psychiatric disorders accompanied by certain neurological effects such as extrapyramidal signs. *Anxiolytic sedatives* (formerly called minor tranquilizers) are substances which reduce pathological anxiety, tension and agitation without therapeutic effects on cognitive or perceptual processes. *Antidepressants* are drugs effective in the treatment of pathological depressive states. (They have sometimes been called psychic energizers and thymoleptics). *Psychostimulants* are substances which increase the level of alertness and/or motivation. *Psychodysleptics* are drugs which produce abnormal mental phenomena, particularly in the cognitive and perceptual spheres.

The WHO (1967) also emphasized that as soon as the use of drugs such as lithium (in acute manic states or as a prophylactic in manic-depressive cycles), cyclazocine and methadone (in narcotic addiction), disulfiram (in chronic alcoholism) becomes better established, new categories will have to be created.

C. PSYCHODYNAMIC FORMULATIONS

The term psychodynamic denotes the relations and interactions of psychic phenomena entirely within the realms of symbolic, conceptual, perceptual and emotional representation. This is represented in psychopharmacology via three approaches (Lehmann, 1966).

One of these is mainly concerned with the economic aspects of psychodynamics, *i.e.*, with the shift in the availability and distribution of psychic energy (Ostow, 1960); another focuses on the structural aspects of psychodynamics and on the changes in cathexis and object relations, *i.e.*, on the shift of focus from superego to id forces and on the change from the schizophrenic personality organization to that of a manic-depressive (Azima, 1959, 1961); and the third approach deals with the dynamic aspects or shifts and changes of psychic defense mechanisms (Sarwer-Foner, 1957, 1960).

1. "Economic" Approach

The "economic" approach as formulated by Ostow (1960, 1962) is based on the hypothesis that a quantum of psychic energy is attached to the intrapsychic representations of instinctual needs. They distinguished between the archaic nucleus of the ego, aiming for an immediate gratification of instincts serving the pleasure principle and its "supplementary segment," which serves as a model of the external world and as such represents the reality principle. In this frame of reference psychoactive drugs were subdivided into tranquilizers, psychic energizers, ego intoxicants and ego tonics.

Tranquilizers (phenothiazines, reserpine, tetrabenazine) are those drugs whose principal action is to decrease the libido content of the ego. Consequently they are substances which ameliorate mania and incipient schizophrenia but aggravate melancholia. On the other hand, *psychic energizers* (MAOI's, imminodibenzyl derivatives, deanol) are substances which provide for large amounts of energy for the ego enabling it to accomplish its functions adequately. Thus psychic energizers can result in a sense of joy and optimism. With increasing dosage, however, the id drives become threatening to the integrity of the ego at a certain point. This may result in a feeling of anxiety. And if the dosage of the drug is further increased, the id pressure may finally cause a rupture of the ego defenses, resulting in a neurotic or psychotic reaction. Consequent to this hypothesis, psychic energizers alleviate melancholia but may bring about mania or schizophrenia.

Ego intoxicants (meprobamate, chlordiazepoxide, also reserpine) are those agents which impair, and *ego tonics* (*e.g.*, amphetamines) those which improve ego functions directly and consequently have rather prompt pharmacological action. They can be utilized to strengthen the ego when its function is impaired by toxins, physical illness, insomnia, etc.

2. Structural Approach

Azima (1959, 1961) suggested that the beneficial effects of neuroleptics in the schizophrenias are the result of the replacement of pathological defenses of withdrawal and splitting by a "movement towards external objects." Simultaneously there is a shift from the schizophrenic organization, comparable to Klein's (1948) paranoid position of infantile development, to a manic-depressive-like organization, comparable to Klein's (1948) depressive position, which replaces the paranoid position in the development.

Within this same frame of reference, the beneficial effects of antidepressants were interpreted as a result of a shift of the invested psychic energy from the superego to the ego and id. This shift leads to a decrease in anxiety and guilt and may possibly result in the appearance of manic symptoms. Such a shift also represents a change in cathexis related to internal objects or superego elements (Lehmann, 1966).

Based on the structural approach is Azima's (1960) concept of the action mechanism of pharmacologically induced sleep in a variety of psychopathological conditions. According to him, pharmacologically induced sleep results in ego-split with an inactivation of part of the ego system. He postulated that the regression produced "is therapeutic in this particular setting because it allows a return to and beyond pathological fixation points and through gratification of those need frustrations which originally had resulted in fixation."

3. Drugs and Psychic Defenses

The third approach is concerned with the drug-induced changes of psychic defense mechanisms. This was first formulated by Sarwer-Foner (1957, 1960). He emphasized that patients characterized by passivity and doubt about their masculinity have a strong urge for overt activity. Rendering these cases more passive by major tranquilizing drugs makes them acutely anxious. This was interpreted by Sarwer-Foner (1957) as a "brutal chemical interference with long-standing defensive modes of expression" which acutely threatens the ego. As a consequence of this ego threat, sudden crises of anxiety, thought disorder, body image changes and increased depression may be seen.

On the other hand, he also revealed that in certain patients with a different and particular kind of psychodynamic constellation the effect of a major tranquilizer is a protection from the overwhelming aggressive and sexual impulses, the comfort of which outweighs the discomfort induced by passivity. It is in this type of patient that the most beneficial effects of drug therapy are observed.

Within the same frame of reference Lehmann (1956, 1966) brought to attention that minor tranquillizers mobilize different kinds of defenses. According to him, the defense mechanisms which become manifest through the effects of minor tranquilizers (anxiolytic sedatives) are mainly regression, denial and projection, in contradistinction to the defense mechanisms which become manifest under the effects of major tranquilizers (neuroleptics), *i.e.*, isolation, rationalization and sublimation.

According to Lehmann (1966), the concept of psychodynamics cannot be restricted to the psychoanalytical system but should extend to any system concerned with psychological regulation. This includes the experimental findings and intervening variables of learning theory and the hypothetical constructs of existentialism. In this extended frame of reference Lehmann (1966, 1967) differentiated anxiolytic, antipsychotic, stimulant and antidepressant drugs.

Anxiolytic sedatives in the psychoanalytic frame of reference are characterized by their ability to mobilize preconscious material, by producing disinhibition and, consequently, reducing superego dominance. They may also facilitate transference phenomena. In the frame of reference of learning theory these drugs reduce anxiety and improve performance. They also produce an increased tolerance to conflicting stimuli and reduce differentiation (*i.e.*, internal inhibition). In the existentialist frame of reference they decrease anxiety and increase the "probability encounter."

Neuroleptics from the psychoanalytic point of view are drugs which induce a depletion of psychic energy; produce a shift in the basic personality organization from the paranoid to the manic-depressive; and constitute a threat through their interference with activity-passivity defenses. From the point of view of learning theory they decrease defensive unconditional responses and improve differentiation. From an existential viewpoint they reduce anxiety, but also initiative and emotional involvement.

Stimulants, in the psychoanalytic frame of reference, are drugs which increase activity and in certain conditions security, too, with or without an improvement in object relations. In other cases, these drugs increase anxiety. In the frame of reference of learning theory these drugs increase drive strength and increase central self-stimulation; and in the "existential" frame of reference they increase initiative, provide motivation to be authentic and increase the possibility for encounters.

Finally, antidepressant drugs in the psychoanalytic perspective were described as substances which changed the direction of aggression from inward to outward; from the point of view of learning theory they increase hypothalamic self-stimulation; and in the "existential" frame of reference they characteristically decrease guilt feelings (Lehmann, 1966, 1967).

REFERENCES

Azima, H. Imipramine (tofranil): a new drug for the depressed. Canad. Med. Ass. J., *80:* 535 (1959).

Azima, H.: Psychodynamic alterations concomitant with tofranil administration. Canad. Psychiat. Ass. J., *4:* 172 (1959).

Azima, H.: Psychodynamic and psychotherapeutic problems in connection with imipramine (tofranil) intake. J. Ment. Sci., *101:* 74 (1961).

Azima, H., Azima, F., and Durost, H.: Psychoanalytic formulations of effects of reserpine on schizophrenic organization. Arch. Gen. Psychiat. (Chicago), *1:* 662 (1959).

Azima, H., Durost, H., and Arthurs, D.: The effect of R 1625 (haloperidol) in mental syndromes: a multiblind study. Amer. J. Psychiat., *117:* 546 (1960).

Azima, H., and Vispo, R. H.: Effects of imipramine (tofranil) on depressive states. Arch. Neurol. Psychiat., *81:* 658 (1959).

Azima, H., and Vispo, R. H.: The problem of regression during prolonged sleep treatment. In: The dynamics of psychiatric drug therapy (ed., Sarwer-Foner, G. J.). (Charles C Thomas, Springfield, 1960.)

Azima, H., *et al.*: The effect of RO-5-0831/1 (marplan) in depressive states. Amer. J. Psychiat., *116:* 453 (1959).

Benson, W. M., and Schiele, B. C.: Tranquillizing and antidepressive drugs. (Charles C Thomas, Springfield, 1962.)

Delay, J.: A reveiw of psychotropic drugs. Whats New, *129:* 8 (1961).

Fabing, H. D.: Designation of tranquillizing agents in neuropharmacology. J.A.M.A., *158:* 1461 (1955).

Gerard, R. W. (1956): In: Hoffer, A.: Enzymology of hallucinogens. In: Enzymes in mental health (eds., Martin, G. J., and Kisch, B.). (Lippincott, Philadelphia, 1966.)

Gerard, R. W.: Drugs for the soul; the rise of psychopharmacology. Science, *125:* 201 (1957).

Himwich, H. E.: Some drugs used in the treatment of mental disorders. Amer. J. Psychiat., *115:* 756 (1959).

Himwich, H. E.: Stimulants. Ass. Res. Nerv. Ment. Dis., *37:* 356 (1959).

Hoffer, A.: D-Lysergic acid diethylamide

(LSD): a review of its present status. Clin. Pharmacol. Ther., *6:* 183 (1965).

Hoffer, A., and Osmond, H.: The association between schizophrenia and two objective tests. Canad. Med. Ass. J., *87:* 641 (1962).

Hoffer, A., and Osmond, H.: Malvaria: a new psychiatric disease. Acta Psychiat. Scand., *39:* 335 (1963).

Hoffer, A., and Osmond, H.: How to live with schizophrenia. (University Books, New York, 1966.)

Hoffer, A., Osmond, H., and Smythies, J.: Schizophrenia: a new approach: result of a year's research. J. Ment. Sci., *100:* 20 (1954).

Kautz, H. D.: Report of the council; psychotropic drugs. J.A.M.A., *166:* 1040 (1958).

Klein, M.: Contributions to psychoanalysis 1921–1945. (Hogarth, London, 1948.)

Kline, N. S.: Psychopharmaceuticals: Effects and side effects. Bull. Wld. Health Org., *21:* 397 (1959).

Kline, N. S. (ed.): Psychopharmacology frontiers. (Little, Brown, Boston, 1959.)

Lehmann, H. E.: A dynamic concept of the action of chlorpromazine at physiological and psychological levels. Encephale, *4:* 1113 (1956).

Lehmann, H. E.: Tranquillizers and other psychotropic drugs in clinical practice. Canad. Med. Ass. J., *79:* 701 (1958).

Lehmann, H. E.: New drugs in psychiatric therapy. Canad. Med. Ass. J., *85:* 1145 (1961).

Lehmann, H. E.: Selection, screening and testing of new psychiatric drugs. (Presented at the Proceedings of the Third World Congress of Psychiatry, Montreal, 1961.)

Lehmann, H. E.: Psychopharmacology: a discussion of current problems, Ohio State Med. J., *59:* 1091 (1963).

Lehmann, H. E.: Problems of evaluation and classification in psychophramacology. In: Psychopharmacological methods (eds. Votava, Z., *et al.*) (Pergamon Press, London, 1963).

Lehmann, H. E.: Methodology of clinical studies of psychotropic drugs. (Presented at the World Health Organization Scientific Group on Research in Psychopharmacology, Geneva, 1966.)

Lehmann, H. E.: Psychodynamic aspects of psychopharmacology. (Presented at the Fourth World Congress of Psychiatry, Madrid, 1966.)

Lehmann, H. E.: Discussion of L. Bellak's paper on ego function patterns as clinical indices. (Presented at the meeting of ECDEU, Montreal, 1967.)

Lehmann, H. E.: The emotional basis of illness. Dis. Nerv. Syst., *28:* 12 (1967).

Osmond, H.: A review of the clinical effects of psychotomimetic agents. Ann. N.Y. Acad. Sci., *66:* 418 (1957).

Ostow, M.: The effects of the newer neuroleptic and stimulating drugs on psychic function. In: The dynamics of psychiatric drug therapy. (ed., Sarwer-Foner, G. J.). (Charles C Thomas, Springfield, 1960.)

Ostow, M.: The psychic function of depression. A study in energetics. Psychoanal. Quart., *29:* 355 (1960).

Ostow, M.: The use of drugs to overcome technical difficulties in psychoanalysis. In: The dynamics of psychiatric drug therapy (ed., Sarwer-Foner, G. J.). (Charles C Thomas, Springfield, 1960.)

Ostow, M.: Drugs in psychoanalysis and psychotherapy. (Basic Books, New York, 1962.)

Sarwer-Foner, G. J.: Psychoanalytic theories of activity-passivity conflicts and of the continuum of ego defences: experimental verification using reserpine and chlorpromazine. Amer. Med. Ass. Arch. Neurol. Psychiat., *78:* 413 (1957).

Sarwer-Foner, G. J.: The transference and nonspecific drug effects in the use of the tranquillizing drugs and their influence on affect. Psychiat. Res. Rep., Amer. Psychiat Ass., *8:* 153 (1957).

Sarwer-Foner, G. J., and Koranyi, E. K.: Transference effects, the attitude of treating physician and countertransference in the use of the neuroleptic drugs in psychiatry. In: The dynamics of psychiatric drug therapy (ed., Sarwer-Foner, G. J.). (Charles C Thomas, Springfield, 1960.)

Sarwer-Foner, G. J., *et al.*: Depressive states and drugs. Med. Serv. J. Canada, *15:* 539 (1959).

Schiele, B. C.: Newer drugs for mental illness. J.A.M.A., *181:* 126 (1962).

WHO, Research in Psychopharmacology. World Health Organization Technical Report Series No 371, W.H.O. Geneva, 1967.

Twenty

General Therapeutic Principles

A. PHARMACOLOGICAL SUBSTANCES AND PHYSICAL TREATMENTS

1. Fever Therapy

In 1887 Wagner von Jauregg suggested that fever could be therapeutic in the treatment of psychiatric disorders. He first produced high temperatures by inoculating tuberculin; later he used typhoid vaccine and found the fever induced by both substances therapeutic for patients suffering from general paralysis (GPI).

Typhoid vaccine (0.2 to 2 ml. intravenously) treatment is still used in penicillin-resistant GPI cases. Fever occurs within 30 to 90 minutes and may last 2 to 3 hours. The course of treatment consists of a total of eight to twelve "fevers." Treatments are usually given every second or third day.

Twenty years later Lundvall, H. (1907) succeeded in producing therapeutic fever by the administration of sodium nucleinate.

Fever is produced by the subcutaneous administration of 50 to 100 ml. of sodium nucleinate from a 2 per cent solution. A course of treatment consists of eight to twelve injections. Drug administration can only be repeated after the fever and the dermatological reaction of the first injection has subsided (Nyirö, 1962).

Fever therapy with malarial blood was first tried by Wagner von Jauregg (1917) in the treatment of GPI with dramatic therapeutic success. Until the introduction of penicillin this treatment with tertian malaria remained the standard therapy for this condition.

There are several accepted procedures. One method (Mayer-Gross *et al.*, 1960) is to inoculate the patient by the bite of a mosquito infected with plasmodium vivax (benign tertian malaria); another is to give an intramuscular injection of 2 to 5 ml. of blood from an infected donor; and a third is to give an intravenous injection of 5 to 10 ml. from the infected donor. There is approximately a 10-day incubation period, and then rigors develop, at first every other day and thereafter at daily intervals. Treatment is terminated after 10 rigors by quinine hydrochloride given in a dosage of 600 mg. twice a day (for 3 days) and in the same amount once a day for a fortnight (Nyirö, 1962).

Other means of inducing fever are the administration of sterilized milk, vaccines, killed *Escherichia coli* suspension, pyrifer (and other preparations consisting of various bacilli) or sulfur in oil (Buscaino, 1951; Gregory, 1961; and Kalinowsky and Hoch, 1961).

Sulfur in oil was first used by Schroeder (1924), who gave one to three series (each consisting of ten injections) of sulfosin (1 per cent) to patients suffering from GPI. Claude *et al.* (1933) also used non-specific organic substances (*e.g.*, colloidal gold) and "sulfur in oil" in the treatment of schizophrenias. They reported a recovery rate of 10 per cent and improvements in 30 per cent of their cases.

More recently, Lehmann (1960) successfully treated some therapy-resistant depressive patients with a combination of artificially induced fever and imipramine.

2. Insulin Therapy

a. Insulin Coma Therapy

Insulin coma therapy in the treatment of schizophrenic patients was introduced by Sakel (1936). It is recommended to commence treatment with the administration of 5 units of crystalline insulin subcutaneously. If there is no undesired reaction this dosage can be increased daily by 10 to 20 units until the coma-inducing amount (an average of 150 to 200 units) is reached. Coma sets in approximately 3 hours after insulin administration and is usually permitted to last from 20 to 40 minutes. It is terminated by the administration of glucose either by esophageal tube or intravenously. A full course of treatment consists of 40 to 60 comas (Valentine, 1962).

Angyal (1937) delineated six successive stages in insulin coma. The first is characterized by irritability, slight psychomotor excitement and euphoria. This is followed by somnolence and muscular hypotonia. The third stage begins with clonic movements and ends in sopor, giving place to dissociated torsion spasms in the fourth, hyporeflexia in the fifth and areflexia with deep coma in the sixth. He also described four different types of reactions: the frontopolar, the parietooccipital, the parietopostcentral and the temporal.

Although there is no conclusive evidence that it is inferior to some of the other treatments used in schizophrenics (Saarma, 1964), insulin coma is used infrequently, and its application is almost entirely restricted to cases resistant to antipsychotic drugs.

b. Modified Insulin Therapy

The sedative effects of small, subcoma, doses of insulin were first utilized by Klemperer (1926), Steck (1932) and Schuster (1937). Somewhat later Sargant and Craske (1941) found it useful in the treatment of certain cases of war neuroses.

At first 5 units of crystalline insulin is given subcutaneously or intramuscularly to the fasting patient. Dosage is raised by 10 units daily to a maximum of 100 units, provided that the patient remains conscious for 3 hours after drug administration. If at any time during the 3-hour treatment period there are signs of slipping into coma, therapy for that day is immediately terminated, and the insulin dose is reduced by 10 units the next day. Treatment is usually continued until the patient regains his normal weight or is stabilized on an initial large weight gain (Sargant and Slater, 1963).

Although modified insulin therapy has been used in the functional psychoses by Polatin *et al.* (1940, 1946), Rennie (1943) and Greaves *et al.* (1955) and in the organic brain syndromes by Tomlinson (1943), the primary indication of this treatment is anxiety irrespective of its etiology (Bernath, 1959).

3. Convulsive Therapy

Improvement in a catatonic schizophrenic patient after camphor injection-induced convulsions and the hypothetical antagonism between schizophrenia and epilepsy led Meduna (1933) to the pharmacological induction of cerebral seizures for therapeutic purposes.

Although the rationale was erroneous, the treatment itself proved to be a success and is considered to be the antecedent not only of other pharmacological convulsive therapies but also of electroshock treatment.

a. Camphor-Induced Convulsions

Camphor-induced convulsions were first used in the treatment of psychiatric patients by Meduna (1933). Because of the unpredictability of seizures with this substance, it was soon replaced by pentetrazol in convulsive treatment.

b. Pentetrazol-Induced Convulsions

Five to 10 ml. of a 10 per cent solution of pentetrazol is administered by rapid intravenous injection. In the absence of convulsions (within 60 seconds) a second injection is immediately given. In case of "second failure" a third and last attempt is made (Meduna, 1937, 1938). Although there are some indications that pentetrazol-induced convulsions are superior therapeutically to the electrically induced ones (Bianchi and Chiarello, 1944) and that combined pentetrazol and insulin treatment is more effective than when ECT and insulin are combined (Polonio, 1951, 1952), convulsion therapy with pentetrazol is only infrequently used because of the great fear the patient experiences in the course of this treatment.

c. Acetylcholine-Induced Convulsions

These were introduced by Fiamberti (1937), who administered 600 mg. of acetylcholine bromide intravenously to schizophrenics. Equivocal findings with somewhat lower doses were reported in psychoneurotics by Fasanaro (1947), Ibor (1952), Maria *et al.* (1960), Pare (1956) and Hawkins and Tibbets (1956).

d. Flurothyl-Induced Convulsions

The convulsion-inducing properties of flurothyl (Indoklon) were first recognized by Krantz (1957). It was first used in convulsive therapy by Esquibel *et al.* (1958) by inhalation, but more recently it has been given intravenously (Krantz, 1959).

Flurothyl convulsions resemble pentetrazol-induced seizures. The loss of consciousness is followed by myoclonic, tonic and finally clonic movements. The substance itself is not metabolized in the body, and irrespective of the route of its administration it is excreted unchanged in the exhaled air.

There is no fear with flurothyl and there are fewer adverse effects than with other convulsive treatments; in fact, Kalinowsky *et al.* (1958) noted a slight euphoria after consciousness is regained. Kurland *et al.* (1959) found flurothyl therapeutically equal to ECT. According to them it produces less confusion and memory impairment than the electrically induced seizures.

e. Convulsions Induced by Other Drugs

There are a number of other substances used in convulsive treatment. Among them, picrotoxin, cyclohexylethyltriazole and tetramethylsuccinimide are infrequently used (Berg and Robbins, 1959; Kalinowsky and Hoch, 1961; and Mayer-Gross and Walk, 1938), but none of them has become an accepted method of treatment.

B. PHARMACOLOGICAL SUBSTANCES AND PSYCHOLOGICAL TREATMENTS

1. Chemically Induced Abreactions

Lindemann (1932) recognized that slowly given barbiturates produce sedation and a lack of inhibition, together with a psychomotor discharge. Since then, barbiturates have gained great importance in both psychiatric diagnosis and treatment.

The two most frequently used narcotherapies are narcoanalysis and narcosynthesis, introduced by Horsley (1943) and Grinker and Spiegel (1945), respectively. The main therapeutic objective in narcoanalysis is to abreact and spontaneously "discharge" the pathology-producing emotional material. In narcosynthesis the patient is encouraged to reexperience the intense emotion accompanying the event which precipitated the anxiety attack (Henderson and Gillespie, 1955; and Sim, 1963).

For practical therapeutic purposes Sargant and Slater (1963) suggested narcotherapies be subdivided according to the three techniques used: that is, into "techniques with barbiturates" particularly useful in the treatment of recently implanted conversion symptoms; "techniques with intravenous methamphetamine" recommended for cases in which a series of problems in the past and present life of the patient has to be "quietly worked over" (valuable also in monosymptomatic obsessional phobic states and obsessional personalities with mild depersonalization symptoms); and "excitatory abreactions" especially beneficial for relief of tension and hysterical symptoms.

a. Techniques with Barbiturates

The two most extensively used barbiturates for this purpose are amobarbital sodium and thiopental sodium, the former a hypnotic and the latter an anesthetic. Amobarbital sodium produces relief of tension at a dosage considerably lower than the hypnotic dose. With thiopental sodium the relaxation-inducing amount for all practical purposes coincides with the dosage at which clouding of consciousness begins. This may be the reason that the former substance results in "merely emotional and verbal expression and ventilation," while the latter drug leads to more dramatic abreactions in words and action (Alexander *et al.*, 1949; and Alexander, 1953).

i. Amobarbital Sodium. Amobarbital sodium (1000 mg.) is prepared in 10 ml. of double-distilled water, *i.e.*, in a 10 per cent solution, which is given intravenously at a rate of 1 ml. per minute. Not more than 300 to 500 mg. of the substance are usually needed. When the therapeutic dosage is reached patient begins, with very little prodding, to give vent to his feelings. If the patient becomes sleepy or falls asleep in the course of the session he is easily awakened by intravenous administration of 10 to 40 mg. of amphetamine sulfate.

ii. Thiopental Sodium. Thiopental sodium (1000 mg.) is prepared in 40 ml. of double-distilled water, *i.e.*, in a 2.5 per cent solution, which is given intravenously at a rate of 1 ml. per 15 seconds, *i.e.*, 100 mg. per minute. Indications that the therapeutic dosage is reached are a sudden change (relaxation) in the facial expression of the patient, a glassy stare and delay (or confusion) in counting backward. Since thiopental sodium may induce motor abreaction, Alexander (1953) suggests that it should be administered through an infusion canula with a rubber tube of sufficient length to allow for gross movements.

A combination of narcosuggestive and narcocathartic procedures under the influence of barbiturates is recommended as a form of short term psychotherapy (Kalinowsky and Hoch, 1961). At first a hypnosis-like state is produced in which suggestions are given with the purpose of directly influencing neurotic symptomatology (narcosuggestion). This is followed by a period in which free associations are encouraged and the emotional material is "discharged." A combination of narcotherapy with barbiturates and insulin shock treatment was introduced by Levy and Perry (1947).

b. Techniques with Methamphetamine

The only extensively used amphetamine preparation for diagnostic and therapeutic purposes is methamphetamine. It was first used for diagnostic purposes by Simon and Taube (1946) and was found useful as an aid in psychotherapy by Levine *et al.* (1948). Shorvon (1953) was first in describing it as an abreactive agent.

Ten to 40 mg. of methamphetamine are given by a rapid intravenous injection. Indications that the therapeutic dosage is reached are a feeling of lightheadedness, relief of tension, increased wakefulness, elimination of fatigue, decrease in sensitivity to pain, some restlessness, overtalkativeness and a dramatic recall of emotionally charged material. Cases of overexcitement can be easily controlled by barbiturates.

Methamphetamine (10 to 20 mg.) is occasionally given in combination with barbiturates (500 mg. of thiopental sodium) in treatment. This was recommended by Sargant and Slater (1954) for obsessional patients whose condition was seen to be aggravated by excitatory abreactions with ether or carbon dioxide.

c. Excitatory Abreactions

i. Ether. The possible diagnostic and therapeutic applications of this substance were first recognized by Schilder and Weissmann (1927). It was reintroduced for the treatment of war neuroses by Palmer (1945) and Sargant and Shorvon (1945).

Ether is administered by inhalation. It is dropped gently onto an open mask. It stimulates the patient to talk. Under the influence of ether forgotten memories are visibly experienced with excitement which rises to a crescendo followed by a sudden silence (Sim, 1963). Essential for therapeutic success is the "ultraparadoxical phase of excitation" which may occur several times in the course of treatment (Sargant and Shorvon, 1945). This can be recognized when the patient becomes transiently mute with a vacant facial expression suggestive of a faint smile.

ii. Trichloroethylene. This was recommended by Rees *et al.* (1950) as a therapeutic aid in psychotherapy. It has a fast onset and short duration of action without producing nausea or other after-effects (Kalinowsky and Hoch, 1961).

iii. Carbon Dioxide. Carbon dioxide was introduced in the therapy of psychiatric patients by Meduna (1947, 1950). In the classical procedure 25 per cent CO_2 with 75 per cent O_2 is inhaled at first and gradually replaced—as soon as the patient relaxes and is breathing deeply—by pure CO_2. After about 20 inspirations, there is a short period of loss of consciousness with motor excitement. Patient usually recalls vivid dreams after each session.

More recently, another procedure was introduced in which 30 per cent CO_2 with 70 per cent O_2 is inhaled. After 30 to 40 inhalations a state of altered consciousness sets in characterized by motor restlessness, increased communicativeness and abreaction.

Moriarty (1954) considered CO_2 treatment beneficial in anxiety-tension and phobic reactions, and Shorvon (1952) found it effective in depersonalization states. On the other hand, Hawkins and Tibbetts (1956), in a controlled clinical trial, could not differentiate between the therapeutic results with this substance and an inactive placebo, and Hargrove *et al.* (1954) found psychotherapy alone more effective in certain cases than when combined with CO_2 treatment.

2. Facilitation of Psychotherapy by Psychotomimetics

There are three ways in which psychotomimetics are used in psychiatric treatment. Most frequently they are used as abreactive agents; less often, in specific psychotherapeutic procedures such as psycholytic and psychedelic treatment; and occasionally they are given with the intention of inducing a toxic psychosis for therapeutic purposes.

a. Psychotomimetic-Induced Abreactions

i. Lysergic Acid Diethylamide. This was first used in psychiatric treatment by Condrau (1949) and Sandison *et al.* (1954). Their pioneering work caused considerable interest in LSD_{25} therapy in various clinical psychopathological conditions. No concensus in regard to the therapeutic indications and efficacy has yet been reached. Sandison *et al.* (1954) and Cutner (1959) suggest that it has its greatest value in obsessional and anxiety states accompanied by psychic tension, while others maintain that the best results are obtained in the treatment of personality disorders. In a group of psychoneurotic patients Robinson *et al.* (1963) were able to demonstrate that as an abreactive agent LSD_{25} produces slightly better therapeutic results than those obtained, for example, with methamphetamine. While passive dependent patients usually show an unfavorable response to this treatment (Paterson, 1963), cases with anxiety-hysteria are likely to be helped (Sargant and Slater, 1963).

The starting dose of LSD_{25} is 25 mcg. given orally in 5 ml. of water. If there is no reaction to this amount, the dose is gradually raised by 25 mcg. a day. The characteristic manifestations usually occur within 30 to 60 minutes after 75 to 150 mcg. are given and reach a peak after 3 to 4 hours of drug administration. Preceding the abreaction are the autonomic, perceptual and affective changes. The average duration of LSD_{25} effects is 6 hours, but they may last as long as 1 to 3 days. Not infrequently LSD effects can only be terminated by chlorpromazine (Sargant and Slater, 1963).

II. Phencyclidine. Phencyclidine is 1-(1-phenlcyclohexyl)piperidine, usually referred to as Sernyl. While Luby *et al.* (1959) suggested that phencyclidine may have anxiolytic effect, Davies (1960) found that it facilitates the flow of thought in certain therapy-resistant severe obsessional cases. For abreactive purposes Davies (1960) used 5 to 10 mg. of the substance orally, which induced the desired effect in about 30 minutes and lasted 1 or 1½ hours. (Because of its potential dangers, the use of this substance in abreaction has practically been abandoned.)

b. Specific Psychotherapeutic Procedures

Among these Leuner (1965) considers psycholytic and psychedelic therapy the most important.

i. Phycholytic Therapy. This is based on the activation of unconscious and repressed memories and complexes by LSD_{25} or psilocybin, as first described by Busch and Johnson, (1950). According to them, under the influence of these drugs neurotic patients are temporarily "transported" into a period of early childhood and with frightening reality relive traumatic childhood experiences. While psycholysis is contraindicated in infantile personalities and in patients with "low ego strength," it is recommended in character neuroses (including criminal and aggressive psychopaths), anxiety neuroses, borderline cases, obsessional neuroses and certain psychosomatic conditions, *e.g.*, migraine, rheumatism, ulcerative colitis (Leuner, 1965).

The dose applied in psycholytic therapy is below that used in eliciting experimental psychotic features. Psycholytic therapy is not a pure form of pharmacotherapy but a therapy based on depth analysis, which is facilitated by the effects of the psychotomimetic drug.

ii. Psychedelic Therapy. This is based on eliciting profound cosmic-mystic experiences by the administration primarily of LSD_{25} or psilocybin. Because of this, psychedelic therapy—named by Osmond (1957)—has also been referred to as "mind-expanding" treatment. Psychedelic therapy is considered to be useful in alcoholism (MacLean *et al.*, 1965; Jensen, 1963; Hoffer, 1965; and Savage and Stolaroff, 1965). In contrast to the psycholytic method, in psychedelic therapy high dosages of the psychotomimetic substance are needed (Leuner, 1965).

c. Toxic Psychoses in Treatment

i. Atropine Therapy. This was recommended by Forrer (1951) for the treatment of anxiety and agitation regardless of etiology. Treatment consists of intramuscular administration of atropine sulfate in a dosage of 32 to 200 mg. per day. The injection induces dry mouth, acceleration of pulse, excitement, confusion, hallucinations and coma, from which there is spontaneous recovery (Kalinowsky and Hoch, 1961).

ii. Ditran Therapy. The chemical structure of Ditran is 1-ethyl-3-piperidyl cyclopentylphenylglycolate. It is an anticholinergic substance which produces atropine-like actions. Even in small 5- to 10-mg. doses it induces hallucinations with a delirium-like confusional state, with marked physical weakness for a period of 12 to 24 hours followed by euphoria. Because of this particular feeling of well being, Ditran has been tried as an antidepressant with equivocal success (Meduna and Abood, 1959).

Treatment consists of oral administration of Ditran in a dosage of 20 mg. a day. The drug induces dry mouth, dilation of pupils, clouding of consciousness, confusion, disorientation and hallucinations. Whereas the toxic psychopathological manifestations subside within 2 to 6 hours, the anticholinergic effects persist for almost a day.

3. Behavior Therapies

The use of drugs in behavior therapy was reviewed by Wolpe and Lazarus (1966), who distingusihed among symptomatic, adjuvant or specific use of pharmacological substances in the course of treatment.

a. Symptomatic Uses

The use of imipramine in the control of enuresis (also encopresis) and the application of thioridazine, diazepam and phenelzine (also imipramine) in the treatment of premature ejaculation are important.

i. Enuresis Nocturna. The control of enuresis by imipramine was demonstrated by Destounis (1963) and confirmed by Drooby (1964). The dosage is usually 50 to 75 mg. a day given in two or three divided doses. Some investigators give the total dosage at bedtime. Treatment becomes effective within days and after it has been used for a year it remains effective after drug withdrawal in 30 per cent of the cases.

ii. Encopresis. The possible control of encopresis by imipramine was recognized by Abraham (1963). Treatment follows the same principles as in enuresis. Controlled studies are, however, lacking.

iii. Premature Ejaculation. The combination of anxiolytic substances such as diazepam (to curb anxiety) with ergotamine (to delay ejaculation) has been used in this condition (Singh, 1963; and Drooby, 1965). Successful performance of sexual intercourse by interfering with anxiety by drugs may lead to a condition in which the "healthy" sexual arousal (by reciprocal inhibition and without drugs) interferes with the pathology.

b. Adjuvant Uses

If "active relaxation" fails, drugs are used to obtain an optimal condition for desensitization treatment. The combination of barbiturates with amphetamines, chlordiazepoxide, hydroxyzine and ethchlorvynol are the drugs most frequently used, but occasionally the administration of phenothiazines, *e.g.*, chlorpromazine, prochlorperazine and trifluoperazine, are essential for successful treatment. In cases of free-floating anxiety, inhalation (1 to 4 inspirations) of a mixture of 65 per cent carbon dioxide and 35 per cent oxygen prior to treatment is considered to be the most effective measure.

c. Specific Uses

The infrequent use of meprobamate in stuttering and the extensive application of emetin or apomorphine in the aversion therapy of alcoholics are specific behavior therapeutic procedures in which pharmacological means are used.

i. Stuttering. Successful therapeutic results were reported in stutterers by the use of meprobamate, 1200 mg. per day (Maxwell and Paterson, 1958). Under the influence of this substance, ordinarily disturbing, *i.e.*, anxiety, and stuttering-provoking stimuli are neutralized. This effect is carried over after the discontinuation of treatment. Nevertheless, strong anxiety in these cases is expected to lead to relapse (Wolpe and Lazarus, 1966).

ii. Alcoholism. The use of emetine and apomorphine in the aversion therapy of alcoholics is one of the most extensively used behavior therapeutic procedures. It consists of the administration of emetine or apomorphine followed by alcohol consumption. The association with the nausea induced by these chemicals renders the alcohol distasteful to the patient (Williams, 1952).

α. Emetine. Emetine is given in graduated injections. To enhance its unpleasant effects, administration is preceded by a dose of amphetamine and followed by injections with pilocarpine and ephedrine. After the onset of perspiration, salivation and tachycardia, alcohol (*e.g.*, one ounce of whisky) is given. This is repeated when nausea develops and once again before vomiting commences (Sargant and Slater, 1954; Kalinowsky and Hoch, 1961; and Sim, 1963).

β. Apomorphine. Apomorphine was originally used in the treatment of acute alcoholism. Five to 10 mg. given subcutaneously have a transient central stimulating effect on the medullary vomiting center and produces emesis. This is followed by narcosis similar to that seen with morphine. The unpleasant aspects of the vomiting episode were utilized as a form of treatment, and apomorphine administration became the model of aversion therapies based on conditioning principles (Alexander, 1953). Aversion treatment with apomorphine is conducted by the administration of 3 mg. of the substance intramuscularly (or subcutaneously) followed by alcohol consumption. Vomiting begins approximately 5 to 10 minutes after the injection, but unless combined with ipecacuanha the discomfort produced is shortlasting. This gives it an advantage over emetine in outpatient treatment (Sargant and Slater, 1963).

C. SINGLE AND COMBINED PHARMACOLOGICAL TREATMENTS

1. Single Drug Therapy

With the increasing information available on the clinical action of psychotherapeutic substances and with the lack of comparable progress in our understanding of the etiology of the various psychiatric disorders, three phases of drug therapy are being increasingly delineated. These are the emergency management of the acutely disturbed patient; the active treatment period; and maintenance therapy.

a. Management of Emergencies

Several conditions may require emergency measures. Among them are hysterical manifestations, agitation in depressed or schizophrenic patients, catatonic or manic excitement and acute brain syndromes.

Excitement and agitation can be controlled by various preparations. The once popular paraldehyde—given intramuscularly in 10- to 15-ml. doses—is less and less frequently used. Hyoscine and apomorphine or hyoscine, morphine and atropine preparations are likewise only rarely administered. On the other hand, barbiturates are still extensively used. Intravenous injections of amobarbital sodium in the dosage of 180 to 450 mg. or thiopental sodium in the dosage of 250 to 500 mg. are frequently given. While the former substance does not produce "unconsciousness" but "secures" "a relative calm," the latter compound induces sleep immediately (Sargant and Slater, 1963).

The most widely used substance in psychiatric emergencies is chlorpromazine. Fifty to 100 mg. of this drug when given intramuscularly are sufficient to control most of the psychiatric emergencies. Injection may have to be repeated at intervals of 4 to 6 hours for 1 to 3 days (not infrequently in the first 12 hours four or five times) to maintain control.

Others suggest the administration of thioproperazine or haloperidol in excited states (Durost, 1965); and St. Jean *et al.* (1967) found propericiazine useful in these conditions.

Another substance frequently used in psychiatric emergencies is chlordiazepoxide in a high (50 to 100 mg.) parenteral dosage repeated at intervals like chlorpromazine. Whereas chlordiazepoxide is most effective in controlling agitation associated with acute brain syndromes, chlorpromazine seems to be especially effective in the management of manic, schizophrenic and catatonic excitement. Furthermore, the barbiturates are considered to be of primary importance when immediate sedation is required.

In all of these conditions it is essential to prevent dehydration and acidosis by forcing fluid intake; to promote elimination by catharsis, colonic irrigation and if necessary gastric lavage; and to provide for essential vitamin needs by oral or parenteral administration (Pearson, 1963). In certain already dehydrated cases, hypodermic or intravenous saline administration (Larson, 1939) is a lifesaving procedure which can not be replaced by intravenous glucose before 24 hours because the vitamin depletion must first be corrected (Middleton, 1966). Similarly it is only after 24 hours that digitalization, with a rapidly acting digitalis preparation, should commence if signs of cardiac failure are present.

b. Active Treatment

Continuous and discontinuous therapy are the two principal therapeutic procedures in the active treatment period.

i. Continuous Therapy. This consists of administration of the therapeutic substance at regular intervals (1 to 6 times a day) over a well defined (short or long) period of time.

α. Therapy with Antipsychotics. The dosage of the antipsychotic drug is gradually increased until the desired therapeutic effect is produced or a significant side-effect occurs. For chlorpromazine it has been noted that 600 mg. (in extreme cases, 1000 mg.) are the maximum initial daily dosage tolerated. This, however, is related to body size, the nature of the psychopathology and the extent of the psychopathological disturbances. Although the dosage of chlorpromazine may have to be raised to 2000 mg. before becoming effective, the average dosage in acute hospitalized schizophrenics, according to Appleton (1967), is from 400 to 800 mg. a day.

β. Therapy with Antidepressants. The dosage of the antidepressant drug is gradually increased until the desired therapeutic effect is produced or the "therapeutic ceiling" is reached. This differs for each substance. For example with imipramine, treatment commences with 75 mg. a day, which is raised by 25- or 50-mg. increments daily until a maximum of 150 to 300 mg (Appleton, 1967).

γ. Therapy with Anxiolytics. The dosage of the anxiolytic drug is progressively increased from a low starting dosage until the therapeutic ceiling is reached. Then it is reduced to the minimum effective daily dosage to lessen the occurrence of dependency. For example, the daily amount of chlordiazepoxide may promptly be raised from 10 mg. to 90 mg. a day and reduced to a daily total of 60 mg.

ii. Discontinuous Therapy. Alternating periods of drug administration with drug-free intervals is often referred to as discontinuous treatment. It has been successfully used—with thioproperazine—in the treatment of chronic schizophrenic and acute manic cases. The dosage of thioproperazine is promptly raised from 15 mg. to a maximum of 240 mg. a day (first day, 15 mg., second day, 30 mg.; third day, 60 mg.; fourth day, 120 mg.; fifth day, 180 mg.; and sixth day, 240 mg.) or up to the dosage at which extrapyramidal hypertonus sets in. After 5 days of parkinsonian manifestations the drug is suddenly withdrawn for a 5- to 7-day period by which time all the neurological signs remit. As a rule three courses of this treatment are given (Denham and Carrick, 1961; Ban *et al.*, 1962; and Paterson, 1963).

More recently, discontinuous therapy was tried in chronically disturbed mental defectives with diazepam (Galambos, 1964). The encouraging findings need to be confirmed.

c. Maintenance Therapy

There is sufficient evidence to believe that continuation of treatment is essential in the treatment of the schizophrenias and manic-depressive psychoses after remission of the acute symptomatology. The maintenance dosage is considerably lower, sometimes only one-fifth of that required in the acute period of the illness, and is given only once or twice a day (Appleton, 1967).

Intermittent pharmacotherapy in the maintenance period of treatment was recommended recently by Ayd (1967). This consists of drug holidays, *i.e.*, 1, 2 or 3 days of the week or 1 week per month when the patient does not take his regular medication. According to Ayd (1967), 90 per cent of the patients can be maintained on drug holidays for 1 to 14 days, 75 per cent from 3 to 4 weeks and 25 per cent for a period of 8 to 12 weeks.

Nicotinic acid in the maintenance treatment of schizophrenics and lithium carbonate in the maintenance treatment of manic-depressives are at present under study.

2. Therapy with Drug Combinations

An excellent review of this topic was recently presented by Freeman (1967). He discussed combinations of major tranquilizers; major and minor tranquilizers; energizers; energizers and major tranquilizers; energizers and minor tranquilizers; and energizers and amino acids.

a. Combinations of Major Tranquilizers

Frequently used combinations are chlorpromazine with trifluoperazine and CPZ with reserpine in the treatment of schizophrenic patients (Casey, 1960; Smith-e-Incas *et al.*, 1960; Childers, 1961; Mann, 1963; Salzberger, 1963; Jenkins and Samborski, 1964; McNichol and Seale, 1964; Morton-Gore, 1964; Talbot, 1964; Barsa and Kline, 1955; Hewat *et al.*, 1955; Eiber, 1955; Lemere, 1955; Barsa and Kline, 1956; Hollister *et al.*, 1956; Leoconte and Barbier, 1956; Rance *et al.*, 1956; Feldman, 1957; and Tuteur, *et al.*, 1957). According to Freeman (1967), neither of these combinations has any advantage over its constituents.

In a recent study, chronic schizophrenics maintained on phenothiazine drugs were given haloperidol, triperidol or an inactive placebo in addition to their regular medication. While no statistically significant difference was seen, some patients on both of the active combinations markedly benefited from the addition of the butyrophenone substance (Lehmann, *et al.*, 1967).

b. Combinations of Major and Minor Tranquilizers

Successful therapeutic results were reported with the combination of promazine (and also of chlorpromazine) with meprobamate in the psychoneuroses, schizophrenias and organic brain syndromes (Barsa and Kline, 1956; Becker and Israel, 1961; Kozlowski, 1961; Splitter, 1961; Thimann and Gauthier, 1961; Bradley, 1962; Pennington, 1962; Faretra and Gozun,

1964; Greene, 1964; and Pennington, 1965). While beneficial effects were seen with a combination of chlorprothixene (and also chlorpromazine) with chlordiazeproxide in the treatment of various depressions (and destructive schizophrenics), the combined administration of diazepam with various phenothiazines remained unsuccessful (Burdine, 1964; Dye, 1961; Forcada, 1961; and Freeman, 1967). Controlled studies in this area are lacking.

c. Combinations of Energizers

There have been combinations of two tricyclic antidepressant substances, or two MAOI antidepressants or an MAOI with a tricyclic drug (Eichborn, 1961; English, 1961; Gayral *et al.*, 1963; Sargant, 1963; Enoch and Barker, 1964; Richmond and Roberts, 1964; and Gander, 1965).

In spite of the favorable findings in some of these studies, Freeman (1967) maintains that there is no clear-cut evidence that antidepressant combinations are superior to single antidepressant drugs. The danger particularly with a tricyclic and MAOI, combination (of hyperpyrexia, convulsions and death), outweighs the possible therapeutic benefit (Ayd, 1961; Himwich and Petersen, 1961; and Barker and Enoch, 1963).

d. Combinations of Energizers and Major Tranquilizers

There are three frequently used combinations: tranylcypromine with trifluoperazine, imipramine with chlorpromazine and amitriptylene with perphenazine.

i. Tranylcypromine with Trifluoperzine. Numerous studies in psychoneuroses, depressions and schizophrenias have been conducted with this combination (Bacsick, 1960; Schiele, 1960; Marksfield, 1961; Orchow, 1961; Joseph, 1962; Sulzer and Schiele, 1962; Litkewitch, 1963; Collins, 1963; Buki, 1964; Winkelman, 1965; Lesse, 1961; Meller, 1962; Milligan, 1962; Chu and Fogel, 1963; Janecek *et al.*, 1963; Lingl, 1964; Tejedor *et al.*, 1964; Bucci, 1962; and Hordern *et al.*, 1962). According to Freeman (1967), in neurotic depressions the combination is somewhat more effective than its constituents. This is not the case in psychotic depressions and in the schizophrenias.

ii. Imipramine with Chlorpromazine. Studies in the depressions and in the schizophrenias have been conducted with this combination (Krakowski, 1962; Pollack, 1962; Schnetzler and Lamand, 1962; Pöldinger, 1963; Cabral and Luskoff de Casal, 1961; and Demartis, 1961). Freeman (1967) has suggested that the therapeutic efficacy of the combination is not superior to imipramine alone.

iii. Amitriptyline and Perphenazine. This combination does not seem to have any advantage over its constituent drugs when given to psychoneurotic (Mattey, 1963; Bowes, 1964; Coffee, 1964; McLaughlin *et al.*, 1964) or depressive patients (Barsa and Saunders, 1961; and Dorfman, 1963). However, on the basis of studies by Karacan *et al.* (1963), Kennedy and Miller (1963), Kris and Gerst (1964), Pennington (1964), Feldman (1965) and Smith-e-Incas (1965), Freeman (1967) recognized that it is a highly effective and superior combination when given to schizophrenics with depressive manifestations.

e. Combinations of Energizers and Minor Tranquilizers

Combinations of MAOI's (isocarboxazid, phenelzine, phenoxypropazine and tranylcypromine) with benzodiazepines (chlordiazepoxide and diazepam) did not effect a significantly superior therapeutic action when given to psychoneurotic patients than its constituents (Freeman, 1967).

f. Combinations of Energizers with Amino Acids

In the *schizophrenias* aggravation of psychopathology was seen with combined administration of methionin (also tryptophan) with an MAOI antidepressant (Lauer *et al.*, 1958; Bailey *et al.*, 1959; Pollin *et al.*, 1961; Alexander *et al.*, 1962, 1963; Berlet *et al.*, 1964; and Bull *et al.*, 1964). On the other hand, Heath *et al.* (1966) were able to show that the antimetabolite of methionine (*dl*-methionine-*dl*-

sulfoximide) caused improvement in schizophrenic patients.

In *depressions* Kline *et al.* (1963, 1964) suggested that the addition of tryptophan to already established MAOI treatment may have a dramatically beneficial effect. This was also the finding of Coppen *et al.* (1965) in a placebo-controlled study.

3. Sleep Treatment

Prolonged sleep treatment (or narcosis) by administration of pharmacological substances was first applied by MacLeod (1900), who used primarily bromides, and Wolff (1901), who used methylsulfonal. Since this pioneering work, sleep treatment has been extensively utilized on the basis of various therapeutic rationales and for various therapeutic indications.

At first it was based on the ancient belief that sleep *per se* has curative values (MacLeod, 1900; Ragg, 1900; and Wolff, 1901). This was followed by the idea that it prevents the production of hypnotoxins (Epifanio, 1915) and, its counterpart, that it renders the patient helpless and dependent, which can be utilized therapeutically (Kläsi, 1922). Then prolonged narcosis was considered for inducing or facilitating the psychotherapeutic intervention by Furrer (1924), Boss (1935), Heldt (1948), Clapp and Loomis (1950), Brisset *et al.* (1951, 1953, 1956, 1957), Azima (1955, 1958), Richter (1957) and Rosman (1958). Simultaneously, on the basis of Pavlovian principles, drug-induced sleep was considered as a process which strengthens protective inhibition and influences corticovisceral reflexes (Ivanov-Smolenskii, 1939; Ischlondsky, 1955; and Ivanov, 1958).

a. The Means of Treatment

Historically, the first chemical substances used in sleep treatment were bromides (MacLeod, 1900; and Ragg, 1900), which were soon replaced by methylsulfonal (Wolff, 1901) and later on by long acting barbiturates (Epifanio, 1915). Somnifen (an equal combination of diethyl and allysopropyl barbituric acid) was used by Kläsi (1922), allobarbital by Mueller (1925) and paraldehyde with scopolamine by Wiethold (1925). Another preparation which has been used is the Cloetta mixture (Cloetta and Maier, 1934). It contains paraldehyde, amylhydrate, chloralhydrate, alcohol, isopropylallylbarbituric acid, digalene and ephedrine.

The preparations most frequently used at present are combinations of short and long acting barbiturates in addition to phenothiazines as introduced by Ey *et al.* (1954, 1956, 1957) and also used by Brisset (1957). One of the most potent combinations is that of Azima (1955) and Cameron (1958). They used a combination of secobarbital (100 mg.), pentobarbital (100 mg.), barbital (150 mg.), phenobarbital (200 mg.) and chlorpromazine (50 mg.) given three to four times a day. They later omitted the phenobarbital but increased the chlorpromazine to 100 mg.

b. The Procedures

One of the classical procedures with diethylamine barbiturate (Somnifen) consists of the intramuscular administration of the substance in a total of 6 (maximum, 8) ml. a day in three divided doses. Along with each injection 10 to 18 units of insulin are given subcutaneously (to facilitate oxidation of the tissues) and one to one and a half ounces of glucose rectally to prevent dehydration and the occurrence of toxic symptoms. This treatment induces approximately 20 hours of sleep a day. The duration of treatment is usually 14 days.

Azima (1955) applied a triple (8 A.M. 2 P.M. and 8 P.M.) and a double (8 A.M. and 8 P.M.) waking technique procedure. His patients slept 20 to 22 hours a day up to a maximum of 60 days (optimal treatment period appeared to be 15 to 20 days). While awake they were cleaned and fed (1500 calories and 2000 ml. of fluids a day), and their vital signs were checked (blood pressure, pulse rate and respiration).

c. Indications and Contraindications

i. Indications. These include psychoneuroses (MacCowan, 1936; Bobon, 1956; Delay, *et al.*, 1956; Deniker, 1957); schizophrenias (Kläsi, 1922; Cloetta and Maier, 1934; and Brisset, 1957); both phases of manic-depressive psychoses (Hennelly, 1936; Gillespie, 1939); and acute and chronic organic brain syndromes (MacLeod, 1900; Epifanio, 1915; Demole, 1921; Mueller, 1925; Deschamps, 1956). Other conditions in which prolonged sleep has been used are hypertension, dermatoses and peptic ulcer.

Sargant and Slater (1963) consider continuous sleep the treatment of choice for the youthful patient suffering from a severe agitated depression or manic state in which the overactivity and the reduced food intake are causing rapid exhaustion. While the results with this treatment in the depressions are controversial, it is a valuable tool in the management of manic excitement.

Others consider schizophrenic conditions with "bland" symptomatology as primary indications for prolonged narcosis. Ivanov-Smolenskij (1939), for example, found sleep therapy superior to insulin treatment in this type of patient. Nevertheless, prolonged sleep therapy is probably most extensively used in the psychoneuroses with prevailing—high level—anxiety.

ii. Contraindications. Prolonged narcosis therapy is contraindicated in cardiovascular (excluding hypertension), bronchopulmonary (including tuberculosis), genitourinary, hepatobiliary and metabolic diseases (Kläsi, 1922; Furrer, 1924; and Gillespie, 1939). Cloetta and Maier (1934) considered somatic illnesses in general as contraindications.

d. Complications: Prevention and Treatment

Toxic complications may occur at an early stage of treatment, which can be prevented or controlled by adequate hydration and environmental manipulation (soothing atmosphere, dark room and warm temperature). Urinary retention is counteracted by carbachol injection or catheterization and constipation by the continuous administration of mild laxatives or, if needed, by enemas. Minor pyrexia, pulse rate changes and vomiting may all be indicators of dehydration, but if they occur with adequate fluid intake they are signals for reduction or withdrawal of medication.

More severe complications are cardiovascular collapse, which calls for intravenous fluids (50 to 100 ml. of 30 per cent glucose) and occasionally for bemegride administration; venous thrombosis; and pneumonia. All three necessitate immediate termination of treatment. Withdrawal delirium and seizures are successfully reduced by gradually tapering off the medication.

A review of the literature on continuous sleep treatment was presented by Clapp and Loomis (1950). More recently, Pivnicki (1959) discussed the place of prolonged narcosis in psychiatry in its historical perspective. Nevertheless, the superiority of sleep treatment over single pharmacological means still remains to be seen.

REFERENCES

Abraham, D.: Treatment of encopresis with imipramine. Amer. J. Psychiat., *119:* 891 (1963).

Alexander, L.: Treatment of mental disorder. (Saunders, Philadelphia and London, 1953.)

Alexander, L., Winston, M. R., and Berman, H.: The electroencephalogram during sodium amytal and sodium pentothal narcosis and during resuscitation with benzedrine sulfate in normal and schizophrenic subjects. Electroenceph. Clin. Neurophysiol., *1:* 255 (1949).

Alexander, F., *et al.:* Effects of amino acids and tranylcypromine on schizophrenic behavior. Fed. Proc., *21:* 417 (1962).

Alexander, F., *et al.:* L'methionine and l-tryptophan feedings in non-psychotic and schizophrenic patients with and without tranylcypromine. J. Nerv. Ment. Dis., *137:* 135 (1963).

Angyal, L.: Über die Motorischen und Tonischen Erscheinungen des Insulin Schocks. Z. Ges. Neurol. Psychiat., *157:* 35 (1937).

Appleton, W. S.: Guide to the use of psychoactive agents. Dis. Nerv. Syst, *28:* 609 (1967).

Ayd, F. J.: A survey of drug-induced extrapyramidal reactions. J.A.M.A., *175:* 1054 (1961).

Ayd, F. J.: Drug holidays: intermittent pharmacotherapy for psychiatric patients. Med. Sci., *1:* 60 (1967).

Azima, H.: Prolonged sleep treatment in mental disorder. Some new psychopharmacological considerations. J. Ment. Sci., *101:* 593 (1955).

Azima, H.: Sleep treatment in mental disorders. Dis. Nerv. Syst., *19:* 523 (1958).

Bacsick, E. J.: Treatment of depression-anxiety in office patients with combination of tranylcypromine and trifluoperazine. Dis. Nerv. Syst., *21:* 626 (1960).

Bailey, S., *et al.:* Comparison of iproniazid with other amine oxidase inhibitors. Ann. N.Y. Acad. Sci., *80:* 652 (1959).

Ban, T. A., *et al.:* Clinical studies with thioproperazine (majeptil). Compr. Psychiat., *3:* 284 (1962).

BARKER, J. C., AND ENOCH, M. D.: Combining the antidepressant drugs. Lancet, *2:* 691 (1963).

BARSA, J. A., AND KLINE, N. S.: Combined reserpine-chlorpromazine in treatment of disturbed psychotics. Amer. Med. Ass. Arch. Neuropsychiat., *74:* 280 (1955).

BARSA, J. A., AND KLINE, N. S.: A comparative study of resprine, chlorpromazine, and combined therapy. Arch. Neurol. Psychiat., *76:* 90 (1956).

BARSA, J. A., AND SAUNDERS, J. C.: Amitriptyline (elavil), a new antidepressant. Amer. J. Psychiat., *117:* 739 (1961).

BECKER, G. S., AND ISRAEL, P.: Integrated drugs and psychotherapy in the treatment of alcoholism. Quart. J. Stud. Alcohol, *22:* 610 (1961).

BERG, S., AND ROBBINS, E. S.: A pharmacological report on PM-1090. J. Neuropsychiat., *1:* 32 (1959).

BERLET, H. H., *et al.:* Endogenous metabolic factor in schizophrenic behavior. Science, *144:* 311 (1964).

BERNATH, A. K.: Modification of anxiety subsequent to insulin-induced mild hypoglycemia. In: Insulin treatment in psychiatry (ed., Rinkel, M.). (Philosophical Library, New York, 1959.)

BIANCHI, J. A., AND CHIARELLO, C. J.: Shock therapy in the involutional and manic-depressive psychoses. Psychiat. Quart., *18:* 118 (1944).

BOBON, J.: Chlorpromazine et la cure de sommeil. Encephale, *45:* 421 (1956).

BOSS, M.: Die Psychische Dynamik der Schlafkur bei Schizophrenen. Schweiz. Arch. Neurol. Psychiat., *36:* 209 (1935).

BOWES, H. A.: Some experiences with a combination of amitriptyline and perphenazine in severe psychiatric syndromes. Psychosom. Med., *5:* 44 (1964).

BRADLEY, W. F.: Adjunctive use of promazine in somatic illness. Ohio Med. J. *58:* 765 (1962).

BRISSET, C.: Reflexions sur la cure de sommeil et les therapeutiques, voisines. Evolut. Psychiat. (Paris), *1:* 241 (1957).

BRISSET, C., ET GASCHKEL, V.: La cure de sommeil. Presse Med., *59:* 465 (1951).

BRISSET, C., *et al.:* La cure de sommeil comme therapeutique psychosomatique. Evolut. Psychiat (Paris), *1:* 387 (1953).

BRISSET, C., *et al.:* Position actuelle des problèmes du sommeil. Evolut. Psychiat. (Paris), *1:* 51 (1956).

BUCCI, L.: Phenomenological versus nosological approach in early therapy of mental illness. Dis. Nerv. Syst., *23:* 461 (1962).

BUKI, R.: A treatment program for homosexuals. Dis. Nerv. Syst., *25:* 304 (1964).

BULL, C., *et al.:* Hypertension with methionine in schizophrenic patients receiving tranylcypromine. Amer. J. Psychiat., *121:* 381 (1964).

BURDINE, W. E.: Diazepam in general psychiatric practice. Amer. J. Psychiat., *121:* 589 (1964).

BUSCAINO, V. M. (1951): In: Kalinowsky, L. B., and Hoch, P. H.: Somatic treatment in psychiatry. (Grune and Stratton, New York, 1961.)

BUSCH, A. K., AND JOHNSON, W. C.: LSD-25 as an aid in psychotherapy: preliminary report of a new drug. Dis. Nerv. Syst., *11:* 241 (1950).

CABRAL, C. A., AND LUSKOFF DE CASAL, O.: Chlorpromazine combined with imipramine in the treatment of chronic illnesses. Sem. Med. (B. Air.), *68:* 438 (1961).

CAMERON, D. E.: The use of nucleic acid in aged patients suffering from memory impairment. Amer. J. Psychiat., *114:* 943 (1958).

CASEY, J. F. (1960): In: Freeman, H.: The therapeutic value of combinations of psychotropic drugs: a review. Psychopharmacology, *4:* 1 (1967).

CHILDERS, R. T.: Controlling the chronically disturbed patient with massive phenothiazine therapy. Amer. J. Psychiat., *118:* 246 (1961).

CHU, J., AND FOGEL, E. J.: Clinical evaluation of the thymoleptic effect of tranylcypromine. J. Indian Med. Ass., *56:* 40 (1963).

CLAPP, J. S., AND LOOMIS, E. A.: Continuous sleep treatment. Amer. J. Psychiat., *196:* 821 (1950).

CLAUDE, H., COSTE, F., AND DUBLINEAU, J.: Etude comparée des pyretothérapies parasitaires, bactériennes, organiques et chimiques dans le traitement de la démence précoce. (Presenté á la Premiere Congres Francais de Therapeutique, Paris, 1933.)

CLOETTA, M., AND MAIER, H.: Über eine Verbesserung der Psychiatrischen Dauernarkosebehandlung. Z. Neurol., *150:* 146 (1934).

COFFEE, H. L.: Combined amitriptyline and perphenazine in combined depression and anxiety. J. Med. Ass. Georgia, *53:* 107 (1964).

COLLINS, J. H.: Combination therapy for depression and anxiety. Psychosom., *4:* 390 (1963).

CONDRAU, G.: Klinische Erfahrungen an Geisteskranken mit Lysergsaurediathylamid. Acta Psychiat. Neurol., *24:* 9 (1949).

COPPEN, A., *et al.:* Changes in 5-hydroxytryptophan metabolism in depression. Brit. J. Psychiat., *111:* 105 (1965).

CUTNER, M.: Analytic work with LSD-25. Psychiat. Quart., *33:* 715 (1959).

DAVIES, B. M.: A preliminary report on the use of sernyl in psychiatric illness. J. Ment. Sci., *106:* 1073 (1960).

DELAY, J., *et al.:* A new neuroleptic phenothiazine: methopromazine (4632 RP). (Presented at the 54th Congress of Psychiatrists and Neurologists of France, Bordeaux, 1956.)

DEMARTIS, D.: Pharmacologic therapy of chronic schizophrenia. Giornate psichiatriche di Torino. Rass. Stud. Psichiat., *50:* 515 (1961).

DEMOLE, V.: Essai de traitement de la demence précoce par somnifen. Schweiz. Arch. Neurol. Psychiat., *8:* 134 (1921).

DENHAM, J., AND CARRICK, D. J. E. L.: Therapeutic value of thioproperazine and the importance of the associated neurological disturbances. J. Ment. Sci., *107:* 326 (1961).

DENIKER, P.: Hibernothérapies et médicaments neuroleptiques en therapeutique psychiatrique. Encephale, *46:* 1 (1957).

DESCHAMPS, A.: Quelques resultats des cures de sommeil. Encephale, *45:* 412 (1956).

DESTOUNIS, N.: Enuresis and imipramine. Amer. J. Psychiat., *119:* 893 (1963).

DORFMAN, W.: Combined drug treatment. Amer. J. Psychiat., *120:* 275 (1963).

DROOBY, A. S.: A reliable truce with enuresis. Dis. Nerv. Syst., *25:* 97 (1964).

DROOBY, A. S. (1965): In: Wolpe, J., and Lazarus, A. A.: Behavior therapy techniques. (Pergamon Press, Oxford, 1966.)

DUROST, H. B.: Excited states. (Presented at the New Brunswick Psychiatric Association, St. John, 1965.)

DYE, E. N.: Dual pharmacotherapy in grossly disturbed psychotic patients. Amer. J. Psychiat., *118:* 548 (1961).

EIBER, H. B.: Chlorpromazine (thorazine) Rauwolfia combination in psychiatry—preliminary report. Amer. Med. Ass. Arch. Neurol. Psychiat., *74:* 36 (1955).

EICHBORN, O.: Beitrag zur Frage der Inkompatibilitat bei Kombination Verschiedener Psychoaktiver Wirkstoffe. Wien. Med. Wschr., *111:* 553 (1961).

ENGLISH, D. C.: A comparative study of antidepressants in balanced therapy. Amer. J. Psychiat., *171:* 865 (1961).

ENOCH, M. D., AND BARKER, J. C.: Combining the antidepressant drugs. Lancet, *1:* 44 (1964).

EPIFANIO, G.: D'ipnosi farmacologica prolungata e sua aplicatione per la cura di alcune psicopatio. Riv. Pat. Nerv. Ment., *20:* 273 (1915).

ESQUIBEL, A. J., *et al.:* Hexafluorodiethyl ether (indoklon): its use as a convulsant in psychiatric treatment. J. Nerv. Ment. Dis., *126:* 530 (1958).

EY, H.: Les diverses methodes d'emploie de la chloropromazino en therapeutique psychiatrique et leurs indications. Encephale, *45:* 361 (1956).

EY, H.: Discussion: cure de sommeil. Evolut. Psychiat. (Paris), *1:* 268 (1957).

EY, H., *et al.:* Les nouvelles techniques de cures de sommeil dans pratique psychiatrique. Evolut. Psychiat., (Paris), *1:* 641 (1954).

EY, H., *et al.:* Les paroxysmes oniriques et anxioux au cours et au décours de la cure de sommeil, vers une socialisation de la cure. Evolut. Psychiat. (Paris), *1:* 753 (1954).

FARETRA, G. AND GOZUN, C.: The use of drug combinations in pediatric psychiatry. Curr. Ther. Res., *6:* 340 (1964).

FASANARO, G.: La prognosi nella schizophrenia con le moderne terapie. Acta Neurol. (Napoli), *2:* 813 (1947).

FELDMAN, P. E.: The personal element in psychiatric research. Amer. J. Psychiat., *113:* 52 (1956).

FELDMAN, P. E. (1957): In: Freeman, H.: The therapeutic value of combinations of psychotropic drugs: a review. Psychopharmacology, *4:* 1 (1967).

FELDMAN, P. E.: Perphenazine and amitriptyline hydrochloride. J.A.M.A., *194:* 24 (1965).

FIAMBERTI, A. M.: Proposta di una tecnica operatoria modificata e semplificata per glia interventi alla Moniz sui lobi prefrontali in malati de mente. Rass. Stud. Psichiat., *26:* 797 (1937).

FORCADA, C. A.: La combinacion librium tarasan en el tratemento de las depressiones. Actas Luso Esp. Neurol. Psiquiat., *20:* 195 (1961).

FORRER, G. R.: Atropine toxicity in the treatment of mental disease. Amer. J. Psychiat., *108:* 107 (1951).

FREEMAN, H.: The therapeutic value of combinations of psychotropic drugs: a review. Psychopharmacology, *4:* 1 (1967).

FURRER, J.: Unsere Erfahrungen mit Sommifendauernarkose der Psychosen. Schweiz. Med. Wschr., *54:* 275 (1924).

GALAMBOS, M.: An interesting observation in the treatment of chronic psychiatric patients. Amer. J. Psychiat., *121:* 273 (1964).

GANDER, D. R.: Combining the antidepressant drugs. Brit. Med. J., *1:* 521 (1965).

GAYRAL, M. L., *et al.:* Note sur l'emploi de la propériciazine, 8909 RP (neuleptil) pour le traitement des troubles du caractére chez les enfants et les adolescents. (Paper presented at the Sixty-first Congress of French Speaking Psychiatrists and Neurologists, Nancy, 1963.)

GILLESPIE, R. D.: Narcosis therapy. J. Neurol. Psychopathol., *2:* 45 (1939).

GREAVES, D. C., REGAN, P. F., AND WEST, L. J.: An evaluation of subcoma insulin therapy. Amer. J. Psychiat., *112:* 135 (1955).

GREENE, M. J.: Evaluation of combined meprobamate and promazine therapy in general practice. Clin. Med., *71:* 1764 (1964).

GREGORY, I.: Psychiatry—biological and social. (Saunders, Philadelphia, 1961.)

GRINKER, R. R., AND SPIEGEL, J. P.: Men under stress. (Blakiston, Philadelphia, 1945.)

HARGROVE, E. A., BENNET, A. E., AND STEELE, M.: Investigation of CO_2 as adjunct to psychotherapy in some neuroses. Amer. J. Psychiat., *110:* 844 (1954).

HAWKINS, J. R., AND TIBBETTS, R. W.: CO_2 in halation therapy in neuroses—controlled clinical trial. J. Ment. Sci., *102:* 52 (1956).

HAWKINS, J. R., AND TIBBETTS, R. W.: Intravenous acetylcholine therapy in neurosis. J. Ment. Sci., *102:* 45 (1956).

HEATH, R. G., *et al.:* D-1-Methionine-d-1-sulfoximine effects in schizophrenic patients. Arch. Gen. Psychiat. (Chicago), *14:* 213 (1966).

HELDT, F. J.: Therapeutic use of prolonged sodium amytal narcosis. Amer. J. Psychiat., *104:* 27 (1948).

HENDERSON, D. K., AND GILLESPIE, R. D.: A textbook of psychiatry. (Oxford Medical Publications, Oxford, 1955.)

HENNELLY, T. J.: Prolonged narcosis in manic-depressive psychosis. J. Ment. Sci., *82:* 608 (1936).

HEWAT, S. K., *et al.:* Chlorpromazine, reserpine and isoniazid treatment in mental disorder; a preliminary communication. Brit. Med. J., *2:* 1119 (1955).

HIMWICH, W. A., AND PETERSEN, J. C.: Effect of combined administration of imipramine and monoamine oxidase inhibitor. Amer. J. Psychiat., *117:* 928 (1961).

HOFFER, A.: D-Lysergic acid diethylamide (LSD): a review of its present status. Clin. Pharmacol. Ther., *6:* 183 (1965).

HOLLISTER, L. E., *et al.:* Treatment of anxious patients with drugs. Dis. Nerv. Syst., *17:* 288 (1956).

HORDERN, A., SOMERVILLE, D. M., AND KRUPINSKY, J.: Does chronic schizophrenia respond to a combination of a neuroleptic and an antidepressant? J. Nerv. Ment. Dis., *134:* 361 (1962).

HORDERN, A., *et al.:* Amitriptyline in depressive states: phenomenology and prognostic considerations. Brit. J. Psychiat. *109:* 815 (1963).

HORSLEY, J. P.: Narco-analysis. (Oxford University Press, London, 1943.)

IBOR, J. L.: Anxiety states and their treatment by intravenous acetylcholine. Proc. Roy. Soc. Med., *45:* 511 (1952).

ISCHLONDSKY, M. D.: The inhibitory processes in the cerebrophysiological laboratory and the clinic. J. Nerv. Ment. Dis., *121:* 5 (1955).

IVANOV, V.: Le traitment de certaines psychoses par le sommeil de longue durée et interrompu. Psychiat. Neurol. (Basel), *136:* 380 (1958).

IVANOV-SMOLENSKIJ, A.: Observations on insulin and prolonged narcosis therapy in schizophrenia. Sovetsk. Psikhonevrol., *15:* 16 (1939).

JANECEK, J., *et al.:* The effects of withdrawal of trifluoperazine on patients maintained on the combination of tranylcypromine and trifluoperazine: a double-blind study. Curr. Ther. Res., *5:* 608 (1963).

JENKINS, S. B., AND SAMBORSKI, A. H.: Symptom specificity of antipsychotic drugs. J. Mich. Med. Soc., *63:* 187 (1964).

JENSEN, S. E. (1963): In: Leuner, H.: Effects of psychotomimetic drugs. In: Psychopharmacology (eds., Kline, N. S., and Lehmann, H. E.). (Little, Brown, Boston, 1965.)

JOSEPH, S. R.: Combined antidepressant tranquillizer therapy in somatic and psychosomatic illnesses. Arizona Med., *19:* 239 (1962).

KALINOWSKY, L. B., AND HOCH, P. H.: Somatic treatments in psychiatry. (Grune and Stratton, New York, 1961.)

KALINOWSKY, L. B., *et al.:* A new inhalant convulsive therapy with hexafluorodiethyl ether (indoklon). (Presented at the First International Congress of NeuroPharmacology, Rome, 1958).

KARACAN, I., *et al.:* Evaluation of combined antidepressant and tranquillizing drug (amitriptyline-perphenazine) in the treatment of hospitalized chronic schizophrenic patients. Amer. J. Psychiat., *120:* 500 (1963).

KENNEDY, R. E., AND MILLER, J. J.: Amitriptyline-perphenazine in the treatment of schizophrenia. Amer. J. Psychiat., *119:* 1092 (1963).

KLÄSI, J.: Über die Therapeutische Anwendung der Dauernarkose, mittels Somnifen bei Schizophrenen. Z. Ges. Neurol. Psychiat., *74:* 557 (1922).

KLEMPERER, E.: Versuch einer Behandlung des Delirium Tremens mit Insulin. Psychiat.-Neurol. Wschr., *50:* 549 (1926).

KLINE, N. S., *et al.:* Further studies on: One day treatment of depression with 5-HTP. Amer. J. Psychiat., *121:* 379 (1964).

KLINE, N. S., AND SACKS, W.: Relief of depression within one day using an MAO inhibitor and intravenous 5-HTP. American J. Psychiat., *120:* 274 (1963).

KOZLOWSKI, V. I.: Meprobamate-promazine therapy for aged psychiatric patients with chronic brain syndrome associated with arteriosclerosis: a preliminary report. J. Amer. Geriat. Soc., *9:* 376 (1961).

KRAKOWSKI, A. J.: Treatment of depression with imipramine (tofranil) and imipramine combined with promazine. J. New Drugs, *2:* 56 (1962).

KRANTZ, J. C., *et al.:* New pharmaco-convulsive agent. Science, *126:* 353 (1957).

KRANTZ, J. C., *et al.:* The availability of hexafluorodiethyl ether by intravenous injection as a convulsant in psychiatric treatment. J. Nerv. Ment. Dis., *129:* 92 (1959).

KRIS, E. B., AND GERST, D.: Combined perphenazine-amitriptyline as adjuvant therapy in psychiatric aftercare. Amer. J. Psychiat., *121:* 498 (1964).

KURLAND, A. A., *et al.:* Comparative study of hexafluorodiethyl ether (indoklon) and electroconvulsive therapy. J. Nerv. Ment. Dis., *129:* 95 (1959).

LARSON, C. P.: Fatal cases of acute manic-depressive psychosis. Amer. J. Psychiat., *95:* 971 (1939).

LAUER, J. W., *et al.:* Observations on schizophrenic patients after iproniazid and tryptophan. Arch. Neurol. Psychiat., *80:* 122 (1958).

LEHMANN, H. E.: Combined pharmaco-fever treatment with imipramine (tofranil) and typhoid vaccine in the management of depressive conditions. Amer. J. Psychiat., *117:* 356 (1960).

LEHMANN, H. E., AND BAN, T. A.: Comparative pharmacotherapy of the aging psychotic patient. Laval Med., *38:* 588 (1967).

LEHMANN, H. E., BAN, T. A., AND LEE, H.: The effectiveness of combined phenothiazine and butyrophenone treatment in chronic schizophrenic patients. Curr. Ther. Res., *9:* 36 (1967).

LEMERE, F.: Combined chlorpromazine-reserpine therapy of psychiatric disorders. Amer. Med. Ass. Arch. Neurol. Psychiat., *74:* 1 (1955).

LEOCONTE, M., AND BARBIER, A.: Guerison par l'association chlorpromazine-reserpine d'un grave syndrome hebephrenicatatonique datant de 10 ans. Ann. Medico Psychol. (Paris), *114:* 637 (1956).

Lesse, S.: Combined use of tranylcypromine and trifluoperazine in ambulatory treatment of patients with agitated depressions. Amer. J. Psychiat., *117:* 1038 (1961).

Leuner, H.: Effects of psychotomimetic drugs. In: Psychopharmacology (eds., Kline, N. S., and Lehmann, H. E.). (Little, Brown, Boston, 1965.)

Levine, J., Rinkel, M., and Greenblatt, M.: Psychological and physiological effects of intravenous pervitin. Amer. J. Psychiat., *105:* 429 (1948).

Levy, S., and Perry, H. A.: Narcosynthesis immediately following insulin shock. J. Nerv. Ment. Dis., *106:* 137 (1947).

Lindemann, E.: Psychological changes in normal and abnormal individuals under the influence of sodium amytal. Amer. J. Psychiat., *11:* 6 (1932).

Lingl, F. A.: Combined drug therapy compared with electric shock in psychotic depressions. Amer. J. Psychiat., *120:* 808 (1944).

Litkewitch, H.: Antidepressant-tranquillizer regimen in menopausal patients: drug report. J. Amer. Med. Wom. Ass., *18:* 819 (1963).

Luby, E. D., *et al.:* Study of a new schizophrenomimetic drug—sernyl. Amer. Med. Ass. Arch. Neurol. Psychiat., *81:* 363 (1959).

Lundvall, H. (1907): In: Gregory, I.: Psychiatry. (Saunders, Philadelphia, 1961.)

MacCowan, P. K.: Somnifen narcosis: indications. J. Ment. Sci., *82:* 437 (1936).

MacLean, P. D., *et al.* (1965): In: Leuner, H.: Effects of psychotomimetic drugs. In: Psychopharmacology (eds, Kline, N. S., and Lehmann, H. E.). (Little, Brown, Boston, 1965.)

MacLeod, N.: The bromide sleep. A new departure in the treatment of acute mania. Brit. Med. J., *1:* 134 (1900).

Mann, J.: The initiation of treatment of unmanageable psychotics with intramuscular administration of trifluoperazine combined with chlorpromazine. Amer. J. Psychiat., *120:* 74 (1963).

Maria, B., Böhm, T., and Adorjani, F.: La terapia acetilcolinica negli ammalati di mente con speciale riguardo al meccanismo d'azione. Riv. Sper. Freniat., *84:* 746 (1960).

Marksfield, W. C.: Tranylcypromine and trifluoperazine in the treatment of psychosomatic complaints. Psychosom., *11:* 130 (1961).

Mattey, W. E.: Combination therapy for relief of anxiety and depression. Curr. Ther. Res., *5:* 310 (1963).

Maxwell, R. D. H., and Paterson, J. W.: Meprobamate in the treatment of stuttering. Brit. Med. J., *1:* 873 (1958).

Mayer-Gross, W., and Walk, A.: Cyclohexylethyltriazol in the convulsion treatment of schizophrenia. Lancet, *1:* 1324 (1938).

Mayer-Gross, W., *et al.:* Clinical psychiatry. (Cassell, Oxford, 1960.)

McLaughlin, B. E., *et al.:* Clinical trials with amitriptyline and perphenazine among psychiatric outpatients. Dis. Nerv. Syst., *25:* 169 (1964).

McNichol, R. W., and Seale, A. L.: Treatment of outpatients with a combination of chlorpromazine and trifluoperazine. Dis. Nerv. Syst., *25:* 240 (1964).

Meduna, L. J. (1933): In: Gregory, I.: Psychiatry. (Saunders, Philadelphia, 1961.)

Meduna, L. J.: Die Konvulsionstherapié der Schizophrenie. (Carl Marhold, Halle, 1937.)

Meduna, L. J.: General discussion of the cardiazol therapy. Amer. J. Psychol., *94:* 40 (1938).

Meduna, L. J.: Pharmaco-dynamic treatment of psychoneurosis. Dis. Nerv. Syst., *8:* 2 (1947).

Meduna, L. J.: Oneirophrenia—the confusional state. (University of Illinois Press, Chicago, 1950.)

Meduna, L. J., and Abood, L. G.: Studies of a new drug (ditran) in depressive states. J. Neuropsychiat., *1:* 20 (1959).

Meller, R. L.: Treatment of depression with combined drug therapy. Minnesota Med., *45:* 24 (1962).

Middleton, P.: Memo to the staff. Interim physician policy manual—unpublished. (Provincial Mental Hospital, Essondale, 1964.)

Middleton, P.: Memo to the staff. Interim physician policy manual—unpublished. (Provincial Mental Hospital, Essondale, 1965.)

Middleton, P.: Memo to the staff. Interim physician policy manual—unpublished. (Provinical Mental Hospital, Essondale, 1966.)

Milligan, W. L.: Treatment of depression by a combination of tranylcypromine and trifluoperazine. Med. Proc., *8:* 237 (1962).

Moriarty, J. D.: Evaluation of CO_2 inhalation therapy. Amer. J. Psychiat., *110:* 765 (1954).

Morton-Gore, N.: Combined tranquillization in the treatment of adolescents exhibiting the schizophrenic syndrome. J. Ment. Subnorm., *18:* 53 (1964).

Mueller, M.: Die Dauernarkose mit Somnifen in der Psychiatrie. Z. Neurol., *96:* 653 (1925).

Nyirö, G.: Psychiatria. (Medicina, Budapest, 1962.)

Orchow, H. S.: Emotional disturbances in general practice. Treatment with a new tranquillizer-antidepressant combination. Amer. Practit. Dig. Treatment, *12:* 286 (1961).

Osmond, H.: A review of the clinical effects of psychotomimetic agents. Ann. N.Y. Acad. Sci., *66:* 418 (1957).

Palmer, H. A.: Abreactive techniques: ether. J. Roy. Army Med. Corps., *84:* 86 (1945).

Pare, C. M. B.: Acetylcholine as therapeutic agent in mild psychiatric disorders. J. Ment. Sci., *102:* 847 (1956).

Paterson, A. S.: Electrical and drug treatment in psychiatry. (Elsevier, Amsterdam, 1963.)

PEARSON, M. M.: Strecker's fundamentals of psychiatry. (Lippincott, Montreal, 1963.)

PENNINGTON, V. M.: Combined psychopharmaceutical treatment in 460 neuropsychiatric patients. Amer. J. Psychiat., *118:* 935 (1962).

PENNINGTON, V. M.: The phrenotropic action of perphenazine-amitriptyline. Amer. J. Psychiat., *120:* 115 (1964).

PENNINGTON, V. M.: Single and multiple psychotropic medication in neuropsychiatric patients compared. Int. J. Neuropsychiat., *1:* 173 (1965).

PIVNICKI, D.: Prolonged narcosis in psychiatry. (Diploma thesis. Department of Psychiatry, McGILL University, Montreal, 1959.)

PÖLDINGER, W.: Comparison between imipramine and desipramine in normal subjects and their action in depressive patients. Psychopharmacologia (Berlin), *4:* 302 (1963).

POLATIN, P., AND SPOTNITZ, H.: Effects of combined ambulatory insulin and electroshock therapy in the treatment of schizophrenia. New York J. Med., *46:* 2648 (1946).

POLATIN, P., SPOTNITZ, H., AND WEISEL, B.: Ambulatory insulin treatment of mental disorders. New York J. Med., *40:* 843 (1940).

POLLACK, B.: Imipramine-promazine therapy for depression. Amer. J. Psychiat., *118:* 842 (1962).

POLLIN, W., *et al.:* Effects of amino acid feeding in schizophrenic patients treated with iproniazid. Science, *133:* 104 (1961).

POLONIO, P.: L'insuline et l'insuline-cardiazol dans les maladies mentales. Ann. Portug. Psiquiat., *3:* 87 (1951).

POLONIO, P.: L'insuline et l'insuline-cardiazol dans les maladies mentales. International Psychiatric Congress Proceedings. (Hermann, Paris, 1952.)

RAGG, P. M.: The bromide sleep in a case of mania. Brit. Med. J., *2:* 1309 (1900).

RANCE, A. M., *et al.:* Reflexions sur le traitement par le largactil et le serpasil. Ann. Medico psychol., *114:* 320 (1956).

REES, L., ANNEAR, M. W., AND CROSSE, G.: Trichlorethylene narcosis as a therapeutic aid in psychiatry. J. Ment. Sci., *94:* 502 (1950).

RENNIE, T. A. C.: Prognosis in manic-depressive and schizophrenic conditions following shock treatment. Psychiat. Quart., *17:* 642 (1943).

RICHMOND, P. W., AND ROBERTS, A. H.: A comparative trial of imipramine, amitriptyline, isocarboxazid and tranylcypromine in outpatient depressive illness. Brit. J. Psychiat., *110:* 846 (1964).

RICHTER, D.: Biochemical aspects of schizophrenia. In: Schizophrenia: somatic aspects (ed., Richter, D.). (Pergamon Press, London, 1957.)

ROBINSON, J. T., DAVIES, L. S., AND SACK, E.: A controlled trial of abreaction with LSD-25. Brit. J. Psychiat., *109:* 46 (1963).

ROSMAN, N. P.: Prolonged sleep therapy in the treatment of mental disorders. McGill Med. J., *27:* 44 (1958).

SAARMA, J. M.: Prognostic prediction of the insulin therapy of schizophrenia based on data on the higher nervous activity. (Presented at the First International Congress of Social Psychiatry, London, 1964.)

SAKEL, M.: Zur Methodik der Hypoglykamiebehandlung von Psychosen. Wien. Klin. Wschr., *49:* 1278 (1936).

SALZBERGER, G. J.: Combined chlorpromazine and trifluoperazine on a readmission service. Dis. Nerv. Syst., *24:* 558 (1963).

SANDISON, R. A.: Psychological aspects of the LSD treatment of the neuroses. J. Ment. Sci., *100:* 508 (1954).

SANDISON, R. A., SPENCER, A. M., AND WHITELAW, J. D.: The therapeutic value of lysergic acid diethylamide in mental illness. J. Ment. Sci., *100:* 491 (1954).

SARGANT, W.: Combining the antidepressant drugs. Lancet, *2:* 634 (1963).

SARGANT, W., AND CRASKE, N.: Modified insulin therapy in war neuroses. Lancet, *2:* 212 (1941).

SARGANT, W., AND SHORVON, H. J.: Acute war neuroses. Arch. Neurol. Psychiat., *54:* 231 (1945).

SARGANT, W., AND SLATER, E.: An introduction to physical methods of treatment in psychiatry. (Livingstone, Edinburgh, 1954.)

SARGANT, W., AND SLATER, E.: An introduction to physical methods of treatment in psychiatry. (Livingstone, London, 1963.)

SAVAGE, C., AND STOLAROFF, M. J.: Clarifying the confusion regarding LSD-25. J. Nerv. Ment. Dis., *140:* 218 (1965).

SCHIELE, B. C.: The unique therapeutic properties of tranylcypromine and trifluoperazine (parstelin). Amer. J. Psychiat., *117:* 245 (1960).

SCHILDER, P., AND WEISSMANN, M.: Atherisierung Gesteiskranker. Ztschr. Ges. Neurol. Psychiat., *11:* 779 (1927).

SCHNETZLER, J. P., AND LAMAND, J. C.: La thoridazine dans le traitement des etats depressifs. Ann. Medico psychol., *120:* 609 (1962).

SCHROEDER, K. (1924): In: Kalinowsky, L. B., and Hoch, P. H.: Somatic treatment in psychiatry. (Grune and Stratton, New York, 1961.)

SCHUSTER, J.: Zur Entdeckung der Insulinshocktherapie bei Akuten Geisteskrankheiten Insbesondere bei der Schizophrenie. (Schuster, Budapest, 1937.)

SHORVON, H. J.: Psychopathologie de la dépersonalisation. Comptes rendues de Premier Congres Mondial de Psychiat. (Hermann, Paris, 1952.)

SHORVON, H. J.: Abreactions. Proc. Roy. Soc. Med., *46:* 158 (1953).

SIM, M.: Guide to psychiatry. (Livingstone, Edinburgh, 1963.)

SIMON, J. L., AND TAUBE, H.: A preliminary study of the use of methedrine in psychiatric diagnosis. J. Nerv. Ment. Dis., *104:* 593 (1946).

SINGH, H.: Therapeutic use of thioridazine in premature ejaculation. Amer. J. Psychiat., *119:* 891 (1963).

SMITH-E-INCAS, J.: Combined amitriptyline and perphenazine in the treatment of severe emotional disorders. Int. J. Neuropsychiat., *1:* 220 (1965).

SMITH-E-INCAS, J., *et al.:* Treatment of psychotic patients with trifluoperazine and trifluoperazine-chlorpromazine combination. Canad. Psychiat. Ass. J., *5:* 185 (1960).

SPLITTER, S. R.: Treatment of office patients in a general practice with a meprobamate-promazine combination. Int. Rec. Med., *174:* 289 (1961).

STECK, H.: Die Behandlung des Delirium Tremens mit Insulin. Schweiz. Arch. Neurol. Psychiat., *29:* 173 (1932).

ST. JEAN, A., *et al.:* Clinical studies with propericiazine. Dis. Nerv. Syst., *28:* 526 (1967).

SULZER, E. S., AND SCHIELE, B. C.: The prediction of response to tranylcypromine plus trifluoperazine by the MMPI. Amer. J. Psychiat., *119:* 69 (1962).

TALBOT, D. R.: Are tranquillizer combinations more effective than a single tranquillizer? Amer. J. Psychiat., *121:* 597 (1964).

TEJEDOR, P., *et al.:* Combined antidepressant tranquillizer regimen in depressed psychotics. Biol. Assoc. Med. P. Rico, *56:* 291 (1964).

THIMANN, J., AND GAUTHIER, J. W.: Promazine-meprobamate compound: a medication in the treatment of alcohol addicts. Med. Times, *89:* 1035 (1961).

TOMLINSON, P. J.: Insulin and electric therapy in general paresis. Psychiat. Quart., *18:* 413 (1943).

TUTEUR, W., *et al.:* Treatment of regressed schizophrenics with chlorpromazine, reserpine and a combination of both drugs. Dis. Nerv. Syst., *18:* 100 (1957).

VALENTINE, M.: An introduction to psychiatry. (Livingstone, Edinburgh, 1962.)

WAGNER, VON JAUREGG, J.: Über die Einwirkung Fieberhafter Erkranrungen auf Psychosen. J. b. Psychiat. Neurol., *7:* 94 (1887).

WAGNER, VON JAUREGG, J.: Die Einwirkung der Malaria auf die Progressive Paralyse. Psychiat.-Neurol. Wschr., *20:* 132 (1918).

WAGNER, VON JAUREGG, J. (1917): In: Gregory, I.: Psychiatry. (Saunders, Philadelphia, 1961.)

WIETHOLD, F.: Weitere Erfahrungen mit der Dauernarkosebehandlung Geisteskranker. Munchen. Med. Wschr., *72:* 1461 (1925).

WILLIAMS, L.: A review of 200 chronic alcoholics. Lancet, *1:* 787 (1952).

WINKELMAN, N. W.: Three evaluations of a monoamine oxidase inhibitor and phenothiazine combination. Dis. Nerv. Syst., *26:* 160 (1965).

WOLFF, O.: Trionalkur. Zbl. Nervenheilk, *26:* 281 (1901).

WOLFF, O.: Trionalkur. Zbl. Nervenheilk, *30:* 128 (1907).

WOLPE, J., AND LAZARUS, A. A.: Behavior therapy techniques. (Pergamon Press Oxford, 1966.)

Twenty-one

Treatment of Psychiatric Disorders

A. PATHOLOGICAL DEVELOPMENTS OF THE PERSONALITY

Jaspers (1913, 1945) considers the development of the personality "an understandable sequence of changes." According to him, there is a continuous scale of transitions between normality on the one hand and mental deficiency (a subnormality of intellectual development) and psychopathic personality (a subnormality of character development) on the other.

1. Mental Deficiencies

a. Preventive Treatment

i. Chromosomal Aberrations. There is no causal pharmacological treatment in the majority of mental deficiencies. Apart from genetic preventive measures, the therapy of the various chromosomal aberrations has remained essentially unsuccessful. Pituitary and thyroid extracts have been given in mongolism (Langdon and Down, 1866) without success. The anticonvulsants administered in epiloia (tuberous sclerosis) and neurofibromatosis have been found to be useful, but only to control the cerebral seizures.

ii. Inborn Errors of Metabolism. *α. Protein Metabolism.* The recognition of a variety of "inborn errors of metabolism" has led to the prevention of mental subnormality in some conditions. Certain disorders of amino acid metabolism can successfully be controlled by dietary intervention. Phenylketonuria (Følling, 1934), a condition characterized by an inability to convert phenylalanine to tyrosin, is treated with a low phenylalanine diet (Bickel, 1954; and Woolf *et al.*, 1955). The therapy of maple syrup disease (Menkes, 1954 and Holt, 1957) (an inability to decarboxylate leucine, isoleucine and valine) is a diet which is low in the three amino acids involved; of Hartnup disease (Baron *et al.*, 1956) (a blockade of conversion of tryptophan to kynurenic acid or nicotinic acid), the administration of nicotinic acid and neomycin; of the diseases of the urea cycle (citrullinuria, hyperammonemia, argininosuccinic aciduria), a low protein diet; and of homocystinuria, the addition of cystine to the food intake (Cytryn and Lourie, 1967).

β. Lipoid and Carbohydrate Metabolism. While there are no known therapeutic measures in the disorders of fat metabolism, some of the disorders of carbohydrate metabolism can be treated if recognized early. In galactosemia (Kalckar, 1956), a galactose-free diet, in fructose intolerance a sucrose- and fructose-free diet, and in leucine-sensitive hypoglycemia, a leucine-deficient diet are therapeutic. In McQuarri type of hypoglycemia the administration of adrenocorticotropic hormone and glucagon is indicated.

γ. Other Metabolic Aberrations. Other inborn metabolic disorders leading to mental deficiency are idiopathic hypercalcemia (treated with cortisone); hypoparathyroidism and pseudohypoparathyroidism (treated with calcium and vitamin D); hypothyroidism, myxedema, cretinism (treated with thyroid); pyridoxine dependency (treated with vitamin B_6); and Wilson's disease (treated with penicillamine, dimercaprol and trisodium edetate).

iii. Perinatal Disturbances. Among these are kernicterus and erythroblastosis fetalis, successfully treated by exchange transfusions.

iv. Postnatal Disturbances. *α. Congenital Lues.* Particularly if recognized at an early stage, this condition can be successfully treated by the administration of crystalline procaine penicillin G (100,000 units/kg. of body weight in two or three divided doses given at 2- or 3-day intervals) or by an intramuscular injection of benzathine penicillin G (50,000 units/kg. of body weight at once). If it is recognized only at a later stage a total of 9 million units of benzathine penicillin is needed (given in three divided doses at three daily intervals). Erythromycin or tetracycline may be used in penicillin-sensitive cases.

β. Miscellaneous. Purulent meningitis, viral meningoencephalitis and toxoplasmosis are treated with steroids, antibiotics and chemotherapy with questionable success; cerebral seizures, by anticonvulsants; and infantile spasms, by adrenocorticotropin.

b. Symptomatic Treatment

There are numerous pharmacological substances used with more or less success in the symptomatic treatment of mentally deficient cases. For several years particular effectiveness was attributed to the administration of glutamic acid (Nyirö, 1962). This did not fulfill the expectations. Similarly, tocopherol, a vitamin preparation (Houze *et al.*, 1964), is only infrequently used nowadays. On the other hand, various stimulant and antidepressant drugs, tranquilizers and antipsychotic compounds have become increasingly favored. Successful therapeutic results have been reported with phacetoperane, deanol, nialamide and imipramine (Fleming and Orlando, 1962; Pilkington, 1962; Beaujard, 1963; Ghosh, 1963; MacKay *et al.*, 1963; Krupanidhi *et al.*, 1964; and Jacobs, 1965) and with captodiamine, carphenazine, chlorpromazine, fluphenazine, perphenazine, propericiazine, thioridazine, trimeprazine, chlordiazepoxide and haloanisone (Carter, 1961; Sylvestre, 1961; Gurtler and Goralsky, 1961; Grambert *et al.*, 1963; Mises and Beauchesne, 1963; Roux *et al.*, 1963; Waites and Keele, 1963; Gayral *et al.* 1964; Zapletalek and Komenda, 1964; Ban, 1967; Davidova and Zapletalek, 1965; and Roy *et al.*, 1966).

There are only a few systematic expositions on the symptomatic treatment of mental deficiencies. From a practical point of view, Kielholz's (1965) review is one of the most valuable. He proposed the use of phenothiazines (particularly chlorpromazine and/or levomepromazine) for restless and agitated; piperidyls (*e.g.*, methylphenidate) and amphetamines (*e.g.*, dextroamphetamine) for excitable; and centrophenoxine for the torpid patients.

There may be a relationship between the observation that certain mental deficiencies respond therapeutically to an "excitatory" while others respond to an "inhibitory" type of substance and the finding that mentally deficient cases cannot be characterized by homogenous response patterns when exposed to conditioning procedures. While a weak orienting reflex is characteristic of the majority of these patients, there is at least one subgroup which is distinguished by the persistence of their orienting responses. Similarly, while conditional reflex formation is slightly impaired in the majority of mental deficiencies, there is at least one subgroup which is characterized by "facilitated" defensive conditional reflex formation. Other subgroups show resistance to extinction of established conditional reflexes, impairment of conditional stimulus discrimination and/or absence of conditional reflex delay (delayed reflex formation) (Ban, 1967).

There are some indications that, for patients with a predominant disturbance of the orienting reflex, stimulants are the drugs of choice; with a weak orienting reflex, centrophenoxine; and for those with a persistent orienting reflex, dextroamphetamine. On the other hand, for patients with a prevailing disturbance of "internal inhibition" (*i.e.*, conditional reflex delay, extinction and conditional stimulus differentiation), antipsychotics are suggested.

2. Psychopathic Personalities

Practically all new psychopharmacological preparations have been tried empirically in the treatment of psychopathic personalities, but none of them has proved to be consistently successful. For a while, hormone preparations, *e.g.*, stilbestrol, were recommended, but they did not fulfill expectations and have been almost entirely abandoned.

A rational basis of drug treatment in psychopathic personalities has been suggested on the basis of conditioning studies. Franks (1954, 1955, 1956) reported that psychopaths are extroverted and poor conditioners. Subsequently criminals with a high extroversion score on the Eysenck Personality Inventory and with a low conditionability were suggested to be psychopaths by Eysenck (1964). This was supported by psychopharmacological evidence, namely, by the finding that alcohol, which is a depressant substance, reduces conditional reflex formation, increases extroversion and not infrequently precipitates criminal behavior (Franks, 1961). While the relationship between extroversion and reduced conditionability was challenged, the lowered conditionability of psychopaths and criminals was confirmed by Quay (1965).

Quay (1965) saw in psychopathy a pathological quest for stimulation and explained the reduced conditionability of psychopaths as an inability of the unconditional stimulus to produce a sufficiently strong "excitatory process," which is the prerequisite for conditional reflex formation.

Quay's (1965) hypothesis was supported by Schachter and Latane (1963), who in psychopharmacological experiments found that the conditionability of a group of sociopaths (in avoidance learning) improved under the stimulant adrenalin, whereas the conditionability of the controls decreased under the administration of the same substance.

Subsequently it was suggested that psychopathic personality in general and criminal behavior in particular might be classified, on the basis of conditioning, into two broad subcategories. The asocial low conditioners who are unable to learn from experience were separated into one group and the antisocial ones into a second group. The latter are not poor conditioners, but their conditioned patterns are acquired from their undesirable environment, and consequently their conduct is undesirable in general and delinquent or criminal in particular.

In a therapeutic perspective the asocial (extroverted) type was further characterized by failure—due to their low conditionability—to be inculcated by the "taboos" of the society (usually labeled as moral-ethical feelings) concerning other individuals or the entire society. These asocial psychopaths are unresponsive to psychic education, psychotherapy, group therapy, or particular training techniques, *i.e.*, behavior therapy. On the other hand, they can be successfully treated by increasing their conditionability by appropriate drugs, along with educational training and treatment procedures. Of the available compounds the amphetamines (*e.g.*, dextroamphetamine), piperidyls (*e.g.*, methylphenidate) and various trimethylxanthine preparations (*e.g.*, caffeine citrate) are particularly effective in this respect. As the "inhibitory process" (particularly differential and retarded inhibition) plays a prominent role in the development of moral, ethical and social emotions (Nyirö, 1958), facilitation of the activity of the inhibitory process has proved to be useful in a considerable number of cases. Whether this is achieved by propericiazine, a hydroxypiperidyl phenothiazine substance found to be useful in character disorders (Ban, 1965), remains to be seen.

In contradistinction to the asocial is the antisocial type with normal conditionability and physiologically functioning inhibitory process. Differential reinforcement of punishment and withholding of reward for behavior that is inappropriate or incorrect have been used successfully in some of these cases (Burchard and Tyler, 1965). There is no conclusive evidence that the administration of LSD_{25} is of any therapeutic value in these patients.

B. EXOGENOUS REACTIONS

1. Exogenous Biological Reactions

a. Brain Syndromes Associated with Infections

Varga (1966) has calculated that the ratio of exogenous psychoses to endogenous psychoses in 1910 exceeded that of 1960. This is at least in part related to the introduction of preventive (vaccination) and therapeutic (chemotherapeutic and antibiotic) measures in the treatment of the various infectious diseases.

i. Infections and Delirium. Delirium may occur in the course of systemic infections, meningitis and encephalitis. Treatment of these deliria is directed to the underlying physical condition by the administration of antibiotic and chemotherapeutic agents. For the immediate control of the psychopathological manifestations intramuscular chlordiazepoxide or chlorpromazine are most frequently used. Among the older preparations paraldehyde (5 to 10 ml.) or chloralhydrate (600 to 1200 mg.) is recommended, while treatment with bromides, barbiturates and morphia is discouraged (Mayer-Gross *et al.*, 1960).

ii. Syphilis and General Paralysis. Syphilis of the central nervous system manifests itself in three major forms: meningovascular syphilis (chronic syphilitic meningitis, endarteritis and periarteritis), periradicular syphilitic meningitis (tabes dorsalis) and parenchymatous syphilis (general paralysis). Parenchymatous syphilis is of great psychiatric importance. Prior to 1940, 8 to 10 per cent of the first admissions committed to mental hospitals in the United States were suffering from this condition. As a result of a decrease in the occurrence of syphilis and of earlier and more adequate treatment, the admission rate of general paralysis declined to 2 per cent by 1961 (Noyes and Kolb, 1961).

The primary treatment of all forms of syphilis of the central nervous system is the administration of antibiotics in general and penicillin in particular. The results of treatment depend on the amount and nature of brain damage (Mulder and Dale, 1967). According to Mayer-Gross *et al.* (1960), 30 per cent of all patients with general paralysis treated with penicillin are discharged from hospital and resume work in society and in approximately 90 to 95 per cent of cases the progress of the disease is arrested. Noyes and Kolb (1961) assert that general paralysis can be arrested in 70 to 80 per cent of the cases, and with early treatment 50 per cent of the patients can return to their former occupation.

Treatment with mercury, bismuth, arsenobenzols and potassium has been almost entirely replaced by penicillin alone or combined with pyrexial methods. The classical procedures in which the administration of mercury salicylate was followed by arsenobenzol compounds (Salvarsan or, more frequently, tryparsamide) prior to fever treatment or in which bismuth (bismostab), penicillin and fever therapy were followed by the administration of arsenobenzols (neoarsphenamine, Mapharsen, Acetylarson) have been completely abandoned.

The stages of treatment of general paralysis are as follows.

α. Antibiotic Treatment. The most frequently used antibiotic is penicillin (a total dosage of 6 to 15 million units). Only in penicillin-sensitive patients is there need to use erythromycin (25 to 60 gm.) or tetracycline (30 to 80 gm.).

To prevent the Jarisch-Herxheimer reaction (fever, exacerbation of psychosis or epileptic attack), it is advisable to commence penicillin treatment with the administration of 80,000 units in four divided doses on the first day. This is followed by injections every 3 hours of 100,000 units of crystalline penicillin until a total of approximately 10 million units of the drug has been administered. More recently, crystalline penicillin has been replaced by procaine penicillin G (in oil with aluminum monostearate), of which 600,000 units are administered daily over a period of 20 days.

With successful treatment cell count in the spinal fluid decreases within 2 months and protein within 3. If cell count and protein remain high, antibiotic treatment has to be repeated.

β. Fever Therapy. In cases of persistent failure, antibiotics are supported by fever therapy induced by malaria, pyrogenic preparations (*e.g.*, typhoid vaccine) or inductotherm. It is usually considered that a minimum of ten pyrexias are essential for a successful therapeutic outcome.

In case of malarial treatment, rigors commence after an average of 10 days' incubation period. Jaundice, cardiac failure and renal damage are among the possible complications. Infection is terminated by the administration of 1200 mg. of quinine hydrochloride given in two divided doses daily over a 3-day period and then once a day for a fortnight. The infection can be terminated immediately by the intramuscular administration of 100 mg. of bismuth sodium thioglycollate.

γ. *Symptomatic Control.* For patients with acute motor excitement, delirious states or who are violent and uncooperative, phenothiazines are given alone or in combination with electroshock. Similarly, in cases with depressive manifestations, tricyclic antidepressants are recommended alone or in combination with convulsive treatment. Memory impairment and dementia cannot be directly influenced by drugs.

b. Brain Syndromes Associated with Intoxication

Although the incidence of brain syndromes associated with infections is declining, the incidence of brain syndromes associated with intoxication remains fairly constant.

i. Alcohol and Alcoholism. Alcohol is primarily a nutritive substance which produces 7.1 calories per gram and which in large doses increases the vitamin requirements of the organisms. Alcohol is promptly absorbed from the stomach and small intestine, and some of it is excreted unchanged via the lungs, kidneys and the skin. The rest is metabolized in the liver to acetaldehyde by a diphosphopyridine nucleotide-dependent enzyme and to acetate by a diphosphopyridine nucleotide-dependent aldehyde dehydrogenase (Redlich and Freedman, 1966).

The absorbed alcohol enters the brain and exerts a depressant effect on the central nervous system. It produces abnormal behavior when blood alcohol concentration reaches 0.15 per cent (Greenberg, 1955).

Under the influence of alcohol, impairment of inductive reasoning with no change or improvement in the performance of deductive tasks was shown by Carpenter (1961). There is also a decrease of (intellectual) inhibition (Wikler, 1952); and interference with motor skills, judgment and driving (Bjerver and Goldberg, 1950).

Chronic alcoholism leads to dependency, personality changes, psychopathological manifestations and also to neuropathological damage.

In 1951 there were more than 350,000 alcoholics in England and Wales, of whom 86,000 had psychiatric and/or physical complications. There are 500,000 persons in the United States who have an adverse effect from alcohol during their lives, and at least 12,000 alcoholics die each year from chronic alcoholism. Thus alcoholism, besides being a psychiatric concern, is also a major public health problem (Noyes and Kolb, 1961; and Sargant and Slater, 1963).

α. *Treatment of Acute Alcoholism.* Insulin in a dose of 40 to 60 units is the accepted way of initial treatment. If this fails to induce somnolence, thirst and diaphoresis, 20 additional units may be given. The relaxation and sleep induced by insulin should be maintained over a 2½-hour period (unless convulsions or coma necessitate earlier intervention) and then terminated either by the intravenous administration of glucose or by the oral administration of fruit juice with sugar. In dehydrated cases the administration of 1000 to 2000 ml. of 5 per cent glucose in saline is needed. Drowsiness and somnolence can be counteracted by caffeine sodium benzoate, dextroamphetamine, methamphetamine or methylphenidate (Noyes and Kolb, 1961).

β. *Treatment of Delirium Tremens and Alcohol Hallucinosis.* Withdrawal of alcohol in chronic alcoholism leads to physical and psychological manifestations. Within the first 12 hours tremor, weakness, perspiration, nausea, anorexia, insomnia and irritability may develop. Hallucinations appear within 24 hours, convulsions within 48 hours, and delirium tremens usually commence on the third or fourth day (Sargant and Slater, 1963).

Chlordiazepoxide and chlorpromazine are most useful in preventing delirium tremens and alcohol hallucinosis. Both drugs (in a dosage of 200 to 400 mg. a day) have a beneficial effect on preventing and controlling the alcohol withdrawal syndrome. Ban *et al.* (1965) suggest that the effect of chlorpromazine appears to be more rapid and less erratic than that of chlordiazepoxide. According to them, chlorpromazine has a more consistent effect on hostility, suspiciousness, aggressiveness and insomnia, whereas chlordiazepoxide is more effective in reducing tremor and improving food and fluid intake.

Although chlorpromazine and chlordiazepoxide are probably the most extensively used, Redlich and Freedman (1966) maintain that the classical treatment with paraldehyde (10 to 40 ml. a day), which has a high margin of safety, is preferable to phenothiazines. The treatment of these conditions with reserpine or barbiturates has been almost entirely abandoned, but magnesium sulfate in a 5 per cent solution is still useful (8000 mg. a day for 3 days and 1000 mg. per day for 2 or 3 more days for cases with a low serum magnesium concentration). Others assuming similar mechanisms in addisonian crises and delirium tremens recommend adrenocorticotropin and cortisone administration (Smith, 1950). Whether the administration of corticotropin in 25-mg. doses at 4-hour intervals helps to bring about a more rapid recovery still remains to be seen. High fluid intake, vitamins and minerals are essential for successful treatment. For sleeplessness chloral hydrate or glutethimide are probably the drugs most frequently prescribed.

γ. Treatment of Chronic Brain Syndromes Due to Alcoholism. Dysmnesic syndrome (Korsakoff, 1890) and "polioencephalitis haemorrhagica superior" (Wernicke, 1882) have been successfully treated with thiamine (100 mg. daily intravenously) in combination with massive doses of vitamin B complex and a high calorie diet. In other alcoholic encephalopathies the administration of nicotinic acid (500 to 1000 mg. a day) or nicotinamide (100 to 200 mg. a day) has proved useful.

δ. Treatment of Chronic Alcoholism. There have been reports that one or two large doses of lysergic acid diethylamide may lead to a profound change in the attitude about drinking (Chwelos *et al.*, 1959; and Smart and Bateman, 1967). Many investigators maintain that disulfiram therapy (Jacobsen and Marten-Larsen, 1949) is very useful (Solms, 1960).

Tetraethylthiuram disulfide (disulfiram) interferes with alcohol metabolism and leads to an accumulation of acetaldehyde in the blood. When the substance is simultaneously ingested with alcohol it produces a reddening of the face, headache, palpitation, lowering of blood pressure, sweating and nausea. Treatment begins with 500 mg. daily which is then reduced to a 250-mg. maintenance dosage.

Apomorphine or emetin is used to "condition" nausea and consequently aversion to alcoholic beverages. Apomorphine also reduces anxiety and craving (Dent, 1955). Dent's (1955) procedure consists of the administration of apomorphine in the "vomiting dose" over a 4-day period. At first 6 mg. are placed in the cheek and dissolved in the saliva without being swallowed for 10 minutes. If this does not cause a feeling of sickness, the dose is doubled in 1 hour, tripled in 2 hours and so on until the "vomiting dose" is reached.

Benzodiazepines, phenothiazines, butyrophenones and tricyclic antidepressants have all been used with more or less success in the treatment of chronic alcoholism. More recently, metronidazole, through its special effects on alcoholic patients (changing the taste of alcohol, decreasing the desire to drink, alleviating anxiety and possibly also decreasing the tolerance for alcohol), is coming to be regarded as a useful addition to the therapy of patients who are well motivated to give up excessive drinking (Ban *et al.*, 1966; Blom, 1967; Bonfiglio and Donadio, 1966; Elusuo, 1966; Friedland *et al.*, 1966; Lehmann *et al.*, 1966; Lehmann and Ban, 1967; Semer *et al.*, 1966; and Taylor, 1965).

It has been suggested that metronidazole may act by occupying the cellular receptors for alcohol, thereby reducing the physical need to drink (Taylor, 1964; and Lehmann *et al.*, 1966). It is also possible that it interferes with the long conditioned sequential chain of events in alcoholics (Lehmann and Ban, 1967). By changing the taste of alcohol and by removing the desire to drink, it removes two conditional stimulus properties with a possible inhibition of the conditioned drive to drink (Lehmann and Ban, 1968).

ii. Morphine and Morphinism. Among the phenanthrene alkaloids of opium are morphine and codeine. In analgesic activity codeine is only one-tenth as potent as morphine, while heroin is two to three times and dihydromorphine is five times as potent as the parent substance. (Among the synthetic compounds methadone is roughly equivalent to morphine, dextropropoxyphene is equivalent to codeine, and meperidine is one-eighth as potent as morphine.) Substitutions on the nitrogen atoms of morphine produce analgesics which are morphine antagonists. Among them, nalorphine is used in the treatment of morphine intoxication (Unna, 1943) and cyclazocine in the maintenance therapy of morphine addicts (Wikler, 1967).

Morphine has a selective depressant action on the conduction of internuncial neurons. This is coupled with excitation which is due to the release from inhibition of the motoneurons. It also inhibits cholinesterase, and its repeated administration results in an increase of brain NE concentration.

A single analgesic dose of morphine induces euphoria with a state of semisomnolence or display of an unaccustomed energy (Wikler and Pescor, 1967). Chronic administration results in personality changes in which "ethical depravity" prevails (Mayer-Gross *et al.*, 1960).

α. Treatment of Morphine Withdrawal. At least three different procedures are used in the treatment of opiate withdrawal. In the most frequently used procedure the patient is stabilized over a 2- to 3-day period on the minimum amount of morphine necessary to prevent withdrawal phenomena. Withdrawal is accomplished within 5 to 10 days by a gradual decrease of the dosage. Simultaneously, intravenous infusions of 5 per cent glucose in saline are given, and provision is made for the symptomatic control of pains and aches, insomnia and autonomic release phenomena. Others prefer to perform drug withdrawal under continuous narcosis (with paraldehyde and barbiturates), with modified insulin therapy or with chlorpromazine treatment.

β. Maintenance Treatment. Administration of cyclazocine (approximately 4 to 6 mg. per day) produces resistance to the euphoric and physiological effects of morphine (also of heroin). Since there are some indications that this morphine antagonist substance interferes with the development of physical dependence, it has been successfully tried as maintenance therapy of addicts after drug withdrawal (Martin, 1966; and Freedman *et al.*, 1967).

There are several other opium derivatives which can induce psychopathological changes and drug dependence. Most important are heroin (which may produce deterioration of the personality with disregard for social and ethical conventions; addiction to this substance is the most difficult to treat); codeine (which has a low grade addiction liability); dihydromorphinone; and methyldihydromorphine. Treatment of psychopathological changes produced by these drugs follows the same lines as with morphine.

iii. Barbiturates and Their Abuse. Abuse of barbiturates (acute intoxication and addiction) is a serious public health problem. Acute intoxication with barbiturates accounts for 25 per cent of all deaths from acute poisoning admitted to general hospitals in the United States.

Acute intoxication may cause manic excitement, delirium or confusional states and coma; whereas chronic intoxication manifests itself in persistent hypomanic excitement interrupted by periods of irritability and restlessness, leading to confusional states and dysmnesic phenomena. Upon withdrawal there is an abstinence syndrome with or without psychosis.

In the treatment of acute intoxication analeptics play an important role (caffeine, amphetamines, pentetrazol, tetrazol, strychnine, etc.), but in chronic intoxication the management of the withdrawal period is of more crucial importance. The usual procedure is replacement of the addiction-producing barbiturate with pentobarbital, a short acting barbiturate, which is then gradually tapered off over a period of 2 to 3 weeks. Administration of benzodiazepines (particularly chloridazepoxide) or a phenothiazine (particularly chlorpromazine) may also be useful, particularly when delirium dominates the clinical picture. In deteriorated cases, thiamine, nicotinic acid, nicotinamide and vitamin B complex are useful.

iv. Amphetamine and Amphetaminism. Amphetamines are a group of sympathomimetic substances widely used in the treatment of obesity, fatigue and narcolepsy (Redlich and Freedman, 1966). Abuses of amphetamines were first reported by Guttman (1939), and addiction to amphetamines has been extensively discussed in the literature (Knapp, 1952; Connell, 1958; and Lemere, 1963).

α. Treatment of Amphetamine Withdrawal. Since there is no physical dependence, immediate withdrawal of the amphetamine drug is the first step in treatment. This is carried out with or without the administration of adjuvant medication.

β. Treatment of Amphetamine Psychoses. In cases of amphetamine psychoses (hallucinosis, paranoid delusions or a condition which closely resembles paranoid schizophrenia), spontaneous recovery may take place only after several months. The administration of antipsychotic phenothiazines can reduce this period considerably.

γ. Treatment of Amphetamine-Induced Organic Changes. The prognosis of these conditions is less favorable. Nevertheless, there is a spontaneous improvement in amphetamine-induced personality changes after drug withdrawal. High doses of thiamin (100 mg. daily) have a beneficial effect on the amphetamine-induced dysmnesic syndrome. Dementia produced by amphetamines alone is rare.

v. Lysergic Acid Diethylamide (LSD_{25}) and Its Abuse. LSD_{25} is a hallucinogen which opened new vistas for experimental psychiatry. Today it is extensively used by thrill seekers. Tolerance, precipitation of functional psychoses (or lasting psychotic episodes) and chromosomal damage have been attributed to its use (Isbell, 1959; Keeler, 1963; Jarvik, 1967; and Cohen, 1967).

Administration of antipsychotic phenothiazines (chlorpromazine in particular) is the accepted treatment of LSD_{25}-induced psychotic manifestations. In phenothiazine-resistant cases butyrophenones (haloperidol) benzodiazepines (diazepam), MAOI's (phenelzine), Rauwolfias (reserpine), and nicotinic acid, have been tried with occasional success.

vi. Other Intoxications. The numerous other chemical intoxications (acute and chronic) may be subdivided into accidental, industrial, medicinal and social categories.

α. Accidental Intoxications. Carbon Monoxide is the major intoxicant of this category. Poisoning may be the result of exposure to exhaust fumes of automobiles in a closed environment or of inhalation of illuminating gas through defective combustion of coal stoves. Since the substance has 250 times the affinity of oxygen for hemoglobin, it displaces oxygen in the red cells. Instead of oxyhemoglobin, carboxyhemoglobin is formed, resulting in oxygen lack and anoxia of the brain. This leads to lowering of efficiency and self-control without insight, culminating in the loss of consciousness. In some cases the loss of consciousness is preceded by reckless, irresponsible behavior or by lack of initiative. The symptoms of acute intoxication may be followed immediately (or after a lucid and symptom-free interval, which may be as long as 3 weeks) by psychosis—usually of a subacute delirious type—from which there is full recovery in a small percentage of cases. In others the toxic psychosis gives place to a neurasthenic syndrome (emotional hyperesthesia with fatiguability), Korsakoff's amnesia or dementia.

Treatment of acute intoxication consists of the inhalation of pure oxygen (under a pressure of two atmospheres), blood trans-fusion and the intravenous administration of 15 per cent saline solution. Subacute delirium can usually be successfully controlled with chlorpromazine (also with chlordiazepoxide), whereas the treatment of the neurasthenic syndrome may respond best to benzodiazepine or propanediol preparations. In Korsakoff's amnesia vitamin (B complex) preparations may lead to at least a partial remission. This has been tried in dementia but has proven much less successful.

β. Industrial Intoxications. Lead poisoning is the most frequent of all the industrial intoxication hazards. Early symptoms are asthenia and lassitude (probably secondary to anemia and malnutrition) followed by peripheral (neuritis) and central (convulsions and coma) neurological symptoms. Encephalopathia saturnina is rare. It may commence with a delirium or a subacute delirious state, from which there may be a full recovery in certain cases. In others the delirium is replaced by emotional hyperesthesia or by Korsakoff's (1890) amnesic syndrome, which may or may not lead to dementia.

Treatment of lead poisoning consists of the administration of calcium disodium ethylenediamine tetraacetic acid, a chelating agent which forms a stable water-soluble complex with metals. It is given in a dosage of 1000 mg./15 kg. of body weight daily (in two divided doses) orally or intravenously (in 250 to 300 ml. of 5 to 10 per cent glucose solution) over a 3-day period. There are indications that it is useful to administer dimercaprol (BAL) initially to increase urinary lead excretion. Others have found the administration of penicillamine of great value in the therapy of lead poisoning cases. Sodium citrate has been used orally in preventing the ill effects of increased lead absorption, and the same substance has been used intravenously in relieving lead colic. In the latter condition antispasmodics such as atropine or intravenous calcium gluconate are also effective. Convulsions and excitement can easily be controlled by barbiturate administration, and delirium, with chlorpromazine or chlordiazepoxide. In the therapy of emotional hyperesthesia, benzodiazepines are particularly helpful, as are vitamin B preparations in the treatment of the amnesic syndrome. At any stage of lead poisoning a high calcium diet and large amounts of vitamin D are recommended (Mayer-Gross *et al.*, 1960; Noyes and Kolb, 1961; Nyirö, 1962; and Hoff, 1967).

Less frequently, industrial poisoning occurs with mercury and manganese. Mercury intoxication usually manifests itself in the form of a neurasthenic syndrome with timidity and lack of self-confidence, which is slowly replaced by apathy leading to Korsakoff's (1890) amnesic syndrome. In the early stage of manganese intoxication psychomotor irritability and impulsive acts are in the forefront of the clinical picture, followed by mental confusion with characteristic aggressiveness.

Although there is no specific therapy for mercury or manganese intoxication, there are indications that the administration of dimercaprol is useful in the early stages. To counteract timidity and lack of self-confidence, prazepam (or other benzodiazepines) should be tried, and in the control of psychomotor irritability and impulsive acts, propericiazine (or other phenothiazines) may be useful. In more advanced stages the administration of vitamins (especially B complex) is recommended.

γ. Medicinal Intoxications. Organic brain syndromes may be causally related to the administration of substances used in psychiatric treatment or of drugs used in the treatment of other conditions. Among the psychotherapeutically applied compounds the various psychopathological reactions to *bromides* have been most extensively explored. Bromide psychosis may manifest itself in four different forms (Levin, 1959). Simple bromide intoxication is characterized by progressive dullness, forgetfulness and irritability as the bromide accumulates in the nervous system (Hoff, 1967). The other forms are "bromide delirium," a condition in which disorientation predominates; "bromide schizophrenia," a condition with resemblance to paranoid schizophrenia; and "bromide hallucinosis," in which perceptual disturbances prevail. Since there is evidence that symptoms of bromide intoxication appear only with high blood bromide concentrations (150 mg./100 ml. and above), the primary treatment of all of these conditions consists of the administration of sodium chloride (6,000 to 12,000 mg. a day) with large quantities of fluid. There are indications that, with the administration of ammonium chloride, bromides are excreted more rapidly than with sodium chloride. Some recommend the addition of deoxycortisone or nicotinamide and others, the administration of mercurial diuretics. Although all this may be sufficient for therapeutic success in simple bromide intoxication, in the other forms of bromide psychosis the administration of paraldehyde, phenothiazines (*e.g.*, chlorpromazine) or benzodiazepines (*e.g.*, diazepam) may be useful. Among the various psychotherapeutically used compounds, chronic administration of *paraldehyde* may lead to delirium tremens or acute hallucinosis, both of which promptly respond to drug withdrawal. *Belladonna alkaloids* (atropine or scopolamine) may induce clouding of consciousness with vivid visual hallucinations, which have been successfully treated with chlorpromazine (Mundy and Zeller, 1958).

While psychopathological reactions to psychotherapeutic drugs (bromides, paraldehyde and belladonna alkaloids) were formerly of major importance, psychopathological reactions to endocrine preparations, antibiotics and antihypertensives are of greater significance nowadays. *Adrenocortical steroids* (cortisone and adrenocorticotropic hormone) may cause euphoria or dysphoria, hypomania or depression, apathy or panic. They may also lead to symptoms of depersonalization, hallucinations or delusions. These changes occur in patients who exhibit sharp and rapid fluctuations in 17-hydroxycorticoid excretion and usually respond well to changing the medication to hydrocortisone or dexamethasone. Toxic psychoses with delirium or confusional state have been described with *antibiotics* (penicillin) and *sulfonamides* but more frequently with antihypertensive *thiocyanates*. The thiocyanate-induced toxic reactions are characterized by confusion, disorientation, auditory and visual hallucinations and occasionally by ideas of persecution. They occur when blood thiocyanate levels exceed 15 mg./100 mg. and usually respond to hydroxycobalamine (vitamin B_{12}). In less severe cases, withholding of the drug and addition of large amounts of chloride to the diet are sufficient (Mayer-Gross *et al.*, 1960; Noyes and Kolb, 1961; and Freedman and Kaplan, 1967).

δ. Social "Intoxication" Problems. The once rather frequent "*cocainism*" appears to be occurring less often. A single dose of this substance may cause a particular kind of "drunkness" in which a short (20 to 30 minutes) hypomanic or manic phase is followed by depression of rather long (several hours) duration. Chronic consumption may lead to "cocaine delirium" or "cocaine hallucinosis" (with tactile hallucinations). Cessation of medication even at this stage may lead to full remission, whereas continuation of drug consumption results in character changes at first and Korsakoff syndrome or dementia later. Delusions of a paranoid nature are not infrequent in cocaine abusers. Since there is no physical dependence, sudden withdrawal of cocaine does not cause abstinence syndrome. In the subacute stage of cocaine withdrawal, electroconvulsive treatment is useful, and in the chronic stage, large doses of vitamins are recommended.

Whereas cocaine dependency is in decline, *marijuana* abuse is on the increase. The reaction to a single dose is a loss of time, disorientation and hallucinations with motor anomalies (hyperkinetic and hypokinetic states). Beringer (1932) distinguished three forms of thought disorder under the influence of this drug. These are fragmentation of "perceptive wholes" through fragmentation of thought processes; a disturbance of memory by which everything is forgotten; and frequent, brief but sudden interruptions of the thought stream. Although there is no physical dependence, chronic abusers of cannabis experience short delirious states with dreamlike hallucinations or twilight states with patchy amnesia (Stringaris, 1933, 1939; and Mayer-Gross *et al.*, 1960). Treatment consists of the discontinuation of the drug and symptomatic measures.

At the present time the occurrence of "accidental" and "industrial" toxic psychopathological reactions is decreasing, "medicinal" reactions are constant, and the incidence of "social" intoxications, particularly with psychotomimetics, is on the increase. Abusers of the last-named substances are primarily individuals in their late teens not infrequently with above average intelligence. This problem calls for attention, probably with as much or even more emphasis on its social implications as on its psychopathological aspects.

c. Brain Syndromes Associated with Deficiencies and Autointoxicants

These may be subdivided into psychopathological changes which are the result of physical exhaustion, avitaminosis, endocrinological diseases and various physical illnesses.

i. Exhaustion. Physical exhaustion with lack of sleep in an anxiety-provoking situation initially produces irritability and hypersensitivity and later a decreased stream of mental activity (thinking and speech) leading to a dazed state of consciousness (Critchley, 1943). Infrequently this picture leads to an acute hallucinatory confusional state and even less often to maniform or schizophreniform manifestations (Nyirö, 1962).

Treatment consists of tranquilization either by anxiolytic or by antipsychotic substances. Probably the most successful is sleep treatment induced by the combination of barbiturates and phenothiazines.

ii. Avitaminoses. *α. Vitamin A.* Deficiency of vitamin A results in night blindness. Sargant and Slater (1963) described night blindness of *hysterical* nature in soldiers during the second world war. They suggested that "hysterical mechanisms are more readily released when the physical state is impaired." In these cases the administration of 5000 international units of vitamin A daily is recommended. On the other hand, excessive doses of vitamin A may result in anorexia, weakness, nervousness, anxiety and headache (Busse, 1967).

β. Vitamin B. Deficiency of *thiamine* results in beriberi, a condition characterized by pathological gastrointestinal, cardiovascular, neurological and psychological changes. Latter consist of irritability, fatigue, anorexia and insomnia, which may lead to delirium. If the deficiency continues, poliencephalitis haemorrhagica superior (Wernicke, 1882) develops with or without Korsakoff's (1890) syndrome. Treatment of these conditions consists of parenteral thiamine administration in daily doses of 50 to 100 mg. This therapy has a striking effect on the ocular palsies and on the milder psychological disturbances (Mayer-Gross *et al.*, 1960).

Deficiency of *nicotinic acid* results in pellagra characterized by the triad of dermatitis, diarrhea and dementia. Early psychoneurotic manifestations with depressive components are followed by delirium, stuporous depression or catatonic excitement. Without therapeutic intervention, Korsakoff's syndrome and/or dementia develops. Treatment consists of nicotinic acid administration in a dosage of 100 to 500 mg. a day depending on the severity of the manifestations. After 2 weeks of active treatment the dosage of vitamin B_3 can be reduced to a maintenance level, which is approximately one-quarter of the amount given during the active treatment period.

Deficiency of *cyanocobalamin* results in pernicious anemia, a serious hematological disease characterized by macrocytic megaloblastic anemia with gastrointestinal discomfort and frequently with psychopathological manifestations. The mental changes are nonspecific and range from irritability and depression through hallucinations and delirium to disorientation and memory defects (Busse, 1967). Treatment consists of parenteral vitamin B_{12} administration in a dosage of 50 to 100 μg. a day. After 2 weeks of active treatment the dosage of vitamin B_{12} is reduced to a maintenance level of a minimum of 60 μg. every four weeks.

γ. Vitamin C. Deficiency of vitamin C (*ascorbic acid*) results in scurvy with or without psychopathological manifestations. The latter occurs mainly in the neurotically predisposed and is present as anorexia, weakness, fatigue, irritability and not infrequently depression. Treatment consists of the administration of 500 to 1000 mg. of ascorbic acid daily over a 3- to 7-day period. The dosage of vitamin C is then reduced to a maintenance level of 100 mg. daily.

δ. *Vitamin D.* Infrequently the lack of vitamin D causes night-terrors in children which can be corrected by the therapeutic administration of the substance. Excessive vitamin D administration, on the other hand, produces anorexia, weakness and nervousness.

iii. Endocrinological Diseases. α. *Specific Hyperfunctions.* Selective hyperfunction of the *pituitary eosinophilic cells* results in *acromegaly* with possible psychopathological manifestations. These include loss of libido, depression and paranoid symptomatology. Whereas attempts to inhibit the pituitary with estrogens have been relatively unsuccessful, X-ray irradiation of the pituitary frequently arrests the disease.

The common psychopathological changes with *thyroid* hyperfunction as in *Graves'* (or *Basedow's*) disease are the neurasthenic syndrome or, in other cases, hyperactivity, euphoria, elation with decreased tenacity and increased vigilance. Frequently present are hysterical, obsessive-compulsive and paranoid manifestations. The association of hyperthyroidism with manic-depressive psychosis is not rare. In thyrotoxicosis delirium or confusional states may be present. Causal treatment includes potassium iodide (5 drops of saturated solution daily), propylthiouracil (150 to 300 mg. daily) or methimazol (30 to 90 mg. daily) administration. Others prefer radioactive iodine therapy or surgical removal of the gland.

Cryptogenic, spontaneous, *idiopathic hypoglycemia* is usually due to an increase in insulin production by the *β cells of Langerhans' islands of the pancreas*, and its manifestations are similar to those produced by an excess in epinephrine production. There is anxiety which may lead to auditory and visual perceptual disturbances and confusion. If no underlying pathology can be detected the maintenance of a steady glucose level by multiple feedings and avoidance of stress situation is the primary goal.

In contradistinction to Cushing's disease which is due to the hyperfunctioning of the *basophilic cells of the pituitary gland*, the Cushing syndrome is the result of hyperfunction of the *adrenal cortex* and the excess production of adrenocortical hormones. Psychopathological changes in this condition are weakness and fatigue, frequently with depression and suicidal ideation. Impulsiveness and paranoid development can occasionally be seen. Causal treatment consists of adrenalectomy, which may aggravate the depressive reaction and, by causing an electrolyte imbalance, often results in delirium. Surgical intervention must therefore be followed by substitution treatment.

β. *Specific Hypofunctions. Pituitary* hypofunction leads to Simmond's disease, with increasing loss of interest, slowing of psychic tempo and in certain cases delirium and confusional states. The picture is somewhat similar to that seen in *thyroid* hypofunction. Both conditions respond to the appropriate hormonal preparation.

In diabetes mellitus, in which a decrease in insulin production of the *cells of the Langerhans' islands of the pancreas* is present, manifest psychopathology is rare, but delirium has occasionally been described. When this occurs, insulin treatment has to be supplemented with phenothiazine or benzodiazepine drugs. On the other hand, psychiatric symptoms are common in chronic *adrenal cortical insufficiency* (Addison's disease). In this condition fatigue, instability, anxiety, depression, a paranoid-hallucinatory syndrome or delirium may be present. All these respond promptly to steroid treatment.

γ. *Premenstrual Psychopathologies.* Commonest are tension states, but occasionally depression or stupor can be seen. From the experience of treating a series of over 300 women with premenstrual disorders, Rees (1966) has suggested that psychotherapy is of limited value and that results with dehydration therapy (restriction of salt and water intake, administration of ammonium chloride, mercurial diuretics or chlorothiazide) are disappointing. The latter enhances physical comfort, but the actual psychopathological manifestations remain. Rees (1966) had the best results with progesterones and recommends the administration of progesterone by intramuscular injection on alternate days for 12 days prior to the expected commencement of the period; or the intramuscular administration of 250 mg. of 17 hydroxyprogesterone capronate in one dose 10 days prior to the onset of menstruation; or orally active progestogens, with preference for ethisterone (10 to 30 mg. daily for 12 days before the period); or 19-norethisterone. He found dimethisterone less effective. According to Sargant and Slater (1963), combined administration of a monoamine oxidase inhibitor (*e.g.*, phenelzine, isocarboxazid) and benzodiazepine (*e.g.*, chlordiazepoxide) drug throughout the cycle (but doubling the dosage 10 to 12 days premenstrually) is also an effective treatment. They maintain that, if other methods have failed, the symptoms can be relieved by giving methyltestosterone sublingually 10 mg. daily for 7 days prior to the expected onset of menstruation.

δ. Involutional Psychopathologies. Involutional psychopathological changes in general do not respond to ovarian or testicular hormones. There is only one group of patients who do greatly benefit from estrogen treatment. This group is characterized by anxiety directly accompanying the onset of menstrual changes, paranoid ideas and fluctuating mood changes. For this group of patients estrin (or stilbestrol) administration is the accepted treatment in doses of 0.5 mg. every other day, reducing at first to three-quarters of this dosage for a 3-month period; to half of the original amount for another month; and by half again for an additional 30 days before treatment is discontinued.

Involutional psychoses as often seen in psychiatric practice are unresponsive to hormonal preparations. They are present as involutional melancholia, paranoia or hysteria and not infrequently as a mixed psychosis characterized by depressive, paranoid and hysterical features. Agitation and intermittent confusional states may also add to the florid picture. In the control of agitation, confusional states and paranoid manifestations, phenothiazines have proved to be helpful. Chlorpromazine and methotrimeprazine are the drugs most frequently used, the former because of its reliable antipsychotic properties, the latter because of its potent tranquilizing and mood-lifting effects. In cases with predominant depression, antidepressants are administered often in combination with phenothiazines. Preference is usually given to tricyclic drugs such as imipramine, amitriptyline and trimepramine. There are indications that diazepam, a benzodiazepine preparation, may have a role in the treatment of these cases. Although a high percentage of the involutional psychotic patients recover within 2 months with active treatment, maintenance drug therapy (in one-fourth or one-fifth of the amount given during the acute phase of the illness) is recommended for at least 2 years after remission of psychopathological symptoms.

iv. Physical Illnesses. *α. Cardiovascular.* There are mental symptoms present in approximately 5 to 10 per cent of the severe *cardiac* cases. Most frequently seen are irritability, "moodiness" and emotional instability, but anxiety with a depressive overtone, insomnia and nocturnal restlessness are also rather common. Occasionally, transient confusional states with auditory and visual hallucinations occur, while delirium associated with cardiac decompensation is rather rare.

Digitalis, with small doses of barbiturates (phenobarbital), was formerly the accepted treatment, while today benzodiazepine preparations, particularly chlordiazepoxide or diazepam, are increasingly used. The advantages of the benzodiazepines over the barbiturates are that they do not aggravate but rather ameliorate the depressive symptoms and that they can also be successfully used in the control of certain psychotic (delirium) manifestations.

β. Pregnancy, Childbirth and Puerperium. Whereas in the first half of *pregnancy* emotional lability, hyperemesis and "pica" may be present (which usually do not require medical intervention), in the second half chorea gravidarum or eclampsia with delirium or confusional states may call for termination of pregnancy if antipsychotic therapy fails. During the same period psychotic depressions, catatonic excitement and schizophreniform psychoses can be successfully treated by convulsive treatment or tricyclic antidepressant and/or phenothiazine antipsychotic drugs. Throughout pregnancy psychoactive drugs should be avoided if possible and given in the lowest effective dosage.

During childbirth psychopathological reactions are usually mild, and if present they are manifested in a transient clouded state of consciousness which requires careful supervision. Confusional states in the puerperium are only rarely seen, and active treatment can prevent the development of Korsakoff's syndrome or dementia. Alternating states of consciousness, schizophreniform, schizoaffective, schizophrenic and affective disorders with jealousy (toward husband) and/or hatred (toward the newborn) are more common. Rees (1966) studied the different methods of treatment in postpartum psychoses and was able to demonstrate the superiority of convulsive therapies to hormonal treatment (with chorionic gonadotrophin and progestogens) and the superiority of electroshock to chemically induced convulsions. Pharmacological therapy with antipsychotic drugs is nowadays increasingly replacing physical treatment.

γ. *Miscellaneous Other Conditions.* These were succinctly summed up by Sim (1963) under the heading of mental changes due to internal poisons. Thus in *respiratory acidosis* (carbon dioxide retention), drowsiness with a decrease of mental activity occurs and the patient appears to be demented. Only occasionally are hallucinations and delusions superimposed on this picture. Although specific treatment is directed to the underlying etiological factor, the perceptual and thought pathology can be controlled by phenothiazine medication. *Respiratory alkalosis* due to neurotic hyperventilation with a characteristic anxiety and panicky reaction usually responds to benzodiazepine drugs.

The main clinical features, which promptly disappear after sodium, potassium or calcium administration, respectively, are, in *hyponatremia*, dysthymic mood changes and delusions with mild confusion; in *hypokalemia*, depression with suicidal ideation or irritability, tension and delirium; and in *hypocalcemia*, irritability, restlessness and confusion.

Among the other physical conditions which may produce psychopathological changes are *gastrointestinal diseases*, not infrequently associated with hypochondriasis and overvalued ideas, in the treatment of which benzodiazepines, particularly diazepam, are useful; *hepatic conditions*, in which dysthymic mood changes and delirium (with the increased concentration of ammonia in the blood confusional states) are common; *uremia*, in which the neurasthenic syndrome is replaced at first by alternating states of consciousness and then by delirium, confusional state and coma; and *carcinosis*, in which delirium and confusional states have been described and, only exceptionally, hallucinatory and/or paranoid psychoses. In the last three conditions (hepatic diseases, uremia and carcinosis) therapy is directed against the underlying pathological conditions, and the psychopathological manifestations are only symptomatically treated.

d. Brain Syndromes Associated with Organic Changes in the CNS

i. Trauma. Posttraumatic acute psychopathological changes may progress in three stages: coma, delirium and Korsakoff's syndrome. The chronic psychopathological changes include posttraumatic cerebrasthenia (reversible), encephalopathy (irreversible), personality changes and dementia. Treatment of the acute stage consists of chlorpromazine or chlordiazepoxide administration, which has been shown to be useful in the therapy of delirium; whereas in the chronic stage vitamins (particularly B complex) are recommended. In the symptomatic control of psychotic and depressive manifestations, antipsychotics and antidepressants are used. Propericiazine or diazepam may be tried in the treatment of pathological personality changes.

ii. Tumor. Approximately 70 per cent of all brain tumors show some psychological disturbances (Walther-Büel, 1951), which are among the early manifestations of the growth. The psychological changes are usually focal (*i.e.*, dependent on the CNS areas involved), and they are generally present along with the headache, vomiting and papilledema. The general psychopathological changes, according to Bleuler (1951), are clouding of consciousness, dysmnesic syndrome and dementia, while occasionally depressive, schizophreniform or neurotic symptomatology becomes manifested. With suddenly developing coma, dehydration may be lifesaving; this can be done by the administration of 75 to 100 mg. of 50 per cent sucrose intravenously or by giving 6 to 10 ounces of 25 per cent magnesium sulfate rectally. Treatment consists of surgical intervention, with symptomatic management of the psychopathological changes.

iii. Multiple Sclerosis. This is a slowly progressing chronic disease of the CNS characterized by disseminated patches of demyelinization in the brain and spinal cord; and clinically by multiple symptoms and signs and by remissions and exacerbations. Although delirium and confusional states may occur in the course of this condition, the most common psychopathological changes commence with lack of attention, increased sexual desire, euphoria, elation and hyperactivity (eutonia sclerotica) followed by increasing lack of judgment and loss of emotional control. Only in very advanced stages is there apathy and intellectual deterioration (dementia sclerotica). Although no causal therapy is available, vitamin preparations (nicotinic acid, B_1, B_{12}) are widely used. Some temporary beneficial effects had been seen with cortisone and corticotropine.

iv. Epilepsy. Epilepsy is a paroxysmal and transitory disturbance of the function of the brain which develops suddenly, ceases spontaneously and exhibits a conspicuous tendency to recur (Brain, 1951). In grand mal sodium diphenylhydantoin and phenobarbital alone or in combination are the most effective. Diphenylhydantoin may be replaced by mephenytoin; and mephobarbital substituted for phenobarbital. In certain cases, however, bromides are more effective than the other drugs. In petit mal ethosuximide is the drug of choice. Other effective substances are trimethadione or paramethadione, acetazolamide and quinacrine. Although phenacetamine seems tc be particularly useful in cases with psychomotor seizures, there is increasing evidence that primidone is one of the most effective drugs in the various epilepsies (Lyght *et al.*, 1966).

Acute and chronic psychopathological changes may occur in epileptic patients. Among the acute psychopathologies, alterations of consciousness and disturbances of associations are the most frequent, and among the chronic psychopathologies, character changes and dementia. Benzodiazepines are used in the treatment of delirium, confusional and twilight states; tricyclic antidepressants are administered in depression; and phenothiazines are the drugs of choice for cases with associational disturbances. There are indications that propericiazine may have a beneficial effect on the character changes in these patients. In a recent study Lehmann and Ban (1968) have shown that the five substances (sulthiame, carbamazepine, diazepam, chlorpromazine and propericiazine) they used had a differential therapeutic effect on various psychopathological symptoms frequently present in hospitalized epileptic patients. They noted that sulthiame raised frustration tolerance and carbamazepine had a favorable effect on disthymic mood changes and psychomotor retardation. The fact that carbamazepine is closely related chemically to the tricylic antidepressant drugs may open vistas in regard to the recognition that at least in one type of patient cerebral seizures may be intimately related to depressive mood changes. It has also been shown that the excitement and hostility so commonly encountered in epileptic patients can successfully and selectively be controlled by diazepam (a benzodiazepine derivative), an anxiolytic substance. Similarly, the opposition and aggressiveness which also are often seen in these patients are favorably influenced by the phenothiazines chlorpromazine and propericiazine, both potent antipsychotic drugs. The latter has been reported as being particularly effective in various personality disorders.

v. Presenile Dementias. Presenile dementias include: Alzheimer's disease (diffuse atrophy of the cerebral cortex), Pick's disease (demarcated atrophy of certain areas of the cerebral cortex), Jacob-Creutzfeldt's disease (cortico-striato-spinal degeneration and spastic pseudosclerosis), Stern's disease (thalamic degeneration) and Kraepelin's disease (atypical depressive psychosis with catatonic features) (Alzheimer, 1907; Pick, 1892; Creutzfeldt, 1920; Jacob, 1921; Stern, 1939; and Kraepelin, 1913). All these conditions represent progressive dementias without any known specific treatment. Therapy consists of the administration of vitamins in general and thiamine and nicotinic acid in particular. To ensure sleep, chloral hydrate is recommended and for the control of agitation, chlorpromazine. Because of their lack of mood-depressant effects, thioridazine or methotrimeprazine are sometimes preferred.

vi. Other Conditions. *α. Wilson's Disease.* This is a rare disease characterized by the degeneration of lenticular nuclei and by nodular cirrhosis of the liver. Since an excessive amount of copper has been found in the brain, liver and urine of patients suffering from hepatolenticular degeneration, it has been suggested that Wilson's disease is the result of abnormal copper metabolism.

Psychiatric manifestations of this condition are irritability, explosive behavior, spasmodic laughter, crying and, in the great majority of cases, progressive dementia. Arrest of both the neurological and the psychiatric features may follow the administration of dimercaprol (200 mg. per day intramuscularly), which increases copper excretion. Recently, a chelating agent, penicillamine (250 mg. per day orally) has proved to be effective.

β. Lupus Erythematosus. Systemic lupus erythematosus is an inflammatory connective tissue disorder with cellular infiltration, fibrinoid necrosis and characteristic bodies of altered nuclear material in and around the small blood vessels. Psychiatric concomitants are neurotic manifestations, delirium, depression or specific psychotic symptoms. Treatment consists of the administration of steroids (cortisone, 150 to 300 mg. a day intramuscularly or orally) if necessary together with antipsychotic phenothiazines or tricyclic antidepressants (Waggoner, 1967).

2. Exogenous Psychological Reactions

a. Paranoid Reactions

The Committee on Nomenclature and Statistics of the American Psychiatric Association defined paranoia and paranoid states (or paranoid reactions) as psychoses without known brain pathology characterized by persistent persecutory or grandiose delusions without hallucinations and with a well preserved intelligence and personality. The paranoid system slowly evolves and is often logically elaborated after a false interpretation of an actual occurrence. Emotional responses and behavior are consistent with the ideas held (American Psychiatric Association, 1952; and Cameron, 1967).

Paranoid reactions are difficult to treat. Psychotherapy, physical treatments (electroshock, insulin coma) and psychosurgery (prefrontal leucotomy) have all been used with limited success. At present therapy usually commences with antipsychotic drugs, which only in refractory cases are complemented with convulsive (or, less frequently, insulin) treatment. Phenothiazines are the most extensively used; among them are the aminoalkyl preparations (*e.g.*, chlorpromazine) in the acute phase of the illness and the piperazinylalkyl preparations (*e.g.*, trifluoperazine) in maintenance. There are indications that piperidylalkyl side chain containing preparations, *e.g.*, thioridazine or propericiazine, may also be useful. Although butyrophenones (*e.g.*, haloperidol) or thioxanthenes (*e.g.*, thiothixene) are therapeutically effective in these cases, they are less frequently used.

b. Psychoneurotic Reactions

Sedatives (*e.g.*, barbiturates), minor tranquilizers (*e.g.*, propanediols and benzodiazepines), neuroleptics (*e.g.*, phenothiazines) and antidepressants (*e.g.*, dibenzazepines) have all been used successfully in various psychoneurotic conditions. It seems, however, that neuroleptics and antidepressants have only limited and specific applications.

Denber (1967) has recently suggested that the muscle relaxing effect of chlordiazepoxide, diazepam and meprobamate is a most useful property for the extremely anxious psychoneurotic patient. This effect is not apparent with the barbiturates. To prevent drowsiness or ataxia, which may affect work performance or driving an automobile, Denber (1967) recommends to commence treatment with small doses (15 mg. of chlordiazepoxide, 6 mg. of diazepam and 1200 mg. of meprobamate a day). This dosage should be slowly increased to the optimum therapeutic level (which is about 30 mg. with chlordiazepoxide and diazepam and 2000 mg. with meprobamate). Because of the addicting properties of these drugs, maintenance dosage should be well below the daily amount used in the period of active treatment, and withdrawal of medication should be gradual (Freedman and Kaplan, 1967).

A most instructive and comprehensive review of the pharmacological treatment of psychoneuroses was presented by Rickels (1967). According to him, minor tranquilizers (often referred to as anxiolytic or antianxiety agents) are the primary choice in the treatment of psychoneurotic patients. Phenothiazines (fluphenazine, prochlorperazine and chlorpromazine) in clinical studies have usually been found to be less effective than benzodiazepine (chlordiazepoxide or diazepam) or propanediol (meprobamate) drugs but more effective than an inactive placebo (Hare, 1963, and Rickels *et al.*, 1959). Since phenothiazines have been successfully used in a large subgroup of neurotics, Rickels *et al.* (1967) maintain that these drugs may appropriately be used as antineurotic agents, particularly when other compounds have proven unsuccessful.

Among the phenothiazines, promethazine is the only generally accepted antineurotic agent. Because of its rather strong drowsiness-producing effects, however, the clinical use of this substance remained rather restricted. More recently, thioxanthene (chlorprothixene and thiothixene) and butyrophenone (haloperidol) preparations in low dosage have been tried in the treatment of psychoneurotic cases. Whether these drugs will obtain a wider application remains to be seen.

Similarly to antipsychotic phenothiazines, sedative barbiturates (phenobarbital sodium and amobarbital sodium) have been found to be less effective than minor tranquilizers (Hollister *et al.*, 1956; Moyer *et al.*, 1958; Rickels *et al.*, 1959; Uhlenhuth *et al.*, 1959; Jenner *et al.*, 1961; Brill *et al.*, 1964; and Capstick *et al.*, 1965) but more effective than an inactive placebo (Raymond *et al.*, 1957; and Rickels *et al.*, 1964). Rickels (1967) suggests the use of these drugs in acute, relatively pure anxiety states, as well as in hospitalized patients, in whom drowsiness is not a great problem (Jenner, 1965; and Wheatley, 1968).

Although the once widely used barbiturates are less and less frequently used in the treatment of psychoneurotic cases, there is a gradual increase in the application of minor tranquilizers. Chlordiazepoxide, diazepam and meprobamate are the three most extensively used drugs. Some give preference to meprobamate in patients with prevailing tension, chlordiazepoxide with anxiety and diazepam when some antidepressant and stronger sedative properties are needed. More recently, a new benzodiazepine, oxazepam and a new propanediol tybamate have been introduced into clinical practice. The last drug seems to be without dependence-producing qualities and is particularly effective in the presence of somatic complaints. There are indications that prazepam (a benzodiazepine in clinical investigation) increases assertiveness.

Among the other minor tranquilizers, chlormezanone and phenaglycodol are occasionally used. Interest has recently been revived in hydroxyzine, particularly in establishing its appropriate antineurotic dosage, and in sodium diphenylhydantoin, an anticonvulsant which seems to be therapeutically useful in certain psychoneurotic cases in which other antineurotic agents failed (Turner, 1967).

Although there are indications that imipramine, protriptyline and amitriptyline can successfully be used as the sole medication in the primarily depressed neurotic patient, the combinations of monoamine oxidase inhibitors with benzodiazepines and of tricyclic antidepressants with propanediols have much wider clinical application.

An important relationship between psychopathological symptom profile and responsiveness to psychotherapeutic agents in psychoneurotic patients has been recognized by Rickels (1967). On the basis of this he subdivided his population into depressed neurotic patients with high and low anxiety level and with an emotional (psychological) *versus* somatic symptom focus. Thus Deprol (meprobamate plus benactyzine) was found to be most effective in the somatizing, anxious and depressed; imipramine, in the less anxious and less somatizing; and fluphenazine, in the more emotionally focused depressives. It has also been shown that meprobamate and chlordiazepoxide are equally effective on both the somatic and the emotional (psychological) neurotic symptoms; that tybamate exerts a beneficial effect only in patients with a "somatic profile;" and that diazepam and phenobarbital sodium (while improving both) are slightly more effective in cases having an "emotional profile" (Rickels *et al.*, 1959, 1964, 1965, 1966; and Hesbacher *et al.*, 1968).

Within the psychoneuroses—on the basis of Pavlovian principles—various patient groups have been differentiated. Attempts were made to treat patients with a weak inhibitory process by the administration of bromides (which strengthen the activity of the inhibitory process that promotes restoration) and to treat patients with a weak excitatory process by the administration of caffeine (a stimulant of the excitatory process). In certain cases the combination of these two substances was tried, and in others sleep therapy was used to prevent further disorganization by protective inhibition (Popov, 1955; and Ban, 1964). Nevertheless, drug treatment of the psychoneuroses on the basis of Pavlovian principles has still not been satisfactorily explored. Similarly, Eysenck's (1961) findings (experimentally supported by various investigators) that depressant drugs produce an increase in hysterical and a decrease in dysthymic symptoms, whereas stimulant drugs increase dysthymic and decrease hysterical symptoms, still need further clinical confirmation.

C. ENDOGENOUS PSYCHOPATHOLOGICAL CONDITIONS

1. Huntington's Chorea

There are numerous genetically determined psychopathological conditions. Idiopathic paralysis agitans, Friedreich's ataxia, Pick's disease and Wilson's disease are considered to be the result of single autosomal dominant genes, whereas in the development of cerebral arteriosclerosis, Alzheimer's disease and senile cortical atrophy, "multiple minor genes" may play an important role (Gregory, 1961). Among the various hereditary organic psychiatric conditions, Huntington's chorea (also called "hereditary chorea" or "chronic chorea") is the most important.

Huntington's chorea is a hereditary disease believed to result from the expression of a single autosomal dominant gene with high penetration resulting in choreiform movements and mental deterioration (Lyght *et al.*, 1966). Its occurrence among parents, siblings and children of affected individuals is approximately 50 per cent with an onset in the majority of cases between the fourth and sixth decades of life. The disease usually commences with slight personality changes (obstinacy, moodiness, lack of initiative) prior to or accompanying the appearance of choreiform movements. In some cases this is followed by a "fatuous euphoria," in others by "spiteful, irascible, destructive and assaultive" behavior. In a more advanced stage, first depressive then paranoid reactions are common, leading to poverty of thought and impairment of attention, memory and judgment. The final stage is characterized by dementia. Although this disease formerly had a continuous and rapid progress which killed the average patient within 15 years from the onset of the first clinical symptoms, nowadays the administration of psychoactive drugs can delay the deterioration considerably.

Although no causal therapy is known, several pharmacological agents ranging from chloral hydrate (250 to 500 mg. three times daily) through scopolamine (60 mg. three or four times a day) are used for palliative purpose with some measure of success. Better therapeutic results have been obtained with antipsychotic phenothiazines (also with Rauwolfia alkaloids). Both chlorpromazine and reserpine are effective in controlling the choreiform movements and also the florid psychotic features (Sim, 1963). On the basis of a systematic study, Lyon (1962) concluded that phenobarbital is most successful among the old preparations in the treatment of these patients. The therapeutic efficacy of the phenothiazine thiopropazate and of the benzodiazepine diazepam, however, surpasses that of the barbiturate drug.

2. Manic-Depressive Psychosis

a. Treatment of the Manic Phase and Maintenance

It was not so long ago that manic patients were almost exclusively treated with various sedative drugs. Among them, bromides, barbiturates and paraldehyde were extensively used, the last mainly as a "sleeping-draught" and the first two for (daytime) sedative purposes (Mayer-Gross *et al.*, 1960).

A great number of psychoactive preparations are now used in the treatment of manic patients. Frequently used are various phenothiazine, Rauwolfia alkaloid, butyrophenone and thioxanthene drugs. Dibenzazepine and dibenzocycloheptene derivatives have occasionally been given with successful therapeutic results. For some time there has been increasing interest in lithium treatment of manic patients. According to Schou (1967), the latter substance is distinguished by its greater specificity for manic conditions. It removes the elation and the hyperactivity of the patients without interfering with their normal mental processes. More recently methysergide was shown to be effective in the treatment of a group of manic patients.

i. Phenothiazines. Chlorpromazine is one of the most frequently used substances in the treatment of manic patients. Lehmann and Hanrahan (1954) recognized its particular usefulness in the control of manic excitement and agitation. Since that time chlorpromazine therapy has become the standard treatment of this condition. The drug has to be given in high dosage (up to 1000 mg. a day or more) before symptoms begin to subside.

Not infrequently, chlorpromazine treatment of the manic patient has to commence with the parenteral administration of the substance. The starting intramuscular dose for females is 25 to 50 mg. and for males, 50 to 75 mg. This can be raised quickly to 300 to 600 mg. a day. As soon as the patient's condition permits, he is switched to peroral medication. To obtain the same effect orally, at least twice (sometimes five times) as much of the effective intramuscular dosage has to be given.

Numerous other phenothiazine preparations are used in the therapy of manic patients. Various aminoalkyl and piperazinylalkyl side chain containing compounds are used, and especially favorable therapeutic results have been reported with discontinuous thioproperazine treatment (Ban *et al.*, 1962).

The dosage of thioproperazine is swiftly raised to produce marked extrapyramidal manifestations. This is followed by a drug-free interval which provides for remission of neurological signs. Therapeutic success requires at least three such courses.

ii. Rauwolfias. Because of its numerous side-effects (including depression), reserpine, although very effective, is less and less frequently used in the treatment of affective disorders. Nevertheless, some still consider this substance one of the most effective psychopharmacological preparations in the control of manic patients. For this purpose, intramuscular (10 mg. a day) and oral (10 mg. daily) medication is combined and, if needed, complemented with barbital.

iii. Butyrophenones. Haloperidol is considered to be one of the most effective drugs in the therapy of mania. In certain cases psychomotor overactivity is brought under control within 3 days after the commencement of haloperidol treatment, and in a considerable percentage of these cases all the symptoms are abolished in 4 or 5 days (Sargant and Slater, 1963).

iv. Thioxanthenes. Among the various thioxanthene preparations, thiothixene was reported to have a therapeutic effect in manic patients (Schiele, 1967; and Filotto *et al.*, 1967).

v. Dibenzazepines. Therapeutic response to imipramine in a "typical endogenous manic" patient was first reported by

Akimoto *et al.* (1961). In a subsequent study, 13 out of 20 manic patients showed complete remission or marked improvement (Akimoto *et al.*, 1961).

Although there are no confirmatory reports based on specially designed and systematically conducted clinical trials in this area, there is at least one other manic patient mentioned in the literature with a favorable and prompt therapeutic response to imipramine treatment (Andersen and Kristiansen, 1959; and Kristjansen, 1962).

vi. Dibenzocycloheptenes. Treatment with amitriptyline has been considered to be effective in certain manic cases (Akimoto, 1962). This was supported by Strömgren and Strömgren (1962), whose patient remained symptom free (her manic as well as her depressive phases disappeared completely) during treatment with amitriptyline.

vii. Lithium. Lithium—a metal—was isolated from the mineral petalite by Arfwedson (1818). The name lithium was derived from the Greek word for stone (Schou, 1957). The first psychiatric application of lithium salts was described by Lange (1897), who claimed beneficial results with the substance in mental depression. It was half a century later before interest in lithium was renewed due to an accidental observation by Cade (1949), who recognized a unique sedative-like action of the substance when it was given to "guinea pigs." After approximately a 2-hour latent period, they became lethargic and unresponsive to stimuli although fully conscious. Cade administered lithium salts (carbonate and citrate) to manic patients, whose condition invariably improved.

The first systematic clinical investigation of the effectiveness of lithium in the therapy of manic patients was conducted by Schou *et al.* (1954). On the basis of a double-blind experiment following a placebo-controlled design, they concluded that "lithium treatment of mania represents a very welcome addition to the therapeutic measures against a disease that is very resistant to most types of treatment or in which the improvement after treatment is frequently rather short-lived." As a result of further studies, Schou (1956) recognized that protracted or frequently recurring manias constitute the main indications for treatment with lithium salts and that kidney and heart diseases as well as conditions leading to a low salt intake are the contraindications. More recently, it has been shown that very acute and severe manic attacks are perhaps better treated with other therapies (*e.g.*, electroconvulsive, haloperidol), whereas lithium seems to be superior to any other therapy in chronic mania, protracted or frequently recurring mania and hypomanic states (Schou, 1963; Strömgren and Schou, 1964; Jacobsen, 1965; and Schou, 1967).

A 300-mg. lithium carbonate tablet has a lithium content of 56 mg. or 8 milliequivalent. The initial dosage is usually 4 to 6 tablets a day given in two to three divided doses. The daily dosage is reduced to 2 to 4 tablets a day after approximately 1 week, and later on this is further reduced to a maintenance level. The maintenance dosage in each case must be individually adjusted to give the proper therapeutic effect with few or no side-effects. Response usually becomes apparent in a few days and reaches a peak between the first and second weeks. The most frequently encountered side-effects are diarrhea, vomiting, tremor, ataxia and giddiness. These can be prevented by keeping the serum lithium concentration below 1.8 milliequivalent. Since lithium replaces the sodium ion in the body, treatment of lithium intoxication consists of giving large amounts of sodium chloride and, if necessary, stopping further lithium intake.

The mechanism by which lithium exerts its action is not fully understood. The "partial resemblance" of lithium to calcium and magnesium yielded the hypothesis that its therapeutic effects are due to an interaction with charged macromolecules in the neuronal membrane, leading to increased stability (Tasaki *et al.*, 1965). Its "partial resemblance" to sodium and potassium indicated a possible interference with electrolyte balance and distribution and consequently with membrane transport and excitability (Schou, 1967). Although abnormally increased neuronal instability during manic phases is not inconceivable, there is already some evidence that a relationship may exist between electrolyte metabolism and mania (Coppen, 1965; Coppen *et al.*, 1965; and Shaw and Coppen, 1966).

On the basis of all the evidence thus far, lithium offers a unitary hypothesis of mania and a specific kind of treatment in contradistinction to the other therapeutically effective drugs, which Schou (1967) asserts are without any specific action on the fundamental derangement of mood. Another possibility is a distinct heterogeneity of manic patients, *e.g.*, a subgroup which responds best to phenothiazines, another with the most favorable response to Rauwolfias and another in which the administration of methyldopa is the most successful.

b. Treatment of the Depressive Phase and Depressions

i. Historical Antecedents. Prior to the recent psychopharmacological era, numerous drug treatments were tried in the various depressive conditions. Bleuler (1924) in his classic textbook suggested the use of tincture of opium and from then until the late nineteen-fifties various opiate derivatives have been used. After Steinberg (1936) reported on the successful treatment of severe depressive cases with hematoporphyrin, the application of this substance remained in the therapeutic armamentarium of the practicing physician until ten years ago (Bruel, 1957). Then amphetamines (Rudolf, 1949) and various hormonal preparations (ACTH, estrogen, testosterone) enjoyed a short-lived popularity (Cleghorn, 1950; Margetts, 1952; and Müller, 1953), being replaced by a variety of other substances such as nicotinic acid (Washburne, 1950; and Thompson and Proctor, 1953) and dinitrile succinate (Gillis and Salfield, 1953). None of these early therapies could compare with convulsive treatment, induced either chemically by pentetrazol or by an electrical current, which from the middle thirties to the middle fifties constituted the only effective therapy in severe depressions (Lehmann *et al.*, 1958; and Lehmann, 1965).

ii. Present Status. *α. Treatment Based on Statistical Evidence.* On the basis of a placebo-controlled study of 389 cases over a period of 5 years, Greenblatt *et al.* (1966) concluded that electroshock produced significantly more improvement (and more rapid improvement) than any of the pharmacological treatment modalities. Second best were imipramine and phenelzine, with imipramine being faster in its therapeutic action. Whereas almost all treatments proved efficacious for psychoneurotic depressive reactions, imipramine and phenelzine proved to be more effective also for manic-depressives and psychotics than isocarboxazid or placebo. In involutional cases imipramine was shown to be particularly useful.

In an extensive clinical study of 137 cases, Hordern (1965) compared the therapeutic activity of amitriptyline with imipramine in hospitalized depressive patients. In the total sample significantly more patients recovered without additional electroconvulsive treatment with amitriptyline than with imipramine. The initial severity of the depressive symptoms was inversely related to the therapeutic outcome with imipramine, and the presence of delusions nullified the effectiveness of the latter drug. On the other hand, severity of the depressive manifestations was unrelated to the therapeutic outcome with amitriptyline, and the presence of delusions only lessened the effectiveness of this drug. It has been noted that for both drugs the response to drug treatment in the first week was significantly correlated with the therapeutic outcome.

β. Treatment Based on Clinical Evidence. The selection of the antidepressant substance and the treatment of the depressed patient have been superbly discussed by Kline (1965) on clinical grounds. With due consideration to Pare *et al.*'s (1962) and Angst's (1964) findings, he asserts that a history of familiar responsiveness to a particular antidepressant drug (or previous responsiveness to a substance by the patient) is an indicator of the drug of choice in treatment. On the other hand, when an antidepressant drug is needed for the first time, Kline (1965) recommends the prescription of a tricyclic preparation because of the somewhat lower incidence of side-effects with these compounds and also because they can be changed more readily to an MAOI drug. Of the various tricyclic antidepressants, he considers imipramine the drug of choice for patients without, and amitriptyline, nortriptyline or desipramine (all in a dosage of 30 to 225 mg. a day) alone or in combination with "psychoinhibitors" for patients with anxiety and agitation.

Other tricyclic antidepressants in clinical use (or investigation) are dibenzepin, dimethracen, melitracen, protriptyline and trimipramine. Of these, melitracen and dimethracin are in the investigational stage (Retboll, 1963; and Guth and Hoffman, 1966), and dibenzepin (Rett *et al.*, 1965), protriptyline (Klerman and Cole, 1965) and trimipramine are already used in clinical practice. The last substance, in the dosage range of 75 to 300 mg. a day, was found to be a potent antidepressant useful also in tense and anxious patients and in geriatric depressive patients (Lehmann *et al.*, 1964; and Kristof *et al.*, 1967).

If treatment with a tricyclic antidepressant fails, *i.e.*, no improvement occurs in 4 to 5 weeks, drug administration has to be discontinued, and after a 2- to 4-day drug-free interval (or even immediately upon discontinuation), treatment with an MAOI is suggested (Kline, 1965). Of the various MAOI's, phenelzine (45 to 135 mg. a day) and tranylcypromine (30 to 60 mg. a day) are the most active, although they produce somewhat more adverse effects than isocarboxazid (30 to 60 mg. a day) or nialamide (150 to 600 mg. a day) (Kline, 1965).

In the course of treatment with an MAOI, antidepressant patients have to be warned not to consume cheese, beer and wine at all or coffee, tea and other beverages in excessive amount. All these substances contain pressor amines, which in combination with MAOI's may precipitate a hypertensive crisis. If the latter occurs it can successfully be treated with phentolamine.

MAOI's potentiate the effect of various amines such as epinephrine and scopolamine; barbiturates; morphine, atropine, 4-aminoquinolines; ganglion-blocking agents; and anesthetics. On the other hand, oral diuretics may potentiate the hypotensive effect of MAOI's. These have to be carefully considered if any other condition of the patient is simultaneously treated.

If this second approach with MAOI's fails within a 3- to 4-week period after commencement of treatment, Kline (1966) suggests a number of other possible therapeutic procedures. Among them are the combination of an MAOI with oral amphetamines (parenteral amphetamines are contraindicated); the combination of an MAOI with tricyclic antidepressants with a very small dose of one in the combination together with a routine substantial dose of the other; and thirdly, the addition of *dl*-5-hydroxytryptophan in a dosage of 25 to 50 mg. (given intravenously) to the patient's routine MAOI treatment (Kline and Sacks, 1963; and Kline *et al.*, 1964).

Other possible treatments consist of the administration of anxiolytic substances (particularly benzodiazepines, *e.g.*, chlordiazepoxide and diazepam) alone (Kline, 1965) or in combination with MAOI (Sargent and Slater, 1963) or tricyclic antidepressant (Rickels, 1967) drugs. Although this is especially recommended in certain neurotic depressive cases, the administration of certain phenothiazines, especially methotrimeprazine and thioridazine, was found to be useful in anxious, agitated, psychotic, depressive patients (Ban and Schwarz, 1963; and Hollister *et al.*, 1967). For therapy-resistant cases Lehmann (1960) used a combined pharmaco-fever treatment with imipramine and typhoid vaccine with considerable success.

The combination of ECT with antidepressant drugs is probably the most frequently used procedure in refractory cases; and more recently, the association of two tricyclic antidepressant drugs (both at half the regular dosage) or the combined administration of reserpine (or tetrabenazine) with an antidepressant is occassionally used.

Lehmann (1965) considers preventive (or maintenance) treatment one of the most important aspects in the pharmacotherapy of depression. Although maintenance therapy in depression is not as successful as in schizophrenias, he asserts that patients maintained on imipraine after recovering from their depression have shown a lower incidence of relapse in the following 6 months than patients who were given a placebo (Imlah *et al.*, 1964). Lehmann (1965) suggests that treatment with the therapeutic dosage should be continued for at least 1 month after the disappearance of depressive symptoms and thereafter for a further 3 to 6 months at a reduced (about one-half or one-third) dosage level.

Side-effects in the course of treatment with antidepressants include postural hypotension, neuralgias and reduced sexual sensitivity; dryness of mouth; and constipation with or without difficulty in micturition. Hypotensive reactions can be counteracted by ephedrine, mephentermine, fludrocortisone and dihydroxyphenylalanine; neuralgias and reduced sexual sensitivity, by pyridoxine and cyanocobalamin; and dryness of mouth, by pilocarpine administration. Saline cathartics are recommended in constipation.

iii. Conceptual Frameworks of Treatment. *α. Clinical Framework.* Overall *et al.* (1964) differentiated three distinctly different profiles in depression: anxious depressed, hostile depressed and retarded depressed. Later it was found that anxious and hostile depressed patients responded better to tranquilizers, and retarded depressed cases, to tricyclic antidepressants.

Rickels *et al.* (1964) described two major dimensions, *i.e.*, emotional (psychological) and a somatic symptom focus, in their depressive cases. They found fluphenazine therapeutically effective in patients with an emotional symptom focus, Deprol in those with a somatic symptom focus and meprobamate or chlordiazepoxide in those with both somatic and emotional symptoms.

Lehmann (1968) has recently suggested that all depressive states show a mixture and interaction of three psychological parameters (drive inhibition, anxiety and depressive mood) and one physical parameter (anorexia, weight loss, insomnia, constipation etc.) He nevertheless considers the depressive mood (feelings of hopelessness, inadequacy, guilt and psychic pain) as the core symptom of any depressive state. Lehmann (1968) has furthermore suggested that with amphetamines and piperidyls psychomotor drive is affected (increased); while with the tricyclic antidepressants (and probably also MAOI's) the depressive mood is specifically ameliorated.

β. Physiological and Biochemical Framework. Eosinophil count in the circulating blood was found to be lower in depressive patients than in normals (Mann and Lehmann, 1952). They also recognized that the number of eosinophils could reflect remissions and relapses in the clinical condition of depressed patients. Since the eosinophil count is mainly regulated by the blood levels of catecholamines and corticosteroids and in view of the alteration in urinary catecholamine excretion (an increase in suicidal cases) in depressive patients, Mann and Lehmann's (1952) original study may be of significance in two important directions of depression research.

There is no single biochemical hypothesis which alone accounts for the multifold phenomena of depression. There is, rather, increasing evidence that, like the clinical varieties, the biochemical changes concomitant with the heterogenous clinical picture are also varied. It is indeed likely that there are numerous depressions in which the norepinephrine-serotonin balance is disturbed. In one of these the therapeutically desired increase in brain norepinephrine levels is achieved by the administration of tricyclic antidepressant drugs, whereas in another the required rise in brain 5-hydroxytryptamine concentration can be produced by the administration of MAOI's. In this frame of reference the serotonin hypothesis of depression (Woolley, 1962) and the catecholamine hypothesis of depression (Schildkraut, 1965) are not mutually exclusive. (Although it may be that the difference in the two pathomechanisms and treatments is that tricyclic drugs interfere with NE uptake while MAOI's interfere with NE breakdown.)

Furthermore, there might be other depressions in which cholinergic mechanisms play a major role. One of these responds to the administration of anticholinergic substances, *e.g.*, Ditran (Abood and Meduna, 1958), while another can only be therapeutically influenced by precursors of acetylcholine, *e.g.*, deanol (Malitz *et al.*, 1967).

Finally, there are depressions with characteristically high (Bunney and Fawcett, 1965) and depressions with characteristically low corticosteroid levels. In the latter group the addition of dexamethasone is an essential prerequisite of successful treatment (McClure, 1967).

There are reports that certain patients with frequently recurring depressions and others with mixed manic-depressive psychosis show a favorable therapeutic response to lithium administration (Baastrup, 1964, 1966; and Hartigan, 1963). This will have to be explored further.

γ. *Psychopharmacological Framework.* There are indications that responsiveness to pharmacological stimuli may differentiate various depressive subgroups. Thus on the basis of blood pressure and pulse rate changes after intravenous injection of epinephrine and mecholyl, ECT responsive and refractory cases were differentiated by Funkenstein *et al.* (1949). The intravenous administration of methamphetamine by Roberts (1959), which intensified the symptoms of psychotic and ameliorated the symptoms of neurotic depressive cases, is considered to have similar prognostic implications. Finally, Shagass (1958) differentiated on the basis of a pharmacological load (sodium amobarbital administration) between two depressions: one with a high (neurotic depression) and the other with a low (psychotic depression) sedation threshold. The pharmacotherapeutic implications of these studies still remain to be seen.

3. Schizophrenias

a. Historical Antecedents

It is not so long ago that there was no successful pharmacological therapy for schizophrenia. For a considerable time morphine and scopolamine (or apomorphine and hyoscine) were used for controlling acutely disturbed cases and bromides and barbiturates alone or in combination in the prevention of disturbed behavior. Oral or parenteral administration of paraldehyde and chloral hydrate were needed to counteract insomnia. In the nineteen-twenties fever therapy induced by the intravenous administration of sulfur preparations was unsuccessfully tried just prior to the first effective treatments by insulin-induced coma and by pentetrazol (or electrically) produced convulsions.

b. Present Status

Today, the treatment of choice for schizophrenia is pharmacotherapy and, according to Lehmann (1965), "no other single therapeutic procedure can compete with it in terms of rapid effectiveness, sustained action, general availability and ease of application." Furthermore, "it compares at least favourably with the shock therapies as far as incidence of side effects, complications and serious risks are concerned." While the rate of spontaneous recovery from this disease has been determined to be about 15 to 25 per cent, modern pharmacotherapy had by 1963 resulted in a recovery rate that lies between 50 and 60 per cent for patients who had been ill for less than 3 years (Pearson, 1963). Today 75 to 80 per cent of all acute hospitalized patients are discharged within a year and more than 50 per cent within 6 months (Lehmann, 1965).

i. Treatment Based on Statistical Evidence. In their review on controlled studies in the treatment of schizophrenic patients Cole *et al.* (1966) established that a large number of phenothiazines, *e.g.*, chlorpromazine, fluphenazine and thioridazine (NIMH-PSC 1964), trifluperazine (Schiele *et al.*, 1961), prochlorperazine and perphenazine (Adelson and Epstein, 1962), are more effective than an inactive placebo. Placebo equaled the active phenothiazine preparation in only 24 studies, while in 71 it was definitely inferior to it. A small patient sample, low drug dosage and/or short treatment duration were common characteristics of the studies in which the superiority of the active substance could not be shown.

None of the studies reviewed showed any of the phenothiazine drugs superior therapeutically to chlorpromazine, whereas in some of the studies promazine (Casey *et al.*, 1960; and Kurland *et al.*, 1961) and also mepazine (Casey *et al.*, 1960) were definitely inferior to it. Promazine and mepazine were also shown to be less effective than perphenazine, prochlorperazine and triflupromazine (Casey *et al.*, 1960; and Kurland *et al.*, 1961).

There is evidence that reserpine is inferior in therapeutic efficacy to chlorpromazine (Simon *et al.*, 1958; and Lasky *et al.*, 1962), and there are indications that, of the butyrophenones, at least haloperidol and triperidol (Lehmann and Ban, 1964) and, of the thioxanthenes, thiothixene (Lehmann and Ban, 1968) equal the activity of the therapeutically effective phenothiazines.

Cole *et al.* (1966) also recognized that the lack of significant difference in the therapeutic activity of effective antipsychotic phenothiazine drugs was the result of the univariate statistical approach (analysis of covariance) most commonly used in the analysis of data. This pitfall in evaluation was corrected by Hanlon *et al.* (1965) by the use of a straight analysis of variance (after converting data into percentage change scores), which showed that chlorpromazine, fluphenazine, perphenazine and prochlorperazine are significantly more effective in the severely ill patients than thioridazine and thiopropazate. On the other hand, there was a trend for thioridazine to be the most effective drug in the less severely ill patients.

With the application of newer multivariate statistical approaches, after defining the two clearest schizophrenic types (the paranoid and the undifferentiated) on the basis of expert ratings, Overall *et al.* (1963) were able to demonstrate that actual schizophrenics resembling the paranoid type did best on acetophenazine, and actual schizophrenics resembling the undifferentiated type did best on perphenazine.

By a somewhat different approach Katz (1965) clustered patients on the basis of "resemblance of their symptom profile." As a result he found that the type which resembles an acute panic state responds significantly better to phenothiazines than the type which is characterized by withdrawal and periodic agitation. Furthermore, he was able to demonstate that fluphenazine was more effective for withdrawn, helpless and suspicious patients, whereas thioridazine was better for the withdrawn, periodically agitated cases.

ii. Treatment Based on Clinical Evidence. The selection of the antipsychotic substance and the treatment of the schizophrenic patient was superbly discussed by Lehmann (1965, 1966) and summed up in a guide by Appleton (1967) based entirely on clinical grounds. Unquestionably, at the present time the phenothiazines are still the drugs of choice in the treatment of both the acute and also the chronic schizophrenic cases. Preference is usually given to one of the aliphatic (aminoalkyl) side chain containing compounds in acute (or acutely exacerbated) excited cases and to piperazinylalkyl side chain containing preparations in stuporous catatonic or chronically withdrawn and apathetic patients. Whatever preparation is chosen, the dosage has to be gradually increased until the desired therapeutic effect is produced, *or* a significant side effect occurs, *or* mild extrapyramidal signs become manifest. Not infrequently, parenteral administration is unavoidable at the commencement of treatment, but this can in most cases be replaced within 3 to 5 days by oral (double or even five times the intramuscular) route. With this treatment one may expect more cooperation from the patient with a reduction of psychomotor excitement within 7 to 14 days; socialization with an improvement of emotional responsiveness within 2 to 6 weeks; and a reduction of major psychotic symptoms involving perceptual and cognitive processes toward the end of the second or beginning of the third month (Lehmann and Ban, 1964).

The average daily dosage of chlorpromazine for an acute hospitalized schizophrenic is 400 to 800 mg. While this can be slowly raised to as high as 2000 mg. a day, 600 (or a maximum of 1000 mg.) of this drug on the first day of treatment should not be exceeded. Taking chlorpromazine as the unit, the approximate dosage ratios of the most frequently used phenothiazines are as follows: acetophenazine, 6 (*i.e.*, the necessary dosage on a milligram basis is six times less than that of chlorpromazine); butaperazine, 5; fluphenazine, 20 to 60; levomepromazine, 1 to 2; perphenazine, 10; prochlorperazine, 2 to 6; proketazine, 3; promazine, 0.5; thiopropazate, 8; thioridazine, 1; trifluoperazine, 20; triflupromazine, 2 to 3; thioproperazine, 30 to 70 (Lehmann, 1965; and Appleton, 1967). It should be noted that the daily dosage of perphenazine should not exceed 64 mg. and of thioridazine, 800 mg. Some recommend regular electrocardiographic checkings whenever the dosage of the latter substance is above 400 mg. a day (St. Jean, 1968; and Lehmann and Ban, 1968).

If therapy with an antipsychotic phenothiazine fails, *i.e.*, no improvement occurs within 4 to 8 weeks after intensive drug treatment has been instituted in an acute patient, a number of electroshocks (eight to ten) or a similar number of insulin comas are suggested. Although antipsychotic drug therapy has to be continued during the period of physical treatment, it is wise to reduce the phenothiazine dosage 1 to 2 days before convulsive or coma treatment and to omit one dose of the drug prior to the ECT. Furthermore, to prevent complications it is important to keep the patient in a lying position for at least 30 minutes after consciousness is regained following electroshock treatment.

It has been noted that cerebral seizures and confusional and hypoglycemic reactions occur more frequently in combined insulin-phenothiazine treatment than if insulin is given alone. On the other hand, the hypotensive action of phenothiazine is intensified by the electroshock. Thus reduction of phenothiazine dosage aims to prevent, or at least reduce the intensity of, these undesired reactions.

If this second approach, *i.e.*, the combination of a phenothiazine with physical treatment (usually ECT) in acute patients fails (or in treatment-resistant acute and chronic cases), other possible therapeutic procedures are needed.

A schizophrenic should not be considered refractory to drug therapy until he has received at least 2000 mg. of chlorpromazine or its equivalent daily dosage for a minimum period of 6 months (Lehmann, 1965) or until he has been treated with phenothiazine for 1 month for every year since the commencement of his illness (Appleton, 1967).

One of the other treatment regimes for the "therapy-resistant" patient consists of the exchange of one phenothiazine for another, usually an aminoalkyl preparation for a piperazinylalkyl compound (or vice versa) or the institution of a discontinuous treatment regime (particularly with thioproperazine) in place of continuous treatment. Another increasingly used regimen is the replacement of phenothiazine therapy by treatment with a butyrophenone (*e.g.*, haloperidol, triperidol), a thioxanthene (*e.g.*, thiothixene, clopenthixol) and less often with a Rauwolfia alkaloid (*e.g.*, reserpine).

Successful therapeutic results in certain treatment-resistant cases have also been obtained by the combination of two different phenothiazine preparations, *e.g.*, one with a piperazine and another with a piperidyl ring on the side chain; by the associated administration of two different antipsychotic drugs, *e.g.*, a phenothiazine with a butyrophenone; by the addition of an antidepressant, *e.g.*, an MAOI or a tricyclic substance to the phenothiazine regime; and by complementing any of the treatments with high dosages of nicotinic acid (Achaintre *et al.*, 1963; and Lehmann and Ban, 1966).

The importance of maintenance therapy cannot be overemphasized when treating schizophrenic cases. There is sufficient evidence to believe that it produces a significant decrease in the number of relapses in the course of the illness. Since there is no way to predict which patient will relapse without maintenance treatment, every recovered schizophrenic should be continued on his medication even after the remission of all the psychopathological manifestations. After the first schizophrenic episode the maintenance period should be not less than a year; after the second, 2 to 3 years; and thereafter it should be for an indefinite period of time. Nevertheless, the dosage of the therapeutic substance may be reduced considerably (to one-third or even one-fifth of the daily amount given in the acute period of the illness). There are definite indications that in most cases it is sufficient to take this dosage once (or at maximum twice) a day.

Among the various side-effects which may occur, transient drowsiness and hypotensive reactions are those which usually appear at an early stage of treatment. In severe hypotensive reactions, norepinephrine and metaraminol bitartrate are the drugs usually used as countermeasures. Some recommend the emergency use of hydrocortisone in these cases. Since phenothiazines are α-adrenergic receptor blockers, the administration of epinephrine is contraindicated.

With continuous treatment other adverse

reactions, *e.g.*, extrapyramidal signs, autonomic atropine-like effects and cerebral seizures, come to the forefront, and very rarely agranulocytosis may develop. Most of the extrapyramidal reactions are successfully treated by antiparkinsonian drugs and only infrequently lead to persistent dyskinesias. Most of the autonomic reactions do not require a countermeasure, whereas cerebral seizures may call for reduction in dosage. In the rare cases of agranulocytosis, early recognition, transfusions and corticoid administration can be lifesaving.

Other complications are photosensitivity and skin rashes, which may require the administration of antihistaminics or corticosteroids; menstrual irregularities which do not call for any intervention; weight gain, which is successfully controlled by restriction of the calorie intake; constipation, which responds to enemas and laxatives; and jaundice (cholestatic type) from which the patient usually recovers spontaneously.

Among the late reactions, pigmentation of the cornea, lens and exposed skin areas can effectively be counteracted by penicillamine administration.

c. *Conceptual Frameworks of Treatment*

There is no single physiological or biochemical hypothesis which applies to all the various schizophrenias. Rather than this, there is increasing evidence that the clinical varieties like the physiological and biochemical changes with the heterogenous clinical pictures are also varied. It is indeed likely that there are numerous schizophrenias, one of which responds best to phenothiazines, *i.e.*, to chemicals which reduce the arousal reaction (related to brain stem reticular formation function), block adrenergic intrareticular mechanisms and decrease the cortial release of acetylcholine. Another responds best to antipsychotic Rauwolfia alkaloids which, unlike the phenathiazines, exert a stimulating effect on the mesodiencephalic alerting system facilitating the transmission of impulses in these areas (Rinaldi and Himwich, 1955), release various amines from their cellular storage sites and decrease brain 5-HT, NE and GABA levels. A third responds best to butyrophenone preparations which, via an inhibitory feedback circuit in the caudate loop, selectively decrease the responsivity of the caudal portion of the reticular formation, produce a dopamine receptor blockade (Rossum, 1965) and possibly by occupying GABA receptors makes them inacessible to glutamic acid. In this frame of reference it is the differential rather than the common characteristics of the various groups of antipsychotic drugs which are stressed to achieve a psychopharmacologically based diagnostic classification.

Furthermore, there might be other schizophrenias associated with an abnormality of methylation processes with the production in the body of some psychotoxic metabolite such as bufotenin or dimethoxyphenylethylamine in which a beneficial effect can be obtained by the methyl acceptor niacin and niacinamide and others again which are related to a positive nitrogen balance in the organism which can be successfully treated by the administration of thyroxin (Gjessing, 1939, 1964).

Finally there are schizophrenias which are characterized by diminished thyroid function and treated by triiodothyronine (Danziger, 1958); others with a positive copper balance and consequently reduced melatonin and increased melanocyte stimulating hormone function, which may respond to penicillamine treatment (Greiner *et al.*, 1964); and others again with a significant decrease in urinary Ca excretion, which may improve on imipramine or ECT.

More than 10 years ago a γ-immunoglobulin fraction was isolated from the sera of schizophrenic patients by Heath *et al.* (1957, 1967). They found that this isolated sera fraction (which they called taraxein) produces a characteristic alteration of brain function by combining with antigenic sites of neural cell nuclei in the septal region. On the basis of this, Heath (1967) has postulated that schizophrenia is an immunological disorder in which the former reaction (probably by interfering with neurohumoral conductors) is responsible for the physiologic changes and behavioral symptoms. There is increasing evidence that at least in one of the schizophrenias this is the pathomechanism involved. Nevertheless, the psychopharmacological implications of taraxein, a substance which exerts anticholinergic effects, still remain to be seen.

D. SPECIAL PSYCHOPATHOLOGICAL CONDITIONS

1. Psychopathology in Children

a. General Principles of Drug Treatment

Childrens' behavioral problems are usually of short duration, and at least 70 per cent of emotionally disturbed children will be significantly improved at the end of 3 months without any kind of treatment. Werry (1967) therefore suggests withholding psychoactive drugs from children at the time of the first visit, except for those conditions which are "serious and marked by psychomotor excitement." When a drug is indicated, Eveloff (1966) recommends starting medication at a very low dosage and raising it gradually until the desired therapeutic response is obtained.

The therapeutic dosage of some of the frequently used drugs for children's psychiatric disorders are as follows (Fish, 1963): amphetamine, 0.2 mg./kg. a day (range, 0.15 to 0.80); diphenhydramine, 4 mg./kg. (range, 2.0 to 10.0); meprobamate, 15.0 mg./kg. (range, 4.0 to 30.0); chlorpromazine, 2.0 mg./kg. (range, 1.0 to 8.0); and trifluoperazine, 0.5 or 0.1 mg./kg. (range, 0.1 to 1.0 or 0.02 to 0.2).

The optimal dosage is the amount of the medication that provides for reduction of the pathological symptoms and for an increase in functioning without causing undesired side-effects (Fish, 1963). On this dosage usually an intermittent (5 days per week or 3 weeks per month) treatment regime is preferred to prevent cumulative effects and minimize the development of tolerance (Werry, 1967). Treatment should continue over a long period of time before it is abandoned as ineffective. Eveloff (1966) suggests a minimum treatment period of 1 month with any of the sedative, anxiolytic, stimulant or antidepressant drugs; and at least 3 months for the major tranquilizers (antipsychotics, neuroleptics). Rosati (1965) recommends an even longer (1 year) therapeutic trial to permit a child to benefit from better concentration, increased social contact, etc. If there is no complete relief of psychopathological symptoms even after this length of time, pharmacotherapy must be continued indefinitely. It is fortunate that there is no disturbance of growth or endocrine development in adolescence even after 5 to 6 years of phenothiazine treatment (Fish, 1963).

b. Drug Treatment of Specific Conditions

i. Historical Aspects. Psychopharmacological treatment in childhood and adolescence is not new. Barbiturates, whiskey-sugar pacifier and paregoric have been given for a considerable period of time, and the anticonvulsants (hydantoins), which are one of the most successful agents for the modification of deviate behavior, cannot be considered as recently developed drugs (Bender, 1959). Amphetamines have been used in child psychiatry since 1940 (Bradley and Bowen, 1940; and Bradley and Green, 1940); and diphenhydramine, and antihistamine particularly useful in the treatment of unorganized, immature behavior, was introduced at child psychiatric clinics well over 10 years ago (Effron and Freedman, 1953; and Silver, 1955).

ii. Selection of the Therapeutic Compound. *α. Treatment of the Neurotic Child.* Sedatives, anxiolytic drugs and antihistaminic substances are used with more or less success. There is no definite evidence that any of these groups is superior to the other, nor is their differential effectiveness clearly established. Whereas Fish (1963) prefers to use diphenhydramine to control anxiety in the very young, Eveloff (1966) recommends chlordiazepoxide as a first choice for neurotic children, and Werry (1967) prescribes phenobarbital to reduce tension. True dependency is exceptionally rare in prepuberty children, unlike adults and adolescents.

Phenobarbital is one of the most frequently used substances in the treatment of the neurotic child. Werry (1967) maintains that there is no clear evidence in favor of the newer sedatives or anxiolytic drugs. He considers *phenobarbital* in a dosage of 3 to 6 mg./kg. a day as the first choice "especially in the less serious conditions" with the exception of children who have "organic brain damage" or "hyperkinetic syndrome."

Fish (1963), on the other hand, does not consider barbiturates particularly effective in prepuberty children. She asserts that barbiturates may in fact increase anxiety and disorganization and prefers chloral-hydrate even when nighttime sedation is needed.

Among the various *anxiolytics* preference is usually given to chlordiazepoxide, hydroxyzine and meprobamate. Successful therapeutic results have been obtained with *chlordiazepoxide* in various neurotic disorders in childhood by Laveck and Buckley (1961), Grant (1962) and Hawke and McGreal (1965); in school phobias by D'Amato (1962); and in the anxiety of mentally retardates by Pilkington (1961). Similar beneficial effects have been reported with *hydroxyzine* in childhood neuroses by Dougan (1962), and Piuck (1963) reported dramatic relief from chronic tic in children who had been refractory to previous treatment. Although in controlled studies (Eisenberg *et al.*, 1961; and Laveck and Buckley, 1961) there was no significant difference between *meprobamate* and an inactive placebo, Bender and Faretra (1961) and also Freed and Friguito (1961) maintain that this drug is therapeutically effective in the mild neurotic disorders of the prepubertal age.

Among the *antihistaminic* substances *diphenhydramine* has been used by Bender and Nichtern (1956), Freedman (1958) and Fish (1960) with great therapeutic success particularly in the control of aggressive-impulsive behavior in childhood. Fish (1963) recognized that below the age of 10 (but not above) it also reduces anxiety without producing drowsiness or lethargy.

There are many other substances used in the behavior disorders of childhood. Although findings with *hydantoins* in behavior disorders associated with nonspecific EEG abnormalities are equivocal (Lindsley and Henry, 1942; Walker and Kirkpatrick, 1947; Pasmanick, 1951; and Freedman, 1958), more recent therapeutic findings with diazepam are encouraging (Gallant, 1967).

β. Treatment of the Nonorganic Hyperactive Child. There is no generally accepted procedure for the treatment of nonorganic hyperactive children. Eveloff (1966), on the basis of the survey of the recent literature, suggests *chlordiazepoxide* as the first choice, *chlorpromazine* or another aminoalkyl side chain containing phenothiazine as the second, and *dextroamphetamine* or *methylphenidate* as the third.

γ. Treatment of Childhood Schizophrenia. Phenothiazines are therapeutically less effective in schizophrenic children than in schizophrenic adults. The drug of choice depends on the prevailing clinical manifestations. In agitated and hyperactive children *aminoalkyl* or *piperidylalkyl* side chain containing *phenothiazine* preparations are the drugs primarily used, whereas in withdrawn (including autistic) children preference is given to compounds with a *piperazine* ring on the side chain. More recently, in the withdrawn group *thiothixene* (a thioxanthene) and *trifluperidol* (a butyrophenone) have also been used successfully. Fish and Campbell (1967) found the latter substance best among the various antipsychotic preparations. According to them it is more stimulating than trifluperazine, and it facilitates speech production, increases motor initiative and reduces withdrawal, affective blunting and psychotic disorganization of language in doses of 0.17 to 0.67 mg. per day.

δ. Treatment of Children with Organic Brain Damage. The drug of choice for the organic brain-damaged child depends on the prevailing clinical manifestations. For severly hyperactive children, Eveloff (1966) recommends the administration of chlorpromazine or thioridazine, although according to Fish's (1963) review, the latter substance has not yet been shown to have any advantage over the former (which would outweigh the possible complication of toxic retinitis). In slightly hyperactive cases dextroamphetamine, methylphenidate and pipradrol and, in the moderately hyperactive, captodiamine (Low and Myers, 1958) and diphenhydramine are the most frequently used. On the other hand, in prevailingly withdrawn children trifluoperazine or, if it fails, perphenazine is suggested.

2. Psychopathology in the Aged

a. General Principles of Drug Treatment

It has been shown that functional disorders of the affective type and neurotic reactions are the prevailing psychiatric disorders in the aged and not, as formerly believed, psychopathological conditions associated with structural changes of the brain tissue or diseases of the cardiovascular system (Roth, 1955; Kral, 1961; and Kral and Papetropoulos, 1965). These findings have led to a more optimistic outlook of treatment in the mental disorders of the older age group.

Nevertheless, it remains true that the aging organism is less resistant to stress than the younger one (Comfort, 1956; and Kral, 1961). This implies that therapeutic measures which induce "harmless" side-effects in the younger age group may act as pathogenic stress in older patients (Kral and Papetropoulos, 1965). Before giving any psychoactive substance to a geriatric patient, the therapeutic and the possible adverse effects must therefore be carefully considered.

b. Drug Treatment of Specific Conditions

i. Treatment Based on Clinical Evidence. Pharmacotherapy in geriatric psychiatry may be subdivided into treatments by substitution or replacement with various metabolic agents, vitamins or hormones; agents influencing cerebral circulation, mainly vasodilators and anticoagulants; central nervous system stimulants and analeptics; minor tranquilizers; antidepressants; and miscellaneous drugs (Lehmann and Ban, 1967). A comprehensive pharmacologically oriented review of this topic has been presented by Lifshitz and Kline (1963); and more recently, a very practical clinically oriented review, by Kral (1967).

α. Neurotic Conditions. These rank highest among the various psychiatric disorders of the aged encountered in the nonhospitalized population. They are frequently characterized by a flat depression with insomnia, anorexia (or obsessive eating), weakness, irritability, hostility (toward family members) and somatic complaints (hypochondriacal fears). Kral (1967) suggests the administration of anxiolytic substances such as benzodiazepines (chloridazepoxide, 15 to 30 mg., or diazepam, 6 mg. a day) or propanediols (meprobamate, 300 to 600 mg. a day) in the treatment of these patients. Not infrequently anxiolytics remain ineffective, whereas small amounts of tricyclic antidepressants (imipramine or amitriptyline, 20 to 30 mg. a day) are very useful.

The possibility of the use of magnesium glutamate hydrobromide in some of these cases needs further exploratory work. The same applies to the newer benzodiazepine and propanediol preparations *e.g.*, oxazepam and tybamate. The administration of barbiturates in the elderly should preferably be avoided and prescribed only if organic (including vascular) cerebral changes are definitely excluded.

β. Affective Disorders. These consitute 50 per cent of all hospitalized geriatric patients (Roth, 1955). The majority are depressed and only a small portion are manic. *Depressions* in the aged are treated just as in the younger groups. Tricyclic antidepressants or MAOI's alone or in combination with various phenothiazines are used. Kral (1967) recommends imipramine (75 to 200 mg. a day) alone or, when anxiety is one of the dominant features, in combination with chlorpromazine (75 to 200 mg. a day), thioridazine (75 mg. to 200 mg. a day) or perphenazine (12 to 32 mg. a day). This treatment lifts depression, improves activity and decreases anxiety. Common but "innocent" side-effects of imipramine in this age group are dryness of mouth and excessive perspiration; while constipation and difficulty of micturition always require careful attention. Absolute contraindications of treatment are cardiac failure or myocardial infarction but not arteriosclerotic heart disease, hypertension or diabetes (Grauer and Kral, 1960). Orthostatic hypotension and somnolence are not infrequent at the onset of treatment and usually subside even if therapy is continued.

Another tricyclic antidepressant frequently used in the aged is amitriptyline (30 to 200 mg. a day), although according to Kral (1967) its side-effects (hypotension, drowsiness, sluggishness, tremor) are not well tolerated. More recently, trimipramine is being increasingly used (Lehmann *et al.*, 1964) as well as methotrimeprazine, particularly in agitated depressive cases.

MAOI antidepressants are well tolerated by geriatric patients. According to Kral (1967), they are particularly useful in retarded endogenous depression and are liked because of their prompt onset of therapeutic action. Nevertheless, their hypotensive (and not the extremely rare hypertensive) action constitutes a great drawback.

Frequently used MAOI's in the aged are tranylcypromine (30 to 60 mg. per day) and phenelzine (45 to 90 mg. per day) alone or in combination with trifluoperazine (3 to 6 mg. per day) or perphenazine (6 to 12 mg. per day).

Manic episodes in the aged are rare but can be successfully controlled by phenothiazine drugs. More recently, as in young adults, haloperidol (a butyrophenone preparation) is being increasingly prescribed in the treatment of these cases and also reserpine, particularly for patients whose psychopathology is associated with hypertension.

γ. *Schizophrenias.* Late paraphrenics and chronologically old schizophrenics can successfully be treated with phenothiazine preparations, *e.g.*, chlorpromazine, trifluoperazine and perphenazine.

δ. *Organic Brain Syndromes.* In acute and subacute confusional states the administration of a 5 per cent glucose (intravenous) infusion and chlorpromazine (or other phenothiazines) has proved to be therapeutically effective. At a later stage treatment may be complemented by an antidepressant (preferably tricyclic) or anxiolytic (preferably benzodiazepine) preparation. In chronic as opposed to acute organic brain syndromes (*e.g.*, senile dementia, arteriosclerotic dementia) vasodilators, hormones, vitamins and procaine hydrochloride have been administered with equivocal success. Symptomatic improvement in these patients may be achieved by tricyclic or MAOI antidepressants and by phenothiazine drugs, especially by thioridazine.

In a series of publications, Cameron *et al.* (1963, 1964) suggested that the administration of ribonucleic acid (RNA) has a beneficial effect on memory function in the aged. Cameron's work was based on Hyden's (1955) demonstration that the amount of nucleic acid decreases with age. Hyden (1955) also asserted that RNA is a possible substrate of memory. The clinical effects of RNA or substances which have an effect on its formation (such as magnesium pemoline) or its destruction still remain to be determined.

ii. Treatment Based on Electroencephalographic Findings. There is sufficient evidence to believe that there are greater EEG differences between the various clinical diagnostic groups in the geriatric population than in the younger age groups (Müller, 1967). An early trial of EEG-based treatment was presented by Müller (1967).

α. *Treatment of Patients with Cerebral Vascular Insufficiency.* The EEG in "persistent" vascular insufficiency is characterized by slow wave or sharp and slow wave abnormalities of a localized type and in "intermittent" vascular insufficiencies by episodic slow wave discharges, most commonly in the left centro-temporal region (Bruens *et al.*, 1960; and Obrist and Busse, 1965). It is this latter group, according to Müller (1967), in which drugs that increase cerebral blood supply may become therapeutically effective.

β. *Treatment of Patients with Cerebral Atrophy.* The EEG in cerebral atrophy is characterized by slowing and later disappearance of background activity. Background activity is replaced by irregular slow waves and in the terminal stages by symmetrical slow wave discharges (Müller and Kral, 1967). There are indications that the early changes are associated with apathy, slowing and disintegration of thought processes or with impairment of memory and orientation (Grunthal and Remy, 1954; and Surwillo, 1964). Müller (1967) suggests that the apathetic patient of this electroencephalographically separated group is a good candidate for treatment with anabolic steroids.

γ. *Treatment of Patients with Functional*

Psychopathology. The EEG in some of these cases shows a well regulated normal alpha activity or low voltage fast activity. In others, there is a pronounced sharpness or "spikiness" of the brain rhythm with or without slow waves. The latter EEG group is usually characterized clinically by more florid psychopathology, agitation and confusion and is expected to be therapeutically responsive to antipsychotic (*e.g.*, phenothiazine), antidepressant (dibenzazepine) or anxiolytic (benzodiazepine) drugs (Müller, 1967).

iii. Treatment Based on Psychopharmacological Findings. Therapeutic responsiveness to pharmacological substances in geriatrics depends upon various factors. There are indications that immediate responsiveness to a pharmacological load, *e.g.*, a sedative (amobarbital), a stimulant (methamphetamine) or a cerebral vasodilator (carbon dioxide), is in this respect the most revealing factor (or at least is more important than the nosological group to which the patient belongs or profiles based on psychopathological symptom assessment and/or psychological test performances). This has been shown for geriatric inpatients in the course of a systematic study (Ban, 1965, 1966; Lehmann and Ban, 1967; Lehmann *et al.*, 1968; Silver *et al.*, 1967; and Debow *et al.*, 1967) in which six drugs were given in increasing dosage over an 8- to 12-week period with the use of a cross-over design. The drugs and dosages were as follows: thioridazine, 75 to 150 mg.; meprobamate, 600 to 1600 mg.; fluoxymesterone, 5 to 20 mg.; nicotinic acid, 300 to 3200 mg.; methylphenidate, 10 to 30 mg.; and amitriptyline, 30 to 150 mg.

The most effective single compound for long term hospitalized geriatric patients was found to be *thioridazine*. It was particularly useful in 65- to 69-year-old organic patients or, independent of age and diagnosis, for those whose performance on psychometric tests deteriorated under the influence of CO_2 and methamphetamine. Arousal, affective (including mood) and organic psychopathology improved under the influence of this phenothiazine drug. Second best in over-all effectiveness was *nicotinic acid*. It was particularly useful for organic patients over 75 years of age or, independent of age and diagnosis, for those whose performance on psychometric tests improved under the influence of CO_2. Affective (including mood) and organic psychopathology improved under the influence of this vitamin preparation. *Fluoxymesterone* was best in males over 70 years of age or in those whose performance improved under the influence of methamphetamine, and *methylphenidate* was most effective in males below 70 years or in those who did poorly after CO_2 or methamphetamine administration. With *meprobamate*, improvement or deterioration paralleled the changes recorded after CO_2 administration; and with amitriptyline, which undoubtedly had a positive effect on mood, clinical deterioration was more often present in those patients whose psychological performance became increasingly impaired after methamphetamine.

REFERENCES

Abood, L. G., and Meduna, L. G. (1958): In: Biel, J. H.: Some rationales for the development of antidepressant drugs. In: Molecular modification in drug design (ed., Gould, R. F.). (American Chemical Society, Washington, 1964.)

Achaintre, A., *et al.*: Actualites de thérapeutique psychiatrique. (Masson, Paris, 1963.)

Adelson, D., and Epstein, L. J.: A study of phenothiazines with male and female chronically ill schizophrenic patients. J. Nerv. Ment. Dis. *134:* 543 (1962).

Akimoto, H., *et al.* (1961): In: Schou, M.: Normothymics, "mood normalizers." Brit. J. Psychiat., *109:* 803 (1963).

Akimoto, H., *et al.* (1962): In: Schou, M.: Normothymics, "mood normalizers." Brit. J. Psychiat., *109:* 803 (1963).

Alzheimer, A.: Über eine Sigenartige Erkrankung der Hirnrinde. Allg. Z. Psychiat., *64:* 146 (1907).

American Psychiatric Association. Diagnostic and statistical manual, mental disorders. (American Psychiatric Association, Washington, 1952).

Andersen, H., and Kristiansen, E. S.: Tofranil treatment of endogenous depression. Acta Psychiat. Scand., *34:* 387 (1959).

Angst, J.: Antidepressiver Effekt und Genetische Factoren. Arzneimittel-forschung, *14:* 496 (1964).

Appleton, W. S.: Guide to the use of psychoactive agents. Dis. Nerv. Syst., *28:* 609 (1967).

Arfwedson, A.: Undersökning af några vid uto jernmalmsbrott förekommande fossilier, och af ett deri funnet eget eldfast alkali. Afhandl. Fysik, Kemi, Mineral, *6:* 145 (1818).

AYD, F. J.: Psychopharmacology in Europe. (Presented at the Annual Meeting of American College of Neuropharmacology, San Juan, 1965.)

Ayd, F. J.: Phenothiazines: skin and eye complications. Int. Drug Ther. Newsletter, *1:* 1 (1966).

BAASTRUP, P. C.: The use of lithium in manic-depressive psychosis. Compr. Psychiat., *5:* 396 (1964).

BAASTRUP, P. C.: Lithium behandlung af maniodepressiv psykos. (Paper presented at the Seventh Scandinavian Congress of Psychopharmacology, Copenhagen, 1966.)

BAN, T. A.: Annual report of the Research Department, Verdun Protestant Hospital, Verdun, 1962.

BAN, T. A.: Conditioning and psychiatry. (Aldine, Chicago, 1964).

BAN, T. A.: The butyrophenones in psychiatry. In: The butyrophenones (eds., Lehmann, H. E., and Ban, T. A.). (Q.P.R.A., Montreal, 1964.)

BAN, T. A.: Annual report of the research department of the Douglas Hospital, Verdun, 1965.

BAN, T. A.: Conditoning and delinquent behavior. (Paper presented at the Meeting of Correctional Psychologists, Montreal, 1965.)

BAN, T. A.: Human pharmacology and systematic clinical studies with a new phenothiazine. In: Preceedings of the Leeds Symposium (ed., Jenner, F. A.). (May and Baker, Dagenham, 1965.)

BAN, T. A.: Annual report of the research department, Douglas Hospital, Verdun, 1966.

BAN, T. A.: Psychophysical deficit-psychiatric diagnoses. (Abstract. Proceedings of the Eighteenth International Congress of Psychology, Moscow, 1966).

BAN, T. A.: Conditioning and Cognitive Pathology. (Presented at the Douglas Hospital Conference on Conditoning and Cognitive Pathology, Montreal, 1967).

BAN, T. A., AND LEHMANN, H. E.: Skin pigmentation, a rare side effect of chlorpromazine. Canad. Psychiat. Ass. J., *10:* 112 (1965).

BAN, T. A., LEHMANN, H. E., AND ROY, P.: Rapport préliminaire sur l'effet thérapeutique de flagyl dans l'alcoolisme. Un Méd. Canada, *95:* 147 (1966).

BAN, T. A., PAPATHOMOPULOS, E., AND SCHWARZ. L.: Clinical studies with thioproperazine (majeptil). Compr. Psychiat., *3:* 284 (1962).

BAN, T. A., AND SCHWARZ, L.: Systematic studies with levomepromazine. J. Neuropsychiat., *5:* 112 (1963).

BAN, T. A., *et al.:* The effect of clopenthixol on chronic psychiatric patients. Amer. J. Psychiat., *119:* 984 (1963).

BAN, T. A., *et al.:* Comparative study of chlorpromazine and chloridazepoxide in the prevention and treatment of alcohol withdrawal symptoms. Clin. Med., *72:* 59 (1965).

BARON, D. N., *et al.:* Hereditary pellagra-like skin rash with temporary cerebellar ataxia, constant renal amino-aciduria, and other bizarre biochemical features. Lancet, *2:* 421 (1956).

BEAUJARD, M.: Phacetoperane in mental retardation in children. In: Psychological and sociological problems in imbecility drug treatment (ed., Stur, O.). (Karger, Bazel, 1963.)

BENDER. L.: Discussion of Leon Eisenberg's paper. In: Child research in psychopharmacology (ed., Fisher, S.). (Charles C Thomas, Springfield, 1959.)

BENDER, L., AND FARETRA, G.: Organic therapy in paediatric psychiatry. Dis. Nerv. Syst., *22:* 110 (1961).

BENDER, L., AND NICHTERN, S.: Chemotherapy in child psychiatry. New York J. Med., *56:* 2791 (1956).

BERINGER, K.: Clinical symptoms of hashish intoxication: psychological disturbances. Nervenarzt, *5:* 346 (1932).

BICKEL, H.: The effects of phenylalanine-free and phenylalanine-poor diet in phenylpyruvic oligophrenia. Exp. Med. Surg., *12:* 114 (1954).

BJERVER, K., AND GOLDBERG, L.: Effect of alcohol ingestion on driving ability. Quart. J. Stud. Alcohol, *11:* 1 (1950).

BLEULER, E.: Textbook of psychiatry. (Macmillan, New York, 1924.)

BLEULER, M.: Psychiatry of cerebral diseases. Brit. Med. J., *2:* 1233 (1951).

BLOM, A.: Some experiences regarding the use of metronidazole in the treatment of alcoholism. Svensk. Lakartidn., *64:* 57 (1967).

BONFIGLIO, G., AND DONADIO, G.: Results of a clinical trial with a new compound, metronidazole, in the treatment of chronic alcoholism. Ill. Laboro Neuropsichiatrico, *38:* 2 (1966).

BORDELEAU, J. M. (ed.): Extrapyramidal system and neuroleptics. (L'Edition Psychiatrique, Montreal, 1961.)

BRADLEY, C., AND BOWEN, M.: School performance of children receiving amphetamine sulfate. Amer. J. Orthopsychiat., *10:* 782 (1940).

BRADLEY, C., AND GREEN, F.: Psychometric performance of children receiving amphetamine sulfate. Amer. J. Psychiat., *97:* 388 (1940).

BRAIN, W. R.: Diseases of the nervous system. (Oxford University Press, Oxford, 1951.)

BRILL, N. O., *et al.:* Controlled study of psychiatric outpatient treatment. Arch. Gen. Psychiat. (Chicago), *10:* 581 (1964).

BRUEL, D.: Behandlung von Depressionszustandes mit Hematoporphyrin. J. Psychiat. Neurol. Basel, *133:* 1 (1957).

BRUENS, H. H., GASTAUT, H., AND GROVE, G.: Electroencephalographic study of chronic vascular insufficiency of the sylvian region in aged people. Electroenceph. Clin. Neurophysiol., *12:* 283 (1960).

BUNNEY, W. C., AND FAWCETT, J. A.: Possibility of a biochemical test for suicidal potential. Arch. Gen. Psychiat. (Chicago), *13:* 232 (1965).

BURCHARD, G., AND TYLER, V.: The modification of delinquent behavior through operant conditioning. Behav. Res. Ther., *2:* 245 (1965).

BUSSE, E. W.: Brain syndromes associated with circulatory disturbances. In: Comprehensive textbook of psychiatry (eds., Freedman, A. M., and Kaplan, H. I.). (Williams and Wilkins, Baltimore, 1967.)

Cade, J. F. J.: Lithium salts in treatment of psychotic excitement. Med. J. Aust., *2:* 349 (1949).

Cameron, D. E.: Treatment of chronic paranoid schizophrenic patients. Canad. Med. Ass. J., *78:* 92 (1958).

Cameron, D. E.: Effects of RNA on memory defect. Amer. J. Psychiat., *120:* 320 (1963).

Cameron, D. E., *et al.:* Ribonucleic acid in psychiatric therapy. In: Current psychiatric therapies, Vol. 6 (ed., Masserman, J. H.). (Grune and Stratton, New York, 1964.)

Cameron, N. A.: Paranoid reactions. In: Comprehensive textbook of psychiatry (eds., Freedman, A. M., and Kaplan, H.). (Williams and Wilkins, Baltimore, 1967.)

Capstick, N. S., *et al.:* A comparative trail of diazepam and amylobarbitone. Brit. J. Psychiat., *3:* 517 (1965).

Casey, J. F., *et al.:* Drug therapy in schizophrenia. A controlled study of the relative effectiveness of chlorpromazine, promazine, phenobarbital and placebo. Arch. Gen. Psychiat. (Chicago), *2:* 210 (1960).

Carpenter, J. A.: Alcohol and higher order problem solving. Quart. J. Stud. Alcohol , *22:* 183 (1961).

Carter, C. H.: Carphenazine in mental defectives: a specific antiemetic. Arch. Pediat., *78:* 349 (1961).

Casey, J. F., *et al.:* Treatment of schizophrenic reactions with phenothiazine derivatives: a comparative study of chlorpromazine, triflupromazine, mepazine, prochlorperazine, perphenazine and phenobarbital. Amer. J. Psychiat., *117:* 97 (1960).

Chwelos, N., *et al.:* Use of d-LSD in the treatment of alcoholism. Quart. J. Stud. Alcohol, *20:* 577 (1959).

Cleghorn, R. A.: A study of the effect of the pituitary ACTH in depressed patients. Canad. Med. Ass. J., *63:* 329 (1950).

Cohen, M. N.: In vivo and in vitro chromosomal damage induced by LSD-25. New Eng. J. Med., *277:* 1043 (1967).

Cole, J. O., Goldberg, S. C., and Davis, J. M.: Drugs in the treatment of psychosis: controlled studies. In: Psychiatric drugs (ed., Solomon, P.). (Grune and Stratton, New York, 1966.)

Comfort, A.: The biology of senescence. (Rinehart, New York, 1956.)

Connell, P. H.: Amphetamine psychosis. (Chapman and Hall, London, 1958.)

Coppen, A.: Mineral metabolism in affective disorders. Brit. J. Psychol., *111:* 1133 (1965).

Coppen, A. J., and Shaw, D. M.: Use of monoamine oxidase inhibitors. Lancet, *1 (7388):* 765 (1965).

Coppen, A., *et al.:* Tryptamine metabolism in depression. Brit. J. Psychiat., *111:* 993 (1965).

Creutzfeldt, H. G.: On a peculiar focal disease of the CNS. Z. Ges. Neurol. Psychiat., *57:* 494 (1920).

Critchley, M. (1943): In: Mayer-Gross, W., *et al.:* Clinical Psychiatry. (Cassell, London, 1960.)

Cytryn, L., and Lourie, R. S.: Mental retardation. In: Comprehensive textbook of psychiatry (eds., Freedman, A. M., and Kaplan, H. I.). (Williams and Wilkins, Baltimore, 1967.)

D'Amato, G.: Chlordiazepoxide in the management of school phobia. Dis. Nerv. Syst., *23:* 292 (1962).

Danziger, L.: Thyroid therapy of schizophrenia. Dis. Nerv. Syst., *19:* 2 (1958).

Davidova, M., and Zapletalek, M.: Some notes on the use of captodiamine in pedopsychiatry. Acta Nerv. Super., *7:* 298 (1965).

Debow, S., *et al.:* Adverse effects of psychoactive drugs in the aged. (Presented at the Q.P.R.A. Symposium on Psychoactive Drugs in the Aged, Quebec, 1967.)

Denber, H. C. B.: Tranquillizers in psychiatry. In: Comprehensive textbook of psychiatry (eds., Freedman, A. M., and Kaplan, H. I.). (Williams and Wilkins, Baltimore, 1967.)

Dent, J. Y.: Anxiety and its treatment: with special reference to alcoholism. (Skeffington, London, 1955.)

Dougan, H. T.: Hydroxyzine syrup (atrarax) in management of paediatric behavior problems. Med. Times, *90:* 9551 (1962).

Effron, A. S., and Freedman, A. M.: The treatment of behavior disorders in children with benadryl. J. Pediat., *42:* 261 (1953).

Eisenberg, L., *et al.:* The effectiveness of psychotherapy alone and in conjunction with perphenazine or placebo in the treatment of neurotic and hyperemetic children. Amer. J. Psychiat., *117:* 1088 (1961).

Elusuo, R.: Metronidazole in the treatment of alcoholism. Suom. Laak., *27:* 2178 (1966).

Eveloff, H. H.: Psychopharmacologic agents in child psychiatry. Arch. Gen. Psychiat. (Chicago), *14:* 472 (1966).

Eysenck, H. J. (ed.): Handbook of abnormal psychology: an experimental approach. (Basic Books, New York, 1961.)

Eysenck, H. J.: Crime and personality. (Routledge and Kegan Paul, London, 1964.)

Filotto, J., *et al.:* Thiothixene in the treatment of effective psychoses: a pilot study. (Presented at the Q.P.R.A. Symposium on Thioxanthenes, Montreal, 1967.)

Fish, B.: Drug therapy in child psychiatry: pharmacological aspects. Compr. Psychiat., *1:* 55 (1960).

Fish, B.: Pharmacotherapy in children's behavior disorders. In: Current psychiatric therapies (ed., Masserman, J.). (Grune and Stratton, New York, 1963.)

Fish, B., and Campbell, M.: Informal ECDEU report from the children's psychopharmacology unit, New York University of Medicine. New York, 1967.

Fleming, J. W., and Orlando, R.: Effect of deanol on attention in the mentally retarded; a reaction time method. J. New Drugs, *2:* 239 (1962).

FØLLING, A.: Über Ausscheidung von Phenylbranztranbensaure in den Harn Alstffwechselanomalie in Verbindung mit Imbezilität. Z. Physiol. Chem., *227:* 196 (1934.)

FRANKS, C. M.: An experimental study of conditioning as related to mental abnormality. (PhD Thesis, University of London, 1954.)

FRANKS, C. M.: The establishment of a conditioning laboratory for the investigation of personality and cortical functioning. Nature (London), *175:* 984 (1955.)

FRANKS, C. M.: Conditioning and personality: a study of normal and neurotic subjects. J. Abnorm. Soc. Psychol., *52:* 143 (1956.)

FRANKS, C. M.: Recidivism, psychopathy and delinquency. Brit. J. Delinquency, *6:* 192 (1956).

FRANKS, C. M.: Conditioning and abnormal behavior. In: Handbook of abnormal psychology (ed., Eysenck, H. J.). (Basic Books, New York, 1961.)

FREED, H., AND FRIGUITO, N.: Tranquillizers in child psychiatry: current status on drugs, particularly phenothiazines. Penn. Psychiat. Quart., *1:* 39 (1961).

FREEDMAN, A. M.: Drug therapy in behavior disorders. (Pediatrics Clinic of North America, Saunders, Baltimore, 1958.)

FREEDMAN, A. M., FINK, M., AND SHAROFF, R.: Cyclazocine and methadone in narcotic addiction. J.A.M.A., *202:* 191 (1967).

FREEDMAN, A. M., AND KAPLAN, H. I. (eds.): Comprehensive textbook of psychiatry. (Williams and Wilkins, Baltimore, 1967.)

FRIEDLAND, P., *et al.:* The use of metronidazole in the treatment of alcoholism: a pilot study. Amer. J. Psychiat., *123:* 722 (1966).

FUNKENSTEIN, D. H., GREENBLATT, M., AND SOLOMON, H. C.: Psychophysiological study of mentally ill patients. I. The status of the peripheral autonomic nervous system as determined by reaction to epinephrine and mecholyl. Amer. J. Psychiat., *106:* 16 (1949).

GALLANT, D. M.: Personal communication. (Montreal, 1967.)

GALLANT, D. M., AND BISHOP, M. P.: The use of imipramine in high dosages: an attempt to elicit antipsychotic activity. Curr. Ther. Res., *9:* 309 (1967).

GAYRAL, R., *et al.:* Etude par les techniques d'expression—notamment picturale—de l'activité thérapeutique de la propériciazine (neuleptil) sur les troubles du comportement chez l'enfant. (Paper presented at the Sixty-second Congress of French-Speaking Neurologists and Psychiatrists, Marseilles, 1964.)

GHOSH, S.: Nialamide in the treatment of mental retardation. Indian J. Child Health, *12:* 347 (1963).

GILLIS, A., AND SALFIELD, D. G.: Treatment of depressive states with dinitrile succinate. J. Ment. Sci., *99:* 542 (1953).

GJESSING, R.: Disturbance of somatic function in catatonic periodic courses and their compensation. J. Ment. Sci., *84:* 608 (1939).

GJESSING, L. R.: Studies of periodic catatonia. II. The urinary excretion of phenolic amines and acids with and without loads of different drugs. J. Psychiat. Res., *2:* 149 (1964).

GRAMBERT, G., *et al.*: Étude clinique du 8909 RP a l'Hopital psychiatrique. (Paper presented at the 61st Congress of French Speaking Psychiatrists and Neurologists, Nancy, 1963.)

GRANT, G. R.: Psychopharmacology in childhood emotional and mental disorders. J. Pediat., *61:* 626 (1962).

GRAUER, H., AND KRAL, V. A.: The use of imipramine (tofranil) in psychiatric patients of a geriatric outpatient clinic. Canad. Med. Ass. J., *83:* 1423 (1960).

GREENBERG, L. A.: The definition of an intoxicating beverage. Quart. J. Stud. Alcohol, *16:* 316 (1955).

GREENBLATT, M., GROSSER, G. H., AND WECHSLER, H.: Drugs in the treatment of depression: controlled studies. In: Psychiatric drugs (ed., Solomon, P.). (Grune and Stratton, New York, 1966.)

GREGORY, I.: Psychiatry—biological and social. (Saunders, Philadephia, 1961.)

GREINER, A. C., NICOLSON, G., AND BAKER, R. A.: Therapy of chlorpromazine melanosis: a preliminary report. Canad. Med. Ass. J., *91:* 636 (1964).

GRÜNTHAL, E., AND REMY, M. (1954): In: Müller, H. F., and Kral, V. A:. The electroencephalogram in advanced senile dementia. J. Amer. Geriat. Soc., *15:* 415 (1967).

GURTLER, J., AND GORALSKY, G.: Experimentation with alimenazine (theralene) in seventy unstable retarded children in an institution. Rev. Neuropsychiat. Infant., *9:* 284 (1961).

GUTH, E., AND HOFFMAN, G. (1966): In: Ayd, F. J.: Int. Drug Ther. Newsletter *2:* 3 (1967).

GUTTMAN, E.: Discussion of benzedrine; uses and abuses. Proc. Roy. Soc. Med., *32:* 388 (1939).

HANLON, T. E., *et al.:* The comparative effectiveness of eight phenothiazines in chronic psychosis. Psychopharmacologia (Berlin), *7:* 89 (1965).

HARE, H. P.: Comparison of diazepam, chlorpromazine and a placebo in psychiatric practice. J. New Drugs, *1:* 233 (1963).

HARTIGAN, G. P.: The use of lithium salts in affective disorders. Brit. J. Psychiat., *109:* 810 (1963).

HAWKE, W. A., AND MCGREAL, D. A.: Tranquillizers. Clin. Pediat. (Phila.) *3:* 192 (1965).

HEATH, R. G., AND KRUPP, I. M.: Schizophrenia as a specific biologic desease. (Presented at the Annual Meeting of the American Psychiatric Association, Detroit, 1967.)

HEATH, R. G., *et al.:* Effect on behavior in humans with the administration of taraxein. Amer J. Psychiat., *114:* 14 (1957).

HESBACHER, P. T., *et al.* (1968): In: Rickels, K.: Antineurotic agents. (Paper presented at the Sixth Annual Meeting of the ACNP, San Juan, 1967.)

HOFF, E. C.: Brain syndromes associated with drug or poison intoxication. In: Comprehensive textbook of psychiatry (eds., Freedman, A. M., and Kaplan, H. I.). (Williams and Wilkins, Baltimore, 1967.)

Hoffer, A., *et al.:* Treatment of schizophrenia with nicotinic acid and nicotinamide. J. Clin. Exp. Psychopath., *18:* 131 (1957).

Hollister, L. E., *et al.:* Treatment of anxious patients with drugs. Dis. Nerv. Syst., *17:* 289 (1956).

Hollister, L. E., *et al.:* Drug therapy of depression. Arch. Gen. Psychiat. (Chicago), *17:* 486 (1967).

Holt, L. E.: Maple sugar urine disease. Penn. Med. J., *60:* 496 (1957).

Hordern, A.: Depressive states. (Charles C Thomas, Springfield, 1965.)

Houze, M., *et al.:* Treatment of mental deficiency with alpha tocopherol. Amer. J. Ment. Defic., *69:* 328 (1964).

Hyden, H. (1955): In: Cameron, D. E., *et al.:* RNA in psychiatric therapy. In: Current psychiatric therapies (ed., Masserman, J.). (Grune and Stratton, New York, 1964.)

Imlah, N. W., Ryan, E., and Harrington, J. A.: The influence of antidepressant drugs on the response to ECT and subsequent relapse rates. (Presented at the Fourth Annual Meeting of the Collegium Internationale Neuropsychopharmacologicum, Birmingham, 1964.)

Isbell, H.: Comparison of the reactions induced by psilocybin and LSD-25 in man. Psychopharmacologia (Berlin), *1:* 29 (1959).

Jacob, A.: On peculiar diseases of the CNS with pathological findings. Z. Ges. Neurol. Psychiat., *64:* 147 (1921).

Jacobs, J.: A controlled trial of deaner and a placebo in mentally defective children. Brit. J. Clin. Pract., *19:* 77 (1965).

Jacobsen, J. E.: The hypomanic alert: a program designed for greater therapeutic control. Amer. J. Psychiat., *122:* 295 (1965).

Jacobsen, J. E., and Marten-Larsen, O.: Treatment of alcoholism with tetraethylthiuram disulfide (antabuse). J.A.M.A., *139:* 918 (1949).

Jarvik, L. F.: LSD and human chromosomes. (Presented at the Annual Meeting of the ACNP, San Juan, 1967.)

Jaspers, K.: Causality and understanding of life and psychosis in dementia praecox. Z. Ges. Neurol. Psychiat., *14:* 158 (1913).

Jaspers, K.: General psychopathology. (Springer, Berlin, 1945.)

Jenner, F. A.: Use of drugs in anxiety states. In: The scientific basis of drug therapy in psychiatry (eds., Marks, J., and Pare, C. M. B.). (Pergamon Press, Oxford, 1965.)

Jenner, F. A., *et al.:* A controlled comparison of methaminodiazepoxide and amylobarbitone in the treatment of anxiety in neurotic patients. J. Ment. Sci., *107:* 583 (1961).

Kalckar, H. M. (1956): In: Cytryn, L., and Lourie, R. S.: Mental retardation. In: Comprehensive textbook of psychiatry (eds., Freedman, A. M., and Kaplan, H. L.). (Williams and Wilkins, Baltimore, 1967.)

Katz, M. M.: A typological approach to the problem of predicting response to treatment. In: Prediction of response to pharmacotherapy (eds., Wittenborn, R., and May, P.). (Charles C Thomas, Springfield, 1965.)

Keeler, M. H.: The use of hallucinogenic, psychotomimetic, psychedelic drugs in North Carolina. N. Carolina Med. J., *24:* 555 (1963).

Kielholz, P.: Diagnose und Therapie der depressionen fur den Praktiker. (Lehmanns Verlag, Munchen, 1965.)

Klerman, G. L., and Cole, J. O.: Clinical pharmacology of imipramine and related antidepressant compounds. Pharmacol. Rev., *17:* 101 (1965).

Kline, N. S.: Recognition and treatment of depression. In: Psychopharmacology (eds., Kline, N. S., and Lehmann, H. E.). (Little, Brown, Boston, 1965.)

Kline, N. S.: Drugs in the treatment of depressions: clinical studies. In: Psychiatric drugs (ed., Solomon, P.). (Grune and Stratton, New York, 1966.)

Kline, N. S., and Lehmann, H. E. (eds.): Psychopharmacology. (Little, Brown, Boston, 1965.)

Kline, N. S., and Sacks, W.: Relief of depression within one day using an MAO inhibitor and intravenous 5-HTP. Amer. J. Psychiat., *120:* 274 (1963).

Kline, N. S., Sacks, W., and Simpson, G. M.: Further studies on: one day treatment of depression with 5-HTP. Amer. J. Psychiat., *121:* 379 (1964).

Knapp, P. H.: Amphetamine and addiction. J. Nerv. Ment. Dis., *115:* 406 (1952).

Korsakoff, S. S.: Über eine Besondere Form Psychischer Störung, Combinirt mit Multipler Neuritis. Arch. Psychiat. Nervenkr., *21:* 669 (1890).

Kraepelin, E.: Psychiatrie ein Lehrbuch für Studierende und Arzte. (Barth, Leipzig, 1913.)

Kral, V. A.: The use of thioridazine in aged people. Canad. Med. Ass. J., *84:* 152 (1961).

Kral, V. A.: Psychotropic drugs in the aged. (Presented at the Q.P.R.A. Symposium on Psychoactive drugs in the aged, Quebec, 1967.)

Kral, V. A., and Papetropoulos, D.: Treatment of geriatric patients. In: Psychopharmacology (eds., Kline, N. S., and Lehmann, H. E.). (Little, Brown, Boston, 1965.)

Kristjansen, P. (1962): In: Gerle, B.: Clinical observations of the side effects of haloperidol. Acta Psychiat. Scand., *40:* 65 (1964).

Kristof, F. E., Lehmann, H. E., and Ban, T. A.: Systematic studies with trimipramine: a new antidepressive drug. Canad. Psychiat. Ass. J., *12:* 517 (1967).

Krupanidhi, I., *et al.:* The use of nialamide in mental retardation in childhood. Indian J. Pediat., *31:* 351 (1964).

Kurland, A. A., *et al.:* The comparative effectiveness of six phenothiazine compounds, phenobarbital and inert placebo in the treatment of acutely ill patients: global measures of severity of illness. J. Nerv. Ment. Dis., *133:* 1 (1961).

Langdon, H., and Down, J. L. H.: Observations

on an ethnic classification of idiots. Clin. Lect. Rep. Lond. Hosp., *3:* 259 (1866).

LANGE, C.: Bidrag til urinsyrediatesens klinik. Hospitalstidende, *5:* 1 (1897).

LASKY, J. J., *et al.:* Drug treatment of schizophrenic patients. Dis. Nerv. Syst., *23:* 698 (1962).

LAVECK, G. D., AND BUCKLEY, P.: The use of psychopharmacologic agents in retarded children with behavior disorders. J. Chronic Dis., *13:* 174 (1961).

LEHMANN, H. E.: Psychoactive drugs and their influence on the dynamics of working capacity. J. Occup. Med., *2:* 523 (1960).

LEHMANN, H. E.: The placebo response and double blind study. In: The evaluation of psychiatric treatment (eds., Hoch, P. H., and Zubin, J.). (Grune and Stratton, New York, 1964.)

LEHMANN, H. E.: Discussion of papers: In: Psychopathology of perception (eds., Hoch, P., and Zubin, J.). (Grune and Stratton, New York, 1965.)

LEHMANN, H. E.: Drug treatment of schizophrenia. In: Psychopharmacology (eds., Kline, N. S., and Lehmann, H. E.). (Little, Brown, Boston, 1965.)

LEHMANN, H. E.: Phenomenology of the depressive illnesses. Canad. Psychiat. Ass. J., *11:* 3 (1965).

LEHMANN, H. E.: Problems of differential diagnosis and choice of therapy in depressive states. Psychosomatics, *6:* 266 (1965).

LEHMANN, H. E.: The pharmacotherapy of the depressive syndrome. Canad. Med. Ass. J., *92:* 821 (1965).

LEHMANN, H. E.: Methodology of clinical studies of psychotropic drugs. (Presented at the W.H.O. Scientific Group on Research in Psychopharmacology, Geneva, 1966.)

LEHMANN, H. E.: Pharmacotherapy of schizophrenia. In: Psychopathology of schizophrenia (eds., Hoch. P., and Zubin. J.). (Grune and Stratton, New York, 1966.)

LEHMANN, H. E.: Experimental psychopathology in depression. (Presented at the symposium on The Depressive Syndrom, Berlin, 1968.)

LEHMANN, H. E., AND BAN, T. A.: Notes from the logbook of a psychopharmacological research unit. I. Canad. Psychiat. Ass. J., *9:* 28 (1964).

LEHMANN, H. E., AND BAN, T. A. (eds.): The butyrophenones in psychiatry. (Québec Psychopharmacological Research Association, Montreal, 1964.)

LEHMANN, H. E., AND BAN, T. A.: Testing new psychoactive drugs. Image, *14:* 13 (1965).

LEHMANN, H. E., AND BAN, T. A.: Early clinical drug evaluation unit Report, Montreal, 1966.

LEHMANN, H. E.: Non-MAO inhibitor antidepressants in clinical perspective. In: Antidepressant drugs of non-MAO inhibitor type (eds., Efron, D. H., and Kety, S. S.). (U.S. Dept. of Health, Education and Welfare, Bethesda, 1966.)

LEHMANN, H. E., AND BAN, T. A.: Chemical reduction of the compulsion to drink with metronidazole: a new treatment modality in the therapeutic program of the alcoholic. Curr. Ther. Res., *9:* 419 (1967).

LEHMANN, H. E., AND BAN, T. A.: Comparative pharmacotherapy of the aging psychotic patient. Laval Med., *38:* 588 (1967).

LEHMANN, H. E., AND BAN, T. A.: Metronidazole in the therapy of alcoholism. In: Current psychiatric therapies, Vol. 7 (ed., Masserman, J.). (Grune and Stratton, New York, 1968.)

LEHMANN, H. E., AND BAN, T. A.: Studies with thioxanthenes. In: The thioxanthenes (eds., Lehmann, H. E., and Ban, T. A.). (Karger, Basel, 1968.)

LEHMANN, H. E., AND BAN, T. A. (eds.): The thioxanthenes. (Karger, Basel, 1968.)

LEHMANN, H. E., AND BAN, T. A.: Studies with new drugs in the treatment of convulsive disorders. Int. J. Clin. Pharmacol., *3:* 231 (1968).

LEHMANN, H. E., AND BAN, T. A. (eds.): Toxicity and adverse reactions with psychoactive drugs. (Q.P.R.A. Montreal, 1968.)

LEHMANN, H. E., AND BAN, T. A.: Clinical use of other antipsychotic agents. In: Principles of psychopharmacology (ed., Clark, W.). (Academic Press, New York, in press.)

LEHMANN, H. E., BAN, T. A., AND DEBOW, S. L.: A clinical pharmacological study with EXP 561. Curr. Ther. Res., *9:* 306 (1967).

LEHMANN, H. E., BAN, T. A., AND KRAL, V. A.: Practice effect in geriatric patients. Geriatrics. *23:* 160 (1968).

LEHMANN, H. E., BAN, T. A., AND LEE, H.: The effectiveness of combined phenothiazine and butyrophenone treatment in chronic schizophrenic patients. Curr. Ther. Res., *9:* 36 (1967).

LEHMANN, H. E., BAN, T. A., AND NALTCHAYAN, E.: Metronidazole in the treatment of the alcoholic. Psychiat. Neurol. (Basel), *152:* 395 (1966).

LEHMANN, H. E., BERTHIAUME, M., AND BAN, T. A. (eds.): Trimipramine, a new anti-depressant. (Q.P.R.A., Montreal, 1964.)

LEHMANN, H. E., CAHN, C. H., AND DEVERTEUIL, R. L.: The treatment of depressive conditions with imipramine (G 22355). Canad. Psychiat. Ass. J., *3:* 155 (1958).

LEHMANN, H. E., AND HANRAHAN, G. E.: Chlorpromazine, a new inhibiting agent for psychomotor excitement and manic states. Amer. Med. Ass. Arch. Neurol. Psychiat., *71:* 227 (1954).

LEMERE, F.: Amphetamine addiction in Japan. J.A.M.A., *185:* 414 (1963).

LEVIN, M.: Toxic psychoses. In: American handbook of psychiatry (ed., Arieti, S.). (Basic Books, New York, 1959.)

LIFSHITZ, K., AND KLINE, N.: Psychopharmacology of the aged. In: Clinical principles and drugs in the aging (ed., Freeman, J. T.). (Charles C Thomas, Springfield, 1963.)

LINDSLEY, D. B., AND HENRY, C. E.: Effect of drugs on behavior and EEG's of children with behavior disorders. Psychosom. Med., *4:* 140 (1942).

LOW, N. L., AND MYERS, G. G.: Suvren in brain-injured children. J. Pediat., *3:* 259 (1958).
LYGHT, C. E., *et al.* (eds.): The Merck manual of diagnosis and therapy. (Merck, Sharp and Dohme Research Laboratories, Rahway, 1966.)
LYON, R. L.: Drug treatment of Huntington's chorea: a trial with thiopropazine. Brit Med. J., *1:* 1308 (1962).
MACKAY, R. I., *et al.:* Monoamine oxidase inhibitors and mental subnormality. J. Ment. Defic. Res., *7:* 107 (1963).
MALITZ, S., *et al.*: A pilot evaluation of deanol in the treatment of anxiety. Curr. Ther. Res., *9:* 261 (1967).
MANN, A., AND LEHMANN, H. E.: The eosinophil level in psychiatric conditions, Canad. Med. Ass. J., *66:* 52 (1952).
MARGETTS, E. L.: Clinical report on use of testosterone in psychiatric syndromes. Canad. Med. Ass. J., *67:* 251 (1952).
MARTIN, W. R.: An experimental study in the treatment of narcotic addicts with cyclazocine. Clin. Pharmacol. Ther., *7:* 455 (1966).
MAYER-GROSS, W., *et al.:* Clinical psychiatry (Cassell, London, 1960.)
MAYR, F., *et al.:* A preliminary report on the results of a clinical investigation with clopenthixol. Wien. Med. Wschr., *122:* 588 (1962).
MCCLURE, D. J.: Presentation at the weekly research conference of the AMI, Montreal, 1967.
MENKES, J. H. (1954): In: Cytryn, L., and Lourie, R. S.: Mental retardation. In: Comprehensive textbook of psychiatry (eds., Freedman, A. M., and Kaplan, H. I.). (Williams and Wilkins, Baltimore, 1967.)
MISES, R., AND BEAUCHESNE, H.: Trial of perphenazine in children and adolescents. Ann. Medico psychol. (Paris), *2:* 89 (1963).
Moyer, J. H., *et al.:* A comparative study of four tranquillizing agents, phenobarbital and inert placebo. Geriatrics, *13:* 153 (1958).
MULDER, D. W., AND DALE, A. J. D.: Brain syndromes associated with infection. In: Comprehensive textbook of psychiatry (eds., Freedman, A. M., and Kaplan, H. I.). (Williams and Wilkins, Baltimore, 1967.)
MÜLLER, C.: Die Implantaschen von Reinsubstänz Östrogen Hormons bei der Frau. Schweiz. Med. Wschr., *83:* 1127 (1953).
MÜLLER, H. F.: Drugs—EEG and the aged. (Presented at the Q.P.R.A. Symposium on Psychoactive drugs in the aged, Quebec, 1967.)
MÜLLER, H. F., AND KRAL, V. A.: The electroencephalogram in advanced senile dementia. J. Amer. Geriat. Soc., *15:* 415 (1967).
MUNDY, L. R., AND ZELLER, W. W.: Acute toxic psychosis due to scopolamine. Dis. Nerv. Syst., *19:* 423 (1958).
NIMH-PSC: Collaborative study group: phenothiazine treatment in acute schizophrenics. Arch. Gen. Psychiat. (Chicago), *10:* 246 (1964).
NOYES, A. P., AND KOLB, L. C.: Modern clinical psychiatry. (Saunders, Philadelphia, 1961.)
NYIRÖ, G.: The structural aspects of mental processes on the basis of reflex mechanisms. In: Psychological studies (ed., Gegessi Kiss, P., *et al.*). (Akademia, Budapest, 1958.)
NYIRÖ, G.: Psychiatria. (Akademia, Budapest, 1962.)
OBRIST, W. D., AND BUSSE, E. W.: The EEG in old age. In: Applications of EEG to psychiatry (ed., Wilson, W. P.). (Duke University Press, Durham, 1965.)
OVERALL, J. E., *et al.:* Benzquinamide in newly admitted schizophrenics: a search for patients best treated with a specific drug. Curr. Ther. Res., *5:* 335 (1963).
OVERALL, J. E., *et al.:* Imipramine and thioridazine in depressed and schizophrenic patients. J.A.M.A., *189:* 605 (1964).
PARE, C. M. B., *et al.:* Differentiation of two genetically specific types of depression by response to antidepressants. Lancet, *2:* 1340 (1962).
PASMANICK, B.: Anticonvulsant drug therapy of behavior problem children with abnormal EEG's Arch. Neurol. Psychiat., *65:* 752 (1951).
PEARSON, M. M.: Strecker's fundamental's of psychiatry. (Lippincott, Montreal, 1963.)
PICK, A.: Über die Beziehungen der Senilen Hirnatrophie zur Aphasie. Prag. Med. Wschr., *17:* 165 (1892).
PILKINGTON, T. L.: Comparative effects of librium and taractan on behavior disorders of mentally retarded children. Dis. Nerv. Syst., *22:* 573 (1961).
PILKINGTON, T.: A report on tofranil in mental deficiency. Amer. J. Ment. Defic., *66:* 733 (1962).
PIUCK, C. L.: Clinical impressions of hydroxyzine and other tranquillizers in a child guidance clinic. Dis. Nerv. Syst., *24:* 483 (1963).
POPOV, E. A.: The significance of the inhibitory phenomena in the clinic of psychiatric diseases. Zh. Vyssh. Nerv. Deiat Pavlov., *5:* 329 (1955).
QUAY, H. C.: Psychopathic personality as pathological stimulating seeking. Amer. J. Psychiat., *122:* 179 (1965).
RAYMOND, M. J., *et al.:* Trial of five tranquillizing drugs in psychoneurosis. Brit. Med. J., *2:* 63 (1957).
REDLICH, F. C., AND FREEDMAN, D. X.: The theory and practice of psychiatry. (Basic Books, New York, 1966.)
REES, W. L.: Endocrine and metabolic studies of post partum and premenstrual psychiatric disorders and reference to treatment by different methods. In: Biological treatment of mental illness (ed., Rinkel, M.). (Ambassador Books, Toronto, 1966.)
RETBOLL, K. (1963): In: Usdin, E., and Efron, D. H.: Psychotropic drugs and related compounds. (PHSP No. 1589, Washington, 1967.)
RETT, A., *et al.* (1965): In: Usdin, E., and Efron, D. H. Psychotropic drugs and related compounds. (PHSP No. 1589, Washington, 1967.)
RICKELS, K.: Antineurotic agents—specific and non-specific effects. (Paper presented at the Sixth Annual Meeting of the ACNP, San Juan, 1967.)

RICKELS, K., *et al.:* Evaluation of tranquillizing drugs in medical outpatients (meprobamate, prochlorperazine, amobarbital sodium, and placebo). J.A.M.A., *171:* 1649 (1959).

RICKELS, K., *et al:* Controlled psychopharmacological research in general practice. J. New Drugs, *4:* 138 (1964).

RICKELS, K., *et al.:* Different populations, different drug responses. Amer. J. Med. Sci., *247:* 328 (1964).

RICKELS, K., *et al.:* A psychopharmacological evaluation of chlordiazepoxide, LA-1 and placebo carried out with anxious neurotic medical clinic patients. Med. Times, *93:* 238 (1965).

RICKELS, K., *et al.:* Personality differences between somatically and psychologically oriented neurotic patients. J. Nerv. Ment. Dis., *142:* 10 (1966).

RICKELS, K., *et al.:* Drug treatment in depression: antidepressant or tranquillizer. J.A.M.A., *201:* 675 (1967).

RICKELS, K., *et al.:* Side reactions on meprobamate and placebo. Dis. Nerv. Syst., *28:* 39 (1967).

RINALDI, F., AND HIMWICH, H. E.: Alerting responses and actions of atropine and cholinergic drugs. Amer. Med. Ass. Arch. Neurol Psychiat., *73:* 387 (1955).

ROBERTS, J. M.: Prognostic factors in the electroshock treatment of depressive states. II. The application of specific tests. J. Ment. Sci., *105:* 703 (1959).

ROSATI, D.: Systematic treatment of psychosis: a seminar on experience with ataractic medicine. Amer. J. Psychiat., *121:* 902 (1965).

ROSSUM, J. M. VAN.: Different types of sympathomimetic-receptors. J. Pharm. Pharmacol., *17:* 202 (1965).

ROTH, M.: The natural history of mental disorders in old age. J. Ment. Sci., *101:* 281 (1955).

ROUX, G., *et al.:* The use of haloanisone in non-epileptic retarded children. Ann. Medico psychol. (Paris), *121:* 84 (1963).

ROY, P. B., *et al.:* La propericiazine dans le controle du comportement antisocial. Uni. Med. Canada, *95:* 1441 (1966).

RUDOLF, G. DEM.: Treatment of depression with desoxyephedrine (methedrine). J. Ment. Sci., *95:* 920 (1949).

SARGANT, W., AND SLATER, E.: Acute war neuroses. Lancet, *2:* 1 (1940).

SARGANT, W., AND SLATER, E.: Physical methods of treatment in psychiatry. Brit. Med. J., *1:* 1315 (1951).

SARGANT, W., AND SLATER, E.: An introduction to physical methods of treatment in psychiatry. (Livingstone, London, 1963.)

SCHACHTER, S., AND LATANE, B.: Crime, cognition and the autonomic nervous system. (Presented at a Collegium at McGill University, Montreal, 1963.)

SCHIELE, B. C., *et al.:* A comparison of thioridazine, trifluoperazine, chlorpromazine and placebo. J. Clin. Exp. Psychopath., *22:* 151 (1961).

SCHIELE, B. C.: Studies with clopenthixol and thiothixene. (Presented at the Q.P.R.A. Symposium on The Thioxanthenes, Montreal, 1967.)

SCHILDKRAUT, J. J.: The catecholamine hypothesis of affective disorders: a review of supportive evidence. Amer. J. Psychiat., *122:* 509 (1965).

SCHILDKRAUT, J. J.: Norepinephrine metabolism in depressed patients treated with imipramine. In: Antidepressant drugs (eds., Garattini, S., and Dukes, M. N. G.). (Excerpta Medica Foundation, Amsterdam, 1967.)

SCHOU, M.: Lithium terapi ved mani praktiske retningslinier. Nord. Med., *55:* 790 (1956).

SCHOU, M.: Biology and pharmacology of the lithium ion. Pharmacol. Rev., *9:* 17 (1957).

SCHOU, M.: Normothymics, "mood normalizers." Brit. J. Psychiat., *109:* 803 (1963).

SCHOU, M.: The metabolism and biochemistry of lithium. In: Antidepressant drugs (eds., Garattini, S., and Dukes, M. N. G.). (Excerpta Medica Foundation, Amsterdam, 1967.)

SCHOU, M., *et al.:* Treatment of manic psychoses by administration of lithium salts. J. Neurol. Neurosurg. Psychiat., *17:* 250 (1954).

SEMER, J. M., *et al.:* The use of metronidazole in the treatment of alcoholism, a pilot study. Amer. J. Psychiat., *123:* 722 (1966).

SHAGASS, C.: Neurophysiological studies of anxiety and depression. Psychiat. Res. Rep. Amer. Psychiat. Ass., *8:* 100 (1958).

SHAW, D. M., AND COPPEN, A.: Potassium and water distribution in depression. Brit. J. Psychiat., *112:* 269 (1966).

SILVER, A. A.: Management of children with schizophrenia. Amer. J. Psychother., *9:* 196 (1955).

SILVER, D., *et al.:* The comparative effectiveness of psychoactive drugs in hospitalized geriatric patients. (Presented at the Q.P.R.A. Symposium on Psychoactive drugs in the aged, Quebec, 1967.)

SIM, M.: Guide to psychiatry. (Livingstone, London, 1963.)

SIMON, W., *et al.:* A controlled study of the short term differential treatment of schizophrenia. Amer. J. Psychiat., *114:* 1077 (1958).

SMART, R. G., AND BATEMAN, K.: Unfavourable reactions to LSD: a review and analysis of the available case reports. Canad. Med. Ass. J., *97:* 1214 (1967).

SMITH, J. J.: The endocrine basis of hormonal therapy of alcoholism. New York J. Med., *50:* 1704 (1950).

SOLMS, H.: On the problem of the mechanism of action of medical methods of therapy in chronic alcoholism: the psychodynamic aspect. Bull. Schweiz. Akad. Med. Wiss., *16:* 88 (1960).

ST. JEAN, A.: General Summary. In: Toxicity and adverse reactions with psychoactive drugs (eds., Lehmann, H. E., and Ban, T. A.). (Q.P.R.A., Montreal, 1968.)

STEINBERG, D. L.: Hematoporphyrin treatment of severe depressions. Amer. J. Psychiat., *92:* 901 (1936).

STERN, K.: Severe dementia associated with bilateral degeneration of thalami. Brain, *62:* 167 (1939).

STRINGARIS, M. G.: Clinical observations in psychoses due to hashish. Arch. Psychiat. Nervenkr., *100:* 522 (1933).

STRINGARIS, M. G. (1939): In: Mayer-Gross, W., *et al.:* Clinical psychiatry. (Cassell, London, 1960.)

STRÖMGREN, E., AND SHOU, M.: Lithium treatment of manic states. Postgrad. Med., *35:* 83 (1964).

STRÖMGREN, L. S., AND STRÖMGREN, E. (1962): In: Schou, M.: Normothymics "mood normalizers." Brit. J. Psychiat., *109:* 803 (1963).

STRÖMGREN, L. S., AND STRÖMGREN, E. (1963): In: Häfliger, F., and Burckhardt, V.: Iminodibenzyl and related compounds. In: Psychopharmacological agents (ed., Gordon, M.). (Academic Press, New York, 1964.)

SURWILLO, W. W.: The relation of decision time to brain wave frequency and old age. Electroenceph. Clin. Neurophysiol., *16:* 510 (1964).

SYLVESTRE, P. E.: Brain weight and mental deficiency. J. Ment. Defic. Res., *5:* 98 (1961).

TASAKI, I., *et al.:* Effects of internal and external ionic environment on excitability of squid giant axon. A macromolecular approach. J. Gen. Physiol., *48:* 1095 (1965).

TAYLOR, J. A.: Metronidazole—a new agent for combined somatic and psychic therapy of alcoholism. Bull. Los Angeles Neurol. Soc., *29:* 158 (1964).

TAYLOR, J. A.: Address to the American Medical Association Convention, New York, 1965.

THOMPSON, L. G., AND PROCTOR, R. C.: Depressive and anxiety reactions treated with nicotinic acid and phenobarbital. N. Carolina Med. J., *14:* 420 (1953).

TURNER, R. A.: Screening methods in pharmacology. (Academic Press, New York, 1965.)

TURNER, W.: Personal communication. (San Juan, 1967.)

UHLENHUTH, E. H., *et al.:* The symptomatic relief of anxiety with meprobamate, phenobarbital and placebo. Amer. J. Psychiat., *115:* 905 (1959).

UNNA, K.: Antagonistic effect of N'allylnormorphine upon morphine. J. Pharmacol., *79:* 27 (1943).

VARGA, E.: Changes in the symptomatology of psychotic patterns. (Academia, Budapest, 1966.)

WAGGONER, R. W.: Brain syndromes associated with diseases of unknown cause. In: Textbook of comprehensive psychiatry (eds., Freedman, A. M., and Kaplan, H. I.). (Williams and Wilkins, Baltimore, 1967.)

WAITES, L., AND KEELE, D. K.: Fluphenazine in management of disturbed mentally retarded children. Dis. Nerv. Syst., *24:* 113 (1963).

WALKER, C. F., AND KIRKPATRICK, B. B.: Dilantin treatment of behavior problem children with abnormal EEG's. Amer. J. Psychiat., *103:* 484 (1947).

WALTHER-BÜEL, H. (1951): In: Mayer-Gross, W., *et al.:* Clinical psychiatry. (Cassell, London, 1960.)

WASHBURNE, A. C.: Nicotinic acid in depressed states; preliminary report. Ann. Intern. Med., *32:* 261 (1950).

WECHSLER, H., GROSSER, G. H., AND BUSFIELD, B. L.: The depression rating scale. Arch. Gen. Psychiat. (Chicago), *9:* 334 (1963).

WERNICKE, C.: Lehrbuch der Gehirnkrankheiten. (Fischer and Kassel, Berlin, 1882.)

WERRY, J. S.: The use of psychoactive drugs in children. Illionois Med. J., *131:* 6 (1967).

WHEATLEY, D.: Effects of doctors and patients attitude and other factors on response to drugs. In: Nonspecific factors in drug therapy (ed., Rickels, K.). (Charles C Thomas, Springfield, 1968.)

WHO Expert Committee: On addiction producing drugs. WHO Techn. Rep. Ser., *116:* 9 (1964).

WIKLER, A.: A critical analysis of some current concepts in psychiatry. J. Psychosom. Med., *14:* 10 (1952).

WIKLER, A.: Mechanisms of actions of drugs that modify personality function. Amer. J. Psychiat., *108:* 590 (1952).

WIKLER, A.: Mechanisms of action of opiates and opiate antagonists: a review of their mechanisms of action in relation to clinical problem. (Public Health Monograph 52, U. S. Dept. Health, Education and Welfare, Public Health Service, Washington, 1958.)

WIKLER, A.: Conditioning factors in opiate addiction and relapse. In: Narcotics (eds., Wilner, D. M., and Kassebaum, G. G.). (McGraw-Hill, New York, 1965.)

WIKLER, A.: Addictions. I. Opioid addiction. In: Comprehensive textbook of psychiatry (eds., Freedman, A. M., and Kaplan, H. I.). (Williams and Wilkins, Baltimore, 1967.)

WIKLER, A., AND PESCOR, F. T.: Classical conditioning of a morphine abstinence phenomenon, reinforcement of opisid-drinking behavior and "relapse" in morphine-addicted rats. Psychopharmacologia (Berlin), *10:* 255 (1967).

WIKLER, A., *et al.:* Electroencephalographic changes associated with chronic alcoholic abstinence syndrome. Amer. J. Psychiat., *113:* 106 (1956).

WIKLER, A., *et al.:* Effects of frontal lobotomy on the morphine abstinence syndrome in man: an experimental study. Amer. Med. Ass. Arch. Neurol. Psychiat., *67:* 510 (1952).

WIKLER, A., *et al.:* Electroencephalograms during cycles of addiction to barbiturates in man. Electroenceph. Clin. Neurophysiol., *7:* 1 (1955).

WOOLF, L. I., *et al.:* Treatment of phenylketonuria with a diet low in phenylalanine. Brit. Med. J., *1:* 57 (1955).

WOOLLEY, D. W.: The biochemical bases of psychoses. (Wiley, New York, London, 1962.)

ZAPLETALEK, M., AND KOMENDA, S.: The effect of thioridazine on activity of serum catalase in oligophrenic and gerontopsychiatric patients. Acta Nerv. Sup., *6:* 227 (1964).

Closing Remarks

By 1920 the foundations of modern clinical psychiatry had been established. On the basis of descriptive classification, psychopathological assessment and psychodynamic analysis a new language—the language of psychiatry—was born. Research in subsequent years was deeply rooted in this classical framework. Contributions were mainly restricted to the exploration of the psychophysical and psychophysiological correlates or the neurophysiological and biochemical basis of the various psychiatric syndromes. This has been rewarding only up to a certain point.

With the advent of psychopharmacology came chemicals with definite therapeutic effects on psychopathological manifestations. Many psychoactive drugs with distinctly different pharmacodynamic properties were synthesized. These new drugs, with well defined behavioral, neurophysiological and biochemical actions, have provided a new means for therapeutically influencing and systematically studying psychopathological conditions.

The findings which have accumulated during the new psychopharmacological era strongly suggest that the classical nosological groups are only in part homogeneous entities. What is becoming obvious is the heterogeneity within these various groups. The recognition of this heterogeneity will inevitably lead to newer concepts, a new language and perhaps a "new" psychiatry.

APPENDIX

Appendix One

Vademecum Psychopharmacologicum

Reference books extensively used in the compilation of the data are Cohen *et al.*'s *Psychochemotherapy* (Western Medical Publications, 1967); Kalinowsky and Hoch's *Somatic Treatments in Psychiatry* (Grune and Stratton, 1961); Marler's *Pharmacological and Chemical Synonyms* (Excerpta Medica Foundation, 1967); Paterson's *Electrical and Drug Treatment in Psychiatry* (Elsevier, 1963); Usdin and Efron's *Psychotropic Drugs and Related Compounds* (United States Public Health Service, 1967); *New Drugs* (American Medical Association, 1967); and *Vademecum International of Canada* (Morgan Jones, 1968).

A. ANTIPSYCHOTIC DRUGS

1. Phenothiazines and Related Compounds

a. Acepromazine

i. Chemical Name. 2-Acetyl-10-(3-dimethylaminopropyl)phenothiazine.

ii. Therapeutic Uses. A weak antipsychotic but effective in the control of overactivity (Ferguson, 1958; Tolan *et al.*, 1959; and Urquhart and Forrest 1959). Simpson (1958) found it of no value in chronic schizophrenics. In combination, with other phenothiazines and barbiturates, it has been successfully used in sleep treatment (Suttel, 1961).

iii. Adverse Effects Reported. Psychiatric (drowsiness, lethargy, excitement, confusional state); neurological (extrapyramidal signs); and local tissue reaction with intramuscular administration.

b. Acetophenazine

i. Chemical Name. 2-Acetyl-10{3-[4-(2-hydroxyethyl)piperazin-1-yl]propyl} phenothiazine.

ii. Therapeutic Uses. Favorable therapeutic effects were seen in chronic schizophrenics (Witton, 1960) and in the treatment of the paranoid symptomatology of geriatric patients (Sheppard *et al.*, 1964). Although it is of limited usefullness in patients whose anxiety is associated with psychosomatic conditions, acetophenazine is a valuable preparation for severe psychoneurotics in whom agitation, anxiety and tension prevail and in the management of patients with chronic brain syndrome (Cook, 1965).

iii. Adverse Effects Reported. Psychiatric (drowsiness, lethargy, weakness, fatigue, motor retardation); neurological (extrapyramidal signs, vertigo); autonomic (blurred vision, pallor, dryness of mouth); cardiovascular (tachycardia, hypotension and paradoxical hypertension); genitourinary (incontinence); allergic (skin reactions, pruritus); hematological (leukopenia); hepatobiliary (transient changes in liver function); and others (*e.g.*, peripheral edema). It potentiates the effect of antihypertensive agents, general anesthetics, hypnotics, alcohol and CNS depressants.

c. Butaperazine

i. Chemical Name. 2-Butyryl-10-[3-(4-methyl-piperazin-1-yl)propyl]phenothiazine.

ii. Therapeutic Uses. Favorable therapeutic effects have been reported in acute schizophrenics and in manics (Moldenhauer, 1961; and Gerz, 1964). In chronic schizophrenics, however, butaperazine is slightly inferior therapeutically to perphenazine or haloperidol (Sharply *et al.*, 1964; and Warnes *et al.*, 1966).

iii. Adverse Effects Reported. Neurological (extrapyramidal signs); autonomic (dry mouth); cardiovascular (hypotension); and hepatobiliary (transient changes in liver function).

d. Carphenazine

i. Chemical Name. 10-{3-[4-(2-Hydroxyethyl) piperazin-1-yl]propyl}-2-propionyl-phenothiazine.

ii. Therapeutic Uses. Favorable therapeutic effects have been reported in acute and chronic schizophrenics (Solomon, 1963; LaSalle, 1964; and Bronsky, 1965). It is comparable in therapeutic effectiveness to chlorpromazine and trifluoperazine in chronic patients (Platz *et al.*, 1966). Carphenazine has a relatively short duration of action.

iii. Adverse Effects Reported. Psychiatric (agitation); neurological (extrapyramidal signs, weakness, dizziness); cardiovascular (hypotension); gastrointestinal (nausea, vomiting); dermatological (rash); allergic (edema and/or puffiness of the eyes); and hepatobiliary (liver dysfunction as indicated by the cephalin flocculation test). It potentiates the effect of antihypertensive agents, general anesthetics, hypnotics, alcohol and CNS depressants.

e. Chlorpromazine

i. Chemical Name. 2-Chloro-10-(3-dimethylaminopropyl)phenothiazine hydrochloride.

ii. Therapeutic Uses. The first antipsychotic drug; it is still one of the most extensively and successfully used phenothiazines in the treatment of acute and chronic schizophrenic patients (Hamon *et al.*, 1952; Delay and Deniker, 1952; and Lehmann and Hanrahan, 1954).

iii. Adverse Effects Reported. Similar to those of other phenothiazines.

f. Chlorprothixene

i. Chemical Name. 2-Chloro-9-(3-dimethylaminopropylidene)thioxanthene.

ii. Therapeutic Uses. An antipsychotic particularly useful for schizophrenics with dysthymic mood changes. It is also used in the treatment of paranoid schizophrenia and severe psychoneuroses (Lehmann and Ban, 1968; Nielsen *et al.*, 1959; Ravn, 1960, 1961; and Remvig and Sonne 1961).

iii. Adverse Effects Reported. Psychiatric (drowsiness, insomnia); neurological (dizziness, convulsions); autonomic (dryness of mouth, nasal congestion); cardiovascular (tachycardia, orthostatic hypotension); gastrointestinal (constipation); genitourinary (anuria); and hematological (granulocytopenia). It produces more drowsiness but less extrapyramidal signs than chlorpromazine.

g. Clopenthixol

i. Chemical Name. 4-[3-(2-Chlorothioxanthen-9-ylidene)propyl]-1-piperazineethanol.

ii. Therapeutic Uses. An antipsychotic with possible usefulness in chronic schizophrenics, especially the hebephrenic type (Anton, 1962; Arnold and Deisenhammer, 1962; Ban *et al.*, 1963; Bartollucci *et al.*, 1966; Lehmann and Ban, 1968; Marx, 1961; Petersen and Nielsen, 1961; Ravn, 1962).

iii. Adverse Effects Reported. Psychiatric (drowsiness); neurological (extrapyramidal signs); autonomic (dry mouth); and cardiovascular (paroxysmal tachycardia).

h. Clothiapine

i. Chemical Name. 2-Chloro-11-(4-methyl-1-piperazinyl)dibenzo[b,f][1,4] thiazepine.

ii. Therapeutic Uses. A major tranquilizer with possible usefulness in the schizophrenias (Gross and Langner, 1966). The place of this substance in psychopharmacotherapy has not yet been established.

iii. Adverse Effects Reported. Needs further assessment.

i. Fluphenazine

i. Chemical Name. 4-[(3,2-Trifluoromethyl)phenothiazine-10-yl]-propyl-1-piperazineethanol.

ii. Therapeutic Uses. A potent antipsychotic drug particularly useful in the schizophrenias. Available also in long acting preparations, *e.g.*, fluphenazine enanthate and decanoate, which are effective over a 14- or 21-day period, respectively (Fouks *et al.*, 1961; Kinross-Wright *et al.*, 1963; Kline and Simpson, 1964; Barsa and Saunders, 1965; Simpson *et al.*, 1965; Bartholomew and Holt, 1966; Denzel, 1966; and Mariatequi, 1966).

iii. Adverse Effects Reported. Similar to those of other phenothiazines.

j. Mesoridazine

i. Chemical Name. 10-[2-(1-Methyl-2-piperidyl)ethyl]-2-methylsulfinyl phenothiazine.

ii. Therapeutic Uses. The sulfoxy derivative of thioridazine—available also for parenteral administration—with a possible usefulness in the schizophrenias (Prusmack *et al.*, 1966; Goldstein and Dippy, 1967; and Ast *et al.*, 1968). The place of this substance in psychopharmacotherapy has not yet been established.

iii. Adverse Effects Reported. Similar to those of thioridazine.

k. Methophenazine

i. Chemical Name. 2-{4-[3-(2-Chlorphenothiazin-10-yl)propyl]piperazin-1-yl}-ethyl-3,4,5-trimethoxybenzoate.

ii. Therapeutic Uses. An antipsychotic with possible usefulness in the treatment of paranoid schizophrenics (Ruck and Schwartz, 1965; and Cagara and Wozniak, 1966). The place of this substance in psychopharmacotherapy has not yet been established.

iii. Adverse Effects Reported. Needs further assessment.

l. Methotrimeprazine

i. Chemical Name. 10[3-(Dimethylamino)-2-methylpropyl]-2-methoxyphenothiazine.

ii. Therapeutic Uses. An antipsychotic which has been successfully used in the treatment of the schizophrenias, agitated depressions and in obsessive-compulsive neuroses (Baker and Thorpe, 1958; Ban and Schwarz, 1963; Baruk *et al.*, 1958; and Sigwald *et al.*, 1956).

iii. Adverse Effects Reported. It produces somewhat more drowsiness but less extrapyramidal signs than chlorpromazine.

m. Methoxypromazine

i. Chemical Name. 10-[3-(Dimethylamino)propyl]-2-methoxyphenothiazine.

ii. Therapeutic Uses. A weak and rather ineffective antipsychotic (Delay *et al.*, 1956; Azima *et al.*, 1958; Gosline *et al.*, 1959; and Kalinowsky and Hoch, 1961).

iii. Adverse Effects Reported. Lower incidence of side-effects than with the other antipsychotic phenothiazines.

n. Perazine

i. Chemical Name. 10-[3-(4-Methyl-1-piperazinyl)propyl]phenothiazine.

ii. Therapeutic Uses. An antipsychotic with a possible usefulness in the maintenance treatment of schizophrenics (Enss and Hippius, 1964; Hippius, 1965; and Laskowska *et al.*, 1966). The place of this substance has not yet been established.

iii. Adverse Effects Reported. Similar to those of other phenothiazines.

o. Perphenazine

i. Chemical Name. 2-Chloro-10-{3-[4-(2-hydroxyethyl)piperazinyl propyl}phenothiazine.

ii. Therapeutic Uses. One of the most

extensively used phenothiazine preparations. It is particularly effective for chronic schizophrenics and in combination with amitriptyline for agitated depressives (Ayd, 1957; Cahn and Lehmann, 1957; O'Reilly *et al.*, 1957; Cohen and Freireich, 1958).

iii. Adverse Effects Reported. Less drowsiness but more extrapyramidal signs than with chlorpromazine.

p. Prochlorperazine

i. Chemical Name. 2-Chloro-10-[3-(4-methyl-1-piperazinyl)propyl]phenothiazine.

ii. Therapeutic Uses. An antipsychotic and antiemetic drug particularly useful in the treatment of chronic simple and hebephrenic schizophrenics (Brousolle *et al.*, 1957; Goldman, 1962; Denber, 1958; Kline *et al.*, 1958; and Milne and Berliner, 1958).

iii. Adverse Effects Reported. Less drowsiness but more extrapyramidal signs than with chlorpromazine.

q. Promazine

i. Chemical Name. 10-[3-(Dimethylamino)propyl]phenothiazine.

ii. Therapeutic Uses. It is particularly useful in the treatment of delirium tremens and in the control of withdrawal symptoms of heroin addicts (Fazekas *et al.*, 1956; Lesse, 1957; Fink and Vlavianos, 1958; Fleming *et al.*, 1959; Gilmore and Shatin, 1959).

iii. Adverse Effects Reported. A lower incidence of hypotensive reactions but a higher incidence of cerebral seizures than with chlorpromazine. Parenteral administration causes less tissue reaction.

r. Propericiazine

i. Chemical Name. 2-Cyano-3-[(4-hydroxy-1-piperidino)-3-propyl]-10-phenothiazine.

ii. Therapeutic Uses. A neuroleptic with particular usefulness in the control of aggressive manifestations (Chanoit *et al.*, 1962; Deshaies, 1962; Berthier *et al.*, 1963; Doussot *et al.*, 1963; Gayral *et al.*, 1964; Gallant *et al.*, 1964; Ban, 1965; Jenner, 1965; and St. Jean *et al.*, 1967).

iii. Adverse Effects Reported. Similar to those of other phenothiazines.

s. Prothipendyl

i. Chemical Name. 10-(3-Dimethylaminopropyl)-1-azaphenothiazine.

ii. Therapeutic Uses. An antipsychotic (with sedative and hypnotic properties) (Koranyi *et al.*, 1958; Schlichtegroll, 1958; Sugerman and Herrmann, 1966) with possible usefulness in the maintenance treatment of schizophrenics (Rondepierre and Ropert, 1961). The place of this substance in psychopharmacotherapy has not yet been established.

iii. Adverse Effects Reported. Needs further assessment.

t. Thiopropazate

i. Chemical Name. 4-[3-(2-Chlorphenothiazin-10-yl)propyl]-1-piperazinethyl.

ii. Therapeutic Uses. One of the fastest acting antipsychotic phenothiazine preparations, particularly useful in paranoid schizophrenic cases (Edisen and Samuels, 1958; and Hollister *et al.*, 1962).

iii. Adverse Effects Reported. Similar to those of other phenothiazines.

u. Thioproperazine

i. Chemical Name. *N,N*-dimethyl-10-[3-(4-methyl-1-piperazinyl)propyl]phenothiazine-2-sulfonamide.

ii. Therapeutic Uses. An antipsychotic particularly useful in the treatment of chronic schizophrenic and manic cases (Ban *et al.*, 1962; Delay *et al.*, 1958; Denber *et al.*, 1959; and Deshaies *et al.*, 1959).

iii. Adverse Effects Reported. Similar to those of other phenothiazines. Relatively high incidence of extrapyramidal signs.

v. Thioridazine

i. Chemical Name. 2-Methylmercapto-10-[2-(*N*-methyl-2-piperidyl)ethyl] phenothiazine.

ii. Therapeutic Uses. An extensively used antipsychotic with particular usefulness in the behavioral problems of children and geriatric patients.

iii. Adverse Effects Reported. Similar to those of other phenothiazines. In high doses, pigmentary retinopathy and electrocardiographic changes have been reported (Ban and St. Jean, 1964; Ban *et al.*,

1965; Barsa and Saunders, 1960; Delay *et al.*, 1959; and Lehmann and Ban, 1968).

w. Thiothixene

i. Chemical Name. *N,N*-Dimethyl-9[3-(4-methyl-piperazinyl)propylidene]thioxanthene-2-sulfonamide.

ii. Therapeutic Uses. An antipsychotic with particular usefulness in the treatment of schizophrenics (Lehmann and Ban, 1968; Oliveros *et al.*, 1967; and Schiele, 1968).

iii. Adverse Effects Reported. Similar to those of thioproperazine but with less severe extrapyramidal manifestations.

x. Trifluoperazine

i. Chemical Name. 10-[3-(4-Methyl-1-piperazinyl)propyl]-2-(trifluoromethyl)phenothiazine.

ii. Therapeutic Uses. An antipsychotic with particular usefulness in the treatment of apathetic chronic schizophrenics. In combination with tranylcypromine, it has been successfully used in the treatment of neurotic depression (Barsa *et al.*, 1959; Gunn, 1958; Kruse, 1959, 1960; and Tolan and Peppel, 1959).

iii. Adverse Effects Reported. Similar to those of other phenothiazines.

y. Triflupromazine

i. Chemical Name. 10-3-(Dimethylamino) propyl-2-(trifluromethyl) phenothiazine.

ii. Therapeutic Uses. An antipsychotic with particular usefulness in the treatment of disturbed schizophrenics (Ayd, 1958; Hegarty and Dabbs, 1959; Ilem and Sainz, 1959; Roebuck *et al.*, 1959; and Walsh *et al.*, 1959).

iii. Adverse Effects Reported. Similar to those of other phenothiazines.

2. Indoles

a. Deserpidine

i. Chemical Name. 11-Desmethoxyreserpine.

ii. Therapeutic Uses. A less potent but faster acting substance than reserpine. Useful in controlling agitation in geriatrics, particularly in cerebral arteriosclerotic cases (Ferguson, 1956; and Cuny *et al.*, 1961).

iii. Adverse Effects Reported. Similar to those of reserpine but a lower incidence.

b. Fenoharman

i. Chemical Name. 1-Benzyl-1,2,3,4-tetrahydronorharman.

ii. Therapeutic Uses. A relatively new preparation synthesized with the purpose of increasing the psychotherapeutic actions of reserpine and to eliminate its autonomic side-effects (Trcka *et al.*, 1961; and Dlabac and Trcka, 1961). This effort remained only partially successful. The place of this substance in psychopharmacotherapy has not yet been established.

iii. Adverse Effects Reported. Needs further assessment.

c. Mepireserpate

i. Chemical Name. Methyl-methyl-18-epireserpate.

ii. Therapeutic Uses. A neuroleptic with possible usefulness in manic exaltation and confusional states (DeMaio, 1964). The place of this substance in psychopharmacotherapy has not yet been established.

iii. Adverse Effects Reported. Needs further assessment.

d. Oxypertine

i. Chemical Name. 5,6-Dimethoxy-2-methyl-3-[2-(4-phenylpiperazine-1-yl)]ethyl indole.

ii. Therapeutic Uses. An antipsychotic which depletes catecholamine stores without affecting serotonin levels (McAuliff *et al.*, 1963). It lifts mood without improving physical performance (Adamson and Finlay, 1965). It is ineffective in the psychoneuroses, but therapeutic in the schizophrenias (Hollister *et al.*, 1963; Kinross-Wright *et al.*, 1963; and Calwell *et al.*, 1964).

iii. Adverse Effects Reported. Needs further assessment.

e. Rescinnamine

i. Chemical Name. 3,4,5-Trimethoxycinnamoylmethylreserpate.

ii. Therapeutic Uses. A psychotropic with particular usefulness in the psychoneuroses (Benson and Schiele, 1962; and Cohen *et al.*, 1967). It is ineffective in the schizophrenias (Malamud *et al.*, 1957).

iii. Adverse Effects Reported. Similar to those of reserpine but with a lower incidence of depression and bradycardia.

f. Reserpine

i. Chemical Name. Methyl-18-*o*-(3,4,5-trimethoxybenzoyl)reserpate.

ii. Therapeutic Uses. A psychotropic with a wide range of actions. Once extensively used in the treatment of functional psychoses (especially in the schizophrenias and mania), psychoneuroses (anxiety and tension states) and also in disturbed general paretics, mental deficients, and alcoholics (Avol and Vogel, 1955; Barett and Hansel, 1955; Drake and Ebaugh, 1955; Ferguson, 1955; Friedman, 1955; Sommerness *et al.*, 1955; Talbot, 1955; Davis and Severinghaus, 1956; Greenfield, 1956; Pearl *et al.*, 1956; Anderson and Kemp, 1957; Jensen, 1957; Kirkegaard *et al.*, 1957; Klinken-Rasmussen *et al.*, 1957; Lyager and Rontorp, 1957; Nielsen, 1957; Schulsinger, 1957; Hoch, 1958; Keyes, 1958; Ayd, 1959; Azima *et al.*, 1959; Goldman and Zamansky, 1959; Kline, 1959; Bellak and Black, 1960; Himwich, 1960; Schwartz and Willis, 1960; Pletscher, 1959; and St. Jean *et al.*, 1965). Reserpine treatment has been increasingly replaced by other psychopharmacotherapies.

iii. Adverse Effects Reported. Psychiatric (depression, insomnia, nightmares, irrational behavior, drowsiness, lassitude); neurological (parkinsonism, headache, dizziness, weakness); autonomic (nasal congestion, dry mouth); cardiovascular (bradycardia, palpitation, hypotension); gastrointestinal (activation and perforation of peptic ulcer); dermatological (skin eruptions); and others (edema, purpura and epistaxis). Contraindications: epilepsy, cardiac failure, peptic ulcer, depression and pregnancy. Reserpine should be discontinued 2 weeks prior to ECT or surgery and should be given cautiously with digitalis or quinidine.

3. Other Heterocyclic and Aromatic Compounds

a. Anisoperidone

i. Chemical Name. 4-Methoxy-4-[1-(4-phenyl)-1,2,3,6-tetrahydropyridino]butyrophenone.

ii. Therapeutic Uses. A neuroleptic butyrophenone which produces a slight increase of GABA concentration in the brain. Beneficial in the schizophrenias (Divry *et al.*, 1959; Waelkens, 1960; and Nodine *et al.*, 1961). The place of this substance in psychopharmacotherapy has not yet been established.

iii. Adverse Effects Reported. Similar to those of other butyrophenones.

b. Azacyclonol

i. Chemical Name. α,α-Diphenyl-α-piperidyl-4-methanol.

ii. Therapeutic Uses. A substance with particular effectiveness in controlling LSD_{25}-induced psychopathology, especially hallucinations (Fabing, 1955; Brown, *et al.*, 1956; Kuziw, *et al.*, 1956; Lehmann, 1958; Bachann, 1960; Decsi, 1961; and Kant and Abele, 1961).

iii. Adverse Effects Reported. Low incidence of adverse effects.

c. Benzperidol

i. Chemical Name. 1-{1-[3-(4-Fluorobenzoyl)-propyl]-4-piperidyl}-2-benzimidazoline.

ii. Therapeutic Uses. An antipsychotic butyrophenone particularly effective in the schizophrenias and in agitated geriatric patients (Bobon *et al.*, 1963; Lambert *et al.*, 1965; and LeBorgne *et al.*, 1966). The place of this substance in psychopharmacotherapy has not yet been established.

iii. Adverse Effects Reported. Similar to those of other butyrophenones.

d. Benzquinamide

i. Chemical Name. *N*,*N*,-Diethyl-1,3,4,6,7,11-*b*-hexahydro-2-hydroxy-9,10-dimethoxy(2H)benzo(*a*)quinolizine-3 carboxamide acetate.

ii. Therapeutic Uses. A serotonin antagonist which reduces anxiety without altering psychomotor performance (Forney and Hughes, 1963; Lapollar, 1963; and Scriabina, *et al.*, 1966). It is successfully used in stress reactions, in the symptomatic management of arousal (agitation) and affective (anxiety) psychopathology, psychoneuroses and schizophrenias (Feldman, 1962; Overall *et al.*, 1963; Sainz, 1963;

Settel, 1963; Smith, 1963; and Holmberg and William-Olsson, 1964). Others found that the toxic behavioral effects of benzquinamide outweigh its therapeutic value (Bishop, *et al.*, 1963; and Barsa and Saunder, 1964). The place of this substance in psychopharmacotherapy has not yet been established.

iii. Adverse Effects Reported. Behavioral toxicity (prevailingly dysthymic mood changes) with or without depressive ideation.

e. Dehydropenzperidol

i. Chemical Name. (1-{1-[4-(*p*-Fluorophenyl)-4-oxobutyl]-1,2,3,6-tetrahydro-4-pyridyl}-2-benzimidazolinone.

ii. Therapeutic Uses. One of the fastest acting antipsychotic butyrophenones with a relatively short duration of action (Janssen, *et al.*, 1963).

iii. Adverse Effects Reported. Similar to those of other butyrophenones.

f. Floropipamide

i. Chemical Name. 4-Carbamoyl-1-[3-(4-fluorobenzoyl)-propyl]-4-piperidyl-piperidine.

ii. Therapeutic Uses. An antipsychotic butyrophenone, somewhat less effective in the schizophrenias than haloperidol and trifluperidol (Bobon *et al.*, 1961; Nutys, 1963; Schwartz *et al.*, 1964; Sugerman, 1964; and Warnes *et al.*, 1964).

iii. Adverse Effects Reported. Similar to those of other butyrophenones.

g. Fluanisone

i. Chemical Name. 4-Fluoro-δ-[4-(2-methoxyphenyl) - 1 - piperazinyl]butyrophenone.

ii. Therapeutic Uses. An antipsychotic butyrophenone. Comparable in its therapeutic effectiveness to chlorpromazine in the schizophrenias (Delay *et al.*, 1960; Paquay *et al.*, 1959; Broussolle *et al.*, 1961; Chauchard and Mazoué, 1961; Fouks, 1961; Janssen *et al.*, 1960, 1966; Kammerer, 1962; Soulairac, 1962; Scherrer, 1962; Deberdt, 1960; Morren *et al.*, 1964).

iii. Adverse Effects Reported. It produces somewhat more drowsiness and hypotension but less extrapyramidal signs than haloperidol.

h. Haloperidol

i. Chemical Name. 4-[4-(*p*-Chlorophenyl)-4-hydroxypiperidino]-4-fluoro-butyrophenone.

ii. Therapeutic Uses. An antipsychotic, particularly useful in the treatment of acute schizophrenics and manics (Delay *et al.*, 1960; Nodine *et al.*, 1962; Paterson, 1963; de Haen, 1964; Lehmann and Ban, 1964).

iii. Adverse Effects Reported. Psychiatric (depression); neurological (extrapyramidal signs); autonomic (perspiration, dehydration, salivation, dry mouth, blurred vision); cardiovascular (orthostatic hypotension); gastrointestinal (dyspepsia, constipation); genitourinary (urinary retention, impotence); and metabolic (hypocholesterolemia).

i. Methyldopa

i. Chemical Name. *l*-2-Amino-3-(3,4-dihydroxyphenyl)-2-methylpropionic acid.

ii. Therapeutic Uses. An antihypertensive with CNS effects with a possible usefulness in the treatment of manics (Sourkes, 1965; St. Jean *et al.*, 1965; and Mosher *et al.*, 1966). The place of this substance in psychopharmacotherapy has not yet been established.

iii. Adverse Effects Reported. Psychiatric (depression, drowsiness); neurological (dizziness, headache, extrapyramidal signs); autonomic (dryness of mouth, nasal stuffiness); endocrinological (breast enlargement, lactation); cardiovascular (bradycardia, postural hypotension, angina pectoris); gastrointestinal (distension, flatus, vomiting, diarrhea); genitourinary (impotence); hepatobiliary (focal liver necrosis); and dermatological (skin rash).

j. Methylperidol

i. Chemical Name. 1-[3-(4-Fluorobenzoyl)-propyl]-4-hydroxy-4-(4-tolyl)piperidine.

ii. Therapeutic Uses. An antipsychotic butyrophenone particularly useful in the maintenance therapy of paranoid schizophrenics (Uytterschaut and Jacobs, 1962;

Table I

Drugs used in the treatment of schizophrenias

Generic name	Trademark			Dosage	
	U.S.A.	Canada	Britain	Intensive treatment	Maintenance treatment
				T.I.D. in mg.	*Q.D. or B.I.D. in mg.*
Acetophenazine	Tindal	Notensil	Notensil	20–80	20–40
Butaperazine	Repoise	Randolectil	NA	25–75	10–30
Carphenazine	Proketazine	NA	NA	50–100	25–50
Chlorpromazine	Thorazine	Largactil	Largactil	150–650	100–150
Chlorprothixene	Taractan	Tarasan	Taractan	100–250	50–100
Deserpidine	Harmonyl	Harmonyl	Harmonyl	2–4	1–2
Fluphenazine	Prolixin	Moditen	Moditen	2–10	2–4
Haloperidol	Haldol	Haldol	Serenace	5–15	2–4
Methotrimeprazine	NA	Nozinan	Veractil	25–100	25–50
Perphenazine	Trilafon	Trilafon	Fentazin	8–40	2–8
Prochlorperazine	Compazine	Stemetil	Stemetil	25–100	25–50
Promazine	Sparine	Sparine	Sparine	200–700	200–250
Reserpine	Serpasil	Serpasil	Serpasil	2–4	1–2
Thiopropazate	Dartal	Dartal	Dartalan	20–30	5–15
Thioproperazine	Majeptil	Majeptil	Majeptil	10–20	2–4
Thioridazine	Mellaril	Mellaril	Mellaril	150–200	100–150
Thiothixene	Navane	Navane	Navane	20–30	10–20
Trifluoperazine	Stelazine	Stelazine	Stelazine	10–20	2–5
Triflupromazine	Vesprin	Vesprin	Vespran	50–200	25–50

Bobon *et al.*, 1963; Gastager and Gruber, 1965; Vinar and Taussigova, 1965).

iii. Adverse Effects Reported. Similar to those of other butyrophenones.

k. Spiroperidol

i. Chemical Name. 8-[3-(4-Fluorobenzoyl)propyl]-4-oxo-1-phenyl-1,3,8-triazaspiro[4,5]decane.

ii. Therapeutic Uses. An antipsychotic butyrophenone with a particular usefulness in the schizophrenias (Bobon *et al.*, 1963; Paquary *et al.*, 1965).

iii. Adverse Effects Reported. Similar to those of other butyrophenones.

l. Tetrabenazine

i. Chemical Name. 1,3,4,6,7,11,*b*-Hexahydro-3-1-isobutyl-9,10-dimethoxy-2H-benzo[*α*]quinolizin-2-one.

ii. Therapeutic Uses. A central parasympatholytic with antipsychotic effects (Bogdansky *et al.*, 1961; and Lingjaerde, 1963). Used in the schizophrenias but particularly useful in the treatment of manic (or hypomanic) patients (Bertolotti and Munarini, 1961; Heinrich, 1961; and Paterson, 1963). The basic properties of tetrabenazine are similar to those of reserpine, but the decrease of brain 5-HT levels and the depression induced are of shorter duration. Consequently it is frequently applied in the screening of psychopharmacological substances in animal pharmacological studies.

iii. Adverse Effects Reported. Similar to those of benzquinamide.

m. Triperidol

i. Chemical Name. 1-[3-(*p*-Fluorobenzoyl)-propyl]-4(*m*-trifluoromethylphenyl)-4-piperidinol.

ii. Therapeutic Uses. An antipsychotic butyrophenone successfully used in the schizophrenias with particular usefulness in chronic cases (Dubois *et al.*, 1963; Warnes *et al.*, 1964; and Hollister *et al.*, 1965).

iii. Adverse Effects Reported. Similar to those of other butyrophenones.

B. ANTIDEPRESSANTS AND STIMULANTS

1. Phenothiazines and Related Compounds

a. Amitriptyline

i. Chemical Name. 5-(3-Dimethylaminopropylidene)-10,11-dihydro(5H)dibenzo(*a*, *d*)-cycloheptene.

ii. Therapeutic Uses. One of the most extensively used antidepressants. It also has some anxiolytic and sedative properties (Ayd, 1960; Dorfman, 1960; Freed, 1960; Dunlop, 1961; Bolzani and Slivar, 1962; Harder, 1962; Karabanov, 1962; Lambert *et al.*, 1962; and Horden *et al.*, 1965).

iii. Adverse Effects Reported. Psychiatric (drowsiness, nervousness, confusional state, activation of latent schizophrenia); neurological (headache, dizziness, weakness, tremor, epileptiform seizures); autonomic (dry mouth, blurred vision); cardiovascular (hypotension); gastrointestinal (constipation) and genitourinary (urinary retention). Its incompatibility with MAOI's was recognized by Harrer (1962). It is contraindicated in glaucoma (Häfliger and Burckhardt, 1964).

b. Carbamazepin

i. Chemical Name. 10,11-Dihydro-5H-dibenz[*b*,*f*]azepine-5-carboxamide.

ii. Therapeutic Uses. An anticonvulsant with mood-lifting properties (Blom, 1963, and Lutz, 1966). It is particularly useful in the treatment of epileptics with depressive symptoms (Ban and Lehmann, 1968). The place of this substance in psychopharmacotherapy has not yet been established.

iii. Adverse Effects Reported. Similar to those of other dibenzazepines.

c. Desipramine

i. Chemical Name. 10,11-Dihydro-5-(3-methylaminopropyl)-5H-dibenz[*b*,*f*]azepine.

ii. Therapeutic Uses. An antidepressant particularly useful in depression in which psychomotor inhibition and lack of drive prevail. Possibly somewhat faster acting than imipramine (Azima *et al.*, 1962; Ban and Lehmann, 1962; Bobon and Goffioul, 1962; Brodie *et al.*, 1961; Mann, 1962; Meduna *et al.*, 1961; Oltman and Friedman, 1962; and St. Jean *et al.*, 1966).

iii. Adverse Effects Reported. Similar to those of other dibenzazepines.

d. Dibenzepin

i. Chemical Name. 10-[2-(Dimethylamino)ethyl]-5,10-dihydro-5-methyl-11H-dibenzo[*b*,*e*][1,4]diazepin-11-one hydrochloride.

ii. Therapeutic Uses. Successfully used as an antidepressant (Rett *et al.*, 1965; and Schigutt and Suchanek-Fröchlich, 1965). The place of this substance in psychopharmacotherapy has not yet been established.

iii. Adverse Effects Reported. Need to be assessed.

e. Dimethacrin

i. Chemical Name. 9,9-Dimethyl-10-(3-dimethylamino)propylacridine tartrate.

ii. Therapeutic Uses. A psychotropic with possible antidepressant properties (Jahn and Häusler, 1966; and Guth and Hofmann, 1966). The place of this substance in psychopharmacotherapy has not yet been established.

iii. Adverse Effects Reported. Need to be assessed.

f. Doxepin

i. Chemical Name. 11-(6H-(3-Dimethylamino-propylidene)-6,11-dihydrodibenz(*b*,*e*)oxepine.

ii. Therapeutic Uses. An anticholinergic with antidepressant properties (Pöldinger *et al.*, 1966; and Schmitt and Schmitt, 1966). Its place in psychopharmacotherapy has not yet been established.

iii. Adverse Effects Reported. Need to be assessed.

g. Imipramine

i. Chemical Name. 2,2-(3-Dimethylaminopropyl-imino)dibenzyl.

ii. Therapeutic Uses. The first tricyclic antidepressant, extensively used clinically. Its primary indications are endogenous depressions, but it is also useful in reactive, neurotic and symptomatic depressions

(Angst, 1961; Ayd, 1959; Azima, 1959; Coirault *et al.*, 1959; Delay *et al.*, 1959; Dunlop, 1962; Fazio *et al.*, 1958; Freyhan, 1960; Hift and Kryspin-Exner, 1959; and Lehmann *et al.*, 1958).

iii. Adverse Effects Reported. Psychiatric (insomnia, activation of schizophrenia, confusional state); neurological (parkinsonism, myoclonia, hyperreflexia, muscular fasciculation, convulsions); autonomic (atropine-like actions); cardiovascular (first-degree atrioventricular block, hypotension); gastrointestinal (constipation); genitourinary (urinary retention); hepatobiliary (jaundice); hematological (leukopenia, eosinophilia); and allergic (urticaria, angioneurotic edema). Contraindicated in glaucoma, coronary artery disease and intraocular tension. It should be combined with thyroid preparations with caution.

h. Imipramine N-Oxide

i. Chemical Name. 5-(3-Dimethylaminopropyl)-10,11-dihydro-5H-dibenz[*b*,*f*]azepine-5-oxide.

ii. Therapeutic Uses. An imipramine metabolite with possible antidepressant properties (Gallant *et al.*, 1965). The place of this substance in psychopharmacotherapy has not yet been established.

iii. Adverse Effects Reported. Need to be assessed.

i. Melitracene

i. Chemical Name. 9,10-Dihydro-10,10-dimethyl-9-(3-dimethylaminopropylidene)anthracene.

ii. Therapeutic Uses. An antidepressant, particularly effective in "vitally inhibited" depressions and in agitated depressions (Bratlund, 1961; and Retboll, 1963). Its place in psychopharmacotherapy has not yet been established.

iii. Adverse Effects Reported. Need to be assessed.

j. Nortriptyline

i. Chemical Name. 5-(3-Methylaminopropylidene)-10,11-dihydro-5H-dibenzo[*a*,*d*]cycloheptene.

ii. Therapeutic Uses. An extensively used antidepressant useful in psychotic, reactive and neurotic depressions (Oltman and Friedman, 1963) and in psychosomatic conditions (Bennett, 1962).

iii. Adverse Effects Reported. Similar to those of amitriptyline.

k. Opipramol

i. Chemical Name. 4-[3-(5H-Dibenz)[*b*,*f*]azepine-5yl]-1-piperazinethanol.

ii. Therapeutic Uses. A psychotropic with slight tranquilizing and mood-lifting properties (Ahmed *et al.*, 1958; and Azima *et al.*, 1962). The place of this substance in psychopharmacotherapy has not yet been established.

iii. Adverse Effects Reported. Similar, but fewer in incidence, than with other tricyclic antidepressants.

l. Proheptatriene

i. Chemical Name. 5-(3-Dimethylaminopropylidene)-5H-dibenzo[*a*,*d*]cycloheptene.

ii. Therapeutic Uses. An antidepressant, therapeutically equal (or superior) to imipramine (Nahunek *et al.*, 1965; and Grof and Vinar, 1965). The place of this substance in psychopharmacotherapy has not yet been established.

iii. Adverse Effects Reported. Need to be assessed.

m. Prothiadene

i. Chemical Name. 11-(3-Dimethylaminopropylidene)-6,11-dihydrodibenzo[*b*,*e*]thiepine.

ii. Therapeutic Uses. A psychotropic with possible usefulness in neurotic depressions (Alapin and Zaborowska, 1966; and Pöldinger *et al.*, 1966).

iii. Adverse Effects Reported. Need to be assessed.

n. Protriptyline

i. Chemical Name. 5-(3-Methylaminopropyl)-5H-dibenzo[*a*,*d*]cycloheptene.

ii. Therapeutic Uses. An antidepressant with psychomotor stimulating effects (Daneman, 1965; Feldman, 1964; Kline and Hackett, 1965; and Krakowski, 1965).

iii. Adverse Effects Reported. Similar to those of the other tricyclic antidepressants.

o. Trimipramine

i. Chemical Name. 1-(3-Dimethylamino-2-methylpropyl)-10,11-dihydro-5H-dibenz-[*b,f*]azepine.

ii. Therapeutic Uses. An antidepressant with sedative and anxiolytic properties (Ban, 1964; Gambs, *et al.*, 1962; Géraud *et al.*, 1962; Kristof *et al.*, 1967; Lambert and Guyotat, 1961; Lehmann *et al.*, 1964; and Sigwald *et al.*, 1961).

iii. Adverse Effects Reported. Similar to those of other dibenzazepines.

2. Indoles

a. Iprindole

i. Chemical Name 5-[3-(Dimethylamino) propyl]-6,7,8,9,10,11-hexahydro-5H-cyclooct[*b*]indole.

ii. Therapeutic Uses. A psychotropic with possible antidepressant properties (Hicks, 1965). The place of this substance in psychopharmacotherapy has not yet been established.

iii. Adverse Effects Reported. Need to be assessed.

3. Other Heterocycles

a. Cyprolidol

i. Chemical Name. α,α-Diphenyl-2-(4-pyridyl)cyclopropylmethanol.

ii. Therapeutic Uses. A psychic energizer with possible therapeutic action in anergic schizophrenics (Lapolla and Nash, 1965; and Nagy and Gershon, 1966).

iii. Adverse Effects Reported. Autonomic side-effects similar to those of imipramine.

b. Isocarboxazide

i. Chemical Name. 1-Benzyl-2-(5-methyl-3-isooxazolylcarbonyl)hydrazine.

ii. Therapeutic Uses. An MAOI antidepressant with particular usefulness in atypical depressions (Pletscher *et al.*, 1960; and Ayd, 1960).

iii. Adverse Effects Reported. Similar to those of other MAOI's. Contraindicated in patients with cardiac decompensation, congestive heart failure, cerebral vascular disease and pheochromocytoma.

c. Levophacetoperane

i. Chemical Name. Phenyl-2-(2-piperidyl)methyl acetate.

ii. Therapeutic Uses. A sympathomimetic with possible therapeutic usefulness in chronic, inactive and apathetic schizophrenics (Sivadon *et al.*, 1959; Ban and St. Laurent, 1961; and Dagirmanjian and Boyd, 1962).

iii. Adverse Effects Reported. Need to be assessed.

d. Methylphenidate

i. Chemical Name. Methyl-α-phenyl-2-pipiridineacetate.

ii. Therapeutic Uses. A stimulant with particular usefulness in the treatment of behavioral problems in children and the aged (Ferguson, 1956; Gruber *et al.*, 1956; Carter and Maley, 1957; Pennington, 1957; Zimmerman and Burgemeister, 1958; Gale, 1958; Wodraska *et al.*, 1958; Darville, 1959; Pargiter, 1959; Kerenyi *et al.*, 1960; and Krueger and McGrath, 1964).

iii. Adverse Effects Reported. Psychiatric (nervousness, insomnia); neurological (headache, dizziness, tremor); and cardiovascular (palpitation, hypertension).

e. Modaline

i. Chemical Name. 2-Methyl-3-piperidinopyrazine.

ii. Therapeutic Uses. An MAOI antidepressant particularly useful when weight gain is undesirable in the course of treatment (Dubnick *et al.*, 1963; Feldman, 1963; Gylys *et al.*, 1963; Dunlop *et al.*, 1964; Nussbaum *et al.*, 1964; and Schaffer *et al.*, 1964).

iii. Adverse Effects Reported. Need to be assessed.

f. Nialamide

i. Chemical Name. *N*-(2-Benzyl-carbamylethyl)isoniazid.

ii. Therapeutic Uses. An MAOI antidepressant; inferior to isocarboxazide or phenelzine in its therapeutic effects (Zbinden *et al.*, 1960).

iii. Adverse Effects Reported. Similar to those of other MAOI's.

g. Pentetrazol

i. Chemical Name. 6,7,8,9-Tetrahydro-5H-tetrazoloazepine.

ii. Therapeutic Uses. A CNS stimulant particularly useful in the treatment of geriatric patients. It may have a beneficial effect on memory (Haydu, 1961; Goldberg and Schuman, 1964; Miller, 1965; Hunt and Krivanek, 1966; and Irwin and Benuazizi, 1966).

iii. Adverse Effects Reported. Cardiac arrhythmia, convulsions and delayed psychotic reactions with overdosage.

h. Pipradrol

i. Chemical Name. α,α-Diphenyl-2-piperidinemethanol.

ii. Therapeutic Uses. A CNS stimulant with particular usefulness in narcolepsy and alcoholism (Levy, 1954; Pomeranze, 1954; Antos, 1955; Andren, 1955; Fabing, 1955; Payne and Moore, 1955; Button, 1956; Cohen, 1956; Gottschalk *et al.*, 1956; Kistner and Duncan, 1956; Proctor, 1956; Lethew, 1957; Martin *et al.*, 1957; and Klingman, 1962).

iii. Adverse Effects Reported. Hyperactivity, insomnia and anxiety with higher dosages. Contraindicated in prepsychotic states, in paranoid and obsessive-compulsive reactions and in chorea.

i. Pyrovalerone

i. Chemical Name. 4-Methyl-2-pyrrolidinyl valerophenone.

ii. Therapeutic Uses. A psychotropic with psychostimulant effects (Heimann and Lukacs, 1965; and Heimann and Vetter, 1965). The place of this substance in psychopharmacotherapy has not yet been established.

iii. Adverse Effects Reported. Need to be assessed.

j. Thiazenone

i. Chemical Name. 5-(2-Dimethylaminoethyl) - 2,3 - dihydro - 2 - phenyl - 1,5 - benzothiazepin-4-(5H)one hydrochloride.

ii. Therapeutic Uses. An antidepressant with possible usefulness in depressions (Horovitz *et al.*, 1963). The place of this substance in psychopharmacotherapy has not yet been established.

iii. Adverse Effects Reported. Need to be assessed.

k. Trioxazine

i. Chemical Name. 4-(3,4,5-Trimethoxy-benzoyl)morpholine.

ii. Therapeutic Uses. A psychotropic with possible usefulness in "exhaustive depressions" (Usdin and Efron, 1967). Its place in psychopharmacotherapy has not yet been established.

iii. Adverse Effects Reported. Need to be assessed.

4. Aromatic Compounds

a. Amphetamine Phosphate

i. Chemical Name. α-Methylphenethylamine phosphate.

ii. Therapeutic Uses. A CNS stimulant, particularly useful for relieving chronic fatigue (Cohen *et al.*, 1967). Its usefulness in psychoneurotic depression, psychosomatic disorders and alcoholism needs to be confirmed.

iii. Adverse Effects Reported. A habit-forming substance. It may produce insomnia, nervousness and gastrointestinal disturbance. It is contraindicated in cardiovascular disease and prepsychotic states.

b. Amphetamine Sulfate

i. Chemical Name. α-Methylphenethylamine sulfate.

ii. Therapeutic Uses. A CNS stimulant particularly useful in narcolepsy, barbiturate poisoning and postencephalitic parkinsonism (Remmen *et al.*, 1962). Its usefulness in psychoneurotic depression and alcoholism needs to be confirmed.

iii. Adverse Effects Reported. Similar to those of amphetamine phosphate.

c. Centrophenoxine

i. Chemical Name. 2-(Dimethylamino)-ethyl-*p*-chlorophenoxyacetate.

ii. Therapeutic Uses. An auxin derivative with possible usefulness in the treatment of chronic brain syndromes, alcohol and narcotic withdrawal (Delay *et al.*, 1960;

Launay and Michelin, 1961; Michon *et al.*, 1961; Gerstenbrand *et al.*, 1963; Denber and Turns, 1964; and Sabbatini, 1964). The place of this substance in psychopharmacotherapy has not yet been established.

iii. Adverse Effects Reported. Need to be assessed.

d. Dextroamphetamine Sulfate

i. Chemical Name. *d*-α-Methylphenethylamine sulfate.

ii. Therapeutic Uses. A CNS stimulant with particular usefulness in narcolepsy and chronic fatigue (Cohen *et al.*, 1967). Its usefulness in depression and alcoholism needs to be confirmed.

iii. Adverse Effects Reported. Similar to those of other amphetamines.

e. Ethamivan

i. Chemical Name. *N*,*N*-Diethyl-vanillamide.

ii. Therapeutic Uses. A respiratory stimulant with analeptic properties. It is the antidote of barbiturate and/or propanediol intoxication. It may also be useful in the treatment of chronic brain syndromes, geriatric cases and depressions (Negwer, 1961; Hamilton and Bennett, 1965; and Silver, 1966). The place of this substance in psychopharmacotherapy has not yet been established.

iii. Adverse Effects Reported. Muscle twitching and cerebral seizures. Contraindicated in epilepsy and incompatible with MAOI's.

f. Fencamfamine

i. Chemical Name. 2-Ethylamino-3-phenyl-norcamphane hydrochloride.

ii. Therapeutic Uses. A CNS stimulant without antidepressant properties (LeGassicke *et al.*, 1964; and Lehmann and Ban, 1966). The place of this substance in psychopharmacotherapy has not yet been established.

iii. Adverse Effects Reported. Activation of psychopathology.

g. Iproclozide

i. Chemical Name. 1-(*p*-Chlorophenoxyacetyl)-2-isopropyl-hydrazine.

ii. Therapeutic Uses. An MAOI with possible therapeutic usefulness in depressions (Fouks *et al.*, 1961; Fournier *et al.*, 1964; and Géraud and Gleizes, 1964). The place of this substance in psychopharmacotherapy has not yet been established.

iii. Adverse Effects Reported. Similar to those of other MAOI's.

h. Mebanazine

i. Chemical Name. 1-(1-Phenylethyl)-hydrazine.

ii. Therapeutic Uses. An MAOI with hypoglycemic properties which induces an increase of nonesterified fatty acid metabolism in drug-responsive depressive patients. It is particularly useful when depression is associated with diabetes (Wickström and Pettersson, 1964; Barker *et al.*, 1965; Gilmour, 1965; and Van Praag and Leijnse, 1966).

iii. Adverse Effects Reported. Similar to those of other MAOI'S.

i. Methamphetamine

i. Chemical Name. dl-*N*,α-Dimethylphenethylamine.

ii. Therapeutic Uses. A sympathomimetic substance with psychomotor stimulating properties with particular usefulness in the treatment of narcolepsy and barbiturate poisoning (Cohen *et al.*, 1967). Its usefulness in depression, apathy, alcoholism and obesity needs to be confirmed.

iii. Adverse Effects Reported. A habit-forming substance (Liddel and Weil-Malherbe, 1953). Contraindicated in cerebral and cardiovascular disease, hyperthyroidism, nephritis and schizophrenia.

j. Pargyline

i. Chemical Name. *N*-Methyl-*N*-propargylbenzylamine.

ii. Therapeutic Uses. An MAOI antidepressant which decreases pigment formation from serotonin *in vitro* (Taylor *et al.*, 1960). Because of its antihypertensive effects it is particularly useful in depression associated with hypertension (Everett *et al.*, 1963).

iii. Adverse Effects Reported. Similar to those of other MAOI's.

k. Phendimetrazine Tartrate

i. Chemical Name. 3,4-Dimethyl-2-phenylmorpholine bitartrate.

ii. Therapeutic Uses. An MAOI with possible antidepressant properties (French and Truelove, 1965; and Dvornik and Schilling, 1965). The place of this substance in psychopharmacotherapy has not yet been established.

iii. Adverse Effects Reported. Similar to those of other MAOI's.

l. Phenelzine

i. Chemical Name. β-Phenethylhydrazine.

ii. Therapeutic Uses. One of the most extensively used MAOI antidepressants (Ayd, 1960; and Zbinden *et al.*, 1960).

iii. Adverse Effects Reported. Similar to those of other MAOI's.

m. Phenoxypropazine

i. Chemical Name. 1-(1-Methyl-2-phenoxyethyl)hydrazine.

ii. Therapeutic Uses. An MAOI antidepressant, therapeutically inferior, but also less toxic than iproniazid (Leahy *et al.*, 1963; Rose *et al.*, 1963; Biel *et al.*, 1964; and McWhinney and Morrell, 1965).

iii. Adverse Effects Reported. Similar to those of other MAOI's.

n. Pivalylbenzhydrazine

i. Chemical Name. 1-Benzyl-2-pivaloylhydrazine.

ii. Therapeutic Uses. An MAOI with antidepressant properties (Zbinden *et al.*, 1960). The place of this substance in psychopharmacotherapy has not yet been established.

iii. Adverse Effects Reported. Similar to those of other MAOI's.

o. Tranylcypromine

i. Chemical Name. 2-Phenylcyclopropylamine.

ii. Therapeutic Uses. A non-hydrazine MAOI antidepressant, particularly useful in the treatment of reactive and psychoneurotic depressions (Atkinson and Ditman, 1965; Freyhan, 1960; English, 1961; Clark, 1961; Agin, 1960; Lemere, 1960: Lurie and Salzer, 1961; Pelzman, 1961; Bartholomew, 1962; Darling, 1962; Dunlop, 1962; Kingston, 1962; Kranzdorf, 1962; Levinson, 1962; Levy, 1962; Lees and Burke, 1963; and MacDonald, 1963).

iii. Adverse Effects Reported. Similar to those of other MAOI's.

C. SEDATIVES AND ANXIOLYTIC DRUGS

1. Phenothiazines and Related Compounds

a. Dixyrazine

i. Chemical Name. 10-[2-Methyl-3-(1-hydroxyethoxyethyl-4-piperazinyl)-propyl]-phenothiazine.

ii. Therapeutic Uses. An anxiolytic particularly useful in the therapy of children with anxiety, restlessness, agitation and lack of concentration (Bensch and Rundberg, 1964, 1965; and Fokstuen, 1965).

iii. Adverse Effects Reported. Similar to those of other phenothiazines.

b. Flupentixol

i. Chemical Name. 2-Trifluoromethyl-9-3-[4-(2-hydroxylethyl)-1-piperazinyl]propylidene thioxanthene.

ii. Therapeutic Uses. A tranquilizer with possible therapeutic action in the psychoneuroses (Holst, 1965; and Ravn and Rud, 1965). The place of this substance in psychopharmacotherapy has not yet been established.

iii. Adverse Effects Reported. Similar to those of other thioxanthenes.

c. Methiomeprazine

i. Chemical Name. 10-(3-Dimethylamino-2-methylpropyl)-2-methylthiophenothiazine.

ii. Therapeutic Uses. A tranquilizer with possible usefulness in the treatment of ambulatory chronic alcoholics (Levy *et al.*, 1961). The place of this substance in psychopharmacotherapy has not yet been established.

iii. Adverse Effects Reported. Need to be assessed.

d. Promethazine

i. Chemical Name. 10-[2-(Dimethylamino)propyl]phenothazine.

TABLE II
Frequently used stimulants and antidepressants

Generic name	Trademark			Dosage	
	U.S.A.	Canada	Britain	Daily dose range	Minimum daily dose
				mg.	*mg.*
Amitriptyline	Elavil	Elavil	Triptizol	150–300	50
Amphetamine sulfate	Benzedrine	Benzedrine	Benzedrine	20–40	10
Desipramine	Norpramin	Pertofrane	Pertofrane	150–300	50
Dextroamphetamine sulfate	Dexedrine	Dexedrine	Dexedrene	20–40	10
Imipramine	Tofranil	Tofranil	Tofranil	150–300	50
Isocarboxazide	Marplan	Marplan	Marplan	20–30	10
Mebanazine	NA	NA	Actomol	20–30	10
Methamphetamine	Desoxyn	Desoxyn	Methedrine	5–15	5
Methylphenidate	Ritalin	Ritalin	Ritalin	30–60	15
Nialamide	Niamid	Niamid	Niamid	300–450	50
Nortriptyline	Aventyl	Aventyl	Allegron	150–300	50
Pargyline	Eutonyl	Eutonyl	Eutonyl	30–50	10
Pentylenetetrazol	Metrazol	Metrazol	Metrazol	300–600	200
Phenelzine	Nardil	Nardil	Nardil	30–60	15
Pipradrol	Meratran	Meratran	Meratran	5–10	2
Protriptyline	Vivactil	Triptil	Concordin	30–60	15
Tranylcypromine	Parnate	Parnate	Parnate	30–60	10
Trimipramine	NA	Surmontil	Surmontil	150–300	50

ii. Therapeutic Uses. An antihistaminic with psychoactive properties. It is particularly useful in the treatment of psychoneurotic patients (Halpern and Ducrot, 1946; Samuels, 1957; and Paterson, 1963).

iii. Adverse Effects Reported. Similar to those of other phenothiazines.

2. Indoles

a. Benanserin

i. Chemical Name. 1-Benzyl-2-methyl-3-(2-aminoethyl)-5-methoxyindole.

ii. Therapeutic Uses. A psychotropic with possible tranquilizing properties (Rudy *et al.*, 1958). The place of this substance in psychopharmacotherapy has not yet been established.

iii. Adverse Effects Reported. Need to be assessed.

b. Benzindopyrine

i. Chemical Name. 4-(1-Benzyl-3-indolylethyl)pyridine.

ii. Therapeutic Uses. A psychotropic with possible tranquilizing properties (Bodi *et al.*, 1959; and Mirsky *et al.*, 1959). The place of this substance in psychopharmacotherapy has not yet been established.

iii. Adverse Effects Reported. Need to be assessed.

3. Other Heterocycles

a. Buclizine

i. Chemical Name. 1-(*p*-tert-Butylbenzyl) - 4 - (*p* - chlorophenylbenzyl)pipera - zine.

ii. Therapeutic Uses. An antihistamine with potent antiemetic and anxiolytic properties (Chinn, 1956; Karnaky, 1956; Olson and Peterson, 1959; Rotherford, 1959; and Morren *et al.*, 1964). The place of this substance in psychopharmacotherapy has not yet been established.

iii. Adverse Effects Reported. Need to be assessed.

b. Captagon

i. Chemical Name. 7-[2-(1-Methyl-2-phenylethylamino)ethyl]theophyllin.

ii. Therapeutic Uses. A psychomotor

stimulant which increases the desire for social contact. It is particularly useful in neurasthenia (Janke and Boss, 1961; Munkelt and Othmer, 1965; and Simka, 1965). The place of this substance in psychopharmacotherapy has not yet been established.

iii. Adverse Effects Reported. Need to be assessed.

c. Chlordiazepoxide

i. Chemical Name. 7-Chloro-2-methylamino-4-phenyl(3H)-1,4-benzodiazepine-4-oxide.

ii. Therapeutic Uses. A potent anxiolytic with primary indications in the psychoneuroses. It is also useful in the treatment of alcohol withdrawal and in the control of the psychological concomitants of cardiovascular and gastrointestinal illnesses (Sternbach *et al.*, 1964).

iii. Adverse Effects Reported. Psychiatric (dependency, drowsiness, ataxia, lethargy, confusion, depersonalization); neurological (ataxia); cardiovascular (syncope); genitourinary (impotence); hepatobiliary (jaundice); and hematological (agranulocytosis).

d. Chlormethazanone

i. Chemical Name. 4H-1,3-Thiazin-4-one-2-(*p*-chlorophenyl)tetrahydro-3-methyl-1,1-dioxide.

ii. Therapeutic Uses. A centrally acting muscle relaxant with anxiolytic properties. It is particularly useful in the treatment of dermatoses of psychological origin and dermatological diseases with superimposed psychological changes (Gessler and Coulston, 1959; and Rogers, 1961).

iii. Adverse Effects Reported. Psychiatric (drowsiness, lethargy); neurological (dizziness); autonomic (dryness of mouth, flushing); and hepatobilary (jaundice).

e. Diazepam

i. Chemical Name. 7-Chloro-1,3-dihydro-1-methyl-5-phenyl-2H-1-4-benzodiazepin-2-one.

ii. Therapeutic Uses. A potent anxiolytic with particular usefulness in the psychoneuroses, involutional melancholia, behavioral disorders of childhood and borderline psychiatric conditions (Randall *et al.*, 1960, 1965).

iii. Adverse Effects Reported. Psychiatric (dependency, paradoxical excitement, depression, hallucinations, drowsiness, fatigue, memory impairment); neurological (dizziness, headache, diplopia, ataxia, tremor, slurred speech); cardiovascular (hypotension); gastrointestinal (constipation); genitourinary (incontinence); and hematological (leukopenia).

f. Glutethimide

i. Chemical Name. 2-Ethyl-2-phenylglutarimide.

ii. Therapeutic Uses. An extensively used hypnotic. Less effective than ethchlorvynol (Ban and McGinnis, 1962) but superior to placebo (Matthews *et al.*, 1964).

iii. Adverse Effects Reported. Chronic administration may lead to dependency.

g. Hydroxyzine

i. Chemical Name. 2-{2-[4-(*p*-Chloro-α-phenyl benzyl)-1-piperazinyl]ethoxy}ethanol.

ii. Therapeutic Uses. An anxiolytic which produces "psychic relaxation" without a "decrease of wakefulness." It is therapeutically useful in the psychoneuroses in general and psychosomatic diseases in particular (Bergouignan, 1956; Ende, 1956; Funfschilling, 1957; Giraud, 1957; Dolan, 1958; Nolan, 1958; Schram, 1959; Golwalla, 1960; Middlefell, 1960; Gibbon, 1961; Trollux, 1961; and Morren *et al.*, 1964). Hydroxyzine has been successfully given in the treatment of alcoholism (Flores, 1957; Van Gasse, 1958; Kulisiewicz, 1959; and McGettigan, 1960); in the behavior disorders of children (Bayart, 1956; Segal, 1957; Freedman, 1958; Bachmann, 1959; Litchfield, 1960; and Maffei, 1961); in geriatrics (Shalowitz, 1956; Negri, 1957; Jouan, 1958; and Rogers, 1959); and in dermatological diseases (Zelger, 1956; Cornbleet, 1960; and Shanon, 1962).

iii. Adverse Effects Reported. Transient drowsiness; chronic administration may lead to dry mouth.

h. Mephenoxalone

i. Chemical Name. 5-(*o*-Methoxyphenoxymethyl)-2-oxazolidinone.

ii. Therapeutic Uses. A muscle relaxant with tension-relieving and anxiolytic properties (Furgiuele *et al.*, 1961; and Martinez and Salas, 1960).

iii. Adverse Effects Reported. Psychiatric (drowsiness, paradoxical insomnia, dependency); neurological (headache, dizziness); and dermatological (rash).

i. Metaxalone

i. Chemical Name. 5-(3,5-Xylyloxymethyl)oxazolidin-2-one.

ii. Therapeutic Uses. A centrally acting muscle relaxant with sedative and tension-relieving properties (Carroll *et al.*, 1961; Kurtzke and Gylfe, 1962; Carter, 1962, 1958; Berger and Ludwig, 1964; and Modell, 1964). The place of this substance in psychopharmacotherapy has not yet been established.

iii. Adverse Effects Reported. Psychiatric (drowsiness, confusional state, nervousness); neurological (dizziness); autonomic (dryness of mouth); gastrointestinal (nausea, vomiting); genitourinary (pyuria, urinary retention); and hematological (transitory leukopenia, anemia).

j. Methaqualone

i. Chemical Name. 2-Methyl-3-*o*-tolyl-4(eH)-quinazolinone.

ii. Therapeutic Uses. A nonbarbiturate hypnotic superior to placebo as a sleep sustainer but not as a sleep inducer (Stein and Moore, 1949; Paterson, 1963; and Tetreault *et al.*, 1965).

iii. Adverse Effects Reported. Chronic administration may lead to dependency (Cohen, 1965; and Martin, 1966).

k. Methyprylon

i. Chemical Name. 3,3-Diethyl-5-methyl-2,4-piperidinedione.

ii. Therapeutic Uses. An effective hypnotic (Pellmont *et al.*, 1955; and LeRiche *et al.*, 1966).

iii. Adverse Effects Reported. Incompatibility with beer consumption (Peters, 1963).

l. Oxanamide

i. Chemical Name. 2,3-Epoxy-2-ethylhexan-amide.

ii. Therapeutic Uses. A tranquilizer with possible usefulness in the treatment of psychoneuroses (to relieve anxiety and tension). It has been successfully used in the control of disturbed cerebral arterioslcerotic patients (Coats and Gray, 1957; Ayd, 1959; Kuhn *et al.*, 1960; Benson and Schiele, 1962; Modell, 1964; and Cohen *et al.*, 1967). The place of this substance in psychopharmacotherapy has not yet been established.

iii. Adverse Effects Reported. Relatively few, mainly drowsiness. Not to be given in endogenous depressions, catatonic schizophrenia, convulsive disorders or kidney and liver disease. The combination of oxanamide with phenothiazines or MAOI's is contraindicated.

m. Oxazepam

i. Chemical Name. 7-Chloro-3-hydroxy-5-phenyl-1,3-dihydro(2H)-1,4-benzodiazepin-2-one.

ii. Therapeutic Uses. An anxiolytic particularly useful in the treatment of psychoneuroses. It has also been successfully given to geriatric cases (Geller, 1964; Gerz, 1964; Beber, 1965; Bobon *et al.*, 1965; Chesrow *et al.*, 1965; Gilbert, 1965; LeGassicke and McPherson, 1965; Sanders, 1965; Scassera, 1965; and Warner, 1965).

iii. Adverse Effects Reported. Similar to those of other benzodiazepines.

n. Prazepam

i. Chemical Name. 7-Chloro-1-(cyclopropylmethyl)-1,3-dihydro-5-phenyl(2H)-1,4-benzodiazepin-2-one.

ii. Therapeutic Uses. An anxiolytic with particular effectiveness in somatized anxiety (Kingstone *et al.*, 1966).

iii. Adverse Effects Reported. Similar to those of other benzodiazepines.

o. Tolboxane

i. Chemical Name. 2-Methyl-2-propyl-1,3-propanediol-*p*-tolylborate.

ii. Therapeutic Uses. A muscle relaxant with tension-relieving and sedative properties (Rickels *et al.*, 1963). The place of this substance in psychopharmacotherapy has not yet been established.

iii. Adverse Effects Reported. Need to be assessed.

4. Aromatic Compounds

a. Adiphenine

i. Chemical Name. 2-Diethylaminoethyl-2,2-diphenylacetate.

ii. Therapeutic Uses. An anticholinergic drug with an inhibitory effect on orienting behavior and with sedative properties (Caldewell, 1958; and Wu, 1961). The place of this substance in psychopharmacotherapy has not yet been established.

iii. Adverse Effects Reported. Atropine-like effects. Contraindicated in glaucoma, prostatic hypertrophy and pyloric obstruction.

b. Benactyzine

i. Chemical Name. β-Diethylaminoethyl benzilate.

ii. Therapeutic Uses. A centrally acting anticholinergic agent which "blockades" certain higher functions of the CNS without prevalent sedation (Jacobsen, 1964). Its therapeutic action in the psychoneuroses is equivocal (Munkvad, 1955; Ostenfeld, 1955; Busscher, 1956; Davies, 1956; Cohen *et al.*, 1957; Gardes and Laulan, 1957; Hargreaves *et al.*, 1957; MacLean, 1957; Pennington, 1959; Seager and Leitch, 1956; Ayd, 1957; Forbes and Earle, 1957; Raymond *et al.*, 1957; Gore and Walton, 1957; and Harrington and Mayer-Gross, 1959). Benactyzine, however, is particularly useful when a neurasthenic syndrome is associated with autonomic manifestations (Nathan, 1958; and Warner, 1958).

iii. Adverse Effects Reported. Atropine-like effects. Contraindicated in glaucoma and prostatic hypertrophy. Should not be combined with electroshock treatment.

c. Captodiame

i. Chemical Name. 2-(*p*-Butylmercaptobenzhydrylmercapto)-*N*,*N*-dimethylethylamine.

ii. Therapeutic Uses. A psychotropic particularly useful in the therapy of psychoneuroses and in the behavior problems of children (Sarro and Cruz, 1956; Sarwer-Foner and Koranyi, 1957; and Davidova and Zapletalek, 1965).

iii. Adverse Effects Reported. Psychiatric (drowsiness); and hepatobiliary (liver impairment). There is a metallic taste in the mouth in the course of treatment.

d. Chlorproheptadiene

i. Chemical Name. 3-Chloro-5-(3-dimethylaminopropylidene)-10, 11-dihydro (5H)dibenzo(*a*, *d*)cycloheptene.

ii. Therapeutic Uses. A psychotropic with possible tranquilizing properties (Votava *et al.*, 1961). The place of this substance in psychopharmacotherapy has not yet been established.

iii. Adverse Effects Reported. Need to be assessed.

e. Deanol

i. Chemical Name. 2-Dimethylaminoethanol-*p*-acetylaminobenzoate.

ii. Therapeutic Uses. A psychostimulant particularly useful in fatigue and possibly in neurasthenia, "mild" depression, "anergic" schizophrenia and mental subnormality (Barsa and Saunders, 1959; Remmen *et al.*, 1962; Jacobs, 1965; and Malitz *et al.*, 1967).

iii. Adverse Effects Reported. Psychiatric (insomnia, nervousness); neurological (headache, cerebral seizures, increased muscle tone); cardiovascular (hypotension); gastrointestinal (constipation); and metabolic (weight loss). Contraindicated in epileptics.

f. Hydroxyphenamate

i. Chemical Name. β-Ethyl-β-hydroxyphenethyl carbamate.

ii. Therapeutic Uses. A muscle relaxant used as an adjunct in the treatment of psychoneuroses for the control of tension (Bastian and Clements, 1961; Bossinger, 1961; Hubarta and Hecht, 1961; Sifferd and Braitberg, 1962; and Berger and Ludwig, 1964).

iii. Adverse Effects Reported. Psychiatric (drowsiness, addiction); cardiovascular (hypotension); and allergic (urticaria).

g. Mefexamide

i. Chemical Name. *N*-(2-Diethylamino-ethyl)-2-(*p*-methoxyphenoxy)acetamide.

ii. Therapeutic Uses. An auxin derivative with possible antidepressant effects. It "tranquilizes" in low, "stimulates" in medium, and "induces convulsions" in high doses (Launay and Maurey, 1965). The place of this substance in psychopharmacotherapy has not yet been established.

iii. Adverse Effects Reported. Psychiatric (activation of psychopathology); and neurological (cerebral seizures).

h. Mephenesin

i. Chemical Name. 3-(*o*-Toloxy)-1,2-propanediol.

ii. Therapeutic Uses. A muscle relaxant once frequently used in the control of anxiety-tension states, alcohol withdrawal and preoperative sedation (Berger and Schwartz, 1948; Remmen *et al.*, 1962; and Cohen *et al.*, 1967).

iii. Adverse Effects Reported. Psychiatric (lassitude, sedation, weakness); neurological (nystagmus, ataxia); gastrointestinal (nausea, vomiting, constipation, diarrhea); allergic (rash, pruritus, anaphylactoid reaction); and hematological (leukopenia, hemolysis, hematuria). Contraindicated in myasthenia gravis and muscular dystrophy.

i. Methocarbamol

i. Chemical Name. 3-(*o*-Methoxy-phenoxy-1,2-propanediol)-1-carbamate.

ii. Therapeutic Uses. A muscle relaxant with tension-relieving and sedative properties (Taeschler and Schlager, 1962).

iii. Adverse Effects Reported. Psychiatric (drowsiness); neurological (headache, vertigo, blurred vision, diplopia, nystagmus, muscular incoordination); autonomic (flushing); and cardiovascular (hypotension, bradycardia). Intramuscular injection may cause local irritation.

j. Orphenadrine

i. Chemical Name. *N,N*-Dimethyl-2-(*o*-methylbenzhydryloxy)ethylamine.

ii. Therapeutic Uses. An antihistaminic successfully used in the treatment of extrapyramidal manifestations. It has a slight euphoriant effect and it has been useful in the treatment of psychasthenic cases (Blair, 1963; Zakrzewska *et al.*, 1965; and Ginzel, 1966).

iii. Adverse Effects Reported. Psychiatric (drowsiness, excitement, hallucinations); neurological (dizziness); autonomic (dryness of mouth, blurring of vision); gastrointestinal (nausea); and dermatological (skin rash). Contraindicated in glaucoma or myasthenia gravis.

k. Phenaglycodol

i. Chemical Name. 2-(*p*-Chlorphenyl)-3-methyl-2,3-butanediol.

ii. Therapeutic Uses. A tranquilizer, equally effective as mephenesin as an anxiolytic, but inferior to meprobamate. Phenaglycodol is particularly useful in the alleviation of nervous tension in patients with tuberculosis and possibly in the control of agitation in geriatrics (Mills *et al.*, 1957; Settel, 1957; Carter, 1958; Friend, 1961; Kalinowsky and Hoch, 1961; Berger and Ludwig, 1964).

iii. Adverse Effects Reported. Drowsiness, mainly with larger doses.

l. Phenprobamate

i. Chemical Name γ-Phenylpropylcarbamate.

ii. Therapeutic Uses. A muscle relaxant with tension-relieving and sedative properties (Garonne *et al.*, 1960).

iii. Adverse Effects Reported. Drowsiness, particularly with higher doses.

5. Aliphatic Compounds

a. Ectylurea

i. Chemical Name. 1-(2-Ethyl-cis-crotonyl)urea.

ii. Therapeutic Uses. An anxiolytic particularly useful in the treatment of mild anxiety and tension, apprehension and emotional stress associated with somatic disorders (Benson and Schiele, 1962; Remmen *et al.*, 1962; and Cohen *et al.*, 1967).

iii. Adverse Effects Reported. Hepatobiliary (jaundice, cholangiolitic hepatitis); and dermatological (skin rash). It is contraindicated in liver or kidney disease, and it should not be used in combination with phenothiazines or MAOI's.

b. Emylcamate

i. Chemical Name. 1-Ethyl-1-methylpropyl carbamate.

ii. Therapeutic Uses. A muscle relaxant with tension-relieving and sedative properties. It is particularly useful for the symptomatic relief of anxiety in a variety of somatic disorders, in premenstrual tension, dermatoses and functional gastrointestinal disturbances (Melander, 1959; Melander and Hanshoff, 1961; Berger and Ludwig, 1964; and Cohen *et al.*, 1967). Emylcamate is superior in the control of the neurotic symptomatology of alcoholics (Martens, 1960).

iii. Adverse Effects Reported. Psychiatric (drowsiness); neurological (headache, dizziness); autonomic (dryness of mouth); gastrointestinal (nausea, vomiting); and dermatological (skin rash).

c. Ethchlorvynol

i. Chemical Name. β-Chlorovinyl ethynyl carbinol.

ii. Therapeutic Uses. A reliable hypnotic useful as a sleep inducer and sustainer (Schwartz, 1957; Ban and McGinnis, 1962; Benson and Schiele, 1962; Remmen *et al.*, 1962; Matthews *et al.*, 1964; and Modell, 1964).

iii. Adverse Effects Reported. Psychiatric (dependency, drowsiness, fatigue, hangover, nightmares, confusional state); neurological (headache, ataxia, vertigo); cardiovascular (hypotension, syncope); and gastrointestinal (nausea, vomiting, bad taste in mouth). It is contraindicated in porphyria.

d. Ethinamate

i. Chemical Name. 1-Ethynylcyclohexanecarboxamide.

ii. Therapeutic Uses. A reliable hypnotic, particularly useful as a sleep inducer (Benson and Schiele, 1962; Falconer and Patterson, 1964; Matthews *et al.*, 1964).

iii. Adverse Effects Reported. Similar to those of other hypnotics.

e. Meprobamate

i. Chemical Name. 2-Methyl-2-propyl-1,3-propanediol dicarbamate.

ii. Therapeutic Uses. One of the clinically most frequently used muscle relaxants with tension-relieving and sedative properties. It is particularly useful for relieving psychic tension in the psychoneuroses (Berger, 1954; Hendley *et al.*, 1954; Benson and Schiele, 1962; Remmen *et al.*, 1962; Paterson, 1963; and Berger and Ludwig, 1964).

iii. Adverse Effects Reported. Psychiatric (dependency, drowsiness, paradoxical insomnia); neurological (headache, ataxia, tremor, convulsion, fever); cardiovascular (syncope); gastrointestinal (stomatitis, nausea, vomiting, constipation); dermatological (rash); allergic (anaphylactoid reaction); and hematological (purpura, aplastic anemia). It is contraindicated in hypersensitivity and capillary fragility.

f. Petrichloral

i. Chemical Name. Pentaerythritolchloral.

ii. Therapeutic Uses. A rapidly acting and relatively safe hypnotic (Fuller, 1958; and Benson and Schiele, 1962).

iii. Adverse Effects Reported. Psychiatric (drowsiness, lethargy, hangover, paradoxic restlessness, excitement); gastrointestinal (nausea, vomiting); and dermatological (skin eruptions).

g. Tybamate

i. Chemical Name. 2-Methyl-2-propyltrimethylene butylcarbamate carbamate.

ii. Therapeutic Uses. A muscle relaxant with greater tension-relieving but less sedative effects than meprobamate (Stern, 1964; Button and Cole, 1965; and Shapiro, 1966).

iii. Adverse Effects Reported. Psychiatric (drowsiness, paradoxical insomnia, hyperactivity or irritability, euphoria or lethargy, fatigue, feeling of unreality, confusion, panic reaction); neurological (dizziness, ataxia, grand mal or petit mal seizures, paresthesias); autonomic (dry mouth, blurred vision); cardiovascular (flushing, tachycardia); and gastrointestinal (glossitis,

Table III

Frequently used hypnotics and anxiolytics

Generic name	Trademark			Dosage
	U.S.A.	Canada	Britain	Daily dosage range
				mg.
Benactyzine	Suavitil	Actozine	NA	2–6
Captodiame	Suvren	Suvren	NA	100–400
Chlordiazepoxide	Librium	Librium	Librium	15–100
Deanol	Deaner	Deaner	Deaner	25–100
Diazepam	Valium	Valium	Valium	10–40
Ectylurea	Levanil	NA	NA	450–1200
Ethchlorvynol	Placidyl	Placidyl	Serensil	200–600
Ethinamate	Valmid	Valmid	Valmidate	500–1000
Glutethimide	Doriden	Doriden	Doriden	500–2000
Hydroxyzine	Atarax	Atarax	Atarax	50–400
Mephenesin	Tolserol	Tolserol	Tolseram	1000–3000
Mephenoxalone	Trepidone	Trepidone	NA	400–1600
Meprobamate	Miltown	Equanil	Miltown	400–1200
Methaqualone	Sopor	Mequelon	Melsedin	150–300
Methocarbamol	Robaxin	Robaxin	Robaxin	500–1500
Methyprylon	Noludar	Noludar	Noludar	200–600
Oxanamide	Quiactin	Quiactin	NA	400–1600
Oxazepam	Serax	Serax	Serenid-D	30–120
Phenaglycodol	Ultran	Acalo	NA	600–1200
Promethazine	Phenergan	Phenergan	Phenergan	10–50
Tybamate	Solacen	Solacen	Solacen	750–1400

constipation). There has been no dependency reported on tybamate.

REFERENCES

Adamson, G. T., and Finlay, S. E.: The effects of two psycho-stimulant drugs on muscular performance in male athletes. Ergonomics, *8:* 237 (1965).

Agin, H. V. (1960): In: Zirkle, C. L., and Kaiser, C.: Monoamine oxidase inhibitors. In: Psychopharmacological agents (ed., Gordon, M.). (Academic Press, New York, 1964.)

Azima, H., and Vispo, R. H.: Imipramine a potent new antidepressant compound. Amer. J. Psychiat., *115:* 245 (1958).

Ahmed, A., *et al.* (1958): In: Usdin, E., and Efron, D. M.: Psychotropic drugs and related compounds. (PHSP No. 1589, Washington, 1967.)

Alapin, B., and Laborowska, E.: Wlasne wyniki leczenia stanow depresygnych prothiadenen. Neurol. Chir. Psychiat. Pol., *16:* 425 (1966).

American Medical Association Council on drugs: New and non-official drugs. (Lippincott, Philadelphia, 1959.)

American Medical Association: New drugs. (AMA, Chicago, 1967.)

Anderson, E., and Kemp, H. (1957): In: Schlittler, E., and Plummer, A. J. Tranquillizing drugs from the Rauwolfia. In: Psychopharmacological agents (ed., Gordon, M.). (Academic Press, New York, 1964.)

Andren, H. E. (1955): In: Krueger, G. L., and McGrath, W. R.: 2-Benzylpiperidines and related compounds. In: Psychopharmacological agents (ed., Gordon, M.). (Academic Press, New York, 1964.)

Angst, J.: A clinical analysis of the effects of tofranil in depression. Longitudinal and follow-up studies. Treatment of blood relations. Psychopharmacologia (Berlin), *2:* 381 (1961).

Anton, A.: Results of clinical investigations with the neuroleptic ciatyl. Med. Welt, *12:* 665 (1962).

Antos, R. J. (1955): In: Krueger, G. L., and McGrath, W. R.: 2-Benzylpiperidines and related compounds. In: Psychopharmacological agents (ed., Gordon, M.). (Academic Press, New York, 1965.)

Arnold, O. H., and Deisenhammer, E.: First experiences with a potent neuroleptic N 746. Wein. Med. Wschr., *112:* 558 (1962).

Ast, H., *et al.*: Mesoridazine in acute psychotic disturbances. Curr. Ther. Res., *9:* 623 (1968).

Atkinson, R. M., and Ditman, K. S.: Tranylcypronine: a review. Clin. Pharmacol. Ther., *6:* 631 (1965).

Avol, M., and Vogel, P. J. (1955): In: Schlittler, E., and Plummer, A. J. Tranquillizing drugs from the Rauwolfia. In: Psychopharmacological agents (ed., Gordon, M.). (Academic Press, New York, 1964.)

AYD, F. J.: The treatment of anxiety, agitation and excitement in the aged. A preliminary report on trilafon. J. Amer. Geriat. Soc., *5:* 92 (1957).

AYD, F. J.: Treatment of ambulatory and hospitalized psychiatric patients with perphenazine. Dis. Nerv. Syst., *18:* 394 (1957).

AYD, F. J.: Fatal agranulocytosis due to triflupromazine hydrochloride. Amer. J. Psychiat., *114:* 940 (1958).

AYD, F. J.: Chemical treatment of depression. Ann. N.Y. Acad. Sci., *80:* 734 (1959).

AYD, F. J.: Fluphenazine: Its spectrum of therapeutic application and clinical results in psychiatric patients. Curr. Ther. Res., *1:* 41 (1959).

AYD, F. J.: Tofranil therapy for depressed states. J. Neuropsychiat., *1:* 35 (1959).

AYD, F. J.: Current status of major tranquillizers. J. Med. Soc. New Jersey, *57:* 4 (1960).

AYD, F. J. (1960): In: Biel, J. H., *et al.*: Monoamine oxidase inhibitors (hydrazines). In: Psychopharmacological agents (ed., Gordon, M.). (Academic Press, New York, 1964.)

AYD, F. J.: Neuroleptics and extrapyramidal reactions. In: Extrapyramidal system and neuroleptics (ed., Bordeleau, J. M.). (Editions Psychiatriques, Montreal, 1960.)

AZIMA, H.: Imipramine (tofranil): a new drug for the depressed. Canad. Med. Ass. J., *76:* 442 (1959).

AZIMA, H., AZIMA, F. G., AND DUROST, H. B.: Psychoanalytic formulations of effects of reserpine on schizophrenic organization. Arch. Gen. Psychiat. (Chicago) *1:* 662 (1959).

AZIMA, H., DUROST, H., AND CAHN, C.: Vesprin and mepazine: two new phenotropic substances. Amer. J. Psychiat., *114:* 747 (1958).

AZIMA, H., *et al.*: The effects of G 33040 in depressive states: a multi-blind study. Amer. J. Psychiat., *119:* 465 (1962).

AZIMA, H., *et al.* (1962): In: Usdin, E., and Efron, D. M.: Psychotropic drugs and related compounds. (PHSP No. 1589, Washington, 1967.)

BACHANN, K. (1960): In: Usdin, E., and Efron, D. H. Psychotropic drugs and related compounds. (PHSP No. 1589, Washington, 1967.)

BACHMAN, H., AND FRIEND, J.: Use of phenaglycodol for alleviation of nervous tension in patients with tuberculosis. Amer. Practit., *9:* 397 (1958).

BACHMANN, W. (1959): In: Morren, H. G., *et al.:* Piperazine derivatives. In: Psychopharmacological agents (ed., Gordon, M.). (Academic Press, New York, 1964.)

BAKER, A. A., AND THORPE, J. G.: Assessing a new phenothiazine. J. Ment. Sci., *104:* 855 (1958).

BAN, T. A.: Trimipramine in psychiatry. In: Trimipramine, a new antidepressant (eds., Lehmann, H. E., *et al.*). (Q.P.R.A., Montreal, 1964.)

BAN, T. A.: Human pharmacology and systematic clinical studies with a new phenothiazine. In: Proceedings of the Leeds Symposium on behavioral disorders (ed., Jenner, F. A.). (May and Baker, Dagenham, 1965.)

BAN, T. A., AND LEHMANN, H. E.: Clinical trial with desmethylimipramine (G-35020)—a new antidepressive compound. Canad. Med. Ass. J., *86:* 1039 (1962).

BAN, T. A., AND MCGINNIS, K.: Comparative clinical study of two hypnotic drugs. Canad. Med. Ass. J., *87:* 816 (1962).

BAN, T. A., PAPATHOMOPULOS, E., AND SCHWARZ, L.: Clinical studies with thioproperazine (majeptil). Compr. Psychiat., *3:* 284 (1962).

BAN, T. A., AND ST. JEAN, A.: The effect of phenothiazines on the electrocardiogram. J. Canad. Med. Ass., *91:* 537 (1964).

BAN, T. A., ST. JEAN, A., AND DESAUTELS, S.: The effects of phenothiazines on the human electrocardiogram. In: Neuropsychopharmacology, Vol. 4 (eds., Bente, D., and Bradley, P. B.) (Elsevier, Amsterdam, 1965.)

BAN, T. A., AND ST. LAURENT, J.: The stimulating effect of RP 8228 on inactive psychiatric patients. J. Neuropsychiat., *3:* 91 (1961).

BAN, T. A., AND SCHWARZ, L.: Systematic studies with levomepromazine. J. Neuropsychiat., *5:* 112 (1963).

BAN, T. A., FERGUSON, K., AND LEHMANN, H. E.: The effect of clopenthixol on chronic psychiatric patients (Clinical Note). Amer. J. Psychiat., *119:* 984, 1963.

BARBER, J. C., *et al.:* A controlled trial of mebanazine (actomol) in depression. Brit. J. Psychiat., *111:* 1095 (1965).

BARETT, B. M., AND HANSEL, F. K. (1955): In: Schlittler, E., and Plummer, A. J.: Tranquillizing drugs from the Rauwolfia. In: Psychopharmacological agents (ed., Gordon, M.). (Academic Press, New York, 1964.)

BARKER, J. C., *et al.:* A controlled trial of mebanazine (Actomol) in depression. Brit. J. Psychiat., *111:* 1095 (1965).

BARSA, J. A., AND SAUNDERS, J. C.: Deanol (deaner) in the treatment of schizophrenia. Amer. J. Psychiat., *116:* 255 (1959).

BARSA, J. A., AND SAUNDERS, J. C.: Thioridazine (mellaril) in the treatment of chronic schizophrenics. Amer. J. Psychiat., *116:* 1028 (1960).

BARSA, J. A., AND SAUNDERS, J. C.: Benzquinamide in the treatment of psychotic patients. Dis. Nerv. Syst., *25:* 620 (1964).

BARSA, J. A., AND SAUNDERS, J. C.: A double blind study of fluphenazine enanthate. Dis. Nerv. Syst., *26:* 496 (1965).

BARSA, J. A., SAUNDERS, J. C., AND KLINE, N. S.: Trifluoperazine in the treatment of chronic schizophrenia. Amer. J. Psychiat., *115:* 812 (1959).

BARTHOLOMEW, A. A.: An evaluation of tranylcypromine (parnate) in the treatment of depression. Med. J. Aust., *149:* 655 (1962).

BARTHOLOMEW, A. A., AND HOLT, W. F.: A long-acting phenothiazine (fluphenazine enanthate): a preliminary communication. Med. J. Aust., *1:* 12 (1966).

BARTOLUCCI, G., *et al.:* Clinical studies with clopenthixol on chronic psychiatric patients. Curr. Ther. Res., *8:* 581 (1966).

BARUK, H., *et al.:* Action therapeutique du 7044 RP dans les nérvoses obsessionelles, les nérvoses digestives et les etats des cénestopathies. Ann. Medico Psychol., *116:* 149 (1958).

BASTIAN, J. W., AND CLEMENTS, G. R.: Pharmacology and toxicology of hydroxyphenamate (listica). Dis. Nerv. Syst., *22:* 9 (1961).

BAYART, J. (1956): In: Morren, H. G., *et al.:* Piperazine derivatives. In: Psychopharmacological agents (ed., Gordon, M.). (Academic Press, New York, 1964.)

BEBER, C. R.: Management of behavior in the institutionalized aged. Dis. Nerv. Syst., *26:* 591 (1965).

BELLAK, L., AND BLACK, B. J. (1960): In: Schlittler, E., and Plummer, A. J.: Tranquillizing drugs from the Rauwolfia. In: Psychopharmacological agents (ed., Gordon, M.). (Academic Press, New York, 1964.)

BENNETT, I. F.: The constellation of depression. I. Criteria for true antidepressant activity. J. Nerv. Ment. Dis., *134:* 561 (1962).

BENSCH, K., AND RUNDBERG, B.: Clinical test of a new neuroplegic, dixyrazine, using double blind procedure and sequential analysis. Acta Neurol. Belg., *67:* 649 (1964).

BENSCH, K., AND RUNDBERG, B.: Clinical trial with a new neuroleptic drug, dixyrazine, with application of a double blind control technique and sequential analysis. Acta paedopsychiat. (Basel), *32:* 83 (1965).

BENSON, W. M., AND SCHIELE, B. C.: Current status of tranquillizing and antidepressive drugs. Lancet, *80:* 579 (1960).

BENSON, W. M., AND SCHIELE, B. E.: Tranquillizing and antidepressant drugs. (Charles C Thomas, Springfield, 1962.)

BENTE, D., *et al.:* Clinical investigations on a neuroleptically active dibenzothiazepine derivative. Arzneimittelforschung *16:* 314 (1966).

BERGER, F. M.: The mode of action of myanesin. Brit. J. Pharmacol., *2:* 241 (1947).

BERGER, F. M.: Spinal cord depressant drugs. Pharmacol. Rev., *1:* 243 (1949).

BERGER, F. M.: The pharmacological properties of 2-methyl-2-N-propyl-1,3 propanediol dicarbamate (Miltown), a new interneuronal blocking agent. J. Pharmacol. Exp. Ther., *112:* 412 (1954).

BERGER, F. M.: The similarities and differences between meprobamate and barbiturates. Clin. Pharmacol. Ther., *4:* 209 (1963).

BERGER, F. M., AND LUDWIG, B. J.: Meprobamate and related compounds. In: Psychopharmacological agents (ed., Gordon, M.). (Academic Press, New York, 1964).

BERGER, F. M., AND SCHWARTZ, R. P. (1948): In: Usdin, E., and Efron, D. H.: Psychotropic drugs and related compounds. (PHSP No. 1589, Washington, 1967.)

BERGER, F. M., STRECKER, H. J., AND WAELSCH, H.: Biochemical effects of psychotherapeutic drugs. Ann. N.Y. Acad. Sci., *66:* 806 (1957).

BERGOUIGNAN, M. (1956): In: Morren, H. G., *et al.:* Piperazine derivatives. In: Psychopharmacological agents (ed., Gordon, M.). (Academic Press, New York, 1964).

BERTHIER, C., *et al.* (1962): Etude clinique d'un nouveau neuroleptique: le 8909 RP. (Paper presented at the Sixty-first Congress of French Speaking Psychiatrists and Neurologists, Nancy, 1963.)

BERTOLOTTI, P., AND MUNARINI, D.: Therapeutic experiences in neuropsychiatry with a derivative of benzoquinolizine. Riv. Sper. Freniat., *85:* 185 (1961).

BIEL, J. H., HORITA, A., AND DRUKKER, A. E.: Monoamine oxidase inhibitors (hydrazines). In: Psychopharmacological agents (ed., Gordon, M.). (Academic Press, New York, 1964.)

BISHOP, M. P., GALLANT, D. M., AND STEELE, C. A.: A controlled evaluation of benzquinamide: behavioral toxicity with high dosage levels in schizophrenics. Curr. Ther. Res., *5:* 238 (1963).

BLAIR, D.: Drugs for depression. Brit. Med. J., *1:* 945 (1963).

BLOM, S.: Tic douloureaux treated with new anticonvulsant. Arch. Neurol. (Chicago) *9:* 285 (1963).

BOBON, J., COLLARD, J., AND BREULET, M.: Oxazepam, or WY 3498, a new myorelaxant tranquillizer in outpatient treatment. Acta Neurol. Belg., *65:* 327 (1965).

BOBON, J., AND GOFFIOUL, F. (1962): In: Häfliger, F., and Burckhardt, V. Iminodibenzyl and related compounds. In: Psychopharmacological agents (ed., Gordon, M.). (Academic Press, New York, 1964.)

BOBON, J., *et al.:* A new neuroleptic with a differential hypnogenic action: dipiperone (R 3345), butyrophenone carbamate. Acta Neurol. Belg., *61:* 64 (1961).

BOBON, J., *et al.*: Benzperidol and promazine: a double-blind comparative study in geriatric medicine with special emphasis on senile mental changes. Acta Neurol. Belg., *63:* 839 (1963).

BOBON, J., *et al.:* Psychopharmacological study of a new methyl derivative of haloperidol: methylperidol or R 1658 (the 9th butyrophenone). Acta Neurol. Belg., *63:* 839 (1963).

BOBON, J., *et al.:* Spiroperidol. Acta Neurol. Belg., *63:* 991 (1963).

BODI, T., *et al.* (1959): In: Usdin, E., and Efron, D. H. Psychotropic drugs and related compounds. (PHSP No. 1589, Washington, 1967.)

BOGDANSKY, D. F., *et al.:* Comparative action of reserpine, tetrabenazine and chlorpromazine on central parasympathetic activity: effects on pupillary size and lacrimation in rabbit and on salivation in dog. J. Pharmacol. Exp. Ther., *132:* 176 (1961).

BOLZANI, L., AND SLIVAR, G. (1962): In: Häfliger, F., and Burckhardt, V.: Iminodibenzyl and related compounds. In: Psychopharmacological agents (ed., Gordon, M.). (Academic Press, New York, 1964).

BOSSINGER, C. D.: Chemistry of hydroxyphenamate. Dis. Nerv. Syst., *22:* 7 (1961).

BRATLUND, H. (1961): In: Psychotropic Drugs and Related Compounds. (eds., Usdin, C., and Efron, D. H.). (U.S. Department of Health, Educ. and Welfare. Washington, 1967.)

BRODIE, B. B., *et al.*: Preliminary pharmacological and clinical results with desmethylimipramine (DMI) G 35020, a metabolite of imipramine. Psychopharmacologia (Berlin), *2:* 467 (1961).

BRONSKY, I.: Carphenazine therapy of acutely psychotic patients in the psychiatric ward of a general hospital. Amer. J. Psychiat., *121:* 1203 (1965).

BROUSSOLLE, P., *et al.*: La prochlorperazine en psychiatrie: expérience tirée de 240 cures. Presse Med., *65:* 1628 (1957).

BROUSSOLLE, P., *et al.*: Use of fluoromethoxy phenylpiperazine butyrophenone chiefly in prolonged treatment (2028 M.D.). Ann. Medico Psychol., *119:* 586 (1961).

BROWN, B. B., *et al.* (1956): In: Usdin, E., and Efron, D. H. Psychotropic drugs and related compounds. (PHSP No. 1589, Washington, 1967.)

BUSSCHER, J. (1956): In: Jacobsen, E.: Benactyzine. In: Psychopharmacological agents (ed., Gordon, M.). (Academic Press, New York, 1967.)

BUTTON, J. C. (1956): In: Krueger, G. L., and McGrath, W. R.: 2-Benzylpiperidines and related compounds. In: Psychopharmacological agents (ed., Gordon, M.). (Academic Press, New York, 1964.)

BUTTON, J. T., AND COLE, W. V.: Treatment of emotional disturbances in clinic patients. J. Amer. Osteopath. Ass., *64:* 812 (1965).

CAGARA, S., AND WOZNIAK, M.: Clinical test of frenolon. Neurol. Neurochir. Psychiat. Pol., *16:* 711 (1966).

CAHN, C. A.: The influence of clopenthixol (sordinol) on the libido of the male. Psychiat. Neurol. Neurochir., *68:* 67 (1965).

CAHN, C. H., AND LEHMANN, H. E.: Perphenazine; observations on the clinical effects of a new tranquillizing agent in psychotic conditions. Canad. Psychiat. Ass. J., *2:* 104 (1957).

CALDWELL, A. E.: Psychopharmaca—a bibliography of psychopharmacology. (PHSP No. 581, Washington, 1958.)

CALWELL, W. P. K., JACOBSEN, M., AND SKARBEK, A.: A comparative study of oxypertine and trifluoperazine in chronic schizophrenia—a new application of the Wing rating scale. Brit. J. Psychiat., *110:* 520 (1964).

CARROLL, M. N., *et al.* (1961): In: Usdin, E., and Efron, D. H. Psychotropic drugs and related compounds. (PHSP No. 1589, Washington, 1967.)

CARTER, C. A., AND MALEY, M. C. (1957): In: Krueger, G. L., and McGroth, W. R.: 2-Benzylpiperidines and related compounds. In: Psychopharmacological agents (ed., Gordon, M.). (Academic Press, New York, 1964.)

CARTER, C. H. (1958): In: Berger, F. M., and Ludwig, B. J.: Meprobamate and related compounds. In: Psychopharmacological agents (ed., Gordon, M.) (Academic Press, New York, 1964.)

CARTER, C. H.: The effect of meprobamate (equanil) on brain damaged patients. Amer. J. Med. Sci., *235:* 632 (1958).

CARTER, C. H. (1962): In: Berger, F. M., and Ludwig, B. J.: Meprobamate and related compounds. In: Psychopharmacological agents (ed., Gordon, M.). (Academic Press, New York, 1964.)

CHANOIT, P., *et al.*: Une indication particulière du 8909 RP: les troubles due caractère. (Paper presented at the Sixty-first Congress of French Speaking Psychiatrists and Neurologists, Antwerp, 1962.)

CHAUCHARD, P., AND MAZOUÉ, H.: Neuroleptic effects of piperazine butyrophenone. Agressologie, *2:* 27 (1961).

CHESROW, E. J., *et al.*: A new psychotherapeutic agent effective in the management of geriatric anxiety, depression and behavioral reactions. J. Amer. Geriat. Soc., *13:* 449 (1965).

CHINN, H. I. (1956): In: Morren, H. G., *et al.*: Piperazine derivatives. In: Psychopharmacological agents (ed., Gordon, M.). (Academic Press, New York, 1964.)

CLARK, J. A.: Side effects of tranylcypromine. Lancet, *1:* 618 (1961).

CLEMENTI, F., *et al.*: α-Methyldopa is not involved in synthesis and storage of catecholamines in rat suprarenal gland. Arch. Int. Pharmacodyn. Ther., *152:* 179 (1964).

COATS, E. A., AND GRAY, R. W. (1957): In: Usdin, E., and Efron, D. H.: Psychotropic drugs and related compounds. (PHSP No. 1589, Washington, 1967.)

COHEN, H. L.: Clinical appraisal of an ataractic agent acetophenazine. Clin. Med. *72:* 1317 (1965).

COHEN, H. L. AND FREIREICH, A. Z.: Trilafon in the treatment of chronically psychotic hospitalized patients. Amer. J. Psychiat., *115:* 452 (1958).

COHEN, J. R. (1957): In: Jacobsen, E.: Benactyzine. In: Psychopharmacological agents (ed., Gordon, M.). (Academic Press, New York, 1964.)

COHEN, S.: Clinical experiences with pipradol and a pipradol-reserpine combination. Intern. Rec. Med., *169:* 751 (1956).

COHEN, S. (1966): In: Cohen, S., *et al.*: Psychochemotherapy (Western Medical Publications, Los Angeles, 1967.)

COHEN, S., DITMAN, K. S., AND GUSTAFSON, S. R.: Psychochemotherapy. (Western Medical Publications, Los Angeles, 1967.)

COIRAULT, R., *et al.* (1959): In: Häfliger, F., and Burckhardt, V.: Iminodibenzyls and related compounds. In: Psychopharmacological agents (ed., Gordon, M.) (Academic Press, New York, 1964.)

COLE, J. O., GOLDBERG, S. C., AND DAVIS, J. M.: Drugs in the treatment of psychosis: controlled studies. In: Psychiatric drugs (ed., P. Solomon). (Grune and Stratton, New York, 1966.)

Cook, R. W.: Use of acetophenazine in office practice. Int. J. Neuropsychiat., *1:* 605 (1965).

Cornbleet, T. (1960): In: Morren, H. G., *et al.:* Piperazine derivatives. In: Psychopharmalogical agents (ed., Gordon, M.). (Academic Press, New York, 1964.)

Cuny, G., *et al.:* Use of 10-chloro-deserpidine in neuropsychic agitation in elderly patients. Thérapie, Paris, *16:* 368 (1961).

Dagirmanjian, R., and Boyd, E. S. (1962): In: Usdin, E., and Efron, D. H. Psychotropic drugs and related compounds. (PHSP No. 1589, Washington, 1967.)

Daneman, E. A.: Clinical experience and a double blind study of a new antidepressant, vivactil hydrochloride. Psychosom., *6:* 342 (1965).

Darling, H. F.: Tranylcypromine on fifty ambulatory psychiatric patients. Dis. Nerv. Syst., *23:* 91 (1962).

Darville, F. T.: Double blind evaluation of methylphenidate (ritalin) hydrochloride. J.A.M.A., *169:* 1739 (1959).

Davidova, M., and Zapletalek, M. Some notes on the use of captodiamine in pedopsychiatry. Acta Nerv. Sup., *7:* 298 (1965).

Davies, E. B. (1956): In: Jacobsen, E.: Benactyzine. In: Psychopharmacological agents (ed., Gordon, M.). (Academic Press, New York, 1964.)

Davis, W. A., and Severinghaus, E. L. (1956): In: Schlittler, E., and Plummer, A. J.: Tranquillizing drugs from the Rauwolfia. In: Psychopharmacological agents (ed., Gordon, M.). Academic Press, New York, 1964.)

Deberdt, R. (1960): In: Morren, H. G.: Piperazine derivatives. In: Psychopharmacological agents (ed., Gordon, M.). (Academic Press, New York, 1964.)

Decsi, L. (1961): In: Usdin, E., and Efron, D. H.: Psychotropic drugs and related compounds. (PHSP No. 1589, Washington, 1967.)

Delay, J., and Deniker, P.: 38 cas de psychoses traites par la cure prolongée et continué de 4568 R.P. Ann. Medico Psychol. (Paris), *110:* 364 (1952).

Delay, J., and Deniker, P.: Le traitment des psychoses par une methode neurolytique dérivée de l'hibernothérapie. (Presenté à la Congrés des médecins alienistes et neurologistes, Luxembourg, 1952.)

Delay, J., and Deniker, P.: Méthodes chimiothérapiques en psychiatrie: les nouveaux médicaments psychotropes. (Masson, Paris, 1961.)

Delay, J., Deniker, P., and Ropert, R.: Four years experience with chlorpromazine in treatment of psychoses. Presse Med., *64:* 493 (1956).

Delay, J., *et al.:* Un neuroleptique majeur non phenothiazinique et non reserpinique, l'halopéridol, dans les traitement des psychoses. Ann. Medico Psychol. (Paris), *118:* 145 (1960).

Delay, J., *et al.:* Cures de sommeil et cures neuroleptiques en psychiatrie. Encephale, *45:* 436 (1956).

Delay, J., *et al.:* Effects psychiques de la nouvelle phénothiazine sulfonidée (7843 RP). Ann. Medico Psychol. (Paris), *116:* 601 (1958).

Delay, J., *et al.:* Essais cliniques d'un nouveau neuroleptique la thioridazine. Ann. Medico Psychol. (Paris), *117:* 724 (1959).

Delay, J., *et al.* (1960): In: Usdin, E., and Efron, D. H.: Psychotropic drugs and related compounds. (PHSP No. 1589, Washington, 1967.)

Delay, J., *et al.:* L'action du halopéridol dans les psychoses. Symposium International sur le haloperidol. Acta Med. Belg., *1:* 21 (1960).

DeMaio, D. (1964): In: Usdin, E., and Efron, D. H.: Psychotropic drugs and related compounds. (PHSP No. 1589, Washington, 1967.)

Denber, H. C. B.: Some preliminary results with a new phenothiazine derivative: prochlorperazine. Psychiat. Res. Rep. Amer. Psychiat. Ass., *9:* 16 (1958.)

Denber, H. C. B., and Turns, D.: Effect of lucidril in abstinence syndrome. (Presented at the Congress of French Speaking Psychiatrists and Neurologists, Marseille, 1964.)

Denber, H. C. B., Rajotte, P., and Kauffman, D.: Clinical experience with a new phenothiazine. Amer. J. Psychiat., *115:* 1116 (1959).

Denham, J.: The use of prochlorperazine (stemetil) in chronic psychotic disorders. J. Ment. Sci., *104:* 1190 (1958).

Denzel, H. A.: Fluphenazine enanthate in the treatment of psychotic patients. Int. J. Neuropsychiat., *2:* 258 (1966).

Deshaies, G.: Les effets cliniques du 8909 RP. Encephale, *6:* 602 (1962).

Deshaies, G., *et al.:* The method of administration of 7843 RP. Ann. Medico psychol. (Paris), *117:* 901 (1959).

Divry, P., *et al.:* Etude et experimentation cliniques du R 1625 ou haloperidol nouveau neuroleptique et "neurodysleptique." Acta Neurol. belg., *59:* 377 (1959).

Dlabac, A., and Trcka, V.: The influence of simpler reserpine models on thermoregulation in connection with other effects. I. Fenoharman. (Presented at the Eighth Pharmacological Meeting, Olomouc, 1961.)

Dolan, M. (1958): In: Morren, H. G., *et al.:* Piperazine derivatives. In: Psychopharmacological agents (ed., Gordon, M.). (Academic Press, New York, 1964.)

Dorfman, W. (1960): In: Häfliger, F., and Burckhardt, V. Iminodibenzyl and related compounds. In: Psychopharmacological agents (ed., Gordon, M.). (Academic Press, New York, 1964.)

Doussot, A., *et al.:* Données expérimentales sur l'action clinique d'un dérivé cyane de la phénothiazine, la propériciazine. Rev. Neuropsychiat. l'Ouest, *1:* 47 (1963).

Drake, F. R., and Ebaugh, F. G. (1955): In: Schlittler, E., and Plummer, A. J.: Tranquillizing drugs from the Rauwolfia. In: Psychopharmacological agents (ed., Gordon, M.). (Academic Press, New York, 1964.)

DUBNICK, B., *et al.:* Inhibition of MAO by 2-methyl-3-piperidino-pyrazine. Ann. N. Y. Acad. Sci., *107:* 914 (1963).

DUBOIS, C., *et al.:* Un nouveau neuroleptique majeur: le triperidol. Schweiz. Med. Wschr., *93:* 1600 (1963).

DUNLOP, E. (1961): In: Häfliger, F., and Burckhardt, V.: Iminodibenzyl and related compounds. In: Psychopharmacological agents (ed., Gordon, M.). (Academic Press, New York, 1964.)

DUNLOP, E. (1962): In: Sternbach, L. H., *et al.:* 1,4-Benzodiazepines. In: Psychopharmacological agents (ed., Gordon, M.). (Academic Press, New York, 1964.)

DUNLOP, E.: The neurotic feeling of inferiority. J. Neuropsychiat., *3:* 79 (1962).

DUNLOP, E., *et al.:* The relationship between monamine oxidase inhibition and improvement of depression: preliminary results with intravenous modaline sulphate (W 3207B). In: Excerpta Medica International Congress, Series 81. Proc. European Soc. Study Drug Toxicity, *4:* 46 (1964).

DVORNIK, D., AND SCHILLING, G.: Stereochemistry of d-3,4-dimethyl-2-phenylmorphaline (phendimetrazine). J. Med. Chem., *8:* 466 (1965).

EDISEN, C. B., AND SAMUELS, A. S.: A clinical evaluation of dartal chemotherapy for emotional disorders. Arch. Neurol. Psychiat., *80:* 481 (1958).

ENDE, M. (1956): In: Morren, H. G., *et al.:* Piperazine derivatives. In: Psychopharmacological agents (ed., Gordon, M.). (Academic Press, New York, 1964.)

ENGLISH, D. C.: A comparative study of antidepressants in balanced therapy. Amer. J. Psychiat., *11:* 865 (1961).

ENSS, H., AND HIPPIUS, H.: Sociopsychiatric aspects of modern psychosis therapy. Deutsch. Med. J., *15:* 529 (1964).

EVERETT, G. M., WEGARD, R. G., AND RINALDI, F. U.: Pharmacologic studies of some non hydrazine MAO inhibitors. Ann. N. Y. Acad. Sci., *107:* 1068 (1963).

FABING, H. D.: Frenquel, blocking agent against experimental LSD-25 and mescaline psychosis. Dis. Nerv. Syst., *16:* 10 (1955).

FABING, H. D.: The dimension of neurology. Neurology (Minneap.) *5:* 603 (1955).

FALCONER, M. W., AND PATTERSON, H. R.: Current drug handbook (Saunders, Philadelphia, 1964.)

FAZEKAS, J. F., *et al.:* Use of dimethylamino-N-propylphenothiazine in the management of patients with acute mental disturbance. Med. Ann. D. C., *25:* 67 (1956).

FAZIO, C., *et al.:* Un nuovo trattamento farmacologio (derivato iminodibenzilico G22355) nella cura degli stati depressivi. Minerva Med., *49:* 3143 (1958).

FELDMAN, P. E.: An analysis of the efficacy of diazepam. J. Neuropsychiat., *3:* 62 (1962).

FELDMAN P. E.,: Clinical evaluation of benzquinamide (P-2647) in the control of tension states and "hypersyndromes." Psychosomatics, *3:* 148 (1962).

FELDMAN, P. E.: Comparison of effect of 2-methyl-3-piperidino-pyrazine on target symptoms of anergic schizophrenics. Ann. N. Y. Acad. Sci., *107:* 1117 (1963).

FELDMAN, P. E.: Protriptyline hydrochloride—a new antidepressant. Psychosomatics *5:* 96 (1964).

FERGUSON, G. A.: Statistical analysis in psychology and education. (McGraw-Hill, New York, 1959.)

FERGUSON, J. T.: Treatment of reserpine-induced depression with a new analeptic: phenidylate. In: Reserpine in the treatment of neuropsychiatric, neurological and related clinical problems (ed., Miner, R. W.). (The Academy, New York, 1955.)

FERGUSON, J. T.: Successful therapeutic regimen for the management of behavior problems in the elderly. J. Amer. Geriat. Soc., *4:* 1080 (1956).

FERGUSON, J. T.: A preliminary evaluation of acepromazine (plegicil). Amer. J. Psychiat., *115:* 548 (1958).

FERGUSON, R. S.: A clinical trial of reserpine in the treatment of anxiety. J. Ment. Sci., *102:* 30 (1956).

FINK, L., AND VLAVIANOS, G.: Clinical impressions of the response to promazine therapy. Amer. J. Psychiat., *114:* 1031 (1958).

FLEMING, B. G., *et al.:* A controlled comparative investigation of the effects of promazine, chlorpromazine, and a placebo in chronic psychosis. J. Ment. Sci., *105:* 349 (1959).

FLORES, M. (1957): In: Morren, H. G., *et al.:* Piperazine derivatives. In: Psychopharmacological agents (ed., Gordon, M.). (Academic Press, New York, 1964.)

FOKSTUEN, T.: Esucos—a new neuroleptic. Int. J. Neuropsychiat., *1:* 294 (1965).

FORBES, H. S., AND EARLE, B. V. (1957): In: Jacobsen, E.: Benactyzine. In: Psychopharmacological agents (ed., Gordon, M.). (Academic Press, New York, 1964.)

FORNEY, R. B., AND HUGES, F. W.: Behavioral effects on the rat of benzquinamide-alcohol combinations. Arch. Int. Pharmacodyn. Ther., *142:* 237 (1963).

FOUKS, L., *et al.:* Fluphenazine, its therapeutic indications. Ann. Medico psychol. (Paris) *119:* 572 (1961).

FOUKS, L., *et al.:* (1961): In: Usdin, E., and Efron, D. H.: Psychotropic drugs and related compounds. (PHSP No. 1589, Washington, 1967.)

FOUKS, L., *et al.:* The clinical use of 2028 M.D. Ann. Medico psychol. (Paris), *119:* 134 (1961).

FOURNIER, A., *et al.:* The association of iproclozide and chlordiazepoxide in the treatment of states of depression. Ann. Medico psychol. (Paris), *122:* 625 (1964).

Freed, H. (1960): In: Häfliger, F., and Burckhardt, V.: Iminodibenzyl and related compounds. In: Psychopharmacological agents (ed., Gordon, M.). (Academic Press, New York, 1964.)

Freedman, A. M. (1958): In: Morren, H. G., *et al.*: Piperazine derivatives. In: Psychopharmacological agents (ed., Gordon, M.). (Academic Press, New York, 1964.)

French, W. N., and Truelove, J. F.: Identification and assay of phendimetrazine in pharmaceutical dosage forms. J. Pharm. Sci., *54:* 306 (1965).

Freyhan, F. A.: Neuroleptic effects: facts and fiction. In: The dynamics of psychiatric drug therapy (ed., Sarwer-Foner, G. J.). (Charles C Thomas, Springfield, 1960.)

Freyhan, F. A.: The modern treatment of depressive disorders. Amer. J. Psychiat., *116:* 1057 (1960).

Friedman, A. P. (1955): In: Schlittler, E., and Plummer, A. J.: Tranquillizing drugs from the Rauwolfia. In: Psychopharmacological agents (ed., Gordon, M.). (Academic Press, New York, 1964.)

Friend, D. G.: Current concepts in therapy: Tranquilizers. III. Meprobamate, phenaglycodol and chlordiazepoxide. New Eng. J. Med., *264:* 870 (1961).

Fuller, H. L. (1958): In: Usdin, E., and Efron, D. H.: Psychotropic drugs and related compounds. (PHSP No. 1589, Washington, 1967.)

Funfschilling, P. (1957): In: Morren, H. G., *et al.*: Piperazine derivatives. In: Psychopharmacological agents (ed., Gordon, M.). (Academic Press, New York, 1964.)

Furgiuele, A. R., *et al.*: Evaluation of certain psychopharmacological compounds. J. Pharm. Sci., *50:* 252 (1961).

Gale, A. S. (1958): In: Krueger, G. L., and McGrath, W. R.: 2-Benzylpiperidines and related compounds. In: Psychopharmacological agents (ed., Gordon, M.). (Academic Press, New York, 1964).

Gallant, D. M., Bishop, M. P., and Sprehe, D. (1965): In: Psychotropic Drugs and Related Compounds (eds., Usdin, E., and Efron, D. H.). (U.S. Dept. of Health, Education and Welfare, Washington, 1967.)

Gallant, D. M., *et al.*: A preliminary evaluation of SKF 20176 (propericiazine) in chronic schizophrenic patients. Curr. Ther. Res., *6:* 597 (1964).

Gambs, P., *et al.*: Aspects cliniques et electroencephalographiques du traitement par le 7162 RP. Ann. Medico psychol. (Paris), *120:* 410 (1962).

Gardes, A., and Laulan, M. (1957): In: Jacobsen, E.: Benactyzine. In: Psychopharmacological agents (ed., Gordon, M.). (Academic Press, New York, 1964.)

Garonne, G., *et al.* (1960): In: Usdin, E., and Efron, D. H. Psychotropic drugs and related compounds. (PHSP No. 1589, Washington, 1967.)

Gastager, H., and Gruber, H.: Clinical experiences with luvatren (methylperidol). Wien. Med. Wschr., *115:* 14 (1965).

Gayral, R., *et al.*: Etude par les techniques d'expression—notamment picturale—de l'activité thérapeutique de la propericiazine (neuleptil) sur les troubles du comportement chez l'enfant. (Paper presented at the Sixty-second Congress of French Speaking Neurologists and Psychiatrists, Marseilles, 1964.)

Geller, I.: Relative potencies of benzodiazepines as measured by their effects on conflict behavior. Arch. Int. Pharmacodyn. Ther., *149:* 243 (1964).

Géraud, J., and Gleizes, L.: Treatment of depressive states with iproclozide. Toulouse Med., *65:* 1286 (1964).

Géraud, J., *et al.*: Notes sur l'emploi de la trimiproprimine (surmontil) pour le traitement de la depression et de la melancolie. Ann. Medico psychol. (Paris), *120:* 258 (1962).

Gerstenbrand, F., Hoff, H., and Prosenz, P.: Therapeutic experiences with lucidril in neuropsychiatric disease pictures. Wien. Med. Wschr., *113:* 539 (1963).

Gerz, H. O.: A preliminary report on a new benzodiazepine in severe depressions. Amer. J. Psychiat., *121:* 495 (1964).

Gerz, H. O.: Evaluation of a new phenothiazine derivative in the treatment of schizophrenia. Amer. J. Psychiat., *121:* 174 (1964).

Gessler, R. M., and Coulston, F. (1959): In: Usdin, E., and Efron, D. H.: Psychotropic drugs and related compounds. (PHSP No. 1589, Washington, 1967.)

Gibbon, J. (1961): In: Morren, H. G., *et al.*: Piperazine derivatives. In: Psychopharmacological agents (ed., Gordon, M.). (Academic Press, New York, 1964.)

Gilbert, M. M.: Clinical trial of a new drug, analogue of chlordiazepoxide, for treatment of anxiety and tension. Int. J. Neuropsychiat., *1:* 556 (1965).

Gilmore, T. H., and Shatin, L.: Quantitative comparison of clinical effectiveness of chlorpromazine and promazine. J. Ment. Sci., *105:* 508 (1959).

Gilmour, S. J. G.: Clinical trial of mebanazine—a new monoamine oxidase inhibitor. Brit. J. Psychiat., *111:* 899 (1965).

Ginzel, K. H.: The blockade of reticular and spinal facilitation of motor function by orphenadrine. J. Pharmacol. Exp. Ther., *154:* 128 (1966).

Giraud, P. A. (1957): In: Morren, H. G., *et al.*: Piperazine derivatives. In: Psychopharmacological agents (ed., Gordon, M.). (Academic Press, New York, 1964).

Goldberg, R. I., and Shuman, F.: Pentamethylenetetrazol, vaso-dilator, vitamin therapy for mentally confused geriatric patients: double blind study. J. Amer. Geriat. Soc., *12:* 589 (1964).

GOLDMAN, A. E., AND ZAMANSKY, H. S. (1959): In: Schlittler, E., and Plummer, A. J.: Tranquillizing drugs from the Rauwolfia. In: Psychopharmacological agents (ed., Gordon, M.). (Academic Press, New York, 1964.)

GOLDMAN, D.: Toxicology of tranquillizers. In: Psychosomatic medicine (eds., Nodine, J. H., and Moyer, J. H.). (Lea and Febiger, Philadelphia, 1962.)

GOLDSTEIN, B. J., AND DIPPY, W. E.: A clinical evaluation of mesoridazine (serentil) in geriatric patients. Curr. Ther. Res., *9:* 256 (1967).

GOLWALLA, A. F. (1960): In: Morren, H. G., *et al.:* Piperazine derivatives. In: Psychopharmacological agents (ed., Gordon, M.). (Academic Press, New York, 1964.)

GORE, C. P., AND WALTON, D. (1957): In: Jacobsen, E.: Benactyzine. In: Psychopharmacological agents (ed., Gordon, M.). (Academic Press, New York, 1964.)

GOSLINE, E., *et al.:* Clinical report on methoxypromazine: a new phenothiazine. Amer. J. Psychiat. *115:* 939 (1959).

GOTTSCHALK, L. A., *et al.* (1956): In: Krueger, G. L., and McGrath, W. R.: 2-Benzylpiperidines and related compounds. In: Psychopharmacological agents (ed., Gordon, M.). (Academic Press, New York, 1964.)

GREENFIELD, A. R. (1956): In: Schlittler, E., and Plummer, A. J.: Tranquillizing drugs from the Rauwolfia. In: Psychopharmacological agents (ed., Gordon, M.). (Academic Press, New York, 1964.)

GROF, P., AND VINAR, O.: Preliminary comparative trial of proheptatriene and imipramine in the treatment of depressions (an intensive and controlled study). Acta Nerv. Sup., *7:* 288 (1965).

GROSS, H., AND LANGNER, E.: The clinical position of 2-chloro-11-(4-methylpiperazin-1-yl)-dibenzo-[b,f] [1,4]-thiazepine (HF-2159) in the group of neuroleptics. Arzneimittelforschung, *16:* 316 (1966).

GRUBER, K., *et al.* (1956): In: Usdin, E., and Efron, D. H.: Psychotropic drugs and related compounds. (PHSP No. 1589, Washington, 1967.)

GUNN, D. R.: Functional psychoses: the role of trifluoperazine in the treatment of refractory mental patients. In: Trifluoperazine. (Lea and Febiger, Philadelphia, 1958.)

GUTH, E., AND HOFMANN, G. (1966): In: Usdin, E., and Efron, D. H. Psychotropic drugs and related compounds. (PHSP No. 1589, Washington, 1967).

GYLYS, J. A., *et al.:* Pharmacological and toxicological properties of 2-methyl-3-piperidinopyrazine, a new antidepressant. Ann. N. Y. Acad. Sci., *107:* 899 (1963).

HAEN, P.: Drugs in research. (Paul deHaen, New York, 1964.)

HÄFLIGER, F., AND BURCKHARDT, V.: Iminodibenzyl and related compounds. In: Psychopharmacological agents, (ed., Gordon, M.) (Academic Press, New York, 1964.)

HALPERN, B. N., AND DUCROT, R. (1946): In: Usdin, E. and Efron, D. H. Psychotropic drugs and related compounds. (PHSP No. 1589, Washington, 1967.)

HAMILTON, L. D., and BENNETT, J. L.: Ethamivan in the management of chronic brain syndrome. J. Amer. Geriat. Soc., *13:* 550 (1965).

HAMON, J., PARAIRE, J., AND VELLUZ, J.: Remarque sur l'action du 4560 RP sur l'agitation maniaque. Ann. Medico psychol., *110:* 331 (1952).

HARDER, A. (1962): In: Häfliger, F., and Burckhardt, V.: Iminodibenzyl and related compounds. In: Psychopharmacological agents (ed., Gordon, M.). (Academic Press, New York, 1964.)

HARGREAVES, G. R., *et al.* (1957): In: Jacobsen, E.: Benactyzine. In: Psychopharmacological agents (ed., Gordon, M.). (Academic Press, New York, 1964.)

HARRER, G. (1962): In: Häfliger, F., and Burchhardt, V. Iminodibenzyl and related compounds. In: Psychopharmacological agents (ed., Gordon, M.). (Academic Press, New York, 1964.)

HARRINGTON, J. A., AND MAYER-GROSS, W. (1959): In: Jacobsen, E.: Benactyzine. In: Psychopharmacological agents (ed., Gordon, M.). (Academic Press, New York, 1964.)

HAYDU, G. G.: Schizophrenic behavior and aspects of pharmacology. (Presented at the conference of the New York Academy of Science on Schizophrenic Behavior, New York, 1961.)

HEGARTY, J. G., AND DABBS, A. R.: A controlled study of the effectiveness of trifluopromazine hydrochloride. J. Ment. Sci., *105:* 811 (1959).

HEIMANN, H., AND LUKACS, G.: Experimental psychological differentiation of the effects of two psychostimulants in man (F-1983 and amphetamine). Psychopharmacologia (Berlin), *8:* 79 (1965).

HEIMANN, H., AND VETTER, K.: Clinical investigations with a new psychostimulant (F-1983). Schweiz. Med. Wschr., *95:* 306 (1965).

HEINRICH, K.: Problems and results of therapy of endogenous psychoses with new psychotropic substances. Med. Welt., *7:* 335 (1961).

HENDLEY, C. D., *et al.:* Effect of 2-methyl-2-N-propyl-1,3-propanediol dicarbamate (Miltown) on central nervous system. Proc. Soc. Exp. Biol. Med., *87:* 608 (1954).

HICKS, J. T.: Iprindole, a new antidepressant for use in general office practice. A double-blind placebo-controlled study. Illinois Med. J., *128:* 622 (1965).

HIFT, S., AND KRYSPIN-EXNER, K. (1959): In: Häfliger, F., and Burckhardt, V.: Iminodibenzyl and related compounds. In: Psychopharmacological agents (ed., Gordon, M.). (Academic Press, New York, 1964.)

HIMWICH, H. E.: Biochemical and neurophysiological action of psychoactive drugs. In: Drugs and behavior (eds., Uhr, L., and Miller, J. G.). (Wiley, New York, 1960.)

HIPPIUS, H.: Dynamics and significance of psychopharmacological intervention in psychiatry. In: Neuro-psychopharmacology, Vol. 4 (eds., Bente, D., and Bradley, P. B.). (Elsevier, Amsterdam, 1965.)

HOCH, P. H. (1958): In: Schlittler, E., and Plummer, A. J. Tranquillizing drugs from the Rauwolfia. In: Psychopharmacological agents (ed., Gordon, M.). (Academic Press, New York, 1964.)

HOLLISTER, L. E.: Nervous system reactions to drugs. In: Evaluation and mechanism of drug toxicity (ed., Whipple, H. E.). (The New York Academy of Sciences, New York, 1965.)

HOLLISTER, L. E.: Toxicity of psychotherapeutic drugs. Practitioner, *194:* 72 (1965).

HOLLISTER, L. E., *et al.:* Controlled comparison of haloperidol with thiopropazate in newly admitted schizophrenics. J. Nerv. Ment. Dis., *135:* 544 (1962).

HOLLISTER, L. E., *et al.:* Evaluation of desipramine in depressive states. J. New Drugs, *3:* 161 (1963).

HOLLISTER, L. E., *et al.:* Triperidol in schizophrenia: further evidence for specific patterns of action of antipsychotic drugs. J. New Drugs, *5:* 34 (1965).

HOLMBERG, G., AND WILLIAM-OLSSON, U.: Effects of benzquinamide, in comparison with chlordiazepoxide and placebo, on subjective experiences and autonomic phenomena in stress experiments. Psychopharmacologia (Berlin), *5:* 147 (1964).

HOLST, B.: N 7009, in the treatment of anxiety states. Acta Psychiat. Scand., *40:* 415 (1965).

HORDEN, A., BURT, C. G., AND HOLT, N. F.: Depressive states: a pharmacotherapeutic study (Charles C Thomas, Springfield, 1965.)

HOROVITZ, Z. P., *et al.* (1963): In: Usdin, E., and Efron, D. H.: Psychotropic drugs and related compounds (PHSP No. 1589, Washington, 1967.)

HUBARTA, J. A., AND HECHT, R. A.: Review of clinical use of hydroxyphenamate in 1759 patients. Clin. Med., *60:* 1594 (1961).

HUNT, E., AND KRIVANEK, J.: The effects of pentylenetetrazole and methylphenoxypropane on discrimination learning. Psychopharmacologia (Berlin), *9:* 1 (1966).

ILEM, P. G., AND SAINZ. A.: The psychiatric application of vesprin. Psychiat. Quart., *33:* 9 (1959).

IRWIN, S., AND BENUAZIZI, A.: Pentylenetetrazol enhances memory function. Science, *152:* 100 (1966).

JACOBS, J.: A controlled trial of deaner and a placebo in mentally defective children. Brit. J. Clin. Pract., *19:* 77 (1965).

JACOBSEN, E.: Investigation into the mode of action of substances acting on the central nervous system. In: Depression (ed., Davies, B. E.). (University Press, Cambridge, 1964.)

JAHN, W., AND HÄUSLER, G. (1966): In: Usdin, E., and Efron, D. H.: Psychotropic drugs and related compounds. (PHSP No. 1589, Washington, 1967.)

JANKE, W., AND BOSS, H.: Experimental studies on the psychic effects of a new psychotonic agent. Arzneimittelforschung, *11:* 783 (1961).

JANSSEN, P. A. J.: Screening tests and prediction from animals to man. In: Animal behavior and drug action (eds., Steinberg, H., DeRenck, A. V. S., and Knight, J.). (Churchill, London, 1964.)

JANSSEN, P. A. J., JAGENEAU, A. H. M., AND NIEMEGEERS, C. J. E.: Effects of various drugs on isolation-induced fighting behavior of male mice. J. Pharmacol. Exp. Ther., *129:* 471 (1960).

JANSSEN, P. A. J., NIEMEGEERS, C. J. E., AND JAGENEAU, A. H. M.: Apomorphine antagonism in rats. Arzneimittelforschung, *10:* 1003 (1960).

JANSSEN, P. A. J., *et al.* (1963): In: Usdin, E., and Efron, D. H.: Psychotropic drugs and related compounds. (PHSP No. 1589, Washington, 1967).

JANSSEN, P. A. J., NIEMEGEERS, C. J. E., AND SCHELLEKENS, K. H. L.: Is it possible to predict the clinical effects of neuroleptic drugs (major tranquillizers) from animal data? III. The subcutaneous and oral activity in rats and dogs of 56 neuroleptic drugs in the jumping box test. Drug Res., *16:* 339 (1966).

JANSSEN, P. A. J., NIEMEGEERS, C. J. E., AND SCHELLEKENS, K. H. L.: Is it possible to predict the clinical effects of neuroleptic drugs (major tranquillizers) from animal data? II. "Neuroleptic activity spectra" for dogs. Arzneimittelforschung, *16:* 2 (1966).

JENNER, F. A. (ed.): Proceedings of the Leeds Symposium on behavioral disorders. (Ray and Baker, Dagenham, 1965.)

JENSEN, E. S. (1957): In: Schlittler, E., and Plummer, A. J.: Tranquillizing drugs from the Rauwolfia. In: Psychopharmacological agents (ed., Gordon, M.). (Academic Press, New York, 1964.)

JONAN, F. (1958): In: Morren, H. G., *et al.:* Piperazine derivatives. In: Psychopharmacological agents (ed., Gordon, M.). (Academic Press, New York, 1964.)

KALINOWSKY, L. B., AND HOCH, P. H.: Somatic treatments in psychiatry. (Grune and Stratton, New York, 1961.)

KALINOWSKY, L. B., AND HOCH, P. H.: Somatic treatments in psychiatry. (Grune and Stratton, New York, 1961.)

KAMMERER, T., *et al.:* Therapeutic results with MD 2028. Ann. Medico psychol. (Paris), *1:* 402 (1962).

KANT, F., AND ABELE, H. B.: Ambulatory psychotherapy for the schizophrenic patient with the aid of drugs. Dis. Nerv. Syst., *22:* 45 (1961).

KARABANOV, O. (1962): In: Häfliger, F., and Burckhardt, V.: Iminodibenzyl and related compounds. In: Psychopharmacological agents (ed., Gordon, M.). (Academic Press, New York, 1964.)

Karnaky, K. J. (1956): In: Morren, H. G., *et al.:* Piperazine derivatives. In: Psychopharmacological agents (ed., Gordon, M.). (Academic Press, New York, 1964.)

Kerenyi, A. B., *et al.* (1960): In: Krueger, G. L., and McGrath, W. R.: 2-Benzylpiperidines and related compounds. In: Psychopharmacological agents (ed., Gordon, M.). (Academic Press, New York, 1964.)

Keyes, B. L. (1958): In: Schlittler, E., and Plummer, A. J. Tranquillizing drugs from the Rauwolfia. In: Psychopharmacological agents (ed., Gordon, M.). (Academic Press, New York, 1964.)

Kingston, W. R. (1962): In: Zirkle, C. L., and Kaiser, C.: Monamine oxidase inhibitors. In: Psychopharmacological agents (ed., Gordon, M.). (Academic Press, New York, 1964.)

Kingstone, E., *et al.:* A clinical study of a new benzodiazepine derivative. Curr. Ther. Res., *8:* 159 (1966).

Kinross-Wright, J., Vogt, A. H., and Charalampoos, K. D. (1963): In: Usdin, E., and Efron, D. H.: Psychotropic drugs and related compounds. (PHSP No. 1589, Washington, 1967.)

Kinross-Wright, J., *et al.:* A new method of drug therapy. Amer. J. Psychiat., *119:* 779 (1963).

Kirkegaard, A., *et al.* (1957): In: Schlittler, E., and Plummer, A. J.: Tranquillizing drugs from the Rauwolfia. In: Psychopharmacological agents (ed., Gordon, M.). (Academic Press, New York, 1964.)

Kistner, R. W., and Duncan, C. J. (1956): In: Krueger, G. L., and McGrath, W. R.: 2-Benzylpiperidines and related compounds. In: Psychopharmacological agents (ed., Gordon, M.). (Academic Press, New York, 1964.)

Kline, N. S. (1959): In: Schlittler, E., and Plummer, A. J.: Tranquillizing drugs from the Rauwolfia. In: Psychopharmacological agents (ed., Gordon, M.). (Academic Press, New York, 1964.)

Kline, N. S., and Hackette, E.: Vivactil (protriptyline): a new and potent antidepressant. Psychosomatics *6:* 330 (1965).

Kline, N. S., and Lehmann, H. E. (eds.): Psychopharmacology (Little, Brown, Boston, 1965.)

Kline, N. S., and Simpson, G. M.: A long-acting phenothiazine in office practice. Amer. J. Psychiat., *120:* 1012 (1964).

Kline, N. S., *et al.:* The use of prochlorperazine (compazine) in a variety of psychiatric conditions. Psychiat. Res. Rep. Amer. Psychiat. Ass., *9:* 2 (1958).

Klingman, W. O.: Clinical use of pipradrol. In: Psychosomatic medicine (eds., Nodine, J. H., and Moyer, J. H.). (Lea and Febiger, Philadelphia, 1962.)

Klinken-Rasmussen, T., *et al.* (1957): In: Schlittler, E., and Plummer, A. J., Tranquillizing drugs from the Rauwolfia. In: Psychopharmacological agents (ed., Gordon, M.). (Academic Press, New York, 1964.)

Koranyi, E. K., Smith, R. L., and Sarwer-Foner, G. J.: Clinical assessment of D-206, a new pyridylamine. Med. Serv. J. Canada *14:* 130 (1958).

Krakowski, A. J.: Suppression of anxiety with oxazepam in a private psychiatric practice. Psychosomatics, *6:* 26 (1965).

Kranzdorf, C. D.: Early recognition and management of depressions. Calif. Clin., *1:* 237 (1962).

Kristof, F. E., Lehmann, H. E., and Ban, T. A.: Systematic studies with trimipramine: a new antidepressive drug. Canad. Psychiat. Ass. J., *12:* 517 (1967).

Krueger, G. L., and McGrath, W. R.: 2-Benzylpiperidines and related compounds. In: Psychopharmacological agents (ed., Gordon, M.). (Academic Press, New York, 1964.)

Kruse, W.: Experience with trifluoperazine in 110 female schizophrenics. Amer. J. Psychiat., *115:* 1031 (1959).

Kuhn, W. L., *et al.:* Effects of oxanamide on the central nervous system. Proc. Soc. Exp. Biol. Med., *103:* 101 (1960).

Kulisiewicz, T. A. (1959): In: Morren, H. G., *et al.:* Piperazine derivatives. In: Psychopharmacological agents (ed., Gordon, M.). (Academic Press, New York, 1964.)

Kurtzke, J. F., and Gylfe, J. C. (1962): In: Berger, F. M., and Ludwig, B. J.: Meprobamate and related drugs. In: Psychopharmacological agents (ed., Gordon, M.). (Academic Press, New York, 1964.)

Kuziw, R., *et al.* (1956): In: Usdin, E., and Efron, D. H.: Psychotropic drugs and related compounds (PHSP No. 1589, Washington, 1967.)

Lambert, P. A. (1965): In: Usdin, E., and Efron, D. H.: Psychotropic drugs and related compounds. (PHSP No. 1589, Washington, 1967.)

Lambert, P. A., and Guyotat, J.: Un nouvel antidepresseur sèdatif dérive de l'iminodibenzyle, le 7162 RP, essais thérapeutiques. Presse Med., *69:* 1425 (1961).

Lambert, P. A., *et al.* (1962): In: Häfliger, F., and Burckhardt, V.: Iminodibenzyl and related compounds. In: Psychopharmacological agents (ed., Gordon, M.). (Academic Press, New York, 1964.)

Lambros, V. S.: The use of reserpine in certain neurological disorders: organic convulsive states, enuresis and head injuries. Ann. N. Y. Acad. Sci., *6:* 211 (1955).

Lapolla, A.: Behavior reaction-time effects of benzquinamide in institutionalized psychotics. Clin. Med., *70:* 1851 (1963).

Lapolla, A., and Nash, L. R.: Two suicide attempts with chlorpromazine. Amer. J. Psychiat., *121:* 920 (1965).

LaSalle, M. W.: Carphenazine in chronic schizophrenia. Amer. J. Psychiat., *121:* 494 (1964).

Laskowska, D., *et al.:* The action of perazine (toxilan). Neurol. Neurochir. Psychiat. Pol., *16:* 433 (1966).

Launay, J., and Maurey, G.: Psychopharmacological animal study and clinical antidepressant tests of a new auxin derivative: mefexamide (A. N. P. 297). Ann. Medico psychol. (Paris), *123:* 141 (1965).

Luanay, J., and Michelin, J.: Action of AWP 235 (lucidril) in the acute and subacute confusional states of chronic alcoholism. Presse Med., *69:* 361 (1961).

Leahy, M. R., *et al.:* A preliminary study of phenoxypropazine in the treatment of depression. Amer. J. Psychiat., *119:* 986 (1963).

LeBorgne, Y., *et al.:* Eighteen months experience with a new neuroleptic "benzperidol." Ann. Medico psychol (Paris), *124:* 365 (1966).

Lees, F., and Burke, C. W.: Tranylcypromine. Lancet, *13:* 7271 (1963).

LeGassick, J., and McPherson, F. M.: A sequential trial of WY 3498 (oxazepam). Brit. J. Psychiat., *111:* 521 (1965).

LeGassicke, J. B., *et al.:* A controlled outpatient trial with fencamfamin. Brit. J. Psychiat., *110:* 267 (1964).

Lehmann, H. E.: Tranquillizers and other psychotropic drugs in clinical practice. Canad. Med. Ass. J., *79:* 701 (1958).

Lehmann, H. E., and Ban, T. A.: Notes from the log-book of a psychopharmacological research unit. I. Canad. Psychiat. Ass. J., *9:* 28 (1964).

Lehmann, H. E., and Ban, T. A.: ECDEU Progress Report. Douglas Hospital, Montreal, 1966.

Lehmann, H. E., and Ban, T. A.: Studies with new drugs in the treatment of convulsive disorders. J. Clin. Pharmacol., *3:* 231 (1968).

Lehmann, H. E., and Ban, T. A. (eds.): The thioxanthenes. (Karger, Basel, 1968.)

Lehmann, H. E., Ban, T. A., and Kral, V. A.: Practice effect in geriatric patients. Geriatrics, *23:* 160 (1968).

Lehmann, H. E., Ban, T. A., and Lee, H.: The effectiveness of combined phenothiazine and butyrophenone treatment in chronic schizophrenic patients. Curr. Ther. Res., *9:* 36 (1967).

Lehmann, H. E., Berthiaume, M., and Ban, T. A. (eds.): Trimipramine: a new antidepressant drug. (Québec Psychopharmacological Research Association, Montreal, 1964.)

Lehmann, H. E., Cahn, C. H., and De Verteuille, R.: The treatment of depressive conditions with imipramine (J. 22355). Canad. Psychiat. Ass. J., *3:* 155 (1958).

Lehmann, H. E., and Hanrahan, G. E.: Chlorpromazine: a new inhibiting agent for psychomotor excitement and manic states. Arch. Neurol. Psychiat., *71:* 227 (1954).

Lehmann, H. E., *et al.:* The effects of psychotropic drugs on biological systems of low complexity. In: Research approaches to psychiatric problems (eds., Tourlentes, T. T., Pollack, S. L., and Himwich, J. E.). (Grune and Stratton, New York, 1962.)

Lemere, F. (1960): In: Zirkle, C. L., and Kaiser, C.: Monoamine oxidase inhibitors. In: Psychopharmacological agents (ed., Gordon, M.). (Academic Press, New York, 1964.)

LeRiche, W., *et al.:* A clinical trial of four hypnotic drugs. Canad. Med. Ass. J., *95:* 300 (1966).

Lesse, S.: An evaluation of promazine hydrochloride in psychiatric practice. Amer. J. Psychiat., *113:* 984 (1957).

Lethew, L. J. (1957): In: Krueger, G. L., and McGrath, W. R.: 2-Benzylpiperidines and related compounds. In: Psychopharmacological agents (ed., Gordon, M.). (Academic Press, New York, 1964.)

Levinson, B. W.: The person behind the pill. Reflections on the new look in depression. Med. Proc., *8:* 374 (1962).

Levy, H. A., *et al.:* A new phenothiazine, methiomeprazine, in the treatment of chronic alcoholism. Curr. Ther. Res., *3:* 11 (1961).

Levy, S. (1954): In: Krueger, G. L., and McGrath, W. R.: 2-Benzylpiperidines and related compounds. In: Psychopharmacological agents (ed., Gordon, M.). (Academic Press, New York, 1964.)

Levy, S. (1962): In: Zirkle, C. L., and Kaiser, C.: Monoamine oxidase inhibitors. In: Psychopharmacological agents (ed., Gordon, M.). (Academic Press, New York, 1964.)

Liddel, D. W., and Weil-Malherbe, H. (1953): In: Usdin, E., and Efron, D. H.: Psychotropic drugs and related compounds. (PHSP No. 1589, Washington, 1967.)

Lingjaerde, O.: Tetrabenazine (nitoman) in the treatment of psychoses. With a discussion on the central mode of action of tetrabenazine and reserpine. Acta Psychiat. Scand., *7:* 109 (1963).

Litchfield, H. R. (1960): In: Morren, H. G., *et al.:* Piperazine derivatives. In: Psychopharmacological agents (ed., Gordon, M.). (Academic Press, New York, 1964.)

Lurie, M. L., and Salzer, H. M.: Tranylcypromine (parnate) in the ambulatory treatment of depressed patients. Amer. J. Psychiat., *118:* 152 (1961).

Lutz, E. G.: Treatment of tic douloureux with G-32883 (carbamazepine). Dis. Nerv. Syst., *27:* 600 (1966).

Lyager, T., and Rontorp, P. S. (1957): In: Schlittler, E., and Plummer, A. J.: Tranquillizing drugs from the Rauwolfia. In: Psychopharmacological agents (ed., Gordon, M.). (Academic Press, New York, 1964.)

Lyght, C. E., *et al.* (eds.): The Merck manual. (Merck and Co., Rahway, 1966.)

MacDonald, R.: Tranylcypromine. Lancet, *269:* 7275 (1963).

MacLean, R. E. G. (1957): In: Jacobsen, E.: Benactyzine. In: Psychopharmacological agents (ed., Gordon, M.). (Academic Press, New York, 1964.)

Maffei, M. (1961): In: Morren, H. G., *et al.:* Piperazine derivatives. In: Psychopharmacological agents (ed., Gordon, M.). (Academic Press, New York, 1964.)

Malamud, W., *et al.:* The evaluation of the effects of derivatives of Rauwolfia in the treatment of schizophrenia. Amer. J. Psychiat., *114:* 193 (1957).

MALITZ, S. (1957): In: Schlittler, E., and Plummer, A. J.: Tranquillizing drugs from the Rauwolfia. In: Psychopharmacological agents (ed., Gordon, M.). (Academic Press, New York, 1964.)

MALITZ, S., *et al.:* A pilot study of deanol in the treatment of anxiety. Curr. Ther. Res., *9:* 261 (1967).

MANN, A. M.: Desmethylimipramine (G 35020) in the treatment of depression. Canad. Med. Ass. J., *86:* 495 (1962).

MARIATEQUI, J.: En say o terapeutico con un derivado fenotiacinico de accion prolongada. El enantato de flufenacina en un grupo de esquizofrénicos cronicos. Rev. Neuropsiquiat., *29:* 33 (1966).

MARLER, I. Pharmacological and chemical synonyms. (Exerpta Medica Foundation, Amsterdam, 1967.)

MARTENS, S. (1960): In: Cohen, S., *et al.:* Psychochemotherapy. (Western Medical Publications, Los Angeles, 1967.)

MARTIN, G. J.: Dependency on methaqualone hydrochloride (melsedin). Brit. Med. J., *2:* 114 (1966).

MARTIN, K. E., *et al.:* Pipradol combined therapy for geriatric and agitated patients. Intern. Rec. Med., *170:* 33 (1957).

MARTINEZ, M., AND SALAS, E. S. (1960): In: Usdin, E., and Efron, D. H. Psychotropic drugs and related compounds. (PHSP No. 1589, Washington, 1967.)

MARX, H. (1961): In: Petersen, P. V., and Nielsen, I. M.: Thioxanthene derivatives. In: Psychopharmacological agents (ed., Gordon, M.). (Academic Press, New York, 1964.)

MATTHEWS, V., LEHMANN, H. E., AND BAN, T. A.: A comparative study of thirteen hypnotic drugs. Appl. Ther., *6:* 806 (1964).

MAY, R. H., *et al.:* Thioridazine therapy: results and complications. J. Nerv. Ment. Dis., *130:* 230 (1960).

MCAULIFF, J. P., *et al.:* Tissue norepinephrine and serotonin levels following graded amounts of 1-[2-(5,6-dimethoxy-2-methylindolyl-3)ethyl]-4-phenylpiperazine (oxypertine). Fed. Proc., *22:* 567 (1963).

MCGETTIGAN, D. L. (1960): In: Morren, H. G., *et al.:* Piperazine derivatives. In: Psychopharmacological agents (ed., Gordon, M.). (Academic Press, New York, 1964.)

MCWHINNEY, I. R., AND MORRELL, D. C.: Treatment of mild endogenous depression with a monoamine oxidase inhibitor: a controlled trial in general practice. J. Coll. Gen. Pract., *9:* 95 (1965).

MEDUNA, L. J., *et al.:* N(γ-methylaminopropyl) iminodibenzyl: a new antidepressant, preliminary report. J. Neuropsychiat., *2:* 232 (1961).

MELANDER, B. (1959): In: Berger, F. M., and Ludwig, B. J. Meprobamate and related compounds. In: Psychopharmacological agents (ed., Gordon, M.). (Academic Press, New York, 1964.)

MELANDER, B. O., AND HANSHOFF, G. (1961): In: Berger, F. M., and Ludwig, B. J. Meprobamate and related compounds. In: Psychopharmacological agents (ed., Gordon, M.). (Academic Press, New York, 1964.)

MICHON, P., *et al.:* Indications and limitations of lucidril (ANP) in reanimating patients. Presse Med., *69:* 1192 (1961).

MIDDLEFELL, R. (1960): In: Morren, H. G., *et al.:* Piperazine derivatives. In: Psychopharmacological agents (ed., Gordon, M.). (Academic Press, New York, 1964.)

MILLER, J. F.: Management of chronic mental patients. Use of pentylenetetrazol with nicotinic acid and team support. Geriatrics, *20:* 789 (1965).

MILLS, J., *et al.* (1957): In: Usdin, E., and Efron, D. H. Psychotropic drugs and related compounds. (PHSP No. 1589, Washington, 1967.)

MILNE, H. B., AND BERLINER, F.: A clinical trial of stemetil (prochlorperazine). J. Ment. Sci., *104:* 873 (1958).

MIRSKY, J. H., *et al.* (1959): In: Usdin, E., and Efron, D. H. Psychotropic drugs and related compounds. (PHSP No. 1589, Washington, 1967.)

MODELL, W. (ed.): Drugs in current use. (Springer, New York, 1964.)

MOLDENHAUER, B.: Butyrylperazin in der Neuropsychiatrie. Med. Welt., *22:* 1217 (1961).

MORIARITY, J. D.: Epinephrine-mecholyl test (Funkenstein test) as a prognostic guide for various physiodynamic therapy. Confin. Neurol., *16:* 105 (1956).

MORIARITY, J. D.: Broad spectrum treatment of the neurotic and the borderline psychotic patient in office practice. J. Neuropsychiat., *1:* 112 (1959).

MORREN, H. G., BIENFET, V., AND REYNTJENS, A. M.: Piperazine derivatives (except phenothiazines). In: Psychopharmacological agents (ed., Gordon, M.). (Academic Press, New York, 1964.)

MOSHER, L. R., *et al.:* A clinical trial of alphamethyldopa in elated states. Amer. J. Psychiat., *122:* 1185 (1966).

MUNKELT, P., AND OTHMER, E.: Influence of psychic stability and lability, and physical constitution of test subjects on the effect of the psychotonic compound: 7-[2'-(1''-methyl-2''-phenylethylamino) ethyl]theophylline HCl. Arzneimittelforschung *15:* 843 (1965).

MUNKVAD, I. (1955): In: Jacobsen, E.: Benactyzine. In: Psychopharmacological agents (ed., Gordon, M.). (Academic Press, New York, 1964.)

NAGY, A., AND GERSHON, S.: Clinical report on IN-1060. Dis. Nerv. Syst., *27:* 257 (1966).

NAHUNEK, K., *et al.:* Some clinical and experimental experience with proheptatriene. Acta. Nerv. Sup., *7:* 291 (1965).

NATHAN, P. W. (1958): In: Jacobsen, E.: Benactyzine. In: Psychopharmacological agents (ed., Gordon, M.). (Academic Press, New York, 1964.)

Negri, F. (1957): In: Morren, H. G., *et al.*: Piperazine derivatives. In: Psychopharmacological agents (ed., Gordon, M.). (Academic Press, New York, 1964.)

Negwer, M.: Organisch-chemische Arzneimittel und ihre Synonyma. (Kunst and Wissen, Stuttgart, 1961.)

Nielsen, J. B. (1957): In: Schlittler, E., and Plummer, A. J.: Tranquillizing drugs from the Rauwolfia. In: Psychopharmacological agents (ed., Gordon, M.). (Academic Press, New York, 1964.)

Nielsen, M. I., *et al.*: On truxal, a new psychotropic drug. Ugeskr. Laeg., *121:* 1432 (1959).

Nodine, J. H., *et al.*: Human bioassay of four butyrophenone derivatives in psychoneurotics. Clin. Res., *9:* 45 (1961).

Nodine, J. H., *et al.*: Modified technique used in human bioassay of four butyrophenone derivatives in psychoneurotic patients. Clin. Pharmacol. Ther., *3:* 432 (1962).

Nolan, F. G. (1958): In: Morren, H. G., *et al.*: Piperazine derivatives. In: Psychopharmacological agents (ed., Gordon, M.). (Academic Press, New York, 1964.)

Nussbaum, K.: "Pseudostimulation" in chronic schizophrenics on placebo. Amer. J. Psychiat., *120:* 1104 (1964).

Nutys, A.: The treatment of chronic psychoses with dipiperon-R 3345. Acta Neurol. Belg., *63:* 326 (1963).

Oliveros, R. F., *et al.*: A clinical trial of thiothixene in schizophrenics. Curr. Ther. Res., *9:* 504 (1967).

Olson, C. W., and Peterson, D. B.: The development of intercurrent disease and injury in the tranquillized psychiatric patient. Amer. J. Psychiat., *116:* 459 (1959).

Oltman, J. E., and Friedman, S.: Preliminary investigation of desmethylimipramine. Amer. J. Psychiat., *119:* 270 (1962).

Oltman, J. E., and Friedman, S.: Evaluation of nortriptyline in the treatment of affective disorders (and comparison with other drugs). Amer. J. Psychiat., *119:* 988 (1963).

O'Reilly, P. O., *et al.*: Perphenazine treatment of psychoses. Canad. Med. Ass. J., *77:* 952 (1957).

Ostenfeld, I. (1955): In: Jacobsen, E.: Benactyzine. In: Psychopharmacological agents (ed., Gordon, M.). (Academic Press, New York, 1964.)

Overall, J. E., *et al.*: Comparison of acetophenazine with perphenazine in schizophrenics: demonstration of differential effects based on computer-derived diagnostic models. Clin. Pharmacol. Ther., *4:* 200 (1963).

Paquay, J., Arnould, F., and Burton, P.: Etude clinique de l'action du R 1625 à doses modérées en psychiatrie. Acta Neurol. Belg., *59:* 882 (1959).

Paquay, J., *et al.*: Spiroperidol (R 5147 in psychiatry). Acta Neurol. Belg., *65:* 720 (1965).

Pargiter, R. A.: Parenteral methylphenidate hydrochloride (ritalin) in chronic underactive schizophrenics. Dis. Nerv. Syst., *20:* 69 (1959).

Paterson, A. S.: Modern techniques for the treatment of acute and prolonged alcoholism. Brit. J. Addict., *47:* 3 (1950).

Paterson, A. S.: Addiction to morphia and allied drugs: some recent developments. Postgrad. Med. J., *30:* 622 (1954).

Paterson, A. S.: Electrical and drug treatments in psychiatry. (Elsevier, Amsterdam, 1963.)

Paterson, A. S., *et al.*: L'hypnose et l'action de drogues ataractiques étudiées par la méthode du reflexe conditionné chez l'homme. (C. R. Congres Psychiat. Neurol. Lang. Franc. Montpellier, 1962.)

Payne, R. B., and Moore, E. W. (1955): In: Krueger, G. L., and McGrath, W. R. 2-Benzylpiperidines and related compounds. In: Psychopharmacological agents (ed., Gordon, M.). (Academic Press, New York, 1964.)

Pearl, D., *et al.*: Effects of reserpine on schizophrenic patients. Amer. J. Psychiat., *112:* 936 (1956).

Pellmont, B., *et al.* (1955): In: Usdin, E., and Efron, D. H.: Psychotropic drugs and related compounds. (PHSP No. 1589, Washington, 1967.)

Pelzman, O.: Tranylcypromine in the office treatment of depression. Psychiat. Quart., *35:* 261 (1961).

Pennington, V. M.: A two year comparative study of ataraxics in neuropsychiatric patients. J. Amer. Geriat. Soc., *5:* 421 (1957).

Pennington, V. M. (1959): In: Jacobsen, E.: Benactyzine. In: Psychopharmacological agents (ed., Gordon, M.). (Academic Press, New York, 1964.)

Peters, V. H.: Chronic methyprylon intoxication and its psychopathology. Arch. Psychiat. Zeitschrift Neurol., *204:* 342 (1963).

Petersen, P. V. and Nielsen, I. M.: Thioxanthene derivatives. In: Psychopharmacological agents (ed., Gordon, M.). (Academic Press, New York, 1964.)

Platz, A. R., Klett, C. J., and Caffey, E. M.: Selective drug action related to chronic schizophrenic subtype: a comparative study of carphenazine, chlorpromazine and trifluoperazine. (Cooperative Studies in Psychiatry, Report No. 68, Perry Point, 1966.)

Pletscher, A.: Biochemical and pharmacological actions of iproniazid on the heart. (Hoffman-La Roche Inc., New York, 1957.)

Pletscher, A.: Alteration of monoamine metabolism caused by drugs acting on the CNS. In: Psychopharmacology frontiers (ed., Kline, N. S.). (Little, Brown, Toronto, 1959.)

Pletscher, A., *et al.* (1960): In: Biel, J. H., Horita, A., and Drukker, A. E.: Monoamine oxidase inhibitors (hydrazines). In: Psychopharmacological agents (ed., Gordon, M.). (Academic Press, New York, 1964.)

Pöldinger, W., *et al.:* Therapeutical experience with the use of a dibenzoxepine derivative in depressive states in five clinics. Arzneimittelforschung, *16:* 650 (1966).

Pomeranze, J. (1954): In: Krueger, G. L., and McGrath, W. R.: 2-Benzylpiperidines and related compounds. In: Psychopharmacological agents (ed., Gordon, M.). (Academic Press, New York, 1964.)

Proctor, R. C.: A new therapeutic approach to certain cases of alcoholism. Southern Med. J., *49:* 73 (1956).

Prusmack, J. J., *et al.:* Mesoridazine (TPS-23) a new antipsychotic drug. J. New Drugs, *6:* 182 (1966).

Randall, L. O.: Pharmacology of methaminodiazepoxide. Dis. Nerv. Syst., *21:* 7 (1960).

Randall, L. O., *et al.:* The psychosedative properties of methaminodiazepoxide. J. Pharmacol. Exp. Ther., *129:* 163 (1960).

Randall, L. O., *et al.:* Zur Pharmakologie von Mogadon, einem Schlafmittel mit Neuartigem Wirkungsmechanismus. Schweiz. Med. Wschr., *95:* 334 (1965).

Ravn, J.: Chlorprothixene: a new psychotropic entity. Amer. J. Psychol., *118:* 227 (1961).

Ravn, J.: Clinical experience with sordinol. Nord. Psykiat. T., *16:* 395 (1962).

Ravn, J.: Further experience with sordinol. Nord. Psykiat. T., *16:* 136 (1962).

Ravn, J. (1961): In: Petersen, P. V., and Nielsen, M. I.: Thioxanthene derivatives. In: Psychopharmacological agents (ed., Gordon, M.). (Academic Press, New York, 1964.)

Ravn, J. (1960): In: Petersen, P. V., and Nielsen, M. I.: Thioxanthene derivatives. In: Psychopharmacological agents (ed., Gordon, M.). (Academic Press, New York, 1964.)

Ravn, J., and Rud, C.: Patients suffering from neuroses treated with flupenthixol. Nord. Psykiat. T., *19:* 66 (1965).

Raymond, M. J., *et al.* (1957): In: Jacobsen, E.: Benactyzine. In: Psychopharmacological agents (ed., Gordon, M.). (Academic Press, New York, 1964.)

Remmen, E., *et al.:* Psychochemotherapy. (Western Medical Publications, Los Angeles, 1962.)

Remvig, J., and Sonne, L.: Chlorprothixene (truxal) compared to chlorpromazine. Psychopharmacologia (Berlin), *2:* 203 (1961).

Retboll, K. (1963): In: Psychotropic Drugs and Related Compounds. (eds., Usdin, E., and Efron, D. H.). (U.S. Department of Health, Education and Welfare, Washington, 1967.)

Rett, A., *et al.* (1965): In: Usdin, E., and Efron, D. H.: Psychotropic drugs and related compounds. (PHSP No. 1589, Washington, 1967.)

Rickels, K.: Antineurotic agents: specific and non-specific effects. (Presented at the Sixth Annual Meeting of the ACNP, San Juan, 1967.)

Rickels, K., *et al.:* Evaluation of tranquillizing drugs in medical outpatients—meprobamate, prochlorperazine, amobarbital sodium and placebo. J.A.M.A., *171:* 1649 (1959).

Rickels, K., *et al.:* Controlled psychopharmacological research in general practice. J. New Drugs, *4:* 138 (1964).

Rickels, K., *et al.* (1963): In: Usdin, E., and Efron, D. H.: Psychotropic drugs and related compounds. (PHSP No. 1589, Washington, 1967.)

Roebuck, B. E., *et al.:* An evaluation of the therapeutic use of trifluopromazine in mental disease. J. Nerv. Ment. Dis., *129:* 184 (1959).

Rogers, E. J.: Treatment of muscle spasm with physical therapy and a central relaxant (chlormezanone). New York J. Med., *61:* 120 (1961).

Rogers, E. J. (1959): In: Morren, H. G., *et al.:* Piperazine derivatives. In: Psychopharmacological agents (ed., Gordon, M.). (Academic Press, New York, 1964.)

Rondepierre, J. J., and Ropert, B.: Experimental and clinical data concerning a new neuroleptic agent, N-3-dimethyl-amino propylthiophenylpyridylamine HCl or dominal. J. Med. Chir. Prat., *132:* 587 (1961).

Rose, J. T., *et al.:* A comparison of phenoxypropazine and amitriptyline in depression. Amer. J. Psychiat., *120:* 393 (1963).

Rotherford, R. N. (1959): In: Morren, H. G., *et al.:* Piperazine derivatives. In: Psychopharmacological agents (ed., Gordon, M.). (Academic Press, New York, 1964.)

Ruck, F., and Schwartz, B.: Experiences regarding the effect of frenolon in cases of schizophrenic psychoses. Psychiat. Neurol. Med. Psychol. (Leipzig), *17:* 341 (1965).

Rudy, L. H., *et al.* (1958) In: Usdin, E., and Efron, D. H. Psychotropic drugs and related compounds. (PHSP No. 1589, Washington, 1967.)

Sabbatini, F.: International meeting on the pharmacy of selective psychostimulants. Minerva Med., *55:* 3215 (1964).

Sainz, A.: Benzquinamide: a preliminary report. Amer. J. Psychiat., *119:* 777 (1963).

Samuels, A. S. (1957): In: Usdin, E., and Efron, D. H.: Psychotropic drugs and related compounds. (PHSP No. 1589, Washington, 1967.)

Sanders, J. F.: Evaluation of oxazepam and placebo in emotionally disturbed aged patients. Geriatrics, *20:* 739 (1965).

Sarro, R., and Cruz, M.: Clinical experience with a new orthothymic drug: covatin (N 68). Medicamenta, *14:* 295 (1956).

Sarwer-Foner, G. J., and Koranyi, E. K.: Clinical investigation of pacatal in open psychiatric settings. Canad. Med. Ass. J., *77:* 450 (1957).

Scassera, B. B.: Place of an antianxiety agent in general practice. Dis. Nerv. Syst., *26:* 511 (1965).

Schaffer, J. W. (1964): In: Usdin, E., and Efron, D. H.: Psychotropic drugs and related compounds. (PHSP No. 1589, Washington, 1967.)

Scherrer, P. (1962): In: Morren, H. G., *et al.:* Piperazine derivatives. In: Psychopharmacological agents (ed., Gordon, M.). (Academic Press, New York, 1964.)

SCHLICHTEGROLL, A. (1958): In: Usdin, E., and Efron, D. H. Psychotropic drugs and related compounds. (PHSP No. 1589, Washington, 1967.)

SCHIELE, B. C.: Studies with clopenthixol and thiothixene. In: The thioxanthenes (eds., Lehmann, H. E. and Ban, T. A.). (Karger, Basel, 1968.)

SCHIGUTT, R., AND SUCHANEK-FRÖCHLICH, H.: Treatment of depression with a new dibenzodiazepine derivative. Wien. Klin. Wschr., *77:* 584 (1965).

SCHMITT, D.: Elektrokardiographische, Untersuchungen, bei der Schock, und Krampfbehandlung der Schizophrenie. Z. Ges. Neurol. Psychiat., *166:* 108 (1939).

SCHMITT, H., AND SCHMITT, H.: Actions cardiovasculaires de l'halopéridol. Arch. Int. Pharmacodyn., *137:* 91 (1962).

SCHMITT, H., AND SCHMITT, H. (1966): In: Usdin, E., and Efron, D.: Psychotropic drugs and related compounds. (PHSP No. 1589, Washington, 1967.)

SCHMITT, W.: Pharmakotherapie Depressiver Psychosen mit einen Iminodibenzyl Derivat. Nervenarzt, *30:* 5 (1959).

SCHRAM, W. S. (1959): In: Morren, H. G., *et al.*: Piperazine derivatives. In: Psychopharmacological agents (ed., Gordon, M.). (Academic Press, New York, 1964.)

SCHULSINGER, F. (1957): In: Schlittler, E., and Plummer, A. J. Tranquillizing drugs from the Rauwolfia. In: Psychopharmacological agents (ed., Gordon, M.). (Academic Press, New York, 1964.)

SCHWARTZ, C. A., AND WILLIS, H. (1960): In: Schlittler, E., and Plummer, A. J. Tranquillizing drugs from the Rauwolfia. In: Psychopharmacological agents (ed., Gordon, M.). (Academic Press, New York, 1964.)

SCHWARTZ, H., *et al.*: Clinicotherapeutic tests of dipiperon, a new derivative of the butyrophenone series. Acta Neurol. Belg., *64:*401 (1964).

SCHWARTZ, D. E., *et al.*: Blood levels after administration of 7-chloro-1, 3-dihydro-1-methyl-5-phenyl-2H-1, 4-benzodiazepine-2-on (diazepam) in various forms. Arzneimittel Forschung *16:* 1109 (1966).

SCHWARTZ, F. R. (1957): In: Usdin, E., and Efron, D. H.: Psychotropic drugs and related compounds. (PHSP No. 1589, Washington, 1967.)

SCHWARZ, L., BAN, T. A., AND SMITH, R.: Clinical trial with cyclopentimine. Amer. J. Psychiat., *118:* 254 (1961).

SCRIABINA, A., *et al.*: Antagonism of 5-hydroxytryptamine by benzquinamide. Int. J. Neuropharmacol., *5:* 367 (1966).

SEAGER, C. P., AND LEITCH, A.: Benactyzine in psychoneurosis: a controlled clinical trial in hospital patients. Brit. Med. J., *2:* 1407 (1956).

SEGAL, L. J. (1957): In: Morren, H. G., *et al.*: Piperazine derivatives. In: Psychopharmacological agents (ed., Gordon, M.). (Academic Press, New York, 1964.)

SETTEL, E.: Clinical observations on the use of hydroxyzine (atarax) in tension states. Amer. Practit., *8:* 1584 (1957).

SETTEL, E.: A clinical evaluation of benzquinamide with observations on the total activity potential. Clin. Med., *70:* 957 (1963).

SHALOWITZ, M. (1956): In: Morren, H. G., *et al.*: Piperazine derivatives. In: Psychopharmacological agents (ed., Gordon, M.). (Academic Press, New York, 1964.)

SHANON, J. (1962): In: Morren, H. G., *et al.*: Piperazine derivatives. In: Psychopharmacological agents (ed., Gordon, M.). (Academic Press, New York, 1964.)

SHAPIRO, I.: Controlled study of the effects of tybamate on the neurotic component in dermatoses. Curr. Ther. Res., *8:* 99 (1966).

SHARPLEY, P., HEISTAD, G., AND SCHIELE, B. C.: Comparison of butaperazine and perphenazine: a double blind controlled study. Psychopharmacologia (Berlin), *5:* 209 (1964).

SHEPPARD, C., *et al.*: Effects of acetophenazine dimaleate on paranoid symptomatology in female geriatric patients: a double blind study. J. Amer. Geriat. Soc., *12 (9):* 884 (1964).

SIEGLER, P. E. (1964): In: Cohen, S., *et al.*: Psychochemotherapy. (Western Medical Publications, Los Angeles, 1967.)

SIFFERD, R. H., AND BRAITBERG, L. D. (1962): In: Berger, F. M., and Ludwig, B. J.: Meprobamate and related compounds. In: Psychopharmacological agents (ed., Gordon, M.). (Academic Press, New York, 1964.)

SIGWALD, J., *et al.*: Le psychoactif 7162 RP (dimethylamino-3'methyl-2'propyl)-5 iminodibenzyle. Proprietes therapeutiques panpsychotropes et antialgiques. Presse Med., *69:* 1780 (1961).

SIGWALD, T., *et al.*: Action of new phenothiazine in psychiatry and neurology: therapeutic properties of maleate acid of 3-levomethoxy (3-dimethylamino-2-methyl-10-propyl) phenothiazine (7044 RP). Presse Med., *64:* 2011 (1956).

SILVER, A. A.: Massive doses of ethamivan in severe phenobarbital and tranquillizer intoxication. Maryland Med. J., *15:* 55 (1966).

SIMKA, A.: Experience with the psychotonic captagon in ambulatory psychiatric patients. Med. Welt., *48:* 2712 (1965).

SIMPSON, G. M., *et al.*: Studies on a second long-acting fluphenazine. Amer. J. Psychiat., *121:* 784 (1965).

SIMPSON, R. W.: The effects of notensil in chronic mental illness. J. Ment. Sci., *104:* 179 (1958).

SIVADON, P., *et al.* (1959): In: Usdin, E., and Efron, D. H.: Psychotropic drugs and related compounds. (PHSP No. 1589, Washington, 1967.)

SMITH, M. E.: The effects of benzquinamide. Dis. Nerv. Syst., *24:* 116 (1963).

SOLOMON, S.: Clinical trial of an antipsychotic agent with a low toxic index: carphenazine. J. Neuropsychiat., *5:* 80 (1963).

SOMMERNESS, M. D., *et al.* (1955): In: Schlittler, E., and Plummer, A. J.: Tranquillizing drugs from the Rauwolfia. In: Psychopharmacological agents (ed., Gordon, M.). (Academic Press, New York, 1964.)

Soulairac, A. (1962): In: Morren, H. G., *et al.:* Piperazine derivatives. In: Psychopharmacological agents (ed., Gordon, M.). (Academic Press, New York, 1964.)

Sourkes, T. L., *et al.:* A clinical and metabolic study of DOPA and methyldopa in Huntington's chorea. Psychiat. Neurol. (Basel), *147:* 7 (1965).

St. Jean, A., *et al.:* The psychophysical effects of butyrophenones in male schizophrenics. In: The butyrophenones in psychiatry (ed., Lehmann, H. E., and Ban, T. A.). (Quebec Psychopharmacological Research Association, Montreal, 1964.)

St. Jean, A., Ban, T. A., and Noe, W.: Psychopharmacological studies with neoserp and aldomet. Int. J. Neuropsychiat., *1:* 491, 1965.

St. Jean, A., Ban, T. A., and Noe, W.: The effect of trimipramine on psychophysical test performance. In: Trimipramine a new antidepressant (eds., Lehmann, H. E., *et al.*). (Quebec Psychopharmacological Research Association, Montreal, 1965.)

St. Jean, A., Ban, T. A., and Noe, W.: The effect of iminodibenzyls in the treatment of chronic psychotic patients. Curr. Ther. Res., *8:* 164 (1966).

St. Jean, A., *et al.:* Clinical studies with propericiazine (RP 8909). Dis. Nerv. Syst., *28:* 526 (1967).

Stein, W. H., and Moore, S. (1949): In: Usdin, E., and Efron, D. H. Psychotropic drugs and related compounds. (PHSP No. 1589, Washington, 1967.)

Stern, F. H.: A new drug (tybamate) effective in the management of chronic brain syndrome. J. Amer. Geriat. Soc., *12:* 1066 (1964).

Sternbach, L. H., Randall, L. O., and Gustafson, S. R.: 1,4-Benzodiazepines (chlordiazepoxide and related compounds). In: Psychopharmacological agents (ed., Gordon, M.). (Academic Press, New York, 1964.)

Sugerman, A. A.: A pilot study of floropipamide (dipiperon). Dis. Nerv. Syst., *25:* 355 (1964).

Sugerman, A. A., and Herrmann, J.: A pilot study of dominal in chronic schizophrenics. Curr. Ther. Res., *8:* 487 (1966).

Suttel, R.: The use of alimenazine tartrate in sleep therapy. Gaz. Med. France, *68:* 955 (1961).

Taeschler, M., and Schlager, E. (1962): In: Usdin, E., and Efron, D. H.: Psychotropic drugs and related compounds. (PHSP No. 1589, Washington, 1967.)

Talbot, M. W. (1955): In: Schlittler, E., and Plummer, A. J. Tranquillizing drugs from the Rauwolfia. In: Psychopharmacological agents (ed., Gordon, M.). (Academic Press, New York, 1964.)

Taylor, J. D., *et al.* (1960): In: Zirkle, C. L. and Kaiser, C.: Monoamine oxidase inhibitors. In: Psychopharmacological agents (ed., Gordon, M.). (Academic Press, New York, 1964).

Tetreault, L., *et al.:* Study of a new non-barbituric hypnotic, methaqualone, in the psychiatric patient. Un. Med. Canada, *94:* 598 (1965).

Tolan, E. J., and Peppel, H. H.: Preliminary observations on trifluoperazine in schizophrenia. Amer. J. Psychiat., *115:* 935 (1959).

Tolan, E. J., *et al.:* Clinical and statistical evaluation of results with plegicil AY-57062 in chronic mental patients. Amer. J. Psychiat., *116:* 69 (1959).

Trcka, V., *et al.:* The reserpine-like action of L-1-benzyl-1,2,3,4-tetrahydronorharman (fenoharman). J. Physiol. (Paris), *53:* 488 (1961).

Trollux, M. (1961): In: Morren, H. G., *et al.:* Piperazine derivatives. In: Psychopharmacological agents (ed., Gordon, M.). (Academic Press, New York, 1964.)

Urquhart, R., and Forrest, A. D.: Clinical trial of promazine hydrochloride and acetylpromazine in chronic schizophrenic patients. J. Ment. Sci., *105:* 260 (1959).

Usdin, E., and Efron, D. H.: Psychotropic drugs and related compounds. (Public Health Service Publication No. 1589, Washington, 1967.)

Uytterschaut, P., and Jacobs, R.: Clinical study of a new neuroleptic: R 1658 or methylperidol. Acta Neurol. Belg., *62:* 677 (1962).

Vademecum International of Canada. (Morgan Jones, Toronto, 1968.)

Van Gasse, J. J. (1958): In: Morren, H. G., *et al.:* Piperazine derivatives. In: Psychopharmacological agents (ed., Gordon, M.). (Academic Press, New York, 1964.)

Van Praag, H. M., and Leijnse, B.: Some aspects of the metabolism of glucose and of the nonesterified fatty acids in depressive patients. Psychopharmacologia (Berlin), *9:* 220 (1966).

Vinar, O., and Taussigova, D.: Clinical experiences with methylperidol. Acta Nerv. Super., *7:* 250 (1965).

Votava, Z., *et al.:* Influence of a new group of tranquillizers, derivatives of dibenzosuberene, on the central nervous system. Biochem. Pharmacol. *8:* 16 (1961).

Waelkens, J. (1960): In: Usdin, E., and Efron, D. H.: Psychotropic drugs and related compounds. (PHSP No. 1589, Washington, 1967.)

Walsh, G. P., *et al.:* The relative efficacy of vespral and chlorpromazine in the treatment of a group of chronic schizophrenic patients. J. Ment. Sci., *105:* 199 (1959).

Warner, H. (1958): In: Jacobsen, E.: Benactyzine. In: Psychopharmacological agents (ed., Gordon, M.). (Academic Press, New York, 1964.)

Warner, R. S.: Management of the office patient with anxiety and depression. Psychosomatics, *6:* 347 (1965).

Warnes, H., Lee, H., and Ban, T. A.: The comparative effectiveness of butyrophenones in chronic psychotic patients. In: The butyrophenones (eds., Lehmann, H. E., and Ban, T. A.). (Q.P.R.A., Montreal, 1964.)

WARNES, H., *et al.*: Butaperazine and haloperidol: a comparative trial of two antipsychotic drugs. Laval Med., *37:* 143 (1966).

WHEATLEY, D.: A report from the British General Practitioner Research Group on mebanazine in the treatment of depression. J. New Drugs, *5:* 348 (1965).

WICKSTRÖM, L., AND PETTERSSON, K.: Treatment of diabetes with monoamine-oxidase inhibitors. Lancet, *2:* 995 (1964).

WITTON, K. (1960): In: Krueger, G. L., and McGrath, W. R.: 2-Benzylpiperidines and related compounds. In: Psychopharmacological agents (ed., Gordon, M.). (Academic Press, New York, 1964.)

WODRASKA, T. W., *et al.* (1958): In: Krueger, G. L., and McGrath, W. R.: 2-Benzylpiperidines and related compounds. In: Psychopharmacological agents (ed., Gordon, M.). (Academic Press, New York, 1964.)

WU, H. J.: Comparative mechanism of action of reserpine and certain tranquillizers. Bull. Eksperimental Biol. Med., *51:* 76 (1961).

ZAKRZEWSKA, F., *et al.*: Electromyographic study of the effect of a single dose of orphenadrine HCL (disipal) or meprobamate on neuroleptic-induced extrapyramidal syndrome. Neurol. Neurochir. Psychiat. Pol., *15:* 107 (1965).

ZBINDEN, G. (1960): In: Biel, J. H., *et al.*: Monoamine oxidase inhibitors (hydrazines). In: Psychopharmacological agents (ed., Gordon, M.). (Academic Press, New York, 1964.)

ZBINDEN, G., RANDALL, L. O., AND MOE, R. A. (1960): In: Zirkle, C. L., and Kaiser, C.: Monoamine oxidase inhibitors. In: Psychopharmacological agents (ed., Gordon, M.). (Academic Press, New York, 1964.)

ZELGER, I. (1956): In: Morren, H. G., *et al.*: Piperazine derivatives. In: Psychopharmacological agents (ed., Gordon, M.). (Academic Press, New York, 1964.)

ZIMMERMAN, F. T., AND BURGEMEISTER, B. B. (1958): In: Krueger, G. L., and McGrath, W. R.: 2-Benzylpiperidines and related compounds. In: Psychopharmacological agents (ed., Gordon, M.). (Academic Press, New York, 1964.)

Index